# ADVANCES IN MINIMALLY INVASIVE GYNECOLOGIC REPRODUCTIVE SURGERY


**Edited by**

**Botros Rizk, MD, MA, FRCOG, FRCS, HCLD, FACOG, FACS**
Medical Director, Elite IVF, Houston, Texas
President of the Middle East Fertility Society
Formerly Professor and Head, Reproductive Endocrinology & Infertility
Department of Obstetrics & Gynecology, University of South Alabama, Mobile, Alabama
Adjunct Professor, Cairo University, Department of Obstetrics & Gynecology
Kasr El Eini Hospital, Cairo, Egypt

**Mostafa I. Abuzeid, MD, FACOG, FRCOG**
Director, Division of Reproductive Endocrinology and Infertility, Department of Obstetrics and Gynecology, Hurley Medical Center, Flint, Michigan
Professor, Michigan State University College of Human Medicine, Flint Campus, Flint, Michigan
Medical and Practice Director, IVF Michigan Rochester Hills and Flint, PC
Rochester Hills, Michigan

**Ibrahim Alkatout, MD, PhD, MA, MaHM**
Professor and Senior Consultant in Obstetrics and Gynecology
University Hospitals of Schleswig-Holstein, Kiel
Director, Kiel School of Gynaecological Endoscopy, Germany

**Liselotte Mettler, MD, PhD, MBBS**
Emeritus Professor in Obstetrics and Gynecology
University Hospitals of Schleswig-Holstein, Kiel, Germany
Senior Consultant, German Medical Center, Dubai Health Care City, UAE
Executive Director, International Academy of Human Reproduction, Dubai, UAE



CRC Press
Taylor & Francis Group
Boca Raton London New York

CRC Press is an imprint of the
Taylor & Francis Group, an **informa** business

CRC Press
Boca Raton and London
First edition published 2022
by CRC Press
6000 Broken Sound Parkway NW, Suite 300, Boca Raton, FL 33487-2742

and by CRC Press
2 Park Square, Milton Park, Abingdon, Oxon, OX14 4RN



CRC Press is an imprint of Taylor & Francis Group, LLC



**Library of Congress Cataloging-in-Publication Data**

Names: Rizk, Botros, editor. | Abuzeid, Mostafa I., editor. | Alkatout, Ibrahim, editor. | Mettler, Liselotte, editor.
Title: Advances in minimally invasive gynecologic reproductive surgery / edited by Botros Rizk, Mostafa I. Abuzeid, Ibrahim Alkatout, Liselotte Mettler.
Description: First edition. | Boca Raton : CRC Press, 2021. | Includes bibliographical references and index. | Summary: "This cutting-edge text for surgeons specializing in Reproductive Medicine details how the latest minimally invasive developments impact on operations in their repertoire. Extensively illustrated throughout, this will be an essential reference in a fast-moving field"– Provided by publisher.
Identifiers: LCCN 2021011668 (print) | LCCN 2021011669 (ebook) | ISBN 9780367188320 (hardback) | ISBN 9781032029368 (paperback) | ISBN 9780429198595 (ebook)
Subjects: MESH: Infertility, Female–surgery | Gynecologic Surgical Procedures–methods | Minimally Invasive Surgical Procedures–methods | Reproductive Techniques
Classification: LCC RG201 (print) | LCC RG201 (ebook) | NLM WP 570 | DDC 618.1/78059–dc23
LC record available at https://lccn.loc.gov/2021011668
LC ebook record available at https://lccn.loc.gov/2021011669

ISBN: 978-0-367-18832-0 (hbk)
ISBN: 978-1-032-02936-8 (pbk)
ISBN: 978-0-429-19859-5 (ebk)

Typeset in Warnock Pro
by KnowledgeWorks Global Ltd.

http://resourcecentre.routledge.com/books/9780367188320

# CONTENTS

# CONTRIBUTORS

**Mostafa I. Abuzeid**
Division of Reproductive Endocrinology and Infertility Department of Obstetrics and Gynecology, Hurley Medical Center
Flint, Michigan
and
Michigan State University College of Human Medicine, Flint Campus
Flint, Michigan
and
IVF Michigan Rochester Hills and Flint, PC Rochester Hills, Michigan

**Omar M. Abuzeid**
Division of Maternal-Fetal Medicine
Department of Obstetrics and Gynecology
Stony Brook University
Long Island, New York

**Huda Afaneh**
Department of Obstetrics and Gynecology
Cleveland Clinic Foundation
Cleveland, Ohio

**Meenu Agarwal**
Morpheus IVF
Pune, Maharashtra

**Ibrahim Alkatout**
University Hospitals of Schleswig-Holstein
Kiel School of Gynaecological Endoscopy
Kiel, Germany

**Tarek Araji**
Faculty of Medicine
American University of Beirut
Beirut, Lebanon

**Andrea Pacheco Arias**
Department of Obstetrics and Gynecology
Hurley Medical Center
Michigan State University College of Human Medicine
Flint, Michigan

**Shima Al Basha**
Department of Obstetrics and Gynecology
Women's Hospital
Hamad Medical Corporation
Doha, Qatar

**Mostafa A. Borahay**
Minimally Invasive Gynecologic Surgery, Gynecology, and Obstetrics
Johns Hopkins Bayview Medical Center
Johns Hopkins University
Baltimore, Maryland

**Anupama Deenadayal-Mettler**
University Clinics of Schleswig Holstein
Kiel, Germany

**Mamata Deenadayal**
Mamata Fertility Hospital
Hyderabad, Telangana

**Damaris Freytag**
Clinic for Obstetrics and Gynecology
UKSH
Campus Kiel, Germany

**Isabella Gottlieb**
Johns Hopkins University Post-Baccalaureate Premedical Program
Los Angeles, California

**Veronika Günther**
Clinic for Obstetrics and Gynecology
UKSH
Campus Kiel, Germany

**Magdi Hanafi**
Gynecology and Fertility Specialists
Atlanta, Georgia

**Candice P. Holliday**
Department of Obstetrics and Gynecology
University of South Alabama
Mobile, Alabama

**Salem K. Joseph**
IVF Michigan Rochester Hills and Flint PC
Rochester Hills, Michigan

**Vishvanath C. Karande**
InVia Fertility Specialists
Hoffman Estates, Illinois

**Jordan S. Klebanoff**
Department of Obstetrics and Gynecology
The George Washington University Hospital
Washington, DC

**Ertug Kovanci**
Houston Assisted Reproductive Technologies
Houston, Texas

**Stephanie Leiva**
Department of Obstetrics and Gynecology
Hurley Medical Center
Michigan State University College of Human Medicine
Flint, Michigan

**Ivo Meinhold-Heerlein**
Zentrum für Frauenheilkunde und Geburtshilfe
Universtitätsklinikum Giessen
Giessen, Germany

**Liselotte Mettler**
Department of Obstetrics and Gynecology
University Hospitals of Schleswig-Holstein
Kiel, Germany
and
German Medical Center
Dubai Health Care City, UAE
and
International Academy of Human Reproduction
Dubai, UAE

**Emad Mikhail**
Department of Obstetrics and Gynecology
University of South Florida
Morsani College of Medicine
Tampa, Florida

**Gaby N. Moawad**
Obstetrics and Gynecology
The George Washington University School of Medicine and Health Science
Washington, DC

**Ahmed S.Z. Moustafa**
Division of Maternal-Fetal Medicine
Department of Obstetrics and Gynecology
University of Mississippi Medical Center
Jackson, Mississippi

**Sara Rahman**
Department of Obstetrics and Gynecology
The George Washington University Hospital
Washington, DC

**Rubin Raju**
Division of Urogynecology
Department of Obstetrics and Gynecology
Mayo Clinic
Rochester, Minnesota

**Botros Rizk**
Elite IVF, Houston, Texas
Middle East Fertility Society
and
Department of Obstetrics and Gynecology
University of South Alabama
Mobile, Alabama
and
Department of Obstetrics and Gynecology
Cairo University
and
Kasr El Eini Hospital
Cairo, Egypt

**Rupinder Kaur Ruprai**
King's College Hospital London
Dubai, UAE

**Mohammed R. Said**
Department of Obstetrics and Gynecology
Hurley Medical Center
Michigan State University College of Human Medicine
Flint, Michigan
and
Kasr El Aini Hospital
Cairo University Medical School
Cairo, Egypt

**Arwa Salehjawich**
Clinic for Obstetrics and Gynecology
UKSH
Campus Kiel, Germany

**Osama Shawki**
Department of Obstetrics and Gynecology
Cairo University
Cairo, Egypt

**Yehia Shawki**
Department of Obstetrics and Gynecology
Cairo University
Cairo, Egypt

**Priyanka Sinha**
Elite IVF
Houston, Texas

**Rooma Sinha**
Department of Gynaecology
Apollo Health City
Hyderabad, Telangana

**Renee Sundstrom**
Central Michigan University College of Medicine and Obstetrics and Gynecology
Covenant Medical Center
Saginaw, Michigan

**Nupur Tamhane**
Department of Obstetrics and Gynecology
University of South Florida
Tampa, Florida

**Brian F.G. Tesler**
Central Michigan University College of Medicine, and Obstetrics and Gynecology
Covenant Medical Center
Saginaw, Michigan

**Aarti Tolani**
Mamata Fertility Hospital
Hyderabad, Telangana

**Rafał Watrowski**
Department of Gynecology and Obstetrics
St. Josefskrankenhaus, Teaching Hospital of the University of Freiburg
Freiburg, Germany
and
Department of Obstetrics and Gynecology
Molecular Oncology Group
Medical University of Vienna
Vienna, Austria

# 1

# LAPAROSCOPIC AND HYSTEROSCOPIC SURGERIES FOR INFERTILITY

**Liselotte Mettler, Meenu Agarwal, and Ibrahim Alkatout**

## Background

Fertility-enhancing surgeries were around long before the introduction of artificial reproductive technologies (ART) like in vitro fertilization and embryo transfer (IVF-ET). They help to diagnose and treat many gynecological conditions that support achieving spontaneous conceptions and also enhance the results of ART. They can slow down the progression of pathologies such as fibroid and endometriosis and improve concomitant symptoms like pain and heavy bleeding.

The role of fertility-enhancing surgeries was adopted and recognized way back in 1970 by Swolin and Gommel [1]. With the advent of minimal invasive surgery route in 1980s, these surgical procedures could be managed laparoscopically giving the patient the benefit of lesser hospital stay, lesser postoperative pain and for the surgeon, better exposure and less postoperative adhesions. Simultaneously, there has been development of technology for imaging and ART. Both surgery and ART are not interchangeable but work in tandem to give the patient the benefit of both for a successful outcome. In this chapter, we report on a few of the surgical possibilities helpful for infertility treatment.

## Laparoscopic cauterization of ovarian surface

Stein and Leventhal, in 1935, reported that several women with metropathia type of bleeding and bulky ovaries underwent wedge resection for ovarian biopsy, experienced a resumption of menstruation and started ovulating. This started the wedge resection as a surgical treatment for polycystic ovarian syndrome (PCOS) so as to reduce the hyperplastic central stroma and for initiation of ovulation. Discovery of clomiphene citrate and gonadotropins decreased the popularity of wedge resection. Ovulation and pregnancy rates increased following electrocautery of ovarian capsule during laparoscopy.

In PCOS patients with clomiphene resistance or failure of ovulation/conception with 3–6 cycles of letrozole, second line of management is either laparoscopic ovarian drilling or ovulation induction with gonadotropins. Laparoscopic ovarian drilling is a one-time procedure with less chances of ovarian hyperstimulation syndrome and multiple pregnancies. This procedure may be preferred over gonadotropins in selected cases. Laparoscopy also helps in diagnosis of associated infertility factors like tubal adhesions and mild-to-moderate endometriosis.

### Technique

- Tubal patency must be checked before starting the procedure.
- The ovary is held with a traumatic grasper and 4 punctures are made with 40 watts current up to a depth of 4 mm.
- Monopolar needle should hit the ovarian surface at an angle of 90° to prevent the surface coagulation of the ovary (**Figure 1.1a**).
- The punctures should be made away from the tubal side of ovary to prevent the occurrence of peritubal adhesions (**Figure 1.1b**).
- Always cool down the ovary before releasing it from the grasper to prevent postoperative adhesions.
- Select the patients well. One should exhaust medical treatment to the fullest before resorting to ovarian drilling.
- Bulky polycystic ovaries seen on a diagnostic laparoscopy should not routinely be drilled.

A complete hormonal profile and all factors for infertility should be ruled out before posting the patient for drilling.

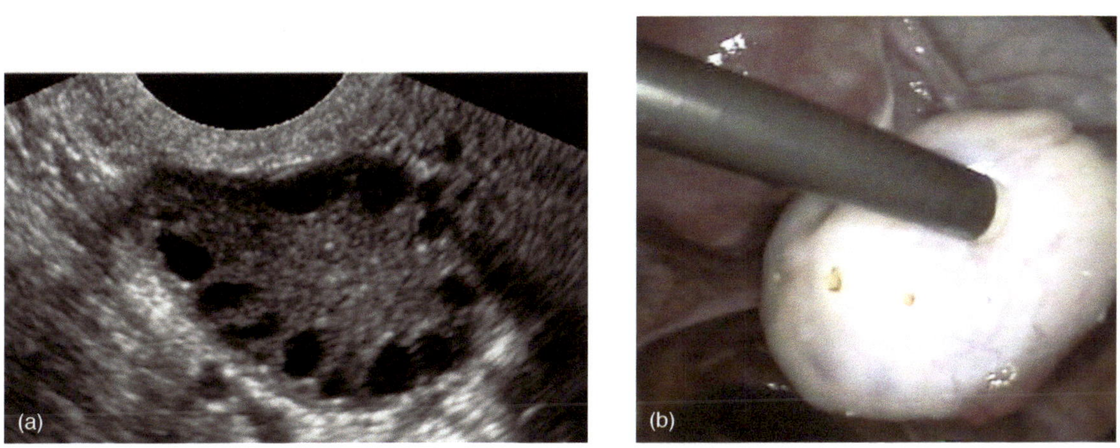

**FIGURE 1.1** (a) Transvaginal ultrasound image of a polycystic ovary. (b) Laparoscopic monopolar drilling of the ovarian cortex.

## Endometriosis

The prevalence of endometriosis among the reproductive age is about 11%. Progressive dysmenorrhea, dyspareunia and infertility are the most common symptoms in women suffering with endometriosis. A 2D/3D transvaginal ultrasound in symptomatic patients can establish a diagnosis of endometriosis. Laparoscopy with the histological evidence of ectopic endometrial glands and epithelium is the gold standard to establish a firm diagnosis.

### Technique

- In patients with mild-to-moderate peritoneal endometriosis, the lesion can be excised with scissors or monopolar needle. In case the lesion is lying over a vital structure like ureter, it can be infiltrated with normal saline just under the lesion to raise it up to protect the underlying structure.
- In cases of scattered nodules, the lesions can be cauterised with bipolar forceps by short spurt of current. Make sure to look at the posterior surface of the ovaries, in the pouch of Douglas and over the uterosacral ligaments for the presence of endometriotic nodules.
- A biopsy must be taken from these nodules to confirm the diagnosis of endometriosis by histopathological examination.
- In cases of endometriotic cyst there is a historical debate between incision and drainage or cystectomy, the former causes an increase in the recurrence rates and the latter might reduce the ovarian reserve.
- Diluted vasopressin is injected between the ovarian surface and cyst wall to get better planes, less bleeding and lesser use of cautery leading to lesser compromise of ovarian reserve.
- In cases of associated infertility factors like bilateral tubal blockage or male factor infertility (these patients may need to directly go for IVF), a judicious decision needs to be taken whether to operate or to go directly for ART.
- Laparoscopic cyst excision in such patients is only required if the cyst size is very large (>5 cm) in size or is coming in the way of Oozyte Pick Up (OPU) or there are multiple implantation failures in young patients (Figure 1.2).
- Young patients with no associated infertility factors should be taken for a laparoscopic cystectomy followed by either OI with Timed Inter Course (TIC)/ Intra Uterine Insemination (IUI) up to 6 cycles failing which a further counselling should be offered to take them in ART program.

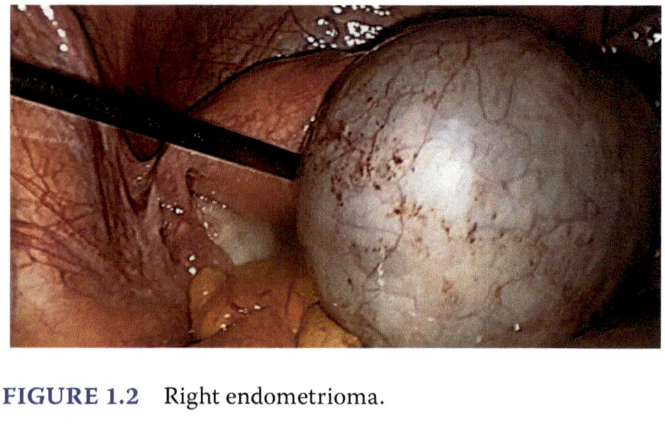

FIGURE 1.2 Right endometrioma.

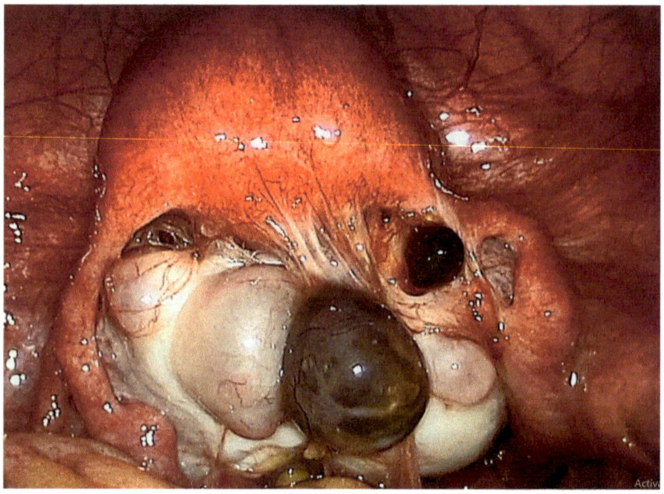

FIGURE 1.3 Endometriosis stage III with frozen pelvis.

- In severe endometriosis (**Figure 1.3**), it is debatable whether to go for surgical clearance followed IUI/TIC or they should be offered straight forward IVF; however, IVF-ET seems to be effective alternative in such cases with a shorter time to pregnancy.
- In cases of previous implantation failures in severe endometriosis, a surgical intervention in the form of laparoscopy is justified. These cases should be handled at tertiary care laparoscopic centers by highly skilled laparoscopic surgeons.
- Ovarian reserve tests (AMH, AFC, Day 2 FSH) must be performed before the surgery, documented and informed to the patient. These tests should be repeated after 3–4 months of surgery.

## Hydrosalpinges

Hydrosalpinges are common findings in infertile patients going for ART. On transvaginal sonography, they appear like fluid-filled cystic cavities which are separated by a thin septa surrounding the ovary and the color Doppler will show poor blood flow. The best time to do an ultrasound scan is at the mid-cycle as the fluid tends to accumulate during the follicular phase. Sometimes the presence of fluid in the endometrial cavity during the follicular phase or at the time of ET may suggest a possibility of subclinical hydrosalpinx and such patients may require a laparoscopic evaluation. The common infections causing hydrosalpinx are gonorrhea and chlamydia; however, in an Indian setting it is not uncommon also to encounter genital tuberculosis as a cause.

Hydrosalpinx reduces pregnancy rate and must be treated before ET. It alters the implantation as well as has direct effect on the embryo. The embryo toxicity occurs due to leakage of fluid from hydrosalpinx to the uterine cavity. This fluid is harmful to the embryo and also has a negative effect on the uterine receptivity and implantation mechanism. The removal of deceased tube not only improves the pregnancy rates but also reduces the rate of miscarriage compared with most of untreated hydrosalpinx.

A Cochrane review confirmed that the odds of pregnancy were increased with laparoscopic salpingectomy for hydrosalpinges prior to IVF (OR = 1.75, 95% CI 1.07 to 2.86), as were the odds of ongoing pregnancy or live birth (OR = 2.13, 95% CI 1.24 to 3.65). All these data demonstrate that laparoscopic salpingectomy for hydrosalpinges is the preferred procedure for improving pregnancy.

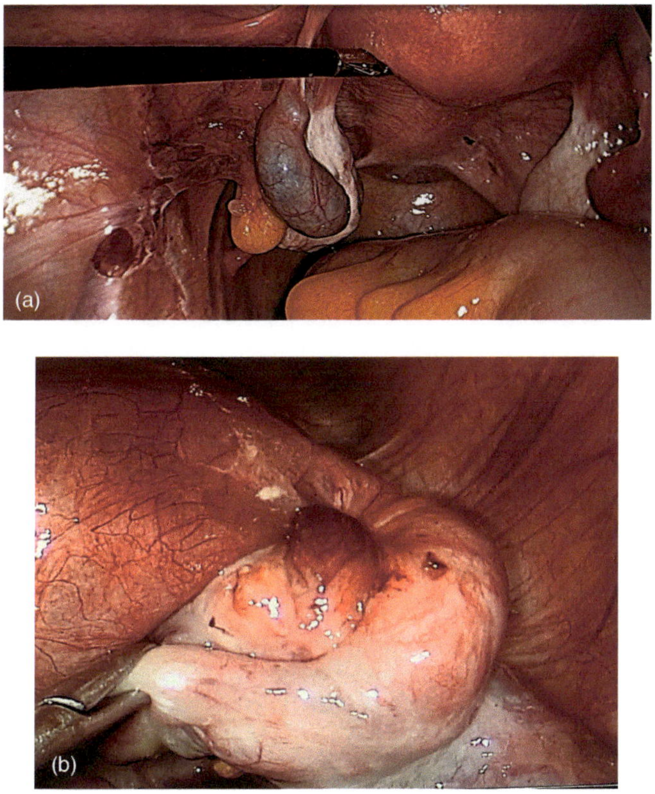

**FIGURE 1.4** (a) Left hydosalpinx with peripheral occlusion after methylene blue injection. (b) Right pyosalpinx with peripheral occlusion.

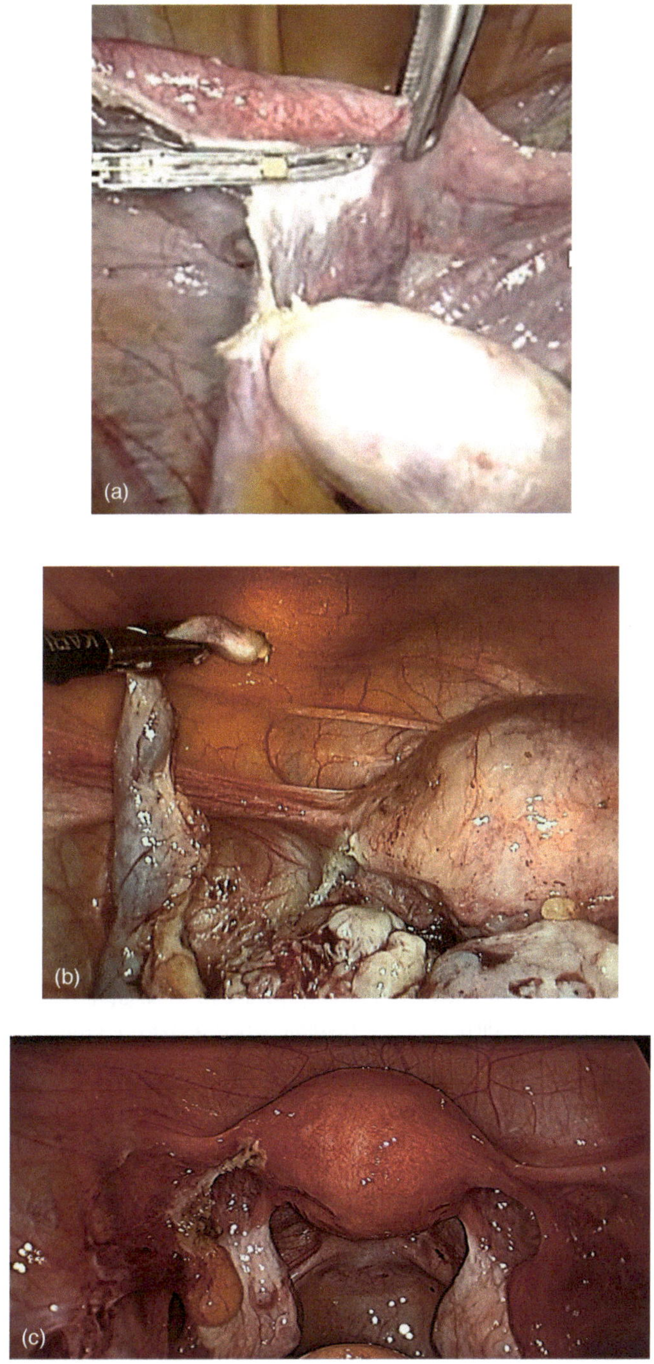

**FIGURE 1.5** (a–c) Steps in left salpingectomy.

### Technique

- The tube is removed entirely through minimally invasive laparoscopic surgery. We use two ipsilateral ports with a primary port in the center at the level of umbilicus.
- The tube is held with a grasper and progressively cauterised and cut at the mesosalphinx closest to the tube.
- It is very important to remain very close to the tube so as to avoid compromising blood supply to ovary so as to preserve the ovarian reserve.
- It is also important to cauterise the stump well after salphingectomy to prevent risk of stump ectopic pregnancy.
- In most of the cases it is possible to do a complete salphingectomy, but in some cases of very large hydrosalphinx with previous history of surgeries, we may find severe bowel adhesions (**Figure 1.5a–c**).
- In such cases intrauterine instillation of methylene blue may help in delineating the dilated tube from the bowel (**Figure 1.4a, b**).
- A possibility of a delinking at the isthmic end with the help of bipolar cautery or scissors can be kept in mind in such cases.

## Myomectomy

Uterine fibroids are the most common benign tumors in women of reproductive age group. Fibroids are present in approximately 5%–10% of the patients presenting with infertility. However, they are found to be the sole identified factor in only 1%–2.4% of the infertile patients [2]. According to Somigliana et al., myomas negatively affect the pregnancy rates [3] and submucosal fibroids strongly interfere with the chance of pregnancy. In patients of infertility associated with fibroid uterus, first other causes of infertility should be ruled out. The prevalence of fibroid in infertile population is about 5%–10%; however, after other causes of infertility are ruled out fibroids are the causative factors in only 1%–2% of infertile patients.

### Which fibroids should be removed?

- All submucous fibroids have a negative impact on pregnancy outcome and should be removed before going for ART.

- Subserous fibroids as expected do not play any role in infertility so need not be removed.
- In intramural fibroids, the effect of surgical intervention is unclear. Those indenting the endometrial cavity and large fibroids (>5 cm) are good candidates for laparoscopic myomectomy.
- Laparoscopic myomectomy may also be considered in patients with intramural fibroids with previous multiple implantation failures or recurrent pregnancy loss even if the myoma is not distorting the endometrial cavity.

### Technique

- Port placement is done depending on the size of fibroid and the surgeon's discretion.
- For ipsilateral secondary ports, a transverse incision is planned as it eases the suturing.
- After initial inspection of the abdomen and fibroid mapping, dilute vasopressin 20 units in 200 mL of NS is injected in subcapsular space.
- Alternatively, in large fibroids we can apply hemostatic clips bilaterally on the uterine arteries and IP ligament, which can be gently removed with the grasper at the end of surgery.
- This reduces the blood loss during surgery and lesser recurrence rate of fibroid is also reported.
- Transverse incision is given on the myoma bulge with monopolar hook/monopolar scissors or the active blade of harmonic scalpel.
- Avoid going close to the cornual end and continue the incision till we find the cleavage plane.
- The myometrial tissue and the fibroid tissue are different in consistency and it is important to find the right plane of dissection. An intra-capsular myomectomy should be achieved (**Figure 1.6**).
- Once the myoma tissue is exposed it is stabilised for traction either with a myoma screw or with a tenaculum (**Figure 1.7**).
- The myometrium is pushed slowly and gently coagulating the tissue as and when required.
- We can use a combination of bipolar and scissors or harmonic scalpel or lotus clamp depending on surgeon preference.
- In large intramural fibroids indenting into the endometrium, it is good to check the integrity of the endometrium by intrauterine injection of methylene blue.
- It is not drastic if the endometrial cavity is breached but we must take precautions not to include the endometrium in the sutures (bluish color of endometrium helps us to delineate from the myometrium), which may lead to increased risk of scar ectopic pregnancy awing to micro-fistulae formation.

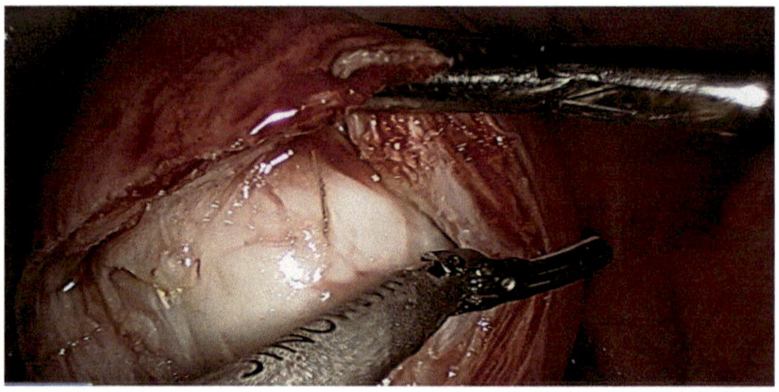

FIGURE 1.6 Myomectomy (endocapsular enucleation of the fibrod).

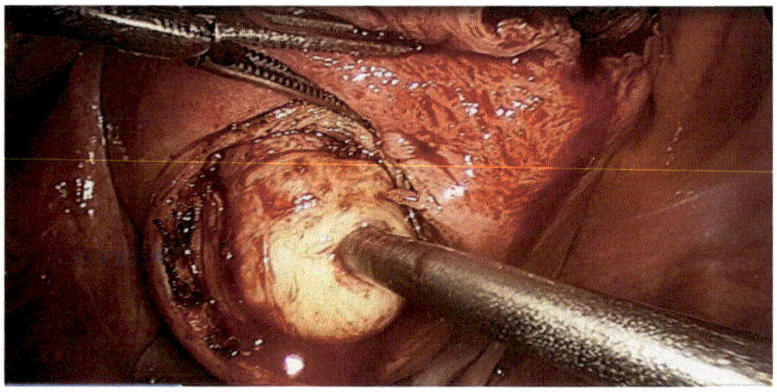

FIGURE 1.7 Myomectomy (grasping the partly enucleated fibrod with the myoma screw for traction).

- The myoma bed is closed in one or two layers with absorbable polygalactin (vicryl) or with barb sutures (viloc) depending on the surgeon's preference.
- The advantage of barb suture is tight sutures and less chances of hematoma formation resulting in a stronger scar.

## Adenomyosis

Transvaginal sonography confirms the diagnosis of adenomyosis in patients with symptomatology of pain, dysmenorrhea, dyspareunia and infertility. First-line management in infertility and pain in adenomyosis is medical management. However, in patients going for ART cycles, a surgical intervention may be required in a large focal adenomyoma and long-standing infertility.

**The surgical option is reserved in patients of**

- Failed medical management.
- Symptomatic patient with chronic pelvic pain and heavy menstrual bleeding.
- Multiple implantation failure and recurrent pregnancy loss.

### Technique

- Although vasopressin is injected at the bulge of the adenomyoma to reduce the intra-operative bleeding, it is difficult to get a definitive plane as there is no capsule.
- So incision is given over the bulge of lesion and a debulking is done in a wedge shape (**Figure 1.8**).

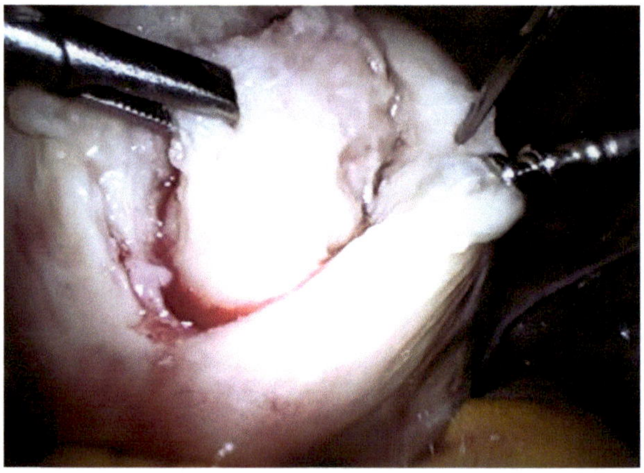

FIGURE 1.8 Adenomyosis resection (no capsule).

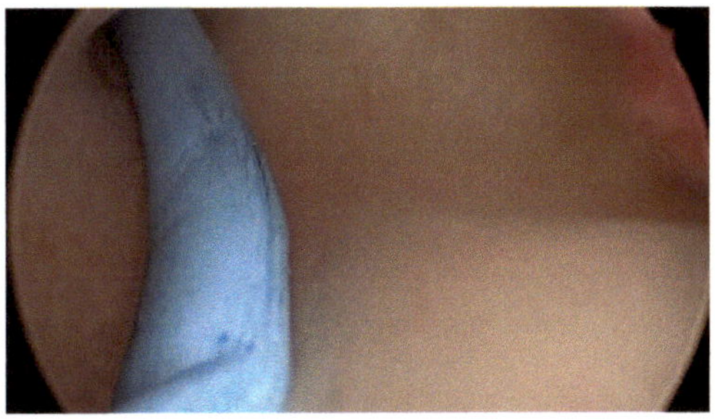

**FIGURE 1.9** Hysteroscopic left tubal canalization.

- Suturing is done with overlapping flap technique so as to get a better strength of the scar for better fertility outcome.

## Hysteroscopic tubal cannulation

The procedure is done in cases of bilateral cornual block under laparoscopic guidance. It is mentioned here as this treatment absolutely needs laparoscopic vision.

### Technique

- A simultaneous laparoscopy and hysteroscopy is performed.
- The conformation of cornual block can be done before starting a procedure by injecting diluted methylene blue solution into the uterine cavity (we use diluted betadine so as to prevent staining of endometrium).
- A 5 French catheter with a obturator is inserted through the operating channel of hysteroscope to reach the ostia.
- Just at the level of ostia, the curved catheter is pushed into the ostia and the obturator is gently pulled out (it is very important not to push obturator in the tubal ostia as it will perforate the cornual end of the tube) (**Figure 1.9**).
- The obturator is to be used only as a guide to reach the ostium.
- After removing the obturator, diluted methylene blue dye is injected through the catheter and free spill is seen from the fimbrial end laparoscopically.
- The same procedure is repeated on the other side.

## Conclusion

1. In endometriosis, laparoscopy is the gold standard to establish the diagnosis. (4) In patients desiring fertility, it is recommended in stages I and II by the American Society of Reproductive Medicine (ASRM). It can be considered in stage III and IV if the patient is young or after several IVF failures. However patients going for ART (for associated infertility factors, long standing infertility, previously operated endometriotic cyst with no spontaneous conception, recurrence of endometriotic cyst, poor ovarian reserve) with endometriotic cyst should not be operated unless the cyst is very large (more than 4 cm), causing pain, coming in the way of Ovum Pick Up or multiple implantation failures especially in young patients.
2. Laparoscopic myomectomy must be carried out by skilled laparoscopic surgeon. Myomas should be removed when they are sub-mucous or indenting the uterine cavity. Large intramural fibroids (>5 cm) should also be considered for surgery especially when there is no other factor affecting fertility.
3. Ovarian drilling should be considered only after exhausting medical management.
4. Patients going for IVF, with hydrosalpinx, should be counseled for salpingectomy to improve the results of ART.
5. For spontaneous conceptions, Laparoscopy should be envisaged when the pathology is treatable and the patient agrees to have 9–15 months interval prior to IVF.

## References


1. Gomel V, Salpingostomy by microsurgery. Fertil Steril. 1978;29(4):380–7.
2. Benecke C, Kruger TF, Siebert TI, et al. Effect of fibroids on fertility in patients undergoing assisted reproduction. A structured literature review. Gynecol Obstet Invest. 2005;59(4):225–30.
3. Somigliana E, Vercellini P, Daguati R, et al. Fibroids and female reproduction: A critical analysis of evidence. Hum Reprod. 2007;13(5):465–76.
4. Alkatout I and Mettler L, *Practical Manual for Laparoscopic and Hysteroscopic. Surgery*, 3rd edition, 2019. Jaypee Brothers Medical Publishers, New Delhi, London, Panama, 798.

# 2

## PRINCIPLES OF LAPAROSCOPIC SUTURING AND ALTERNATIVES

**Ibrahim Alkatout**

### Introduction

Ligatures and suturing techniques represent a safe and, in many cases, the only method of hemostasis in endoscopic surgery and are often better suited than thermal methods. Various suture materials, applicators and needle holders have been developed for this purpose.

Laparoscopic intracorporeal knot tying in minimally invasive surgery requires great manual dexterity. There is a difference between laparoscopic suturing and open or robotic-assisted suturing. Given a skill score of 10 for various surgical modalities, conventional laparotomy requires a score of 2, microsurgery a score of 4, laparoscopy a score of 6 and laparoscopic suturing a score of 8, while robotic laparoscopic suturing returns to the skill level of general laparoscopic surgery with a score of 6. This is due to the limited movement abilities of laparoscopic instruments compared to open and robotic surgery. Furthermore, there is a variety of alternatives including bipolar and ultrasound-based sealing instruments that have replaced intracorporeal ligatures and needle handling. Therefore, the art of suturing also includes the art of proper selection [1, 2].

The lesson is clear; Never underestimate the art of laparoscopic suturing, never get too frustrated and understand that laparoscopic suturing requires repeated training [3].

### High-frequency electricity

#### Physics

Hemostasis can be achieved by using high-frequency electricity in the correct manner. Before the application of electric current in surgery, hemostasis was managed by suturing. Electric current is provided by a high-frequency generator and conducted through a neutral null electrode.

In the majority of endoscopic operations, electric current is used to expose tissue and achieve hemostasis. Knowledge of the underlying physical phenomena is essential in order to use electric current meaningfully as well as estimate and avoid potential risks. The use of electrosurgery is based on the fact that the human body conducts high-frequency alternating current. The flow of electric current through tissue causes the following three specific effects:

1. **Faraday effect**: The flow of electric current stimulates electrically stimulable cells (muscles and nerves), which causes muscle contractions. The application of alternating current at frequencies above 300 kHz prevents this undesirable effect.
2. **Electrolytic effect**: Direct current causes the migration of positive ions to the cathode and negative ions to the anode. In human tissue this effect causes cell damage; however, alternating current at sufficiently high frequencies prevents this effect and causes no more than an occasional ion oscillation.
3. **Thermal effect**: The flow of electric current warms human tissue. This is dependent on tissue resistance, current density and exposure time. The thermal effect is the sole desired effect when using high-frequency electrical current in surgery and is the basis of operative endoscopy.

No relevant cell damage occurs below 40°C. Depending on the duration of exposure, reversible damage to tissue occurs between 40°C and 49°C. Irreversible cell damage occurs at temperatures above 49°C. Such damage is caused by the coagulation of cell proteins. Initially, the cell matrix remains intact although individual cells may already have perished. Such damage can be compensated, depending on the regeneration potential of the tissue. Temperatures above 60°C cause desiccation due to the evaporation of intracellular and extracellular water. As long as water particles are present, the tissue temperature remains below the boiling point of 100°C, it then rises and is followed by carbonization effects (blackish discoloration of tissue) (**Figure 2.1**).

High-frequency electrosurgery employs alternating current of 300,000 to 1,000,000 Hz. The thermal effect is also the therapeutic effect.

#### Electrocoagulation

A coagulation effect occurs when tissue is slowly heated to more than 60°C. Several changes occur during this "boiling" process, such as the denaturation of protein, the evaporation of intracellular and extracellular water and shrinkage of tissue. Depending on the quality of the current and the type of application, a distinction is made in high-frequency electrosurgery between contact coagulation, forced coagulation, desiccation (coagulation through a pierced needle electrode), spray coagulation (fulguration), argon plasma coagulation (APC), bipolar coagulation and bipolar vessel sealing.

#### Electrotomy

A cutting effect is achieved by rapid heating of tissue to 90–100°C. This causes steam in cells which tears the cell walls and then acts as an insulator. Cutting tension is created between the electrode and tissue, causing (renewed) transmission of sparks from about 200 V onward. A very high current density is present at the base points. The surroundings (air and fluid) are of no importance for the formation of this electric arc. Modulation of the electricity (increased voltage with interruptions) causes additional coagulation of the wound margins. Depending on the intensity, a distinction is made between a smooth incision and a scabbed incision. Further thermal effects of electricity (of secondary importance in high-frequency surgery) include carbonization (from about 200°C onward) and vaporization (at several hundred degrees Celsius).

#### Monopolar technique

When using monopolar electric current, the patient's body is within the electric circuit (**Figure 2.2A**). The electric current

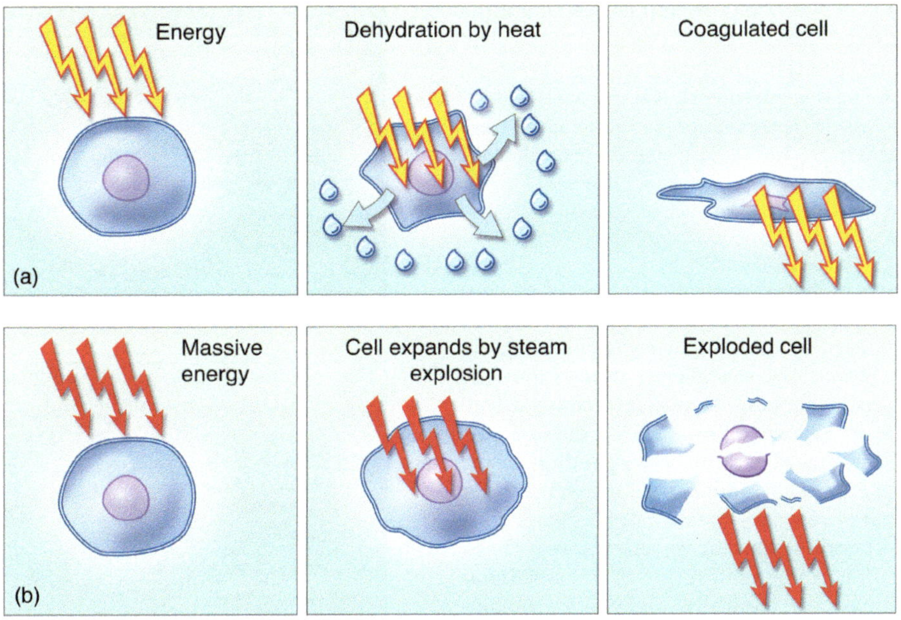


FIGURE 2.1 Effects on the individual cell, depending on the electric current used: (a) coagulation; (b) cutting.

makes contact with the tissue through an active electrode, flows through the body and leaves the body via a neutral electrode. The ratio of surfaces (active electrode and passive electrode) is shifted in favor of the active electrode which enhances the thermal effect of the greater current density at this site. The electric current used for resection has a sinewave vibration of relatively low-voltage amplitude. This causes a very rapid increase of temperature in tissue, followed by cell vaporization and greater permeability of tissue. Coagulation current has greater voltage and is applied in a rapid exchange of on-off phases. After being heated in the on-phase, the tissue is able to cool in the off-phase. This alternation causes slow tissue heating which is manifested as coagulation.

Defects in the insulation of instruments or trocars may cause direct coupling of electricity and undetected tissue damage. Likewise, coagulation in the proximity of thin tissue bridges may cause thermal defects when electric current flows through the tissue bridge. The result is heat and undesirable damage at a considerable distance from the actual area of surgery.

The neutral electrode should be placed at a site where the pathway of the electric current between the active and the neutral electrode is as short as possible and runs longitudinally or diagonally towards the body because muscles in the direction of the fibrils possess greater conductivity. The neutral electrode must be in full contact with the skin because the generated heat is proportional to the surface of the electrode.

## Bipolar technique

Even in bipolar electricity, warmth is produced in an electric circuit. However, the active and the neutral electrode are as close to each other as possible and possess the same mass. Thus, only

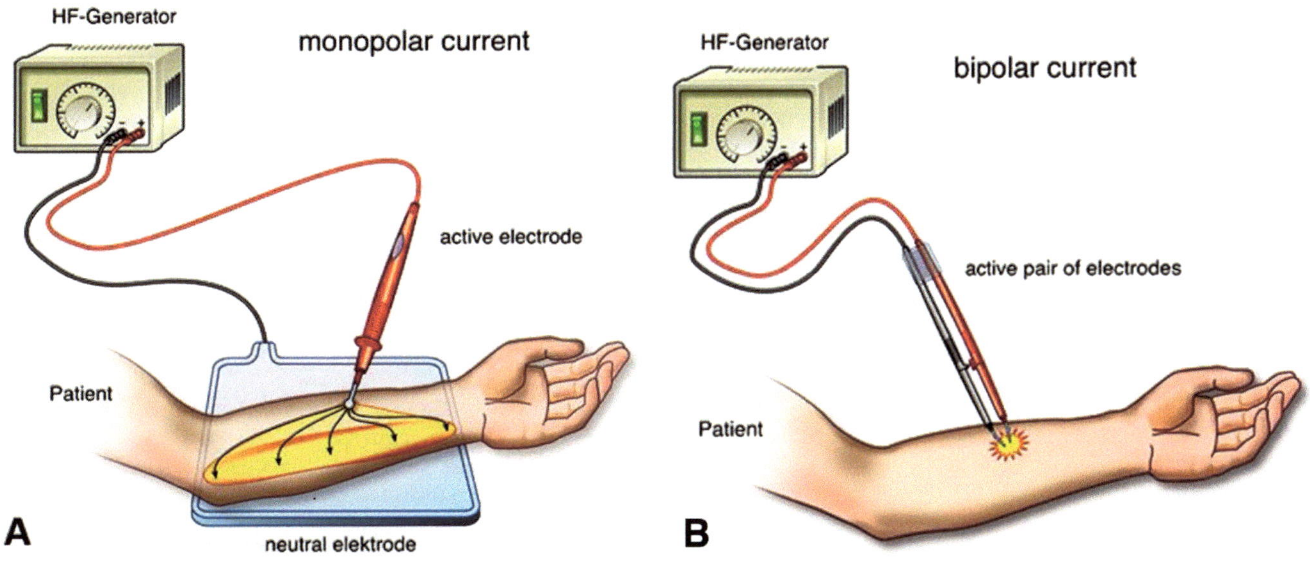


FIGURE 2.2 Principle of (A) monopolar current; (B) bipolar.

the operating field (tissue between the two branches) and not the entire patient is within the electric circuit. Activation of the electric current causes warming of tissue and coagulation. Therefore, the neutral electrode can be dispensed with (**Figure 2.2B**).

The application of excessive thermal energy is liable to damage sensitive organ structures in the immediate vicinity (bowel, bladder, ureter and blood vessels).

### Vessel sealing

Vessels larger than 2 mm in diameter cannot be treated by conventional electrocoagulation. Reliable hemostasis and permanent closure can only be achieved by using bipolar vessel sealing, an ultrasonic scalpel or ligation. The vascular or tissue bundle is grasped with a special instrument and compressed constantly at a predefined pressure level. Several automatically regulated current cycles with variable electrical parameters, depending on the grasped tissue, "fuse" the mutually opposing tissue walls. Exact preparatory visualization of vessels is usually not necessary. One can grasp entire tissue bundles, contain vessels and seal these. Technically, bipolar sealing can be achieved up to a vessel diameter of about 10 mm; it has been clinically validated for a diameter of 7 mm. Due to warming of the instrument tip, it should be performed at a safe distance from sensitive tissue structures. The blade of the ultrasound scalpel becomes much hotter than that of insulated bipolar instruments but produces efficient torsional movement in the waveguide to direct strong compression energy to the target tissue.

Histologically, it was found that in conventional coagulation, shrinkage of the wall and the formation of a thrombus are involved in hemostasis. In contrast, vessel sealing is associated with the denaturation of collagen and the fusion of opposing layers while the elastic internal membrane, whose fibers are denatured at a temperature above 100°C, is largely preserved. There is a transition zone of 1–2 mm with thermal damage, lateral to the sharply margined homogeneous coagulation zone. Immunohistochemical examination revealed a two-fold increase in the width of the transition zone. This is followed by a sterile inflammation due to resorption, especially in the surrounding connective tissue, with no sign of any (even temporary) failure of the sealing. The main advantages of bipolar vessel sealing compared to other procedures, such as ligatures, sutures or the use of clips, are fast exposure, rapid and safe vessel closure, the absence of foreign material remaining in the operating field and lower costs. This results in shorter operating times, less blood loss and less stress for the patient. Therefore, these instruments are now widely used in open surgery and vaginal surgery.

Depending on the type, strength and frequency of the electric current, it exerts an electrolytic (disintegrating), Faradaic (stimulating nerves and muscles) or thermal effect. Alternating currents with a frequency of at least 200 kHz are used in high-frequency surgery and the thermal effect is dominant. It mainly depends on the exposure time, current density and the specific resistance of tissue which, to put it simply, drops with increasing water content or rising perfusion. The quantity of electric current flowing alongside the target site, which may warm and damage other areas, is also important in the practical setting (such as during irrigation, when using the monopolar technique rather than the bipolar one) [4, 5].

Additional substances, such as hemostatic agents, are required in laparoscopy because prolonged active compression cannot be achieved with abdominal surgical belts. Furthermore, electric current should be used as stringently as possible in very sensitive locations (close to the ureter or the bowel). In these regions the surgeon must frequently resort to additives. Carriers developed specifically for laparoscopy can be introduced and used easily; they provide additional protection and safety for the patient (**Figure 2.3**).

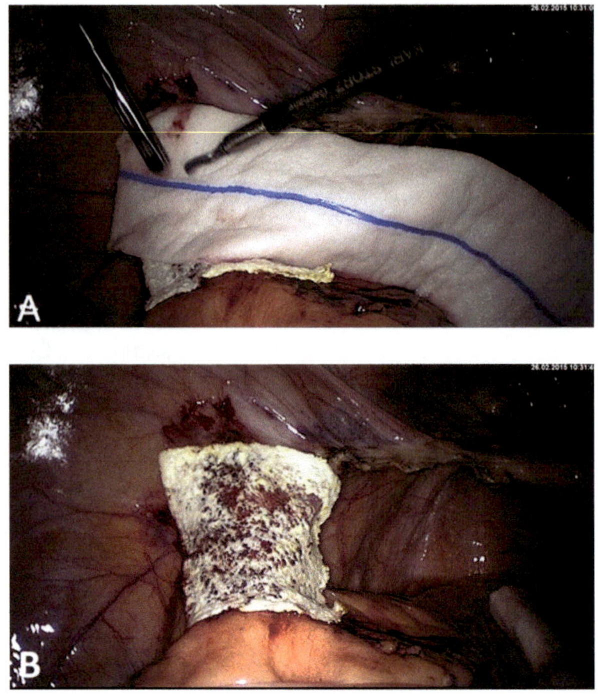


**FIGURE 2.3** Endoscopic use of Tachosil (Takeda Company) on the pelvic wall. (A) Moistened gauze pad pressing the patch onto slightly bleeding tissue until the tissue is fully moistened (B).

## Sutures and suture technique

### Suture material

Sutures are either monofilament or polyfilament/braided and they are either absorbable or non-absorbable depending on whether the body will naturally degrade and absorb the suture material over time. The resorption process includes hydrolysis and proteolytic enzymatic degradation. Depending on the material, the process can take from 10 days to 8 weeks. The suture holds the body tissues together long enough to allow healing, but it will disintegrate so that no foreign material is left. Initially, there is a transient foreign body reaction to the material. After complete resorption only connective tissue remains. Non-absorbable sutures are made of special silk or synthetics. These sutures are used either on skin wound closure, if the sutures can be removed after a few weeks, or in stressful internal environments where absorbable sutures will not suffice. Non-absorbable sutures mostly cause less scarring because they do not provoke immune responses.

Monofilament sutures: These sutures are rigid and the knots are not well positioned on the wound.

Braided sutures: These have a capillary effect and high friction resistance. For an overview on suture materials, see **Table 2.1**.

### Thread thickness/Suture sizes

Suture sizes are defined by the United States Pharmacopeia (USP) and are shown in **Table 2.2**.

**TABLE 2.1: Examples of Suture Materials**

| Suture Material (Examples) | | | |
|---|---|---|---|
| Absorbable | | Non-Absorbable | |
| **Monofilamental** | **Braided** | **Monofilamental** | **Braided** |
| PDS (PD)<br>Maxon (PGS) | Vicryl (G/L)<br>Dexon (G/L) | Ethilon (PA)<br>Prolene (PP) | Ethibond (POE)<br>Mersilene (POE) |

G/L = Glycolid/Lactid
PD = Polydiaxanon
PGS = Polygylcol acid
POE = Polyester
PP = Polypropylene
PA = Polyamid

**TABLE 2.2: Suture Sizes, Defined by the United States Pharmacopeia (USP)**

| USP Designation | Synthetic Absorbable Diameter (mm) | Non-Absorbable Diameter (mm) |
|---|---|---|
| 11-0 | | 0.01 |
| 10-0 | 0.02 | 0.02 |
| 9-0 | 0.03 | 0.03 |
| 8-0 | 0.04 | 0.04 |
| 7-0 | 0.05 | 0.05 |
| 6-0 | 0.07 | 0.07 |
| 5-0 | 0.1 | 0.1 |
| 4-0 | 0.15 | 0.15 |
| 3-0 | 0.2 | 0.2 |
| 2-0 | 0.3 | 0.3 |
| 0 | 0.35 | 0.35 |
| 1 | 0.4 | 0.4 |
| 2 | 0.5 | 0.5 |
| 3 | 0.6 | 0.6 |
| 4 | 0.6 | 0.6 |
| 5 | 0.7 | 0.7 |
| 6 | | 0.8 |
| 7 | | |

### Barbed sutures

To avoid the time-consuming knotting process but still create reliable and fixed sutures, barbed suture threads have been invented. These sutures have small barbs that allow traction in one direction only, thereby preventing the thread from being drawn back. Barbed sutures are used for vaginal cuff closure and also for bowel or bladder surgery. Nevertheless, a higher rate of bowel irritation and infection has been described in some cases in the literature. Furthermore, barbed sutures have a higher price than normal absorbable suture materials. Nevertheless, the existing data and meta-analysis describe the use of barbed sutures as a safe procedure to reduce time and surgical difficulty compared to conventional sutures in vaginal cuff closure. The comparison of barbed suture versus conventional suturing is shown in **Table 2.3** [6, 7].

### Surgical needles

Needles can be reusable (eyed needles). Reusable needles have holes (eyes) and are supplied separately from their suture thread which must be threaded on site. The advantage of these needles is that any thread and needle combination is possible. Needles with integrated thread are used in laparoscopy. They have less traumatic tissue effects and are time efficient but more expensive. Needles may also be classified by their point geometry: taper, cutting, reverse cutting, trocar point or blunt points.

**TABLE 2.3: Comparison of Barbed Suture versus Conventional Suture Material**

| Barbed Suture versus Conventional Suture | |
|---|---|
| Less operative time | Higher costs |
| Less suturing time | Higher rate of bowel obstructions |
| Lower degree of suturing difficulty / technically less demanding | |
| Similar patient outcome | |
| Similar duration of hospital stay | |
| Preferred method based on surgeon's preference | |

**TABLE 2.4: Surgical Needle Types and Variations**

| |
|---|
| Straight |
| 1/4 circle |
| 3/8 circle |
| 1/2 circle: Subtypes include from larger to smaller: CT, CT-1, CT-2 and CT-3 |
| 5/8 circle |
| Compound curve |
| Half-curved (ski needle) |
| Half-curved at both ends of a straight segment (canoe needle) |

There are several shapes of surgical needles. These are listed in **Table 2.4**.

The correct selection of the appropriate suture is essential. Each surgical procedure requires specific needle configurations and needle-suture combinations.

The following suture exercises are described in easy steps:

a. Two extracorporeal knotting techniques, the Roeder and the von Leffern knot (**Figures 2.4** and **2.5**)
b. The step-by-step procedure of intracorporeal knotting using the common techniques of knot tying (**Figures 2.6** and **2.7**)

The primary role of the needle holder/driver is handling the needle although suturing and tissue grasping are also part of its function. The preferred shape of the tip is a slightly spooning curvature. For grasping tissue and looping suture, the tip must be able to reach in almost any direction. The jaws should be finely engineered to grasp fine sutures without slipping and have rounded edges to avoid accidental cutting of the suture as traction is applied. The dominant needle holder should have a lock that the surgeon can activate or inactivate at will. It should be strong and preferably have one moving jaw to reduce suture snagging. The lock on the non-dominant needle holder should preferably be inactivated.

## Tips and tricks

### Loading the needle

First grasp the thread about an inch from the needle with the assisting grasper. Dangle it in a fashion so that the tip of the needle touches the tissue surface. The needle is rotated and pivoted until it lines up in the direction required. It is then grasped with the contralateral needle driver. The needle is loaded up at the junction of middle and proximal third of the shaft of the needle and at the very end of the needle driver.

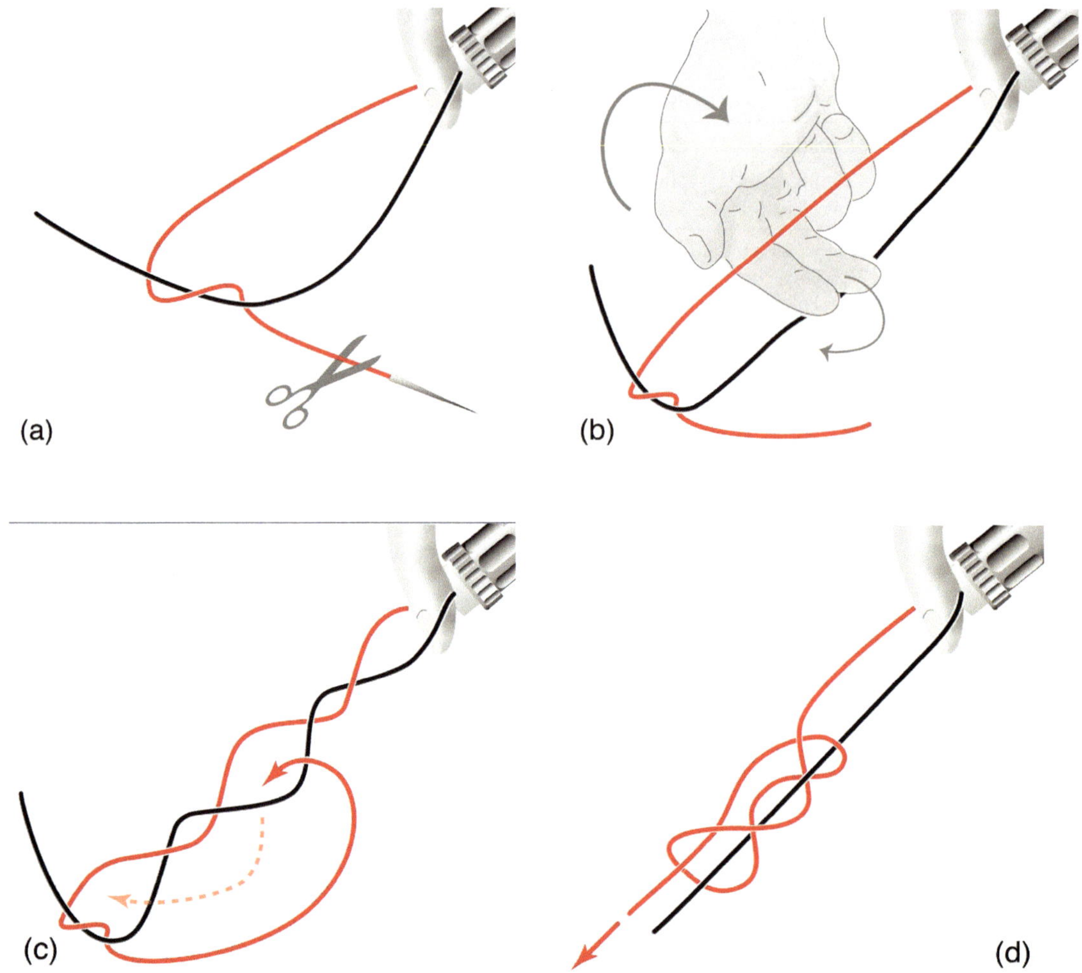


**FIGURE 2.4** *Von Leffern knot*: (a) Pull out the suture, remove the needle and perform a half hitch. (b) The index and middle finger then twist from below in between the sutures and grasp the short end which is led back, exiting before the half hitch. (c) Hold the knot with the left hand and reach over with the right hand; both ends are pulled on gently so that the knot does not slip over but tightens smoothly. (d) Finally, the knot pusher can push the knot onto the leading suture line in the operating field; hold the straight suture and tighten the knot.

Optimal conditions for good suturing include a needle holding angle of 90° and an angle of needle insertion into tissue of 80–100°. This can only be guaranteed if the contralateral hand is flipping the targeted tissue over the needle.

## Adjusting the needle

Adjusting the needle requires good coordination between the left and the right hand. After having grasped the needle at about the middle of the needle rounding, it is held very lightly. The other hand can then readjust by manipulating close to the tip in very deliberate movements.

Alternatively, the needle can be adjusted by holding the suture near the swaged end of the needle and maneuvering it till the needle is aligned perpendicular to the jaws. The other needle holder can then either grasp the needle in the estimated location or the needle is placed on the tissue so that it cannot squeeze out once the free needle holder takes over.

After the ideal position has been reached, the grip on the needle is tightened to lock it into position. Most important for stitching in the right position is that the targeted tissue is pushed over the needle tip at the exact location required. By this means, the limited degrees of freedom of movement in laparoscopy can be overcome even in challenging situations. Nevertheless, these are the steps that require the most time in training.

## Tying the knot

The thread can be held in the right position by either adjusting the needle or the thread itself. It is most important that the thread runs as parallel as possible to the free and rotating needle holder. Rotating then becomes easy in both directions. Tying the knot is easier if the short end is really short (about 3 cm) and if the rotating needle holder grasps the thread at the very end before pulling it out of the loop smoothly using light rotating movements. For the second and the blocking knot, it is important to pull on the long end only so that there is enough thread for the following knots; however, the thread should not be longer than necessary [8].

Intracorporeal knotting techniques are shown in **Figures 2.6** and **2.7**.

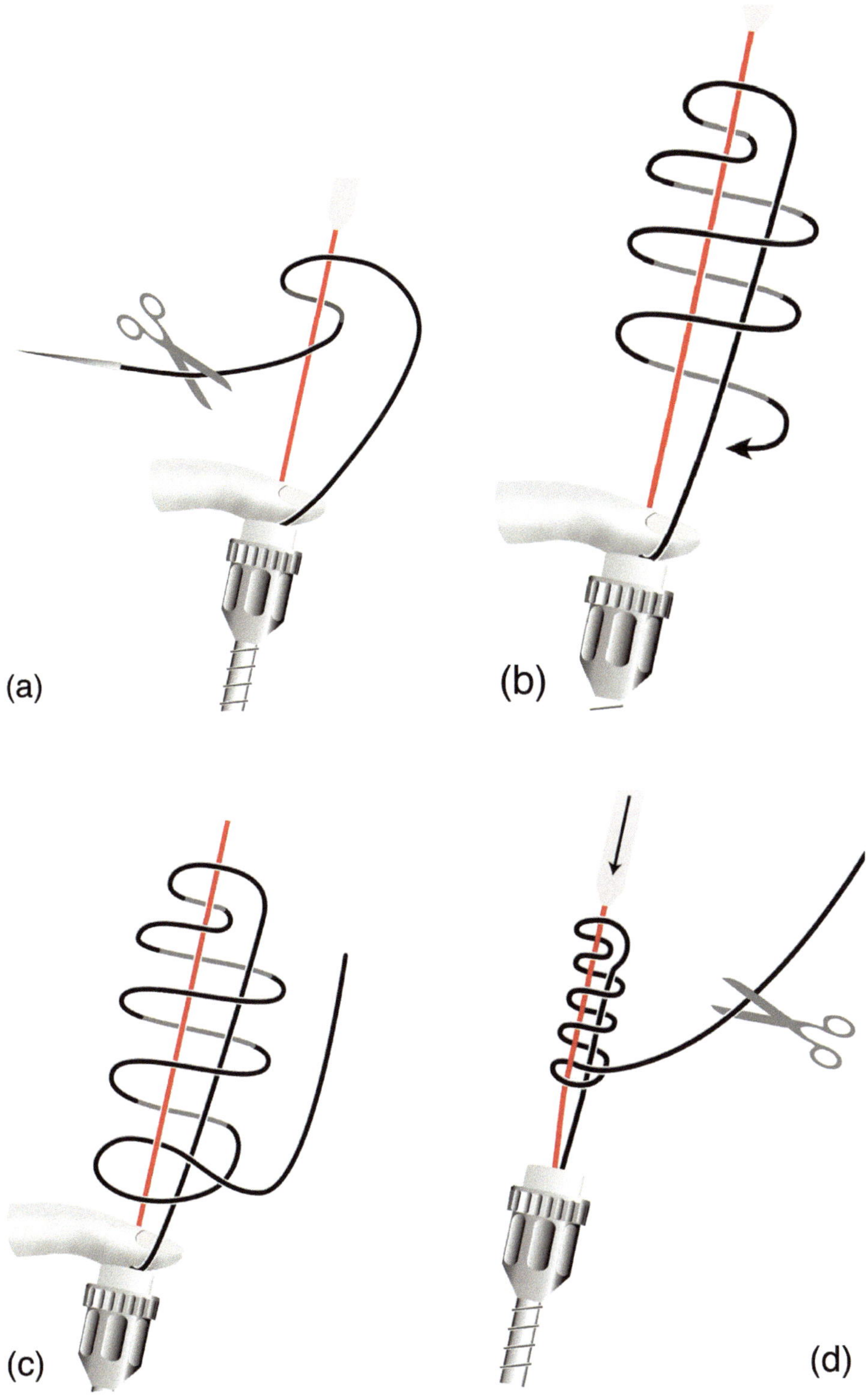


**FIGURE 2.5** *Roeder knot:* (a) Pull out the suture, remove the needle and perform a half-hitch around the post strand (red). (b) The shorter suture is looped three times around both sutures, maintaining tension. (c) The fourth time it is only looped halfway and then pulled through the post strand. Both ends are pulled on gently that the knot does not slip over but tightens smoothly. (d) Finally, the knot pusher can push the knot onto the leading suture line in the operating field; shorten the suture to approx. 2–3 cm and perform intra-abdominal safety knot.

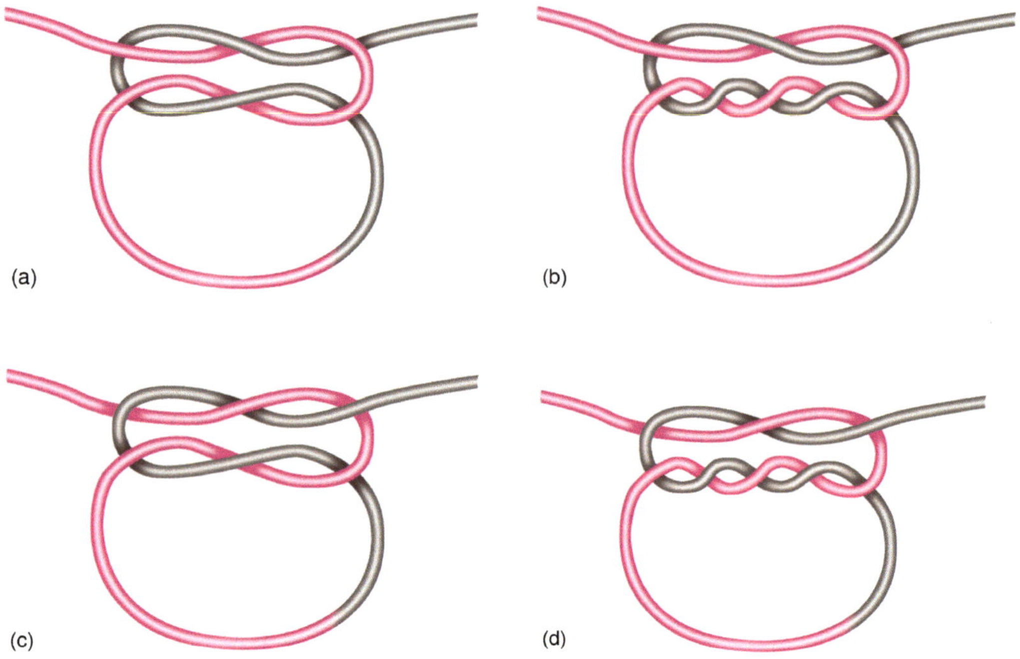

**FIGURE 2.6** (a) The classical *square knot*; (b) the surgical *square knot*; (c) the classical *granny knot* and (d) the surgical *granny knot*.

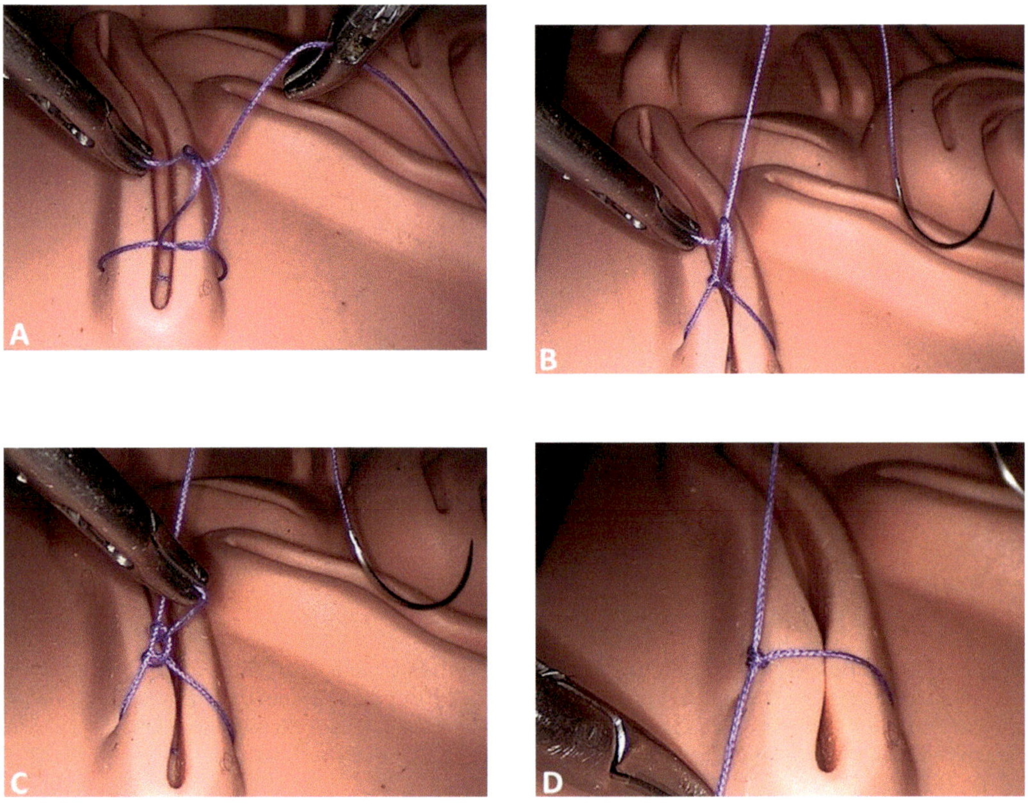

**FIGURE 2.7** *Sliding knot*: (A) After performing a normal half-hitch the initial knot lies directly on the wound. The second hitch is performed in exactly the same manner. (B) It is not essential that the lower knot lies deep in the tissue. The second knot is not straight but torqued. (C) As soon as the right instrument smoothly pulls the thread, the two knots, which are not yet tightened, will twist around the suture line that is being pulled on. (D) It is then possible to slide the complete double knot down to the tissue.

## Conclusion

Laparoscopic suturing courses from beginner to expert for vertical and horizontal suturing, including hands-on training, are offered today all around the world. The advice of our teacher Kurt Semm, that laparoscopic suturing is essential, has been accepted by the endoscopic surgical community. Technical innovations have led to a number of alternatives including bipolar, monopolar or ultrasound-guided energy. Nevertheless, for each individual situation, the right type of treatment needs to be selected, and therefore, it is obligatory that the experienced surgeon is conversant with all types of devices and is able to perform laparoscopic suturing. Otherwise, each surgery can become a jeopardy for both the patient and the surgeon [8, 9].

## References


1. Alkatout, I., et al., *Abdominal anatomy in the context of port placement and trocars.* J Turk Ger Gynecol Assoc, 2015. **16**(4): p. 241–251.
2. Alkatout, I., et al., *Robotic surgery in gynecology.* J Turk Ger Gynecol Assoc, 2016. **17**(4): p. 224–232.
3. Alkatout, I., *Complications of laparoscopy in connection with entry techniques.* J Gynecol Surg, 2017. **33**(3): p. 81–91.
4. Alkatout, I. and L. Mettler, *Hysterectomy* 1/m *A Comprehensive Surgical Approach* 2017: Springer Science. 1639.
5. Mettler, L., et al., *Endometriosis* 1/m *A Concise Practical Guide to Current Diagnosis and Treatment.* First ed. 2017: Endo Press, Tuttlingen.
6. Bogliolo, S., et al., *Barbed suture in minimally invasive hysterectomy: a systematic review and meta-analysis.* Arch Gynecol Obstet, 2015. **292**(3): p. 489–497.
7. Kim, J.H., et al., *Barbed versus conventional 2-layer continuous running sutures for laparoscopic vaginal cuff closure.* Medicine (Baltimore), 2016. **95**(39): p. e4981.
8. Alkatout, I., et al., *Safety and economical innovations regarding surgical treatment of fibroids.* Minim Invasive Ther Allied Technol, 2016. **25**(6): p. 301–313.
9. Alkatout, I., *Communicative and ethical aspects of physician-patient relationship in extreme situations.* Wien Med Wochenschr, 2015. **165**(23–24): p. 491–498.

# 3

# ROLE OF HYSTEROSCOPY IN THE DIAGNOSIS OF INCOMPLETE UTERINE SEPTUM AND SIGNIFICANT ARCUATE UTERINE ANOMALY

**Omar M. Abuzeid, Ahmed S.Z. Moustafa, and Mostafa I. Abuzeid**

## Introduction

Uterine septum is the most common congenital Müllerian anomaly accounting for more than 50% of cases [1]. Such anomalies are associated not only with the worst reproductive outcomes but also with excellent results following hysteroscopic surgical correction [2]. In an extensive review of the literature, it was concluded that the septate uterus is the most common uterine anomaly in the infertile population (3.9%), while the arcuate uterus is the most common anomaly in the general population and in those with recurrent miscarriage [3]. The prevalence of uterine septum and arcuate uterus in infertile patients varies in the literature, but it is estimated to be 3.9% and 2.1%, respectively [3].

The issue of uterine septum and infertility remains controversial, with conflicting data in the literature [3]. However, the stand of the American Society of Reproductive Medicine (ASRM) is that "There is insufficient evidence to conclude that a uterine septum is associated with infertility" [4]. Furthermore, the association of arcuate uterine anomaly (AUA) and reproductive failure remains controversial with most data suggesting that such anomaly is a variant of normal, if the internal indentation length at the fundal midline (IILFM) is < 10 mm [4].

The prevalence of uterine anomalies in patients with recurrent pregnancy loss (RPL) when optimal tests, such as transvaginal 3D ultrasound scan (TV 3D US), are used has been estimated to be 13.3% [5]. Septate uterus is the most common anomaly in this population accounting for approximately 50% [1,5]. Sugiura-Ogasawara et al. (2012) [6] suggested that major uterine anomalies have a negative impact on the reproductive outcome in patients with RPL [6]. Once such anomalies are discovered and surgically corrected, 70%–80% of patients achieve a successful live birth [2].

Parry and Isaacson (2019) [7], in a recent article on the value of hysteroscopy before fertility treatment, indicated that some "nonrandomized prospective trials have shown septate uteri to be associated with 47% lower fecundity (relative to post-transection) and a 67% chance of miscarriage" [7–9]. They also pointed out that there is currently an ongoing randomized trial entitled *The Randomized Uterine Septum Transection Trial* (TRUST), which hopefully will provide us with some answers on the value of hysteroscopic divisions of such uterine anomalies [10].

The purpose of this chapter is to briefly review old and current classification of Müllerian anomalies as it pertains to septate uterus, subseptae uterus, and AUA. We will also briefly review the various radiologic diagnostic methods being used for the diagnosis of such anomalies. However, the main purpose of this chapter is to discuss the role of diagnostic hysteroscopy in detecting subtle incomplete uterine septum (IUS) and AUA in infertile patients and patients with RPL. This chapter is also meant to increase the awareness of the short-comings of TV 3D US in ruling out such subtle anomalies. In brief, although TV 3D US is mandatory in screening for such anomalies, it is not as accurate as most of the current literature indicate.

## Classifications

ASRM classification of Müllerian anomalies is the most accepted and utilized classification, although it has some limitations, among them, the lack of morphometric criteria and its vague description of AUA (class VI) [11]. The latter makes it difficult to distinguish it from subseptate uterus (class Vb) [11]. The new guidelines by ASRM define AUA as a uterus with a "depth from the interstitial line to the apex of the indentation < 1 cm and angle of the indentation > 90°" [4]. Unfortunately, this new definition does not take into account patients with arcuate appearance (angle of the indentation > 90) and an internal indentation length ≥ 1 cm [4]. If one adopts this definition of AUA, many patients who are found to have an appearance of such anomaly on TV 3D US or hysteroscopy, with an internal indentation length ≥ 10 mm, remain unclassifiable. In addition, the new guidelines by ASRM define subseptate uterus "as having a fundal invagination > 1.5 cm with the central point of the septum at an acute angle < 90°" [4]. On the other hand, the new classification of Müllerian anomalies proposed by the European Society of Human Reproduction and Embryology and the European Society for Gynecological Endoscopy (ESHRE/ESGE) do not differentiate between AUA and uterine septum [12]. Instead they adopted a definition of uterine septum, if there is an IILFM > 50% of myometrial wall thickness [12]. Although ESHRE-ESGE classification has been criticized in few reports, it provides the long overdue morphometric criteria needed to make a diagnosis [13–15]. The main criticism is over diagnosis that may lead to over treatment. The ESHRE-ESGE was subsequently modified by the Thessaloniki ESHRE/ESGE, which addressed some of the concerns raised by some investigators [16]. A recent publication suggested ESHRE-ESGE cut-off value overestimates the prevalence of septate uterus while that of ASRM underestimates this prevalence, leaving in the gray-zone most of the uteri that experts considered as septate [17]. The authors of this chapter recommend considering indentation depth ≥ 10 mm as septate or subseptate [depending on whether IILFM reaches the internal or external cervical os (septate) or not (subseptate)], and this criterion is in agreement with expert opinion [17].

### Diagnostic modalities

Hysterosalpingography (HSG) has been used for the diagnosis of congenital uterine anomalies for many decades. HSG also provides valuable information about tubal patency in infertile patients. Other imaging modalities including ultrasonography (US) and magnetic resonance imaging (MRI) have been shown to be useful complementary tools in characterizing and delineating more clearly the exact nature of the Müllerian anomalies [18]. Transvaginal 2D ultrasound scan (TV 2D US) has been used to help in the diagnosis of congenital uterine anomalies for the last four decades. More recently, the role of TV 3D US in the diagnosis of such anomalies has become evident during the last 15 years. TV 3D US has been accepted as a noninvasive, accurate, highly reproducible, and cost-effective diagnostic test for screening at risk patients for congenital uterine anomalies [4,12,19,20]. This can be achieved by the ability of a TV 3D US to assess both internal and external contour of the uterine fundus, as it enables the operator to visualize the uterus in the coronal plane. Thus, TV 3D US enables us to do away with invasive and more costly procedures such as a combined hysteroscopy and laparoscopy or MRI, which were considered the gold standard to make the diagnosis of such anomalies. It is now recommended by ASRM that imaging with hysteroscopy should be used to diagnose uterine septa instead of laparoscopy with hysteroscopy, because this approach is less invasive [4]. In addition, both new ASRM guidelines and ESHRE/ESGE classification require TV 3D US [4,12].

On the other hand, in many parts of the world, especially in developing countries, TV 3D US is not commonly used during the work-up of patients with RPL. Instead, other radiological tests such as TV 2D US and HSG are being used in screening for such anomalies. Although, HSG can detect significant fundal indentation, it cannot differentiate between septate and bicornuate uterus because the image of the cavities may be exactly the same. Similarly, TV 2D US can detect a significant endometrial separation in the transverse plane, but cannot differentiate between septate and bicornuate uterus. In addition, limited data published by our group suggest that HSG and TV 2D US are not accurate in detecting subtle fundal indentation in patients with RPL or infertility [21,22].

Saline infusion sonohysterography (SIH) at the time of TV 2D or 3D US, during the follicular phase, provides optimal imaging of the endometrium and myometrium. Therefore, it clearly outlines the endometrial contour, and allows easy detection of any lesion protruding into the uterine cavity such as endometrial polyps, submucosal fibroid or uterine septum. The overall belief by experts in the field of ultrasonography of uterine cavity disorders is that SIH is highly sensitive in the diagnosis of major uterine malformations; however, it is not sufficiently sensitive in the diagnosis of minor uterine abnormalities [23].

MRI is considered the best radiologic method for detecting all types of Müllerian anomalies. MRI can clearly delineate both internal and external uterine architecture and therefore is very useful in differentiating between the various uterine anomalies. However, several disadvantages make it difficult to apply for routine practice. Such disadvantages include high cost and lack of accessibility in an office setting. Therefore, it is not useful in screening for congenital uterine anomalies, but it is essential for definitive diagnosis of complex Müllerian anomalies [24].

Diagnostic hysteroscopy allows both direct visualization of the uterine cavity and operative intervention when uterine septa are encountered. However, as is the case with HSG and TV 2D US, hysteroscopy cannot evaluate the external contour of the uterus. Concurrent laparoscopy is essential for evaluation of the external contour of the uterus mainly to differentiate between uterine septum and bicornuate uterus. However, one advantage of hysteroscopy is that it can be performed as an office procedure. This procedure provides a relatively low-cost method to evaluate the endometrial cavity for any endometrial lesions including congenital uterine anomalies such as complete uterine septum, IUS, AUA, unicornuate uterus, uterus didelphys, and variant of T-shaped uterus.

## Role of diagnostic hysteroscopy in the diagnosis of subtle subseptate and significant arcuate uterus in the era of TV 3D US

The current literature suggests high sensitivity and specificity of TV 3D US in the diagnosis of uterine septum in patients with infertility and RPL [19,25]. TV 3D US and MRI are the best radiologic tests available to evaluate the fundal contour of the uterus to distinguish bicornuate from septate uteri. Although laparoscopy can also evaluate the fundal contour of the uterus in such patients, it is more invasive and more costly. Therefore, laparoscopy should be reserved to situations in which there is another indication for this surgery. On the other hand, diagnostic office hysteroscopy gives a rapid assessment of the depth of the internal indentation and the conditions anticipated to facilitate operative hysteroscopy [7].

However, some work by our group showed that TV 3D US may not be accurate in detecting subtle internal indentation in patients with infertility or RPL [22,26–28]. Therefore, our group suggested that a diagnostic hysteroscopy should be part of the work-up of infertility and RPL, especially to rule out subtle uterine anomalies such as IUS and significant AUA [21,22,26–28].

Because published data in the literature suggest that TV 3D US is very accurate for the diagnosis of complete uterine septum, IUS, and AUA, it is considered to be the gold standard for the diagnosis of such anomalies [19,20]. However, most of this literature did not differentiate between patients with complete septum and IUS, and between those with subtle and significant IUS [25]. Patients with complete uterine septum and those with significant IUS could arguably be suspected on TV 2D US (in transverse view) [**Figure 3.1**] or even on HSG (**Figures 3.2a** and **b**), albeit such tests cannot differentiate between such anomalies, and complete or incomplete bicornuate uteri because of lack of evaluation of the external fundal contour [29]. In addition, the data in the literature on the use of TV 3D US for the diagnosis of AUA is both limited and confusing. Such studies may have also included patients with subtle AUA of no clinical significance. This is in part due to the fact that when the American Fertility Society Classification was published in 1988, and designated class VI to describe AUA, such classification did not describe the extent of the depth of the internal indentation [11]. Although the recent guidelines published by ASRM came up with a clearer definition of AUA and a determination of the depth of the internal indentation, it failed in including patients who had an internal indentation length ≥ 10 mm [4]. Therefore, as we pointed out

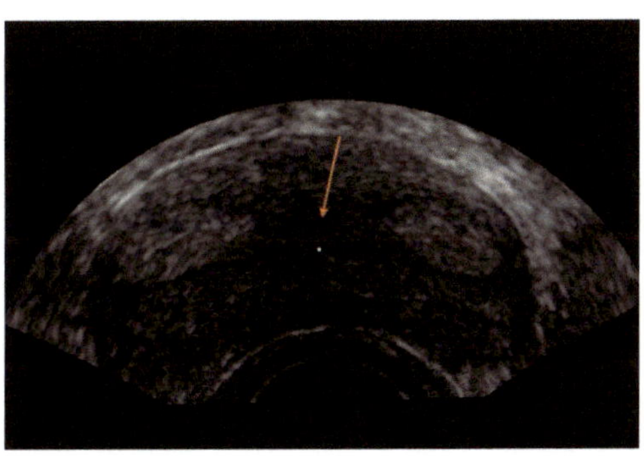

FIGURE 3.1 TV 2D US the phenomena of a significant endometrial separation (orange arrow) in the transverse plane, suggesting a uterine septum vs. bicornuate uterus.

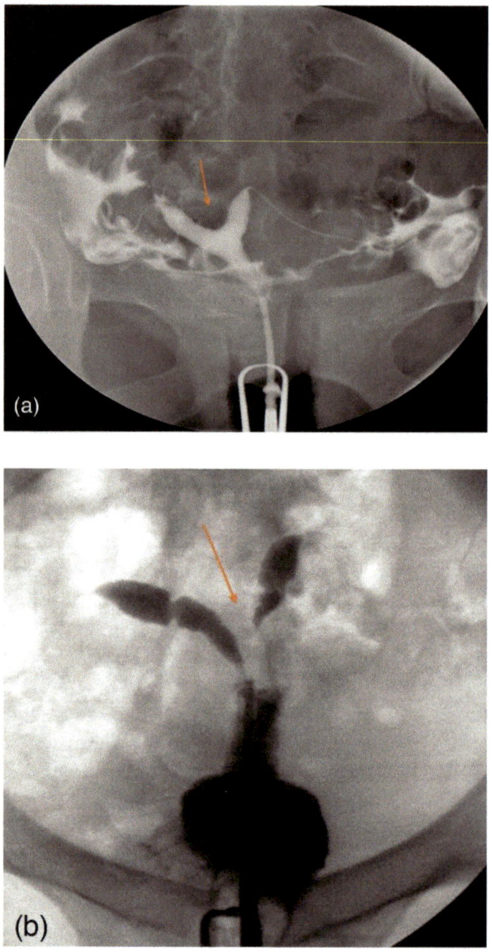


**FIGURE 3.2** (a) HSG picture illustrating a filling defect protruding from the fundal region (orange arrow), differential diagnosis should include IUS/PSUAA vs. incomplete bicornuate uterus. (b) HSG picture illustrating a filling defect protruding from the fundal region down to the internal cervical os (orange arrow), differential diagnosis should include complete uterine septum vs. complete bicornuate uterus.

earlier, such patients, who have a significant AUA, remain unclassifiable [4]. In a study by Graupera et al. (2015) [25], that compared TV 3D US to MRI in diagnosis of Müllerian anomalies, using the ESHRE–ESGE consensus, all patients appeared to have a significant pathology [25]. The authors of this chapter reached to that conclusion based on the fact that Graupera et al. (2015) [25] indicated that these patients were initially suspected to have such pathology on TV 2D US [25]. TV 2D US is usually useful in detecting such pathology when they are significant. Moini et al. (2013) [30] compared the findings on TV 3D US to hysteroscopy and laparoscopy in patients with suspected uterine septum and reported that TV 3D US was more accurate in long complete septum and less accurate in IUS and AUA [30]. The later findings are similar to our results on the value of TV 3D US in screening for IUS and AUA [31].

Several publications, albeit with small sample size, that reported on the accuracy of TV 3D US in diagnosis of IUS or AUA relied on comparison to office hysteroscopy [19,32,33]. Many investigators found office hysteroscopy to be a valuable method to screen for congenital anomalies of the uterine cavity [19,32,33]. However, we believe that such subtle anomalies can be missed if uterine distension is inadequate, as commonly happens during office hysteroscopy to avoid patients' discomfort [34–36]. A recent video abstract, published by our group, suggested that even a diagnostic hysteroscopy, performed under modified general anesthesia, can miss the diagnosis of such anomalies if uterine distension is suboptimal [37]. In addition, the narrow and small view on office hysteroscopy can make the evaluation for such anomalies difficult, especially if the patient is uncomfortable. This can be the case especially if the office hysteroscopy is done by less experienced operators. Furthermore, a study that reported on the reproducibility of diagnosing intrauterine abnormalities through office hysteroscopy, found that the interobserver agreement appeared to be disappointing [38]. In a study by Smit et al. (2013) [35], it was shown that in infertile patients the international agreement on the diagnosis of the septate uterus and arcuate uterus by office hysteroscopy appeared to be rather disappointing [35]. The same findings were found in a subsequent study by the same authors even when some diagnostic criteria were used at time of office hysteroscopy [36]. Therefore, the consensus on the accuracy of office hysteroscopy during assessment of the uterine shape seemed to be poor, especially for the less profound variations. However, the suggestion that office hysteroscopy is less accurate than a diagnostic hysteroscopy under sedation in diagnosis of IUS and AUA can only be confirmed by a prospective comparative study.

Two recent retrospective studies published by our group suggested, for the first time, that TV 3D US is not accurate in estimating the IIL`FM in patients with IUS or AUA when compared to a diagnostic hysteroscopy [39,40]. One study included infertile patients, while the other study included patients with RPL [39,40]. The aim of both studies was to determine the accuracy of measurement of IILFM on TV 3D US in detecting patients with IUS or AUA, based on the actual length as measured on diagnostic hysteroscopy [39,40]. In both studies, we compared the mean IILFM on TV 3D US and on diagnostic hysteroscopy in patients with IUS or a significant AUA [39,40]. The study of infertile population included 546 infertile patients, who were found to have IUS or a significant AUA on a diagnostic hysteroscopy, performed as part of their infertility work up, at our unit in the period between January 1, 2008, and October 31, 2017 [39]. The study of RPL population included 113 patients with an initial diagnosis of unexplained RPL, who were subsequently found to have IUS or a significant AUA on diagnostic hysteroscopy and who had TV 3D US prior to surgery between January 1, 2008, and October 31, 2017 [40]. In both studies hysteroscopy was performed under modified general anesthesia. Medications commonly used during modified general anesthesia included: Propofol, Versed, and Fentanyl. At the time of diagnostic hysteroscopy, in the infertile population paper, the type of uterine anomaly was documented and described according to the ASRM classification [11]. The population was classified based on hysteroscopic findings into patients with IUS (134 patients, 24.5%) [Class Vb] and those with significant AUA (412 patients, 75.5%) [Class VI]. Similarly, at the time of diagnostic hysteroscopy for the RPL population, the type of uterine anomaly was documented and described according to the ASRM classification [11]. The population was classified based on hysteroscopic findings into patients with incomplete uterine septum (34 patients, 30.1%) [Class Vb] and those with significant arcuate uterine anomaly (79 patients, 69.9%) [Class VI]. In 2013, a new classification of Müllerian anomalies was proposed by the European Society of Human Reproduction and Embryology and the European Society for Gynecological Endoscopy (ESHRE-ESGE) [12]. It is now acknowledged by many practitioners that the ESHRE-ESGE classification is more useful in clinical practice than the ASRM classification. Therefore, we reclassified the population in our RPL study according to the ESHRE-ESGE classification [12]. In doing so, all patients with IUS or significant AUA were renamed partial septate uterus (PSU) [12]. The population was reclassified based on hysteroscopic findings into patients who have PSU with the central point of indentation at an acute angle < 90° (PSUAA) [34 patients, 30.1%] and those who have PSU with the central point of indentation at an obtuse angle (PSUOA) [79 patients, 69.9%]. For the purpose of both studies, a diagnosis of an IUS (in the infertile population paper) and PSUAA (in the RPL population paper) were made, if the central point of indentation was at an acute angle (< 90°), did not reach to the region of the internal or external cervical os, and the IILFM measured ≥ 10 mm. While if the central point of indentation was at obtuse angle (> 90°) and the IILFM was ≥ 10 mm, the diagnosis of a significant AUA (in the infertile population paper) and PSUOA (in the RPL population paper) were made. From now on in this chapter, whenever we are discussing the RPL study we will use PSUAA to refer to IUS, and PSUOA to refer to AUA. The internal indentation length was measured using a straight resectoscope loop electrode of the ACMI hysteroscope (**Figure 3.3a**). The black metal tip of the straight resectoscope loop electrode is 5 mm in length, while the yellow insulating portion of the resectoscope loop is 10 mm in length (**Figure 3.3a**). The initial measurement was done by advancing a straight loop electrode on one side of the internal indentation up to the tubal ostium (**Figure 3.3b**). The IILFM was then indirectly calculated to be approximately 60% of that length (according to Pythagorean Theorem in Mathematics). If an IUS/PSUAA or a significant AUA/PSUOA was divided during the same setting, the actual internal indentation length was measured directly (**Figure 3.3c**). Based on internal indentation length on hysteroscopy, the patients (in the infertile population paper) with IUS or significant AUA anomalies were further divided into two main groups, those with moderate internal indentation length (10–14 mm) [52%] and those with significant internal indentation length (≥ 15 mm) [48%].

Before hysteroscopy, a TV 3D US with or without SIH utilizing a Medison Sonace 8000 US machine (Medison, Seoul 135-280, Korea) and an endocavitary probe (RIC5- 9H 5–9 MHz) were used. Any internal indentation in the endometrial cavity was calculated on TV 3D US with or without SIH in the infertility study and only on TV 3D US in the RPL study. This involved measuring the distance from the midpoint of the line joining the internal tubal ostia and the bottom of indentation of the cavity (**Figures 3.4a** and **3.5a** with their corresponding hysteroscopic

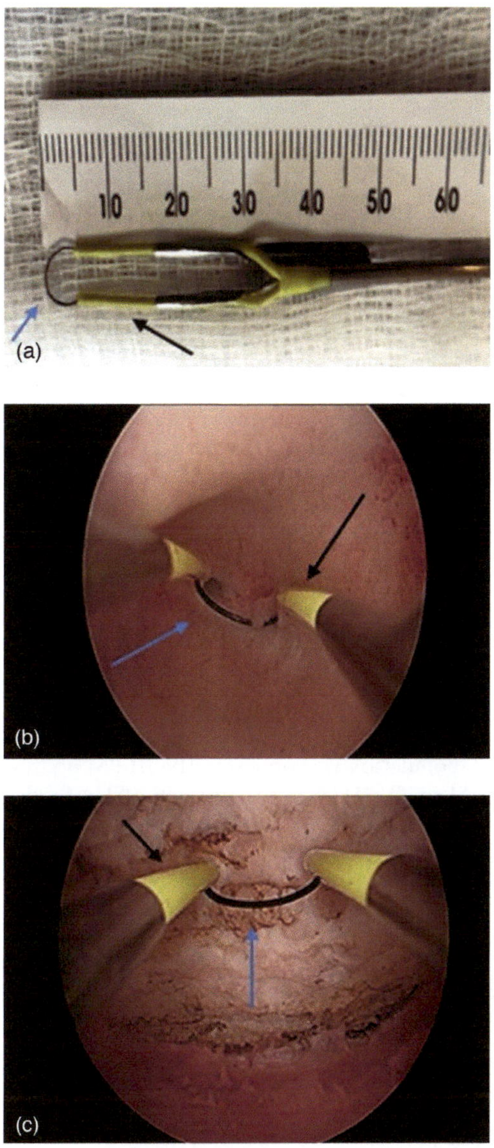


**FIGURE 3.3** (a) The length of various parts of a straight resectoscope loop electrode of the ACMI hysteroscope. (b) A straight resectoscope loop electrode used to indirectly measure the internal indentation length. (c) A straight resectoscope loop electrode used to directly measure the internal indentation length. In all three figures a blue arrow points to the metal electrode (5 mm in length) and a black arrow points to the yellow insulator (10 mm in length after the septum was divided). (From Abuzeid O, et al. (2020) Middle East Fertil Soc J 25:1 [39]. With permission.)

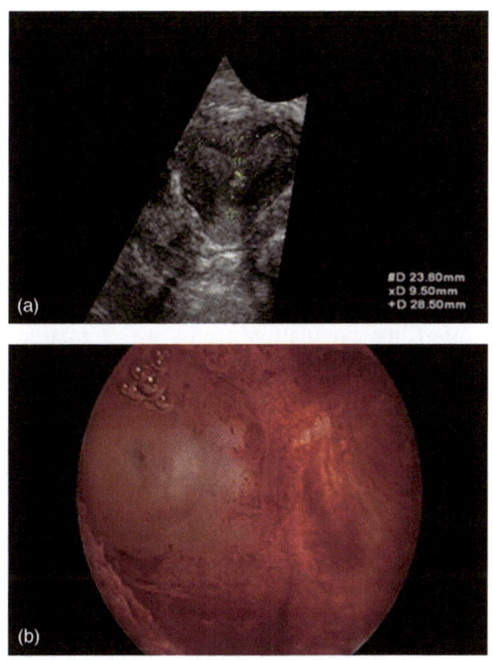


**FIGURE 3.4** (a) The internal indentation length (IILFM) on TV 3D US, measuring the distance from the midpoint of the line joining the internal tubal ostia and the bottom of indentation of the cavity in a patient with an incomplete uterine septum. (b) The corresponding hysteroscopic appearance of the uterine fundus of the patient whose TV 3D US is illustrated in **Figure 4a**. (From Abuzeid O, et al. (2020) Middle East Fertil Soc J 25:1 [39]. With permission.)

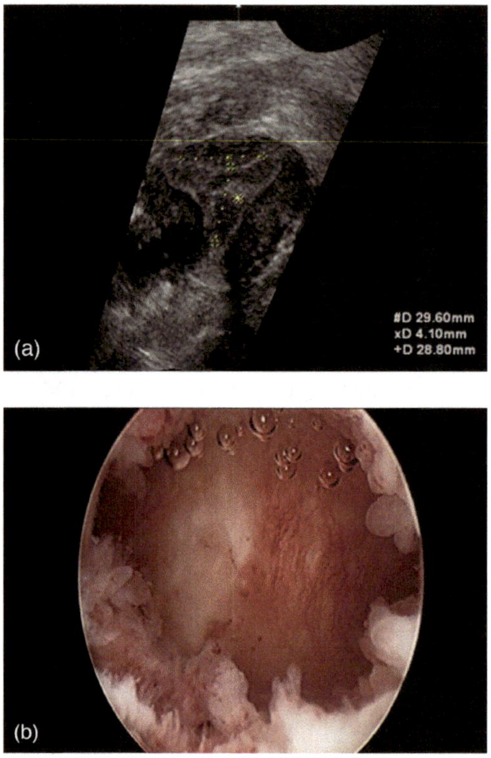


FIGURE 3.5 (a) Internal indentation length (IILFM) on TV 3D US, measuring the distance from the midpoint of the line joining the internal tubal ostia and the bottom of indentation of the cavity in a patient with a significant arcuate uterine anomaly. (b) The corresponding hysteroscopic appearance of the uterine fundus of the patient whose TV 3D US is illustrated in **Figure 5a**. (From Abuzeid O, et al. (2020) Middle East Fertil Soc J 25:1 [39]. With permission.)

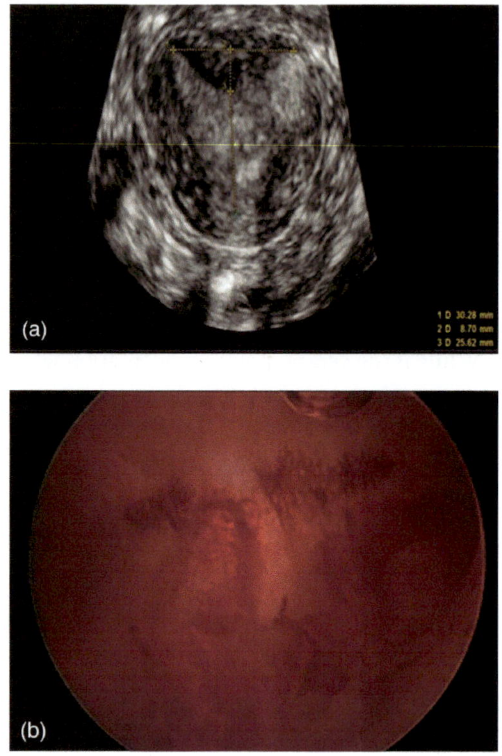


FIGURE 3.6 (a) The IILFM was calculated on TV 3D US by measuring the distance from the midpoint of the line joining the internal tubal ostia and the central point of indentation in a patient with a PSUAA. (b) The corresponding hysteroscopic appearance of the uterine fundus of the patient with PSUAA whose TV 3D US is illustrated in **Figure 6a**. (From Abuzeid O, et al. (2019) Gynecological Surg 16:14 [40]. With permission.)

appearance, **Figures 3.4b** and **3.5b**) in the infertile population paper. This represented the IILFM. In the infertility study, if the two values were available on TV 3D US, and TV 3D US with SIH, a mean value was obtained; otherwise, the one available value was used. Similarly, in the RPL population any internal indentation in the endometrial cavity was calculated on only TV 3D US as described above (**Figures 3.6a** and **3.7a** with their corresponding hysteroscopic appearance, **Figures 3.6b** and **3.7b**).

In the infertility population study, we compared internal indentation length on hysteroscopy to the internal indentation length on TV 3D US with or without SIH in patients with IUS, significant AUA and the overall population. In addition, based on the findings on hysteroscopy, this comparison was repeated for patients with moderate internal indentation length (10–14 mm) and those with significant internal indentation length (> 15 mm). In the RPL population we compared the IILFM on hysteroscopy to the IILFM on TV 3D US in patients with PSUAA, with PSUOA, and in the overall population.

In both studies, based on internal indentation length on TV 3D US, the patients were divided into four subgroups.

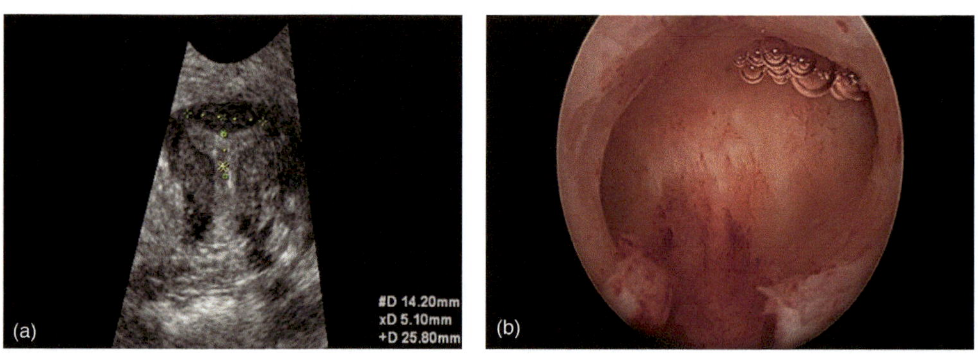


FIGURE 3.7 (a) The IILFM was calculated on TV 3D US by measuring the distance from the midpoint of the line joining the internal tubal ostia and the central point of indentation in a patient with a PSUOA. (b) The corresponding hysteroscopic appearance of the uterine fundus of the patient with PSUOA whose TV 3D US is illustrated in **Figure 7a**. (From Abuzeid O, et al. (2019) Gynecological Surg 16:14 [40]. With permission.)

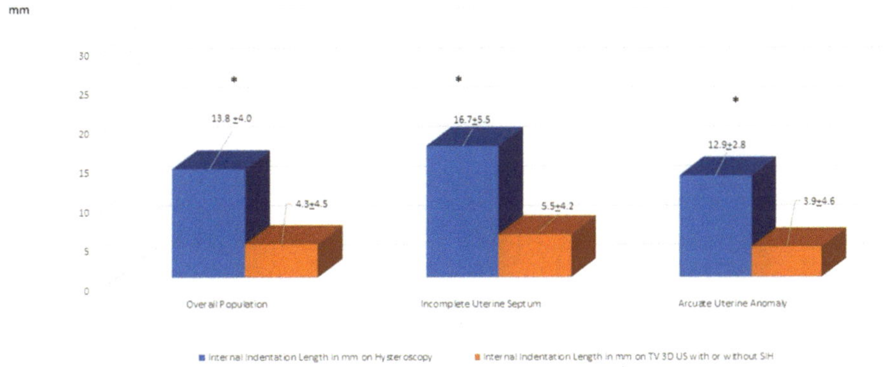


**FIGURE 3.8** Comparison between the mean IILFM measured in mm on hysteroscopy and on TV 3D US with or without SIH, in patients with IUS, significant AUA and in the overall population in all patients. (From Abuzeid O, et al. (2020) Middle East Fertil Soc J 25:1 [39]. With permission.)

The internal indentation length of subgroups 1, 2, 3, and 4 were 0.00 mm, 1–4.9 mm, 5–9.9 mm, and ≥ 10 mm, respectively. In the infertility population study, we calculated the incidence of all subgroups (1–4) in patients with IUS and AUA in the total population, in patients with moderate significant, and in those with significant internal indentation length. In the RPL population study, we also calculated the incidence of all subgroups (1–4) in patients with PSUAA, with PSUOA, and in the overall population.

In the infertility population study, the mean internal indentation length measured in millimeter on hysteroscopy was significantly higher than the mean internal indentation length measured on TV 3D US in patients with IUS, in patients with significant AUA, and in the overall population (**Figure 3.8**). The same findings were obtained when the comparison was limited to patients who had moderate significant internal indentation length (10–14 mm) and those with significant internal indentation length (15–25 mm) [**Figures 3.9** and **3.10**, respectively]. In

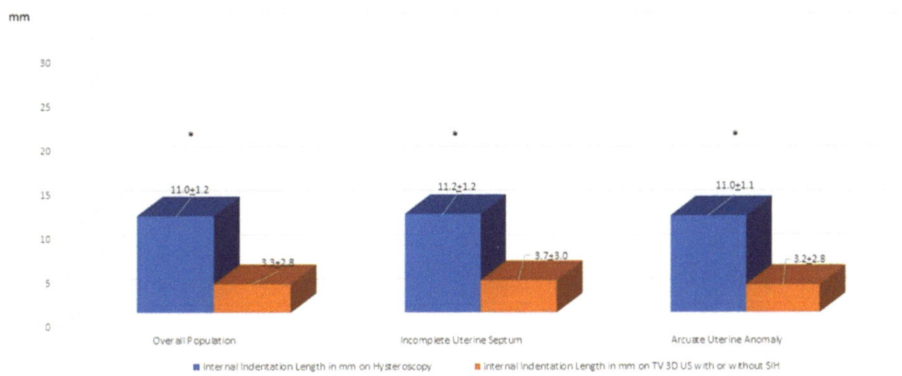


**FIGURE 3.9** Comparison between the mean IILFM measured in mm on hysteroscopy and on TV 3D US with or without SIH, in patients with IUS, significant AUA and in the overall population in patients with moderate internal indentation length (10–14 mm). (From Abuzeid O, et al. (2020) Middle East Fertil Soc J 25:1 [39]. With permission.)

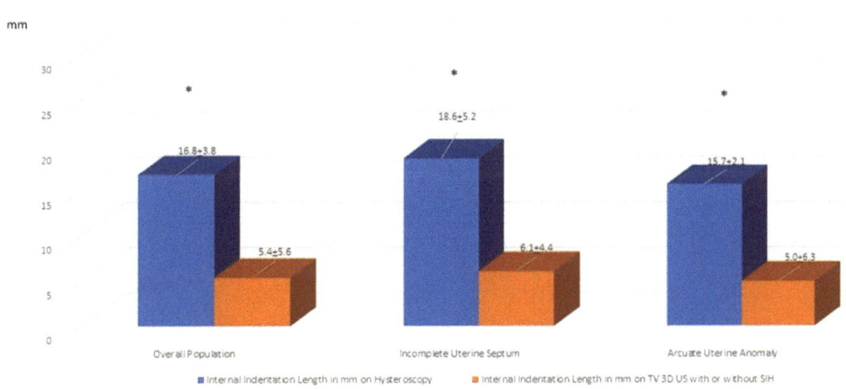


**FIGURE 3.10** Comparison between the mean IILFM measured in mm on hysteroscopy and on TV 3D US with or without SIH, in patients with IUS, significant AUA and in the overall population in patients with significant internal indentation length (>15 mm). (From Abuzeid O, et al. (2020) Middle East Fertil Soc J 25:1 [39]. With permission.)

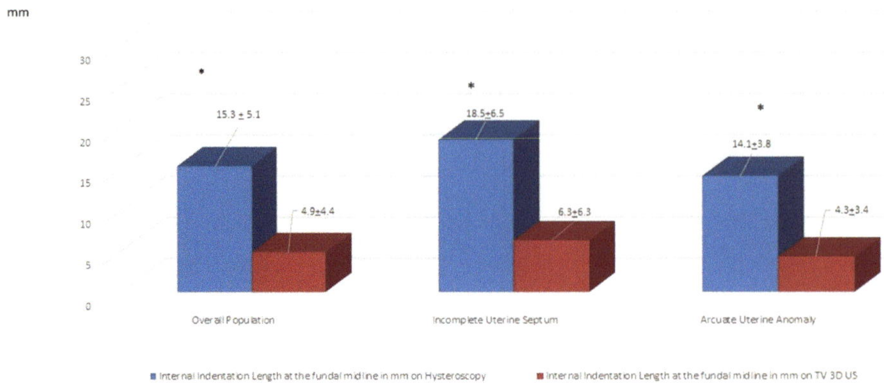


**FIGURE 3.11** Comparison between the mean IILFM measured in mm on hysteroscopy and on TV 3D US in patients with PSUAA, with PSUOA and in the overall population. (From Abuzeid O, et al. (2019) Gynecological Surg 16:14 [40]. With permission.)

the RPL population study, the mean IILFM measured in millimeters on hysteroscopy was significantly higher than the IILFM measured on TV 3D US, in patients with PSUAA, in patients with PSUOA, and in the overall population (**Figure 3.11**).

In the infertility population study, there was no evidence of any internal indentation length (0.00 mm) on TV 3D US with or without SIH in 161 patients (29.5%) [Subgroup 1]. The internal indentation length on TV 3D US with or without SIH was found to be 1–4.9 mm in 159 patients (29.1%) [Subgroup 2], 5–9.9 mm in 199 patients (36.4%) [Subgroup 3], and ≥ 10 mm 27 patients (4.9%) [Subgroup 4]. **Table 3.1** illustrates that in patients with a moderate internal indentation (10–14 mm) on hysteroscopy, there was no significant difference in percentage of patient who had IUS vs AUA irrespective of the length of the internal indentation on TV 3D US in four subgroups (**Table 3.1**). The majority of such patients (71.8%) had either no internal indentation (36.6%) or very subtle internal indentation (1–4.9 mm) [35.2%] on TV 3D US. The remaining patients (28.2%) had an internal indentation on TV 3D US that was between 5 and 9.9 mm (27.1%) or ≥ 10 mm (1.1%). **Table 3.2** illustrates that in patients with a significant internal indentation (≥ 15 mm) on hysteroscopy, there was no significant difference in percentage of patients who had IUS vs AUA irrespective of the length of the internal indentation on TV 3D US in the four subgroups (**Table 3.2**). The majority of such patients (55.7%) had either an internal indentation on TV 3D US that was between 5 and 9.9 mm (46.5%) or ≥ 10 mm (9.2%). The remaining patients (44.3%) had no internal indentation on TV 3D US (21.8%) or very subtle internal indentation (1–4.9 mm) [22.5%].

In the RPL study, **Table 3.3** illustrates the incidence of four subgroups (1–4) based on the IILFM on TV 3D US in patients with PSUAA, with PSUOA, and in the overall population with IILFM ≥ 10 mm on hysteroscopy (**Table 3.3**). There was no evidence of any IILFM (0.00 mm) on TV 3D US in 31 patients (27.4%) [Subgroup 1]. In the overall population, the IILFM on TV 3D US was found to be 1–4.9 mm in 19 patients (16.8%) [Subgroup 2], 5–9.9 mm in 42 patients (37.2%) [Subgroup 3], and ≥ 10 mm in 21 patients (18.6%) [Subgroup 4] (**Table 3.3**). There was no significant difference between the incidence PSUAA (23.5% and 20.6%) and PSUOA (29.1% and 15.2%) in subgroups 1 and 2 respectively (**Table 3.3**). The incidence of PSUAA (20.6%) was significantly lower than the incidence of PSUOA (44.3%) in subgroup 3 (IILFM between 5 and 9.9 mm) [$P < 0.01$] (**Table 3.3**). In addition, the incidence of PSUAA (35.8%) was significantly higher than the incidence of PSUOA (11.4%) in subgroup 4 (≥10 mm) [$P < 0.01$] (**Table 3.3**). The percentage of patients with IILFM < 10 mm in patients with PSUOA (88.6%) was higher than those with PSUAA (64.7%).

It is important to discuss our findings in context with the recent guidelines of ASRM and ESHRE/ESGE [4,12]. Some of the patients, in the infertility study, with AUA and IILFM of 5–9.9 mm and some of the patients, in the RPL study, with PSUOA and IILFM of 5–9.9 mm (Subgroup 3) on TV 3D US would have been diagnosed as arcuate uterus, but it would have been thought to be of no clinical significance, based on the recent ASRM guidelines [4]. On the other hand, all the patients in both studies who had AUA or PSUOA with IILFM ≥ 10 mm on hysteroscopy would have been considered unclassifiable by the recent guidelines of ASRM (2016) [4]. In that context, it is worth noting that some investigators defined AUA as those with arcuate appearance and indentation length to be between 1.0 and 1.5 cm [41]. In contrast, all the patients in our study would have been considered to have an IUS based on ESHRE/ESGE classification [12].

The data in both studies indicate that measurement on TV 3D US consistently underestimates the IILFM compared to the

**TABLE 3.1: Percentage of Patients with IUS and AUA and Moderate Internal Indentation (10–14 mm) on Hysteroscopy in Four Subgroups Based on the Internal Indentation Length on TV 3D US with or without SIH**

| | Incomplete Uterine Septum (IUS) No. = 35 | Significant Arcuate Uterine Anomaly (AUA) No. = 249 | P Value | Overall Total Population No. = 284 |
|---|---|---|---|---|
| **Subgroup 1, IILFM (0.00 mm) on TV 3D US** | 11 (31.4%) | 93 (37.3%) | NS | 104 (36.6%) |
| **Subgroup 2, IILFM (1–4.9 mm) on TV 3D US** | 13 (37.1%) | 87 (34.9%) | NS | 100 (35.2%) |
| **Subgroup 3, IILFM (5–9.9 mm) on TV 3D US** | 9 (25.7% | 68 (27.3%) | NS | 77 (27.1%) |
| **Subgroup 4, IILFM (>10 mm) on TV 3D US** | 2 (5.7%) | 1 (0.4%) | NS | 3 (1.1%) |

*Source:* From Abuzeid O, et al. (2020) Middle East Fertil Soc J 25:1 [39]. With permission.

**TABLE 3.2: Percentage of Patients with IUS and AUA and a Significant Internal Indentation (>15 mm) on Hysteroscopy in Four Subgroups Based on the Internal Indentation Length on TV 3D US with or without SIH**

| | Incomplete Uterine Septum (IUS) No. = 99 | Significant Arcuate Uterine Anomaly (AUA) No. = 163 | P Value | Overall Total Population No. = 262 |
|---|---|---|---|---|
| **Subgroup 1, IILFM (0.00 mm) on TV 3D US** | 18 (18.2%) | 39 (23.9%) | NS | 57 (21.8%) |
| **Subgroup 2, IILFM (1–4.9 mm) on TV 3D US** | 17 (17.2%) | 42 (25.8%) | NS | 59 (22.5%) |
| **Subgroup 3, IILFM (5–9.9 mm) on TV 3D US** | 51 (51.5%) | 71 (43.6%) | NS | 122 (46.5%) |
| **Subgroup 4, IILFM (>10 mm) on TV 3D US** | 13 (13.1%) | 11 (6.7%) | NS | 24 (9.2%) |

*Source:* From Abuzeid O, et al. (2020) Middle East Fertil Soc J 25:1 [39]. With permission.

actual measurement on diagnostic hysteroscopy. Therefore, we believe that the diagnostic accuracy of TV 3D US in patients with such uterine anomalies may need further evaluation. Such findings, in both studies, were confirmed irrespective of the type of the anomaly or the actual length of the internal indentation as measured on diagnostic hysteroscopy [39,40]. Patients in the infertility study, with moderate internal indentation length (10–14 mm) and those with significant internal indentation length (≥ 15 mm) on diagnostic hysteroscopy had such lesions underestimated on TV 3D US with or without SIH. It is not clear as to why the measurement of the internal indentation length of IUS and AUA on TV 3D US is not accurate. However, volume transvaginal ultrasound pictures are computer generated, and therefore, it is possible that the IILFM in the generated pictures is not accurate [39,40].

In turn, our data suggest that there may be an element of uterine factor in some infertile patients that goes undiagnosed if one relies on TV 3D US with or without SIH. Such uterine anomalies may also be found in some patients with unexplained infertility. It may also explain a possible etiology for repeated implantation failure after various infertility treatments including in vitro fertilization/embryo transfer (IVF-ET). The presence of uterine septum has been linked to repeated implantation failure [42]. In addition, our findings may in part explain the variable incidence of uterine septum and AUA in infertile patients in the literature [3]. Similarly, the data in the RPL study suggest that in patients with unexplained RPL, who were found to have PSU on hysteroscopy, IILFM can be underestimated on TV 3D US. We suggest that before a diagnosis of unexplained RPL is made, consideration should be given to a diagnostic hysteroscopy to adequately evaluate the endometrial cavity to rule out PSU.

However, in a prospective study of patients with recurrent pregnancy loss, who were suspected to have septate, subseptate, and AUA, TV 3D US was extremely accurate in making the diagnosis of such anomalies, as confirmed on subsequent diagnostic hysteroscopy and laparoscopy [19]. In the same study, the authors reported that a negative study on TV 3D US was also accurate in ruling out such anomalies as confirmed on subsequent office hysteroscopy [19]. In contrast, 29.5% of the patients, in our infertility study, and 27.4% of the patients, in the RPL study, were found to have no evidence of any internal indentation (IILFM = 0.00 mm) on TV 3D US [Subgroup 1]. Therefore, our findings are not in agreement with those of Ghi et al. (2009) [19]. If the recommendation by Ghi et al. (2009) [19] is followed, 29.5% of the patients, in the infertility study, and 27.4% of the patients in the RPL study (Subgroup 1) would have been considered to have no IUS/significant AUA or PSUAA/PSUOA, respectively, based on TV 3D US [39,40]. In addition, another 29.1% of the patients, in the infertility study, and 16.8% of the patients in the RPL study, with IILFM of 1–4.9 mm (Subgroup 2) would have also been considered normal with respect to such Müllerian anomaly based on TV 3D US [39,40]. Furthermore, an additional 36.4% of the patients in the infertility study, and 37.2% of the patients in the RPL study, with IILFM of 5–9.9 mm (Subgroup 3) would also have been considered a variant of normal based on TV 3D US. This group of patients (Subgroup 3) with IILFM of 5–9.9 mm on TV 3D US would have been considered to have insignificant internal indentation length, irrespective of its appearance, according to recent ASRM guidelines [4]. In such patients, a hysteroscopy would not be recommended, and in turn, the diagnosis would have been missed. On the other hand, these patients (Subgroup 3) would be considered to have an IUS, irrespective of its appearance, according to ESHRE/ESGE classification [12]. All in all, in only 4.9% of patients, in the infertility study, and 18.6% of patients in the RPL study, TV 3D US would have revealed an internal indentation length of ≥10 mm (Subgroup 4), and in turn, a correct diagnosis would have been made according to the criteria used in our study providing that one does not follow the recent ASRM guidelines, which suggest that IUS is defined as an internal indentation length of >15 mm [4,39,40]. While, in 95.4% of the patients in the infertility study, and in 81.4% of patients in the RPL study, TV 3D US would have been most likely interpreted as normal or a variant of normal for such Müllerian anomaly [39,40]. It is worth of note that even if the new classification of ESHRE/ESGE regarding

**TABLE 3.3: Incidence of Four Subgroups (1–4) Based on the IILFM on TV 3D US in Patients with PSUAA, with PSUOA and in the Overall Population with IILFM >10 mm on Hysteroscopy**

| | PSUAA No. = 34 | PSUOA No. = 79 | Overall Total Population No. = 113 |
|---|---|---|---|
| **Subgroup 1, IILFM (0.00 mm) on TV 3D US** | 8 (23.5%) | 23 (29.1%) | 31 (27.4%) |
| **Subgroup 2, IILFM (1–4.9 mm) on TV 3D US** | 7 (20.6%) | 12 (15.2%) | 19 (16.8%) |
| **Subgroup 3, IILFM (5–9.9 mm) on TV 3D US*** | 7 (20.6%) | 35 (44.3%) | 42 (37.2%) |
| **Subgroup 4, IILFM (≥ 10 mm) on TV 3D US*** | 12 (35.8%) | 9 (11.4%) | 21 (18.6%) |

*P < 0.01.

*Source:* From Abuzeid O, et al. (2019) Gynecological Surg 16:14 [40]. With permission.

uterine septum (IILFM > 50% of myometrial thickness) was used in our study, only 41.0% of the patients in the infertility study, and 55.8% of the patients in the RPL study, (Subgroup 3 and Subgroup 4) would have been suspected [12,39,40]. Congenital uterine anomaly is one of the underlying etiologies of RPL. Though emphasis is given to septate uteri, all Müllerian anomalies apart from slight AUA are associated with both increased miscarriage rates and preterm labor [20,43]. Patients with a uterine septum have the highest incidence of RPL (44.3%) followed by bicornuate (36%) and arcuate uteri (25.7%) [1]. Uterine septum accounts for approximately 13.3% of causes of RPL [5]. Hysteroscopic surgical correction of such anomalies has proven to be very successful in achieving live birth in these patients, albeit there is no prospective randomized controlled study to prove this notion until now [2]. Unexplained factors account for more than 50% of the etiology of RPL [44,45]. A large number of these patients are advised to keep trying, have IVF with pre-implantation genetic screening (PGS), or are referred for evaluation for immunological factors of RPL [46]. Such treatment options are expensive and may not be successful, especially if the actual underlying etiology is missed [46]. In addition, in patients with idiopathic RPL, the work by Murugappan et al. (2016) [47] suggested that expectant management of RPL is a successful as IVF-ET with PGS and had a lower median time to pregnancy [47]. However, one recent study reported a 41.1% incidence of abnormal embryonic karyotype in patients who had a negative work-up for RPL, suggesting the true incidence of unexplained RPL to be approximately 24.5% [6]. In addition, a recent study by Hodes-Wertz et al. (2012) [48], the authors suggested that unexplained RPL is mostly caused by chromosomal abnormalities, with only a residual 6.9% miscarriage rate [48]. As mentioned earlier, the prevalence of uterine anomalies in patients with RPL when optimal tests, such as TV 3D US, are used has been estimated to be 13.3% [5]. It has been suggested that septate uterus is the most common uterine anomaly in patients with RPL accounting for approximately 50% [1,5]. Major uterine anomalies have been shown to have a negative impact on reproductive outcome in patients with RPL [6]. After surgical correction of such anomalies, 70%–80% of patients achieve a successful live birth [2].

It should be emphasized that TV 3D US is an essential part of work-up of infertile patients. The value of TV 3D US in the diagnosis of IUS and AUA is well established, and therefore, it is a mandatory step in the assessment of the uterine cavity in patients with a suspected complete uterine septum, IUS, AUA, variant of T-shaped uterus or bicornuate uterus, especially before planning operative hysteroscopy. This noninvasive radiological test is reproducible and can provide information about both the external contour and the uterine cavity at the same time. Unless laparoscopy is used at the same time as hysteroscopy, one cannot differentiate between septate and bicornuate uterus. Therefore, diagnostic hysteroscopy should only be performed after TV 3D US is done in such patients.

## Conclusion

The authors of this chapter suggest that mean IILFM in patients with IUS (PSUAA) or AUA (PSUOA) can be underestimated on TV 3D US. In turn, it is possible that TV 3D US may miss the diagnosis of such subtle uterine anomalies in some patients. It appears that a diagnostic hysteroscopy by an experienced reproductive surgeon is the only gold standard to make the correct diagnosis. However, it is important to stress that TV 3D US is mandatory in evaluation of patients with infertility and RPL prior to office hysteroscopy or diagnostic hysteroscopy. Our findings may have tremendous implications in the management of infertility patients and patients with RPL. However, we believe that additional prospective studies are needed to confirm our findings. In addition, we recommend that patients with unexplained poor reproductive outcome, such as; placental abruption, preterm prelabor rupture of membranes, preterm birth and stillborn should be evaluated with TV 3D US and hysteroscopy to rule out the possibility of such subtle uterine anomalies.

## References


1. Grimbizis G, Camus M, Tarlatzis BC, et al (2001) Clinical implications of uterine malformation and hysteroscopic treatment results. Hum Reprod Update 7(2):161–174.
2. Homer HA, Li TC, Cooke ID (2000) The septate uterus: a review of management and reproductive outcome. Fertil Steril 73(1):1–14.
3. Saravelos SH, Cocksedge KA, Li TC (2008) Prevalence and diagnosis of congenital uterine anomalies in women with reproductive failure: a critical appraisal. Hum Reprod Update 14(5):415–429.
4. The American Society for Reproductive Medicine, Practice Committee of the American Society for Reproductive Medicine (2016) Uterine septum: a guideline. Fertil Steril 106(3):530–540.
5. Chan Y, Jayaprakasan K, Zamora J, Thornton JG, Raine-Fenning N, Coomarasamy A (2011) The prevalence of congenital uterine anomalies in unselected and high-risk populations: a systematic review. Hum Reprod Update 17(6):761–771.
6. Sugiura-Ogasawara M, Ozaki Y, Katano K, Suzumori N, Kitaori T, Mizutani E (2012) Abnormal embryonic karyotype is the most frequent cause of recurrent miscarriage. Hum Reprod 27:2297–2303.
7. Parry JP and Isaacson KB. (2019) Hysteroscopy and why macroscopic uterine factors matter for fertility. Fertil Steril 112(2):203–210.
8. Mollo A, De Franciscis P, Colacurci N, Cobellis L, Perino A, Venezia R, et al. (2009) Hysteroscopic resection of the septum improves the pregnancy rate of women with unexplained infertility: a prospective controlled trial. Fertil Steril 91:2628–2231.
9. Ghi T, De Musso F, Maroni E, Youssef A, Savelli L, Farina A, et al. (2012) The pregnancy outcome in women with incidental diagnosis of septate uterus at first trimester scan. Hum Reprod 27:2671–2675.
10. Rikken J, Kowalik C, Emanuel M, Bongers M, Spinder T, de Kruif J, et al. (2018) The randomised uterine septum transsection trial (TRUST): design and protocol. BMC Womens Health 18:163–167.
11. The American Fertility Society classifications of adnexal adhesions, distal tubal occlusion, tubal occlusion secondary to tubal ligation, tubal pregnancies, Müllerian anomalies and intrauterine adhesions (1988). Fertil Steril 49:944–955.
12. Grimbizis GF, Gordts S, Di Spiezio SA, et al. (2013) The ESHRE/ESGE consensus on the classification of female genital tract congenital anomalies. Hum Reprod 28(8):2032–2044.
13. Knez J, Saridogan E, Van Den Bosch T, et al. (2018) ESHRE/ESGE female genital tract anomalies classification system—the potential impact of discarding arcuate uterus on clinical practice. Hum Reprod 33(4):600–606.
14. Ludwin A, Ludwin I, Kudla M, et al. (2015) Reliability of the European Society of Human Reproduction and Embryology/European Society for Gynaecological Endoscopy and American Society for Reproductive Medicine classification systems for congenital uterine anomalies detected using three-dimensional ultrasonography. Fertil Steril 104(3):688–697.
15. Ludwin A, Ludwin J (2015) Comparison of the ESHRE–ESGE and ASRM classifications of Mullerian duct anomalies in everyday practice. Hum Reprod 30(3):569–580.
16. Grimbizis GF, Di Spiezio SA, Saravelos SH, et al. (2016) The Thessaloniki ESHRE/ESGE consensus on diagnosis of female genital anomalies. Hum Reprod 13(1):1–16.
17. Ludwin A, Martins WP, Nastri CO, et al. (2018) Congenital Uterine Malformation by Experts (CUME): better criteria for distinguishing between normal/arcuate and septate uterus. Ultrasound Obstet Gynecol 51(1):101–109.

18. Carrington BM, Hricak H, Nuruddin RN, et al. (1990) Müllerian duct anomalies: magnetic resonance imaging evaluation. Radiology 176:715.
19. Ghi T, Casadio P, Kuleva M, et al. (2009) Accuracy of three-dimensional ultrasound in diagnosis and classification of congenital uterine anomalies. Fertil Steril 92(2):808–81312.
20. Jurkovic D, Geipel A, Gruboeck K (1995) Three-dimensional ultrasound for the assessment of uterine anatomy and detection of congenital anomalies: a comparison with hysterosalpingography and two-dimensional sonography. Ultrasound Obstet Gynecol 5(4):233–237.
21. Kallia N, Abuzeid O, Ashraf M, Abuzeid M. (2011) Role of hysteroscopy in diagnosis of subtle uterine anomalies in patients with normal hysterosalpingography. Fertil Steril 96(3)S12, O-40.
22. Abuzeid O, Abdullah A, Moustafa ASZ, Hebert J, Rocha F, Abuzeid MI. (2016) Limitations of radiological screening tests in detection of subtle incomplete septum or arcuate uterine anomaly in patients with recurrent pregnancy loss (RPL). Hum Reprod 23(7):S187.
23. Kupesic S (2001) Clinical implications of sonographic detection of uterine anomalies for reproductive outcome. Ultrasound Obstet Gynecol 18:387–400.
24. Mitwally MFM, Abuzeid M. Uterine Septum. (2010) Textbook of Ultrasonography in Ultrasonography in Reproductive Medicine and Infertility. Edited by Botros Rizk. Cambridge University Press, Chapter 18, pp. 141–154.
25. Graupera B, Pascual MA, Hereter L, et al. (2015) Accuracy of three-dimensional ultrasound compared with magnetic resonance imaging in diagnosis of Müllerian duct anomalies using ESHRE–ESGE consensus on the classification of congenital anomalies of the female genital tract. Ultrasound Obstet Gynecol 46(5):616–622.
26. Abuzeid M, Abuzeid O. Three-dimensional ultrasonography of subtle uterine anomalies: correlation with hysterosalpingogram, two-dimensional ultrasonography, and hysteroscopy. In: Ultrasonography in Gynecology. Editors: Botros Rizk and Elizabeth Puscheck. Cambridge University Press 2014, Chapter 8, pp. 66–79.
27. Abuzeid O, Zaghmout O, Corrado J, Hebert J, Ashraf M, Abuzeid M. (2015) Comparison between the findings on transvaginal 3D ultrasound scan and hysteroscopy in patients diagnosed with subtle incomplete uterine septum/arcuate uterine anomaly on hysteroscopy. Fertil Steril 104(3), e28.
28. Abuzeid O, Zaghmout O, Corrado J, Hebert J, Abuzeid M. (2016) Three-dimensional ultrasonography with or without saline infusion sonogram in detecting subtle uterine anomalies: correlation with hysteroscopy. J Minim Invasive Gynecol 23(7):S145.
29. Yu LL, Zhang X, Zhang T, et al. (2014) Detection of congenital uterine malformation by using transvaginal three-dimensional ultrasound. J Univ Sci Technolog Med Sci 34(5):782–784. https://doi.org/10.1007/s11596-014-1352-7
30. Moini A, Mohammadi S, Hosseini R, et al. (2013) Accuracy of 3-dimensional sonography for diagnosis and Classification of congenital uterine anomalies. J Ultrasound Med 32:923–927.
31. Corrado J, Abuzeid O, Ashraf M, Abuzeid M. (2013) The limitations of radiological screening tests in the detection of incomplete uterine septum or arcuate anomaly in comparison to diagnostic hysteroscopy. Fertil Steril 100(3), S384–S385, P-820.
32. Faivre E, Fernandez H, Deffieux X, et al. (2012) Accuracy of three-dimensional ultrasonography in differential diagnosis of septate and bicornuate uterus compared with office hysteroscopy and pelvic magnetic resonance imaging. J Minim Ivasive Gynecol 19(1):101–106.
33. Lagana AS, Ciancimino L, Mancuso A, et al. (2014) 3D sonohysterography vs hysteroscopy: a cross-sectional study for the evaluation of endouterine diseases. Arch Gynecol Obstet 290:1173–1178.
34. Ludwin A, Ludwin I, Kudla M, et al. (2014) Diagnostic accuracy of three-dimensional sonohysterography compared with office hysteroscopy and its interrater/intrarater agreement in uterine cavity assessment after hysteroscopic metroplasty. Fertil Steril 101(5):1392–1399.
35. Smit JG, Kasius JC, Eijkemans MJC, et al. (2013) The international agreement study on the diagnosis of the septate uterus at office hysteroscopy in infertile patients. Fertil Steril 99(7):2108–2113.
36. Smit JG, Overdijkink S, Mol BW, et al. (2015) The impact of diagnostic criteria on the reproducibility of the hysteroscopic diagnosis of the septate uterus: a randomized controlled trial. Hum Reprod 30(6):1323–1330.
37. Abuzeid O, Raju R, Hebert J, et al. (2016) Effect of proper uterine distention on the detection rate of subtle uterine anomalies during hysteroscopy. JMIG 23(7):S134–S135.
38. Kasius JC, Broekmans FJM, Veersema S, et al. (2011) Observer agreement in the evaluation of the uterine cavity by hysteroscopy prior to in vitro fertilization. Hum Reprod 26(4):801–807.
39. Abuzeid O, LaChance J, Zaghmout O, Corrado J, Hebert J, Ashraf M, Abuzeid MI. (2020) The role of diagnostic hysteroscopy in diagnosis of incomplete uterine septum/significant arcuate uterine anomaly in infertile patients in the era of transvaginal 3D ultrasound scan. Middle East Fertil Soc J 25:1.
40. Abuzeid O, LaChance J, Hebert J, Abuzeid MI, Welch R. (2019) The role of diagnostic hysteroscopy in diagnosis of incomplete uterine septum in patients with recurrent pregnancy loss in the era of transvaginal 3D ultrasound scan. Gynecological Surg 16:14.
41. Ludwin A, Ludwin I, Banas T, et al. (2011) Diagnostic accuracy of sonohysterography, hysterosalpingography and diagnostic hysteroscopy in diagnosis of arcuate, septate and bicornuate uterus. J Obstet Gynaecol Res 37(3):178–186.
42. Raga F, Bauset C, Remohi J, et al. (1997) Reproductive impact of congenital Müllerian anomalies. Hum Reprod 12:2277–2281.
43. Chan Y, Jayaprakasan K, Tan A, Thornton J, Coomarasamy A, Raine-Fenning N. (2011) Reproductive outcomes in women with congenital uterine anomalies: a systematic review. Ultrasound Obstet Gynecol 38:371–382.
44. Stephenson M (1996) Frequency of factors associated with habitual abortion in 197 couples. Fertil Steril 66:24–29.
45. Branch DW, Gibson M, Silver RM (2010) Clinical practice: recurrent miscarriage. N Engl J Med. 363:1740–1747.
46. Stephenson M, Kutteh W (2007) Evaluation and management of recurrent early pregnancy loss. Clin Obstet Gynecol 50:132–145.
47. Murugappan G, Shahine LK, Perfetto CO, Hickok LR, Lathi RB (2016) Intent to treat analysis of in vitro fertilization and preimplantation genetic screening versus expectant management in patients with recurrent pregnancy loss. Hum Reprod 31:1668–1674.
48. Hodes-Wertz B, Grifo J, Ghadir S, Kaplan B, Laskin CA, Glassner M, Munne S (2012) Idiopathic recurrent miscarriage is caused mostly by aneuploid embryos. Fertil Steril 98(3):675–580.

# 4

# COMPLICATIONS OF GYNECOLOGICAL LAPAROSCOPY

**Rafał Watrowski**

## Introduction

The well-recognized benefits of laparoscopy are, among others, reduced blood loss, decreased postoperative pain, smaller incision size, reduced risk of adhesion formation, shorter hospital stay, faster return to daily activities, higher patient satisfaction, and lower treatment costs in comparison to open abdominal procedures [1–4]. A magnified view and instrument-only access to body cavities can be further mentioned [2]. For these purposes, laparoscopy gained wide acceptance by surgeons, patients, and public health systems. The popularization of laparoscopy has reciprocally fueled the development of individual surgical skills and technical equipment. In the 21st century, practically all areas of gynecologic surgery (except of cytoreductive procedures for advanced ovarian cancer) can be managed via minimally invasive approach. The advantages of laparoscopy are maintained also in older [3] or obese [4] patients.

Like any surgical treatment, laparoscopic operations can be associated with adverse events. The most frequently reported overall complication rates of laparoscopic procedures are 0.6%–2.0% (range 0.4%–13%), with an overall mortality rate about 0.02% (0.01%–0.03%) [5–17]. The fatalities result most often from injuries of major vessels, followed by bowel injuries. A considerable proportion of complications are due to delayed diagnosis: the majority of bowel and ureter damages are recognized postoperatively. Nevertheless, in comparison to abdominal approach, laparoscopy (both for benign and oncologic indications)—is associated with similar or lower rates of "major" complications (1.4%) [7], and significantly less frequent "minor" complications (4.3%–8.9% vs. 15.2%) [6–8]. The safety of laparoscopic surgery has continuously increased during the last three decades.

Confusingly, it is the minimal transdermal access that encounters both for several advantages, but also for the majority of complications. For this reason, even a simple laparoscopy (e.g., sterilization) can morph into fatality [6, 11, 18]. Additionally, some adverse events are exclusively related to the laparoscopic technique, for example, postlaparoscopic shoulder pain, subcutaneous emphysema, tumor morcellation, trocar port metastases, etc.

Unique challenges of the laparoscopic approach are:

- the (usually) blind entering the abdominal cavity,
- intraoperative vision restriction (field and angle of view, impairment of vision in presence of smoke, fog or bleeding, equipment quality, experience of camera assistant),
- practically not correctable position of trocars,
- lack of tactile feedback,
- effects of intra-abdominal pressure (distension of nerves and liver capsule, impaired ventilation),
- physical and chemical effects of insufflation gas ($CO_2$),
- necessity of specimen fragmentation (morcellation) prior to evacuation.

The recognition of those unique pitfalls can help to prevent complications. The fact that every second surgical adverse event is preventable is valid also in minimally invasive surgery [8, 19]. One avoided complication protects in the first line the patient, but secondary the surgeon and the health systems. In the sometimes dramatically sequel of complications, surgeon has been recognized as "the second victim" [20]. It is of particular importance, since—in turn—a considerable number of adverse events is related to the "human factor"—the surgeon's skills and volume, sleep deprivation, physical fatigue, or distraction. All these conditions significantly impact the complication rate, thus in fact the patient's life, health, and well-being.

From one more perspective, gynecologic surgery accounts for a high proportion of malpractice claims, independent of health and law systems [21–23]. The majority of claims (82%) results from visceral and/or vascular injuries, especially to the bowel (40%) and ureters (20%) [23]. The abdominal entry accounts for 38% of claimed injuries [23–25]. In the Dutch evaluation, a surprisingly high proportion (77%) of the claims was filed after non-advanced procedures. Generally, the most often reason for financial compensation (33%) is delayed diagnosis [23]. In fact, 30%–50% of all bowel injuries and 13%–50% of vascular injuries are first detected postoperatively [5, 15, 25, 26].

## Definition, classification, and incidence of surgical complications

The reporting, comparison, and prevention of surgical complications require a comprehensive and applicable definition. A demarcation against other undesirable surgery-associated events (negative outcomes) has been proposed early by Clavien et al. [27]. The authors grouped negative postoperative outcomes into "complications," "failure to cure," and "sequelae." *Complications* were defined as "any deviation from the normal postoperative course," inclusive "asymptomatic complications such as arrhythmia or atelectasis." A *sequela* is "an 'after-effect' of surgery that is inherent to the procedure (e.g., inability to walk after amputation of the leg)" [28]. The third category of negative outcomes is the *failure to cure*, when—despite uncomplicated surgical course—the intended result of surgery, for example, complete oncological cytoreduction, has not been achieved. "Sequelae" and "failure to cure" should be assessed separately from complications [27, 28]. Sokol and Wilson [29] established the following, widely accepted definition: "A surgical complication is any undesirable, unintended, and direct result of an operation affecting the patient, which would not have occurred had the operation gone as well as could reasonably be hoped" [29]. They argued that, albeit in high-risk procedures complications can be "expected," their distinctive feature is that they are never intended and when the opposite (= an uncomplicated course) is still realistic.

Usually, surgical complications are classified according to their severity grade. This categorization is based on necessary

**TABLE 4.1: European Association of Urology Intraoperative Adverse Incidents Grading**

| Grade | Description |
|---|---|
| 0 | Event requiring no intervention or change in operative approach, no deviation from planned intraoperative steps, no consequence for the patient |
| 1 | Event requiring additional/alternative procedure in planned intraoperative steps, not life threatening or involving part or full organ removal. The event was addressed in a controlled manner with no long-term side effects |
| 2 | Event requiring major additional/alternative procedure in operative approach but NOT immediately life-threatening. The event was addressed in a controlled manner, however may have short- or long-term side effects |
| 3 | Event requiring major additional/alternative procedure in addition to planned intraoperative steps and incident becoming immediately life-threatening but NOT requiring part or full organ removal; may have short- or long-term side effects |
| 4 | Event requiring major additional/alternative procedure in addition to planned intraoperative steps becoming immediately life-threatening and with short- or long-term consequences to patient |
| | A. Requiring part or full organ removal |
| | B. Unable to complete planned procedure as planned due to a technical issue or surgical event and/or required unplanned stoma (change in body image, eg stoma, major skin flap) |
| 5 | A. Wrong site or side for ablative surgery or removal of an organ or wrong patient or no consent |
| | B. Intraoperative death |

*Source:* Adapted from Biyani CS, et al. Eur Urol. 2020;77:601–610 [30].

additional interventions, medications, affected organs, duration of patient's impairment, or eventually life-long disability. An interdisciplinary practicable classification of ***intra***operative complications has been recently proposed by the European Association of Urology (**Table 4.1**) [30].

Two broadly used classifications of ***post***operative complications are the Accordion Severity Classification of Postoperative Complications [31] and the Clavien–Dindo Classification of Surgical Complications [27, 28] (**Table 4.2**). The first of them subdivides complications into "mild," "moderate," severe," and "death," while the latter uses for their grading a 5-point Likert scale. Especially the Clavien–Dindo Classification has become popular across surgical disciplines including gynecology. Those general classifications can be useful for interdisciplinary comparisons or in a number of research questions, but they do not allow for a differentiation between specific types of injury (vascular, intestinal, urological, etc.) nor between typical context of occurrence (e.g., abdominal entry, specimen evacuation or pneumoperitoneum).

The complication rates are highly correlated with surgeon's experience and complexity of the surgical procedure [6, 32, 33]. Unfortunately, the definitions of surgical complexity are not uniform. Laparoscopic boards and societies use (in some variations) for training and certification purposes a four-level classification [34]. The scientific literature describes laparoscopic procedures, sometimes arbitrally, rather as "minor" (or "basic"), "major" (or "moderate"), and "advanced" (sometimes confluent with "major") procedures [32]. Representative examples for both classification systems are shown in **Table 4.3**. Notably, the difficulty of some

**TABLE 4.2: Accordion Severity Classification of Postoperative Complications (Contracted Classification) and Clavien–Dindo Classification of Surgical Complications**

| Severity | Accordion Severity Classification of Postoperative Complications (Contracted Classification) [31] | Clavien–Dindo Classification of Surgical Complications [27, 28] | Grade |
|---|---|---|---|
| 1. Mild complication | Requires only minor invasive procedures that can be done at the bedside such as insertion of intravenous lines, urinary catheters, and nasogastric tubes, and drainage of wound infections. Physiotherapy and the following drugs are allowed–antiemetics, antipyretics, analgesics, diuretics, electrolytes, and physiotherapy. | Any deviation from the normal postoperative course without the need for pharmacological treatment or surgical, endoscopic, and radiological interventions. Allowed therapeutic regimens are: drugs as antiemetics, antipyretics, analgesics, diuretics, electrolytes, and physiotherapy. This grade also includes wound infections opened at the bedside. | Grade 1 |
| 2. Moderate complication | Requires pharmacologic treatment with drugs other than such allowed for minor complications, for instance antibiotics. Blood transfusions and total parenteral nutrition are also included. | Requiring pharmacological treatment with drugs other than such allowed for grade 1 complications. Blood transfusions and total parenteral nutrition are also included. | Grade 2 |
| 3. Severe complication | All complications requiring endoscopic or interventional radiologic procedures or re-operation as well as complications resulting in failure of one or more organ systems. | Requiring surgical, endoscopic or radiological intervention | Grade 3 |
| | | Grade 3a. Intervention not under general anesthesia | |
| | | Grade 3b. Intervention under general anesthesia | |
| | | Grade 4 Life-threatening complication (including CNS complications)* requiring IC/ICU management | Grade 4 |
| | | Grade 4a. Single organ dysfunction (including dialysis) | |
| | | Grade 4b. Multiorgan dysfunction | |
| 4. Death | Complications resulting in death | Death of a patient | Grade 5 |
| | | Suffix "d" if the patient suffers from a complication at the time of discharge, the suffix "d" (for "disability") is added to the respective grade of complication. This label indicates the need for a follow-up to fully evaluate the complication. | |

* Brain hemorrhage, ischemic stroke, subarachnoidal bleeding, but excluding transient ischemic attacks.

**TABLE 4.3: Complexity Classification of Gynecologic Laparoscopic Surgical Procedures**

| | Chapron et al. 1998 [32] | German Association of Gynecologic Endoscopy [34] | |
|---|---|---|---|
| Diagnostic | Diagnostic laparoscopy | Diagnostic laparoscopy,<br>Tubal sterilization, | Type I |
| Minor | Minimal adhesiolysis (as assessed by the surgeon),<br>Destruction of minimal endometriosis,<br>Ovarian biopsies,<br>Ovarian punctures,<br>Tubal sterilization<br>Assisted conception procedures | Chromopertubation,<br>Simple adhesiolysis,<br>Destruction of endometriosis rAFS I,<br>or comparable procedure. | |
| Major | Ectopic pregnancy,<br>Pelvic inflammatory disease,<br>Polycystic ovaries,<br>Benign ovarian cysts,<br>Distal tubal plasty,<br>Uterine suspension,<br>Extended adhesiolysis and<br>Moderate or severe endometriosis | Ectopic pregnancy,<br>Salpingectomy, oophorectomy, adnexectomy<br>Ovarian cystectomy,<br>Myomectomy for pedunculated or subserous myomas (without uterine reconstruction),<br>Hysterectomy,<br>Extended adhesiolysis,<br>Destruction of endometriosis rAFS I/II, Enzian A1/B1,<br>or comparable procedure. | Type II |
| Advanced | Hysterectomy,<br>Myomectomy,<br>Lymphadenectomy,<br>Colposuspension,<br>Tubal sterilization reversal,<br>Genital prolapse,<br>Endometrial and cervical cancer,<br>Retroperitoneal endometriosis | Type II procedures performed in presence of distorted anatomy,<br>Intramural or intraligamentary myomectomy,<br>Destruction of endometriosis rAFS III/Enzian A2/B2/C1,<br>Microsurgical distal tubal reconstruction,<br>Cervico- or colposacropexy,<br>or comparable procedure. | Type III |
| | | Radical hysterectomy,<br>Lymphadenectomy,<br>Destruction of endometriosis rAFS IV/Enzian A3/B3/C2-3/FB/FU/FI,<br>Complexe pelvic floor reconstruction,<br>Microsurgical proximal tubal reconstruction,<br>Reconstructive surgery for congenital malformations,<br>or comparable procedure. | Type IV |

procedures, for example, myomectomy, is differently mirrored within these systems.

The quality and variability of data concerning perioperative adverse events is depending on several confounding factors: differences between reporting criteria, proportion of minor to major procedures, time frame, differences between institutions or—more important but hard to assess—between individual surgeons, unequal and evolving equipment, etc.

Said that, following rates of organ-specific injuries are recommended for the purpose of, for example, informed consent prior to laparoscopy [5–10, 12–16, 32]:

- Abdominal wall vessels: 0.4%–1%
- Large retroperitoneal vessels: 0.2%–1.0%
- Bladder: 0.8%–2%
- Ureter: 0.1%–1.0%
- Gastrointestinal tract: 0.06%–0.5%

According to surgical complexity, undesirable surgical events are reported in 0.08%, 0.4%, and 1.7% of "minor," "major," and "advanced" gynecologic laparoscopies, respectively [8]. Interestingly, if applying the less specific Clavien–Dindo classifications, the general incidence of laparoscopic complications is much higher, for example, 13.1% for gynecologic laparoscopies [33] and 12.5% for general-surgical laparoscopies [35].

As of 2020, the overall mortality of laparoscopic procedures is quoted at 0.02% (0.01%–0.03%), which can be translated into an estimated risk of death in 1 of 6512 (1:3971–1:10,680) laparoscopies. The mortality of laparoscopic hysterectomy (LH) is 0.01% (0.01%–0.02%), corresponding to 1:6799 (1:4109–1:11,249) procedures. Laparoscopic sacrocolpopexy is associated with a higher mortality of 0.07% (0%–5.65%), that is 1:1343 (1:18–1:107,855) procedures [17].

## Entry-related complications

The most risky part of a laparoscopic operation is the placement of the first trocar. About 50% (35%–57%) of all laparoscopic complications, 50%–83% of serious vascular complications, and 41%–50% of all visceral complications occur during entering the abdomen [5, 9, 14, 32]. The landscape of complications related to transdermal endoscopic entry encompasses:

- Injuries to the vessels of the anterior abdominal wall
- Perforation of omental, mesenterial, and large retroperitoneal vessels
- Bowel lacerations – both in presence of its normal position (due to incorrect trocar insertion) or distorted anatomy (when bowel is adherent to the abdominal wall)
- Failed entry/extraperitoneal insufflation
- Subcutaneous emphysema and pneumothorax

as well late complications like:

- Port site herniation
- Tumor implantation in port sites

For this reason, laparoscopic first entry should nether be delegated to unexperienced trainees without advision.

The methods of first abdominal entry can be divided into:

- **I. Closed**
  - *a. Blind*
    - i. With pneumoperitoneum
      - 1. Veres needle
    - ii. Without pneumoperitoneum
      - 1. Direct trocar access
        - a. Normal trocar
        - b. Radially expanding trocar
  - *b. Under view (with or without pneumoperitoneum)*
    - i. Optical Veres needle
    - ii. Optical trocar
- **II. Open**
  - *a.* Hasson technique

Among them, three methods reached the status of standard techniques: Veres needle (VN), direct trocar entry (DTE), and the open access (Hasson technique). Using VN or DTE, the abdominal cavity is entered in a blind manner. The VN was actually developed in the 1930s by the Hungarian internist Janos Veres for pleural punctions [36]. The blunt inner core of the VN is pushed back by the resistance of the skin and soft tissue, which allows the sharp-edged outer sheath to penetrate easily. With the loss of resistance while entering a hollow space (like pleural or abdominal cavity), the inner blunt part of the needle springs forward and prevents injury to the internal organs [36]. Nowadays, 96%–98% gynecologic laparoscopists use the VN for the creation of pneumoperitoneum [11, 37]. Before insertion of the first instrument, the skin of lower abdomen is pulled upward and caudally, what increases the distance between navel and the viscera. A vertical incision at the base of umbilicus is made with scalpel. It is important, not cut too deep, to prevent the bowel, omental vessels or (especially in thin patients) the aorta. The VN is inserted perpendicularly to navels bottom, toward pelvis, strictly within the midline trajectory. Usually, a discrete tactile response (double-click) informs the operator that the fascia and the peritoneum have been passed. The ritual safety tests (aspiration, injection, reaspiration, hanging drop) possess low diagnostic accuracy [37–39]. About correct intra-abdominal position of the VN informs the initial low intra-abdominal pressure (<8 mmHg) associated with unimpeded insufflation flow. An elevation of the abdominal wall should result in a prompt decline of intra-abdominal pressure (positive manometer test). The diagnostic accuracy of the safety tests is compared in **Table 4.4**.

The recommended insufflation pressure for the first entry is about 20 mmHg (up to 25 mmHg in patients without respiratory problems) [40, 41]. The pneumoperitoneum of 20–25 mmHg allows—as compared to 10–15 mmHg—for more distance between abdominal wall and abdominal organs and less insertion forces required for trocar insertion [41, 42]. After insertion of the camera trocar a 360° inspection is mandatory. Provided no evidence for entry-related intra-abdominal injuries or retroperitoneal hematoma, the patient is brought into the Trendelenburg position and 2–3 ancillary trocars are inserted under visual control. In contrast, by use of DTE, the pneumoperitoneum is created first after insertion of the first trocar. For both, VN and trocars, modern variants with integrated camera systems, were developed. Against expectations, the vision-guided entry did not reduce the complication rates [5, 6], so the optical VN and optical trocars reached low popularity yet. If the open access (Hasson technique) is chosen, a small incision (kind of umbilical minilaparotomy) is performed under vision, prior to the insertion of laparoscopic ports. The open access has become increasingly popular in the United States.

Before placement of the primary trocar, a careful examination of the abdomen should inform the surgeon about abdominal scars, hernias, distribution of the subcutaneous fat, abdominal wall laxity, palpable intraabdominal mass etc. After insertion of the camera trocar and before placement of secondary trocars, the identification of the key peritoneal folds covering vascular structures of the abdominal wall helps to prevent injuries of the inferior and superficial epigastric arteries at this stage [41–43].

- Medial umbilical ligament (covering obliterated fetal umbilical artery)
- Lateral umbilical ligament (covering inferior epigastric artery)
- Round ligament entering inguinal ring (the superficial epigastric artery travels from the femoral artery in front of the inguinal ring upward to the umbilical region)

The safe placement of the ancillary ports should occur laterally from these structures. Smaller vessels of the abdominal wall can be identified by use of diaphanoscopy (transillumination) [44]. The linear and rotational forces applied during insertion of the trocar must be controlled, especially by trespassing the fascia. A study showed that novices insert trocars with significantly higher forces when compared to experts [42]. After placement of all trocars a thorough 360° inspection of the whole peritoneal cavity should be carried out to rule out any entry-related injuries (presence of free blood or a retroperitoneal hematoma, intestinal injuries). Then the pneumoperitoneum should be reduced down to 10–15 mmHg. The rules for safe transumbilical VN and trocar insertion are summarized in **Table 4.5** [40, 41, 45].

Entry-related complications are significantly less common in gynecologic than in general surgery (OR 4.3 and 2.8 for bowel and

**TABLE 4.4: Comparison of Safety Tests**

| | Sensitivity (%) | Specificity (%) | Positive Predictive Value (%) | Negative Predictive Value (%) |
|---|---|---|---|---|
| Double click test | 39 | 69 | 19 | 86 |
| Aspiration – injection – reaspiration (Palmers test) | 92 | 50–98 | 98 | 20–83 |
| Hanging drop test | 16 | 89 | 22 | 85 |
| Pressure profile test (initial insufflation pressure 0–9 mmHg) | 79–100 | 63–100 | 32–100 | 75–100 |

*Source:* Adapted from Yoong W, et al. Eur J Obstet Gynecol Reprod Biol. 2010;152:210–13 [37]; Teoh B, et al. J Minim Invasive Gynecol. 2005;12:153–58 [38]; Azevedo OC, et al. Acta Cir Bras. 2006;21:385–91 [39].

**TABLE 4.5: First Access—Rules of Thumb**

| |
|---|
| Palpate the abdominal wall and the aortic bifurcation before VN or DTE |
| Choose the appropriate length and check functionality of the VN |
| Keep the operating table during VN and primary port insertion horizontally (0°) |
| Elevate the skin below umbilicus upward and caudally during VN insertion |
| Start the vertical incision (not to deep!) from the base to the lower margin of the umbilicus |
| Adjust the insertion angle of the first trocar to the abdominal wall thickness |
| Insert instruments through the umbilicus parallel to the long axis of the patient |
| After maximal three failed attempts with VN, consider alternative access points (Palmer, Lee-Huang) or laparotomy |
| Keep the pneumoperitoneum at 20–25 mmHg during access creation |
| Change to Trendelenburg position first after the introduction of the optical trocar |
| Insert the secondary trocars always under vision |

combined bowel/vascular injuries, respectively [9]). Studies from the 20th century comparing open vs. closed entry modes indicated a higher number of vascular injuries with closed techniques as compared to open entry (0.8% vs. 0%), and no significant differences in relation to bowel injuries, gas embolism or perioperative death [5]. The latest Cochrane Review (as of 2019), however, did not find differences between laparoscopic entry techniques in regard to vascular injury, visceral injury, or solid organ injury [46]. Failed entry was less frequent with DTE as compared to VN, and no difference was seen when comparing direct VN with open-entry technique. In conclusion, the evidence was judged to be "insufficient to support the use of one laparoscopic entry technique over another" [46]. Cuss et al. [47] analyzed the recommendations for laparoscopic entry technique published by general-surgical and gynecological societies from all around the world. With one exception, none of the governing bodies found an entry technique being superior to others. Nevertheless, although VN related injuries occur, they can be self-limiting, are seldom deadly and lead less frequent to malpractice claims as lacerations caused by trocar. The latter are larger (2 mm vs. 5–10 mm) and usually associated with serious morbidity and mortality [24]. While complications associated with the blind insertion of the primary trocar cannot be fully eliminated, so seem those related to secondary trocar insertion being completely preventable. Nevertheless, they account for every third of trocar reported injuries [5, 26].

## Anatomical landmarks and anatomical variations

### *Position of the umbilicus*

Umbilicus is the primarily access point in gynecological laparoscopy. The navel is the thinnest part of abdominal wall, relatively weak vascularized, with good fixed parietal peritoneum. Furthermore, the almost invisible scar offers a cosmetic advantage.

The position of the umbilicus is traditionally judged to be exactly in the body midline and slightly cranial to the aortal bifurcation. This is the origin of the classical recommendation, that the transumbilical instrument insertion in non-obese patients should be strictly medial and at 45° to the horizontal supine plane ("toward the pelvis"). However, every surgeon should be aware that the umbilicus, like any other organ, is variable in position (deviance from midline), thickness (older patients, previous laparoscopies etc.), depth (relation to the subcutaneous fat) and—most important—relation to intra-abdominal organs. The latter can result from original patient anatomy as well as from her history (previous surgeries, infections, etc.).

Rohrich et al. [48] demonstrated that only 2% of patients have a truly midline umbilicus. In every second patient the navel is located more than 2% laterally, and in 13% cases more than 4% laterally from the midline.

Respecting the body mass index (BMI) is an important precaution for safe laparoscopic entry [11, 41, 49–51]. Generally, with increasing BMI the umbilicus relatively "drops" caudally and the aortal bifurcation "moves" cranially [49, 50]. The umbilicus is located caudal to the aortic bifurcation in 48%–53% of non-obese, 56% of overweight, and 68% of obese patients [50]. Very thin and very obese women are at elevated risks of visceral and vascular injuries because the angle of insertion of the VN and umbilical trocar vary depending of fat tissue deep [11]. The frequently cited figure from the work of Hurd et al. [51] demonstrates the relation between subcutaneous fat and insertion angle of transumbilical instruments (**Figure 4.1**, with permission).

In the individual patient, the position of the aorta can be palpated through abdominal wall in the majority of cases (85%), including 67% of obese women, and 93% of those with a low or normal BMI who are at higher risk of vascular injury. The routine palpation for the aortic bifurcation can be recommended as a simple means to reduce the risk of injury to a major retroperitoneal

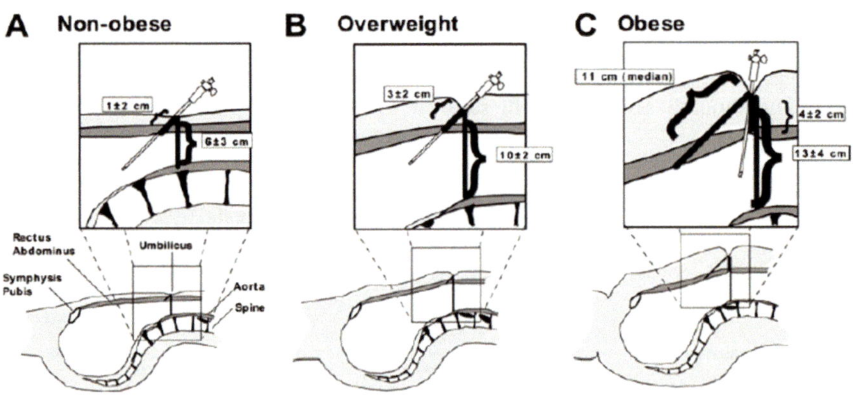


**FIGURE 4.1** The effect of abdominal wall thickness on the laparoscopic approach. (From Pickett SD, et al. Obstet Gynecol Clin North Am. 2010;37:387–397 [41]; Hurd W, et al. J Reprod Med. 991;36:473–476 [51]. With permission).

vessels [52]. The relation between umbilicus and aortic bifurcation, however, can change according to the patient position: in the supine position it lies from 5 cm cranially to 3 cm caudally in relation to the navel, and in the Trendelenburg position from 3 cm cranially to 3 cm caudally [53]. Generally, the aortic bifurcation is located caudally to the umbilicus in only 11% of patients in supine position, but in 33% of patients in the Trendelenburg position [53]. For this reason, the patients should be brought into the Trendelenburg position only after safe placement of the camera trocar and inconspicuous 360° inspection.

### Intraperitoneal adhesions

Intra-abdominal adhesions represent a substantial risk for any kind of laparoscopic complications. Of special importance are adhesions adjacent to the umbilicus—the standard laparoscopic entry site. Adhesions can be asymptomatic or, in turn, be by themselves an indication for surgery as source of chronic pain or fertility problems. Periumbilical adhesions are to be expected in 0.7% of patients with no previous abdominal operations, and in 1.6%, 20%, and 52% of patients after laparoscopy, Pfannenstiel laparotomy, and midline laparotomy in the past, respectively [54, 55]. In women with known risk factors (abdominal operations, endometriosis or pelvic inflammation), following measures can be helpful for choosing the appropriate surgical approach:

- Preoperative sonographic "visceral slide test": absent or minimal (<1 cm) movement of the intestine against abdominal wall is suggestive for adhesions [56, 57]
- Preoperative conventional or dynamic magnetic resonance imaging (MRI, cine MRI) [58]
- Avoiding blind entry via the midline laparotomy scar,
- Using alternative entry sites:
  - *Palmers point* (located 2–3 cm subcostal in the left midclavicular line); well supported by literature and practice, but contraindicated after splenic surgery or after upper-abdominal trauma [59]
  - *Lee–Huang point* (in the mid between navel and xyphoid; especially helpful for enlarged uteri) [60]
  - *Jain's point* (left lateral entry, about 10 cm caudally from the costal margin), in presence of contraindications for Palmers point [61]
- Use of instruments with integrated optical systems (optical VN, optical trocar), if available [43, 62]
- A combination of alternative access site (Palmers point) and optical trocar [63]

Since every surgery can stimulate the development of adhesions, efforts toward reducing the adhesion formation—careful hemostasis, gentle tissue handling, avoiding unnecessary dissection, minimizing desiccation, use of antiadhesive agents—should be taken by surgeons, whenever they actually perform laparoscopy, gynecologic laparotomy or cesarean section [64].

### Failed entry

At first attempt, the peritoneal cavity is usually reached in 85%–87%; two attempts are required in 8.5%—11.6%, three attempts in 2.6%—3.0%, and more than three attempts in 0.3%—0.6% of procedures [38, 65]. However, any misplacing of the VN or first trocar increases the risk of complications like extraperitoneal insufflation, omental and bowel injuries, or conversion to laparotomy. Preperitoneal insufflation was reported in 2.7%, 15%, 44.4%, and 100% of cases of one, two, three, and more than three failed attempts, respectively [38]. The overall complication rates reported in relation to the number of failed attempts are: 0.8% to 16.3% after one attempt; 16.31% to 37.5% after two attempts; 44.4% to 64% after three attempts; and 84.6% to 100% at more than three attempts [38, 65]. From empirical-practical point of view, after three failed attempts, alternative access points should be chosen, provided no evidence that a severe complication has already happened. Amongst alternative entry sites, the left upper quadrant (Palmers point) and the subxiphoid Lee–Huang access are recommendable [41, 43, 62, 65]. In morbidly obese patients without suspicion of pelvic adhesions, a transuterine or transforniceal VN insertion has been associated with less insufflation failure as transumbilical insufflation or open laparoscopy [66]. When a grave entry-related complication is supposed (e.g., feces or blood in VN), an immediate laparotomy is mandatory.

## Vascular injuries

### Abdominal wall vessels

The perforation of the abdominal wall vessels (inferior and superficial epigastric arteries and muscular perforating vessels)—occur almost exclusively due to secondary trocar insertion. This complications is reported in 0.4%—1% procedures. The use of sharp-cutting trocars (0.83%) rather than cone-shaped or blunt ones (0%) elevates the risk [5]. The bleeding can usually be stopped immediately, with an occasional port site hematoma. In rare cases, the bleeding spreads toward vulva and lower limbs [67]. A bleeding from the trocar insertion site should be treated with immediate manual (external) and instrumental (internal) compression. A useful option is the insertion of a Foley catheter. The blocking balloon can be expanded directly within the abdominal port site or used as counterforce after previous inserting into the abdominal cavity. Small identifiable vessels can be coagulated with bipolar. If compression or coagulation are not sufficient or not suitable, hemostatic sutures can be applied either laparoscopically or transabdominally (e.g., out-in/in-out).

### Major vascular injury

Injuries to large retroperitoneal (aorta, vena cava, and the iliac) vessels occur in 0.2%–1.0% of procedures, with the most quoted rate of 0.5% [5, 10, 12, 68]. This kind of complication is associated with high mortality (6%–31%) [11, 12, 14, 68], being responsible for up to 74%–82% of all laparoscopy-related deaths [17, 47, 69]. Although arteries are frequently affected, venous lacerations are those predominantly involved in lethal cases [13]. The difficulty to manage major vascular injuries results from their fulminant course and often co-occurrence with other organ injuries [13, 41]. Every fourth major vascular complication occurs during diagnostic laparoscopy [13].

The right iliac arteries are affected in 41%–48% of cases, followed by the right iliac veins (38%), left iliac veins (29%), aorta (13%–25%), inferior vena cava (6%–11%), and mesenteric vessels (6%–17%) [13, 14, 66]. Since multiple injuries are common, at least one right-sided iliac vessel (regardless vein or artery) is involved in 70%–81% of all vascular complications [13, 14, 41]. Perforations of large veins are commonly accompanied by injuries of the corresponding overlying arteries, including vena cava inferior and aorta [41].

Collateral damage of adjacent structures (small bowel, ureters, nerves, suturing the wrong vessel, etc.) happens concurrently or sequentially in every second case of major vascular injury [14, 24]. In catastrophic events, the immediate cause of death is the exsanguination. Picket et al. reported a mean blood loss 3400 mL, ranging from 1000 mL to 7000 mL, which can occur within few minutes [13]. Also in cured patients, massive blood transfusions are needed [13]. Rarely, fatal outcome can also be related to massive gas embolism [12]. The delayed complications are arterial or venous thrombosis, pulmonary embolism, arterial or venous stricture, compartment syndrome, chronic edema, permanent brain damage, or loss of limb following ischemia [12, 13, 24].

As mentioned in the previous section, 50%–83% of major vascular complications take place during laparoscopic entry [11–14]. In 6%–46% they are caused by VN, in 54%–83% by trocar [5, 9–11, 13, 24, 69], with occasionally reported higher frequency and severity by disposable than by reusable trocars [5, 13]. Peculiarly, 6%–37% of severe vascular events are attributable to the insertion of secondary trocars, despite they are placed under visual control and in presence of maximal pneumoperitoneum [5, 13]. In the analysis of Paśnik and Modrzejewski, 3/51 (6%) of major vascular injuries were created by scalpel at the moment of skin incision [70]. The latter can specifically occur in very thin patients or those with periumbilical adhesions [66]. Furthermore, 10%–20% of severe vascular complications are caused intraoperatively by dissecting instruments, stapling devices, and energy sources [12–14]. Veins have thinner walls compared with arteries, so are the vena cava and its branches at greater risk than the corresponding arteries [8, 12].

### Recognition and management

In case of a serious vascular injury, the time to recognition and immediate reaction are of critical importance. A delay of seconds or minutes can decide about patients survival [5, 11, 18, 68]. Evident vascular injury signs are:

- Blood coming back from the VN or trocar
- Fresh, unexpected hemoperitoneum
- Visible bleeding source in the abdominal cavity
- Hemodynamic instability

A fresh bleeding can be difficult to diagnose in patients undergoing surgery in cases when hemoperitoneum is already present (ectopic pregnancy, hemorrhagic ovarian cyst, etc.). Furthermore, injury to retroperitoneal vessels can expand to a rapidly growing retroperitoneal hematoma, which can be overseen. Baggish reported an alarming high rate of 68% (21 out of 31) grave vascular injuries which were noticed first after the patients developed hemorrhagic shock (hypotony, tachycardia, tachpnea) [13].

The quintessence of management of major vascular injury is obtaining rapid access to the bleeding site and applying direct pressure on the bleeding site, followed by vascular repair and paralleled by patients stabilization or resuscitation [12, 45, 68, 71]. In the most cases, an emergency midline laparotomy is indicated. Based on the location and severity of the injury, a laparoscopic repair is sometime feasible, but should be reserved to extraordinary experienced surgeons [5, 72, 73]. An immediate communication of the problem and tailoring of parallel tasks (calling visceral surgeon and additional personal, application of tranexamic acid and replacing liquids, preparing for blood transfusions, stabilization and resuscitation of the patient) are mandatory [45, 68]. In case of laparoscopic management, additional trocars (allowing for rapid introduction and removal of swabs etc.) as well as avoiding too close distance to the camera (loss of visibility by blood contamination) and too intensive suction are recommended [12, 13, 68]. Gynecologic surgeons should be familiar with the use of local hemostatic agents, like hemostatic patches or flowable hemostats [12, 71, 74, 75]. They application can be helpful even in cases of great vessel lacerations, however, an unreflected use can cause harm. Hemostats should never be applied intravascularly [74]. In case of large venous injuries, a preformed patch should be preferred instead of flowable or pulverized hemostats for preventing inadvertent clot migration into the lumen of large veins. In exceptional situations, it can be useful to leave the penetrating instrument in the vessel until arrival of the vascular surgeon. Blind grasping, clamping or uncontrolled coagulation of the damaged vessel can worsen the situation and should be avoided [5]. Lam et al. proposed the acronym "SAAS" for dealing with vascular injury: **S**top the arterial bleeder immediately; **A**lert the team; **A**ccess the bleeding site by the quickest and safest route; **S**ecure the vascular injury by using an appropriate hemostatic method [71]. Baggish, based on large case series, and Vilos, analyzing only litigated cases, identified any form of delay (delayed diagnosis, delayed communication, delayed involving of the vascular surgeon), performing Pfanennstiel instead of midline laparotomy, and inadequate blood management as the most the typical errors, being relevant both for medical and forensic reasons [11, 13].

### Gas embolism

Carbon dioxide is a soluble gas. Minimal amounts introducing capillary vessels are clinically irrelevant. Kim et al. observed that 100% of patients undergoing total laparoscopic hysterectomy (TLH) had detectable gas in venous blood, with 37.5% of patients demonstrating bubbles filling more than half of the right side of the heart at transesophageal echocardiography. However, no patient in this study developed hemodynamic instability or electrocardiogram changes despite confirmed venous air embolism [76]. However, gas embolism following damage of large retroperitoneal vessels or high-pressure insufflation into the hepatic venous system, although extremely rare has a high fatality rate [9, 12]. Recommended treatment for massive gas embolism can range from stopping insufflation and supportive measures to external chest compression and insertion of a central line to withdraw gas from the right side of the heart [12].

## Intestinal injuries

### Incidence and causes

The incidence of gastrointestinal (GI) complications following gynecological laparoscopies is reported at 0.13% (0.06%–0.5%) [5, 15, 25, 26, 77]. Within this number, the small intestine is with 34%–62% the most frequently damaged part of the GI tract, followed by large bowel (39%–48%), and stomach (1.6%–6%) [15, 25, 26, 77]. Ileum (accounting alone for 48% of GI injuries) is the predominantly affected part of small intestine, whereas sigmoid (with 22%–29%) is the most hit colon segment [25, 26]. About 55% (32%–77%) of all GI injuries occur during the initial set up procedure (VN or trocar insertion, and creation of pneumoperitoneum) [9, 10, 15, 25, 26, 77], with 77% of small intestinal and 41% of large intestinal injuries happing at this step [26]. Disposable trocars are associated with more frequent injuries (47%) as compared to reusable or other trocar types [26]. Further 45% (23%–57%) of GI lacerations happen during the operative procedure, with—unlike in entry-related complications—the large bowel being significantly more frequent involved as compared to small bowel (60% vs. 25%, respectively) [15, 25, 26]. The causative factor for 26%–34% of bowel lesions are energy-based devices, whereas mechanical—dissecting, grasping or morcellating—instruments are involved in 15%–20% mishaps [15, 26, 77]. Among energy-based devices, monopolar instruments are responsible for 43% of bowel injuries [26]. Especially, electrosurgery is a frequent cause of late-presenting complications. The main risk factor for bowel injury are adhesions and/or previous laparotomy, noted in 70%

of respective cases [26, 77]. The risk of laparoscopic bowel injury raises with surgical complexity and is estimated 0.07% (0.05–0.1%) for diagnostic and minor procedures, 0.2% (0.17%–0.24%) for major procedures like endometriosis surgery, 0.39% (0.34%–0.45%) for any form of LH, and 1% (0.43%–2.3%) for laparoscopic sacrocolpoplexy [15]. The overall mortality rate associated with bowel injury at laparoscopy is 0.8% (0.36%–3.6%), almost exclusively resulting from delayed diagnosis [15, 77]. Delayed recognition of bowel injury increases the mortality rate to 3.2%–3.6% [15, 77]. Unfortunately, more than half (41%–84%) of GI injuries is diagnosed postoperatively [15, 25, 26, 77]. About 70% of small bowel and 50% of large bowel perforations are diagnosed > 48 h after surgery [26, 77], with a median time to diagnosis 3 (1–13) days [15].

### Recognition, treatment, and prevention

Immediate manifestations of bowel injury are: gastrointestinal content in VN or trocar, foul smell, visible laceration by VN or trocar, asymmetrical abdominal distention or flautus passage due to insufflation of the bowel [25]. In case of uncertainty, filling the peritoneal cavity with Ringer or saline solutions and a concurrent transanal air insufflation ("bubble air test"), transanal application of diluted povidone-iodine solution ("brown enema"), or toluidine blue dye ("blue enema") can facilitate the diagnosis. A further possibility is the intraoperative coloscopy.

Uncomplicated bowel puncture with the VN can be managed conservatively, however, a perioperative antibiotic prophylaxis and postoperative controls of C-reactive protein (CRP) on 1st and 3rd postoperative days are mandatory. In any other case, the intraoperative repair is indispensable. Depending on localization, severity and mode of injury, the repair is performed laparoscopically or per laparotomy [77]. Simple incisional injuries are treated by closing the defect in two layers with absorbable sutures, while large, irregular or thermal injuries require usually segmental resection with endo-to-end anastomosis [26, 71]. Postoperative CRP monitoring and antibiotic treatment do not differ from common post-anastomotic care, but generally, intraoperatively recognized and repaired injuries are associated with low morbidity [26]. Unfortunately, the majority of postoperative GI injuries is recognized postoperatively, the most of them 2–3 or more days after surgery. The symptomatology can be unspecific and at can partially overlap with normal postoperative signs and symptoms, for example, abdominal pain and tenderness, or nausea [2, 25, 78]. However, given the mostly rapid recovery after laparoscopic interventions, deviations from the usual postoperative course associated with fever, abdominal pain and distension, nausea/vomiting, or CRP exceeding 100 mg/dl on 3rd or later postoperative day, should be alarming [15, 26]. Unrecognized bowel perforations inevitably lead to peritonitis and in one of 30 patients' death. When the diagnosis is delayed 48 hours or more, 100% of colonic, and every second small bowel perforation is complicated by sepsis [26, 77]. For this reason, in each suspected case, a computed tomography scan with contrast should be early performed. Contrast medium extravasation is the most reliable sign, accompanied by intra-abdominal air or fluid collections or other radiologic peritonitis markers [2, 78]. Of note, low-volume intraperitoneal air retention is possible in the early postoperative period and has little diagnostic value in absence of symptoms. The surgical treatment requires usually a midline laparotomy and refers to localization and severity of lacerations. The postoperative treatment can require intensive care unit and depends on infection severity and critical organ function. Because the bowel injuries are often intraoperatively not evident or overseen, the best prophylaxis is to maximize protective measures at entry, for example, consider alternative entry points, create a larger pneumoperitoneum, limited use of monopolar instruments, avoiding blunt adhesiolysis, and careful inspection of the surgical field before leaving abdomen [78].

## Urinary tract injuries

### Incidence and predisposing factors

Gynecological surgeries are responsible for the majority (52%–82%) of all iatrogenic urinary tract injuries (UTI) [79–81]. A systematic review of 136 studies published between 1975 and 2015 including 140,444 gynecologic laparoscopies for benign indication revealed an overall incidence of UTIs of 0.33%. Bladder injury occurs three times more common than ureteral injury (0.24% vs. 0.08%, respectively). LH and laparoscopically assisted vaginal hysterectomy (LAVH) represent with 1.8% and 1.0%, respectively, the highest rates of UTI [82]. Fortunately, the urologic complication rates continuously drop paralleling the evolution and popularization of laparoscopy. If restricted to publications from 2003–2013, an overall incidence of UTI after LH was estimated at 0.73%–0.84%. The bladder injury rates range from 0.05% to 0.66% across procedure types, and the ureteral injury rate ranged from 0.02% to 0.4% across procedure type [16]. The TLH and LAVH are associated with a higher proportion of bladder to ureteral injuries, whereas the laparoscopic supracervical hysterectomy (LASH) is complicated relatively more frequent by ureteral as by bladder injury [16]. Laparoscopic radical hysterectomy is associated with significantly higher risk of urological complications at 3.8%, with injuries to the bladder occurring in 2.5%, and to the ureter in 1.3%–1.8% of surgeries [83]. This risk is higher (OR 1.35–1.4) than with abdominal approach. Bladder injuries are diagnosed at the time of surgery in 45%–85%. In contrast, the intraoperative diagnosis of ureteral injuries is made in only 3%–12% (0%–40%) of cases [16, 82, 84, 85]. The delayed diagnosis contributes to a long-term sequelae of ureteral injury.

Monopolar, bipolar or ultrasonic devices are responsible for 45% and 33%–48% of bladder and ureteral injuries, respectively [82, 84]. Thermal damage promotes delayed necrosis with perforation (bladder) or tear off (ureter), as well as swelling, scarring, temporary or chronic stricture, or fistula formation [86, 87].

Adhesions, including post-cesarean adhesions, are the most relevant risk factor for bladder injury, and endometriosis is considered the most important risk factors for ureter injury. The risk of UTI is further increased in patients with broad ligament fibroids, pelvic malignancy, and being operated by low-volume surgeon [16, 82, 84].

### Bladder injury

In the analysis of Baggish [84], 64% of all bladder injuries resulted from the operative procedure, whereas 36% were entry-related. Separating the bladder from the uterus at hysterectomy or during adhesiolysis accounted for 42% of all bladder injuries, followed by primary (30%), and secondary trocars insertion (6%) [84]. The superior margin of the bladder is highest in the midline, blending into the median umbilical fold (obliterated remnant of the fetal urachus). Importantly, it can lie much higher as expected in presence of adhesions, for example, after prior cesarean delivery. For the safe placement of the suprapubic ancillary trocar, it is useful to recognize bladder boundaries before insertion of the middle ancillary trocar, for example, by backfilling the bladder via Foley catheter [78]. As a rule of thumb, the suprapubic trocar should be placed at least 2 fingers above symphysis.

An bladder laceration is often evident intraoperatively: visible defect, visible balloon of the Foley catheter, macrohematuria, air in the Foley catheter, intra-abdominal urine extravasation, and vaginal urine leakage [84, 86]. Bladder injuries caused by the suprapubic trocar can be initially asymptomatic, since the trocar prevents the urine leakage. In case of uncertainty, the integrity of the bladder can be easily proven by filling the bladder with indigo carmine or toluidine blue dye. Intraoperative cystoscopy additionally increases the rate of correct diagnosis to 95% [79, 88].

An inadvertent punction of the bladder with VN usually do not require any repair out of Foley catheter for 24 hours. Some authors opt for conservatively only management also in case of small defects less than 10 mm (e.g., 5-mm trocar injury) with bladder drainage for 5–10 days, depending on the extent of injury [89]. In any other case, when thermal damage is not suspected, the bladder defect the should be closed with resorbable two-layer suture, followed by catheterization and antibiotics for one week. When laceration occurs in the proximity to ureteral ostium, an ureteral double-J catheter is indicated for preventing its fibrotic stenosis. When a thermal injury without loss of bladder integrity is noted, the area of injury can be sewn over and a prolonged Foley catheter can be considered. In the event of severe thermal injury, a partial cystectomy can be necessary [84, 86, 89]. Difficult bladder complications should be managed by urologist. Generally, bladder lacerations, when recognized and repaired intraoperatively, have an excellent prognosis. The late manifestation of bladder injury are urinoma (urinary ascites), abdominal pain, subfebrile or febrile temperatures, and escalating peritonitis. The diagnosis is confirmed by radiologic investigations, usually with computed tomography with contrast medium. The inadvertent bladder injury can be minimizing by preoperative emptying of the bladder, insertion of the suprapubic trocar at least 3–4 cm above the superior margin of the pubic bone, working nearer the uterus or vagina than the bladder during dissection, and cautious use of monopolar energy.

### Ureteral injury

The majority (70%) of the ureteral injuries occur at the level of cervix, approximately 2–4 cm from the ureteral orifice [85]. This predisposed localization results from the anatomical proximity of the ureter to the cervix—the ureter runs $2.3 \pm 0.8$ cm (range, 0.1–5.3 cm) laterally to the cervix [90]. Notably, in 12% of women, this adjacency is less than 0.5 cm [90]. Although the mean distance between cervix and ureter is 3–4 mm closer on the right side, 70%–80% of ureteral injuries occurs on the left side [91]. Bilateral ureteral injuries have been reported in up to 21% of cases [84].

Intraoperatively, ureteral injury can be direct visualized in case of, for example, transection with urinary extravasation. However, the clinical presentation of ureteral injury often results from inadvertent ligation, thermal damage with delayed tear off or fibrosis, temporary or chronic stricture caused by swelling and scarring, etc. In the face of the discouraging recognition rate of ureteric complications, their prevention is even more crucial. A simple and effective way for observing the ureter's course and peristalsis is its transperitoneal visualization, which is usually unproblematic in thin patients without peritoneal or retroperitoneal fibrosis. Of note, the maintained peristalsis of the ureter does not guarantee its integrity. In fact, an obstructed ureter can pulsate more vigorously than a normal one [78]. The identification of the ureter should begin at the level of the pelvic brim, where it enters the pelvis overcrossing the infundibulopelvic ligament [81]. Importantly, this localization is also the second most frequent injured site of the ureter, commonly in course of oophorectomy. Newly, transurethral application of indocyanine green into the bladder provides a safe and feasible method for ureter localization under near-infrared light even in problematic surgical fields [92]. Prophylactic ureteral stenting can improve its intraoperative detection and immediate repair in selected cases, for example, after prior pelvic radiation or known distorted anatomy [81], however, a prophylactic ureteral catheterization prior to "difficult" surgery is not recommended [93]. When a ureter injury is suspected a cystoscopy can be useful [79]. Hematuria or lacking urine jet from the ureteral ostium can enhance the diagnosis; however, normal intraoperative cystoscopy findings did not exclude the presence of ureteral injury [85]. If detected during surgery, the appropriate management of ureteral injury can reach from deligation or oversewing to segmental excision, reconstruction and reimplantation. Whereas the former steps can be performed by experienced gynecological surgeon, the latter should be reserved for urology specialist.

Unfortunately, up to 90% of ureteral injuries are detected postoperatively. In case of bilateral ureteral transection or occlusion, anuria and flank pain will develop within first hours after surgery. Otherwise, ureteric injury typically becomes symptomatic on the 7th–11th (range 2nd–30th) postoperative day [85]. The clinical presentation is nonspecific and variable, with abdominal and loin pain, dysuria, nausea, fever, and bloating as the most frequent symptoms, and abdominal distention and tenderness, decreased bowel sounds, hematuria, and transvaginal urine leakage being the most common signs [84, 87, 89]. On ultrasound, intraperitoneal free fluid can usually be seen. The definitive diagnosis is made by a pyelography or CT scan with contrast medium [84, 88]. Unlike during surgery, the postoperative cystoscopy does not improve the diagnosis of ureteral injury [79]. In more favorable cases, the management of ureteral injury can be less invasive, for example, with endourologic retrograde balloon dilation, ureterotomy, stenting, or with percutaneous nephrostomy. However, in more than every second case at least one repeat surgery is necessary, for example, open ureteral anastomosis, ureteroneocystostomy, vesicopsoas hitch, etc. [80, 87, 89].

### Genitourinary fistula, and rare urological complications

Genitourinary fistulas can occur immediately during operation or develop in the late postoperative period. Vesicovaginal fistulas accounts for 3.44% and ureterovaginal fistulas for 2.35% of urological complications after LH [16]. Adequate dissection of the vesicovaginal space far from the urinary bladder, proper placement of vaginal cuff sutures, immediate identification and—when appropriate—placement of indwelling ureteral stent decrease the risk of developing both ureteral and bladder fistulas [86, 94].

Injuries to other parts of urinary tract (urethra, kidney) in connection with gynecologic laparoscopic procedures are very rare. Direct kidney laceration was described after inappropriate morcellator use [95]. Rupture of the renal pelvis can develop as a late complication of postoperative occlusion of the distal ureter [87].

## Neurological complications

Central nervous injuries in connection with gynecological laparoscopy are almost always secondary to anesthesiological or severe surgical complications, for example, cerebral ischemia following exsanguination [24] or gas embolism [12], both resulting from major vessel injury. Much higher (1.1%–1.9%) is the rate of peripheral neuropathies related to patient malpositioning, insertion of trocars or closure of lower lateral trocar sites, intraoperative nerve entrapment, transection or thermal damage, or nerve compression following hematoma formation [96–98]. Inappropriate patient positioning is by far the commonest cause. Nerves of the lower limb (1.5%–1.8%) are more frequent affected as those of the upper limbs (0.02%–0.16%). Injuries occurring intraoperatively include the femoral, ilioinguinal, pudendal, obturator, lateral cutaneous, iliohypogastric and genitofemoral nerves [97]. A compression of the femoral nerve (running under the inguinal ligament) and the lateral femoral cutaneous nerve (coursing over the iliacus muscle), can both easily be prevented by avoiding excessive flexion, extreme abduction, and external rotation of the hips in the lithotomy position [98].

The pre-existing risk factors for peripheral nerve injury during gynecologic laparoscopy include but are not limited to preexisting peripheral neuropathies, diabetes mellitus, peripheral vascular disease, extreme body mass index. Modifiable or avoidable surgical factors are nerve stretch or compression due to malpositioning, use of candy cane stirrups for leg support in lithotomy position, and prolonged surgical times [96]. Fortunately, the most nerve injuries related to gynecologic laparoscopy are self-limiting or resolving with physiotherapy. Nevertheless, iatrogenic sensory and motor deficits can negatively impact patient recovery, sometimes require additional pharmacological treatments, and elevate therapy costs. Severe motor disability persist after one out of 3600 gynecologic laparoscopies [96].

To minimize the risk of neurological injuries one should pay attention to following positioning rules: arms tucked by the sides in a neutral position with the thumb pointing up, the angle of hip abduction maximal 90° (measured between from inner thighs) to minimize strain on the obturator nerve, hip flexion between 60° and 170°, possibly minimal external hip rotation for protecting the femoral, obturator, or sciatic nerves (and therefore voidance of candy cane stirrups). The knee flexion should be between 90° and 120° degrees and the knee should be padded around to reduce the pressure on the common peroneal nerve [96, 99].

## Instrument-related complications: energy

Energy-based surgical devices (ESD) are the first choice for dissection and hemostasis in laparoscopy. The ESD comprise electrosurgical, ultrasonic, hybrid (electrosurgical and ultrasonic), and laser-based instruments, whereas the latter are less popular in gynecology. The majority of ESD-related complications is preventable and related to inappropriate use of such devices. Nevertheless, studies exploring gynecologic surgeon's knowledge about application of thermal energy, deliver repeatedly alarming results. Gynecologists seem to present significant "knowledge gap in the safe and effective use of surgical energy devices," which "is not improved with experience" [100–102]. Independent authors attest the gynecologists a regular "ignorance" about appropriate electrosurgery use [101], and conclude that surgeons literally "don't know what they don't know about the safe use of energy in surgery" [103]. In fact, up to 82% of surgeons are not familiar with basic information about electrosurgical devices and two third of them uses diathermy in a manner which can be dangerous to patient [101, 103].

### Function principles of energy-based surgical devices

*Electrosurgery* (also called diathermy or radiofrequency surgery) uses the thermal effects of high-frequency alternating current travelling through body tissues. Electro surgical units (ESUs) produce alternating currents in the frequency range between 200 kHz and 5000 kHz, a bandwidth corresponding to the frequency of radio waves. Within these bandwidth no side-effects on muscle or nerve function may be expected [104–106]. Electrosurgery requires the presence of a circuit for current to flow. By use of *monopolar* instruments, electrons travel from the tip of the active electrode (where the current density it greatest) throughout the patient's body to the dispersive electrode (conductive adhesive grounding pad applied to the patient). Additionally, the argon "plasma" beamer can be considered as an offspring of monopolar instruments: the argon gas streams over a monopolar electrode, becoming fully ionized and allowing the current to arc from the electrode to the underlying tissue. A diffuse superficial coagulation occurs within the area reached by the column of argon gas [107].

When using *bipolar* instrumentation, electrons trespass only the tissue placed between two electrodes [106]. In advanced bipolar systems (BiClamp, Ligasure, EnSeal), this electron flow is controlled by an integrated tissue-impedance feedback mechanisms [104, 105].

When the high-frequency electrical current passes through tissue, the rapid movement of electrons through the cytoplasm of cells results in intracellular temperature rise [107]. Up to 45°C tissues can restore their structure and function after recovery to the normal temperature. Above this level, the proteins become denatured—their structure and function becomes irreversibly destroyed. For instance, cellular death occurs within 6 minutes at 50°C, and immediately at 60°C. At temperatures between 60°–95°C cells rapidly retract and desiccate, similar to heating the egg white. This effect is called "white coagulation." An explosive vaporization of intracellular water, resulting in cell membrane disintegration and cell separation, occurs when the cells are rapidly heated to 100°C. Above 200°C, the solid organic phase of the tissue is carbonized, which presents as "black coagulation" [105–108].

Although from biological point of view all these processes mean tissue damage, if used intentionally and in a controlled manner, they are the principal effects of ESDs. The thermal denaturation and desiccation are used for "coagulation" (required for clotting of blood or agglutination of tissue), while the vaporization for "cutting" tissues. The black coagulation of oozing surfaces, achieved by the electrical arc sparking to the tissue, is named "fulguration" or "spray mode." "Termofusion" or "copative coagulation" is an combined effect of mechanical forces (clamping) and impendance-controlled application of bipolar coagulation of a bleeding vessel (up to 7 mm in diameter), resulting in its "sealing" by collagen weld [104, 106, 109]. According to international standards, the activation of the cutting mode occurs on all electrosurgical instruments by pressing the *yellow* switch, while coagulation by activation of the *blue* switch.

The tissue effects described above differ in detail according to the current density, voltage, and waveform. They are programmed in modern ESUs and offered to the surgeon as pre-set or adjustable electric wave modulations. In the cutting mode of monopolar devices, a continuous, low-voltage, and high-current output is delivered to the tip of the electrode for rapid heating the tissue above the boiling point, causing its vaporization and allowing for a clean incision with minimal hemostasis and little lateral thermal damage (100–400 microns) [106]. Exactly the opposite is happens in the coagulation mode: an interrupted, high-voltage (4000–1000 V) current is compensated (according to the Ohms law) with its low density. Because of the lower current density, tissue heating is slower and more moderate. As a result, denaturation of proteins (required for hemostasis and tissue agglutination), but also greater thermal spread are obtained [106]. Several "blended" modes provide combinations of cutting and coagulation forms in various proportions. While the pure "coagulation" mode means an interrupted high-voltage current being delivered in only 6% of the activated time, so consist the mixed modes of, for example, "80% cut and 20% coagulation," "60% cut and 40% coagulation" or "50% cut and 50% coagulation" blends. Proportionally to the rate of the coagulation in a blend, the proportion of interrupted to continuous and the peak-voltage increase. The "blends" are needed for concurrent cutting and hemostasis [104–107].

In the bipolar mode, a low-voltage (under 1000 V) and high-amperage current is continuously delivered 100% of the duty cycle. Because the current flows between two electrodes situated very close to each other, several risks are reduced or not present [106, 108, 109].

Ultrasonic devices (e.g., Harmonic Scalpel®, Harmonic ACE®, Ultracision, SonoSurg) heat adjacent tissues to 80°C by converting electrical energy into vibrations of piezoelectric crystals at frequencies of 55,000 per second or higher, which leads to protein denaturation, desiccation, and coaptive coagulation of tissues [104, 109]. In turn, the cutting effect of ultrasonic instruments is obtained by mechanical shearing forces produced by oscillating and non-oscillating jaws and applied to the tissue [109].

## Incidence and causes of ESD-related complications

The overall complication rate related to energy based devices is 0.2%–0.5% [107–110] of all laparoscopic procedures. One of four laparoscopic complications is caused by inadvertent energy release, making them the second most common after entry-related complications. In fact, 26%–29% of bowel injuries and 33%–50% of ureter injuries are associated with the use of ESD [15, 26, 77, 84, 110]. Peculiarly, 70% of injuries created with ESD are recognized first in the postoperative period [108]. Unlike non-thermal injuries, they often require excision of the tissue margin surrounding laceration. Lacerations caused with monopolar instruments are usually larger than those from bipolar and ultrasonic instruments, and they are also associated with larger collateral injury as ultrasonic scalpel [111]. Unique for monopolar instruments is, that they can cause iatrogenic effects not only within their activation area but also at places distant from surgical field (direct, indirect, and capacitive coupling; return electrode failure) [104–106, 108, 110]. In direct comparisons, advanced bipolar and ultrasonic devices are superior to conventional monopolar or bipolar instruments in terms of safety and efficiency of coagulation and obtaining hemostasis, as well as because of less lateral thermal damage and less adjacent histological inflammatory reaction [104, 109, 112].

## The mechanisms of energy-related trauma

The complications resulting from ESD use are caused by:

- Thermal spread to adjacent tissues
- Direct application (inadvertent activation, residual heat)
- Direct coupling
- Insulation failure
- Capacitive coupling
- Return electrode failure

## Thermal spread to adjacent tissues

All types of ESD produce thermal effects. Ideally, the effects are limited to the target tissue with no significant lateral temperature spread. However, a margin of thermal damage is always present and depends on tissue properties, instrument type, power setting and application time [105, 113, 114]. Generally, monopolar instruments on coagulation mode are associated with the greatest degree of lateral thermal spread, whereas advanced bipolar instruments (like Ligasure or BiClamp) as well as ultrasonic devices are associated with less thermal damage [109, 114]. This is in accordance with the mean working temperatures: 100–300°C (70–400°C) for monopolar instruments, circa 100 (80–120°C) for bipolar instruments, 80–90 (60–100°C) for advanced bipolar, about 80°C (60–200°C, depending on modus) for ultrasonic devices, and 100–220°C for Thunderbeat [109, 115]. The usual thermal spread range is 2–22 mm for monopolar instruments and 2–6 mm for conventional bipolar instruments. Advanced bipolar systems seal vessels up to 7 mm in diameter, and their lateral thermal spread is reported at 1.8–5.1 mm for Ligasure, 1.1–1.7 mm for Enseal and 1.3–6.3 mm for PK PlasmaKinetics. Among ultrasonic devices, Harmonic Scalpel produces 1–4 mm lateral spread, and the hybrid device Thunderbeat 2–3 mm [104, 111, 113–116].

The unintended lateral effect can reach from edema through desiccation to black coagulation. This collateral effect can cause immediate injury of adjacent organs (bowel, bladder, ureter) or delayed effects due to tissue necrosis and scarring (e.g., delayed bladder perforation or ureteral stenosis). Knowing the working temperature range and expected thermal spread of surgical devices can help the surgeon to tailor their use and minimize the risk of adverse events.

## Direct application

It results in a similar tissue effects (cutting, coagulation, etc.) as in the event of intended application, but it occurs at not the right place and not the right time.

It can be result of surgeons fatigue, distraction, insufficient training, or non-familiarity with the equipment, etc. Because of the heterogeneity of reasons this kind of failure is hardly preventable, but in turn, it is almost always human error—and as that but preventable and prone to malpractice litigation.

Simple measures for preventing inadvertent direct application are that [104, 108, 110]:

- ESD should always remain visible in the surgical field (whether activated or no)
- ESD should be activated solely by the surgeon
- ESD should not be routinely used for grasping non-targeted tissues
- Touching of vital structures with the tip of ESD should be avoided at least 15 seconds after deactivation

The latter recommendation is based on the fact that active tips of all ESD need time for cooling. Until the safe residual tip temperature sink beyond 45°C can last more than 15 seconds. The longest cooling times are reported for tips of ultrasonic devices, although their working temperatures are comparably low.

## Direct coupling

This condition occurs when one conductor (the active electrode) touches another secondary conductor (another metal instrument, camera telescope etc.). Current from the active electrode flows to the second conductor and cam cause unintended burns to adjacent tissues. Similarly to inadvertent direct activation, harm caused via direct coupling is almost always preventable and therefore responsibility of the surgeon. Risk reduction can be achieved by following regarding similar rules. Additionally, the attention should be paid as to none of the instruments comes in direct contact with the active electrode. Energy can never be activated until the monopolar instrument is within the metal trocar and its tip is not in view [104–106, 108, 110].

### Insulation failure

Insulation failure is a common cause of ESD-related complications [110, 117]. In presence of insulation defect, the monopolar current uses an alternate pathway to complete the circuit between ESU and neutral electrode. Because of the high-power density and the high temperature of the sparks (plasma) of 700–1000°C, the thermal injuries to the adjacent organs (e.g., bowel) are often beyond the surgical field, severe and irreversible. The smaller the insulation defect, the higher the stray current density and the more severe the iatrogenic burn. One hundred percent of the energy can be delivered to unintended tissue when both layers of insulation are defect [110].

Full-thickness insulation failures are reported in 20% of reusable and in 3% of reusable disposable instruments. Macroscopically invisible leaks are detected in 50% of all laparoscopic instruments [110, 117]. In 71% of reusable sets at least one instrument has an insulation failure, and one in four reusable laparoscopic instruments has more than one insulation leak [117]. The defects are localized predominantly (54%) at the distal third of the instrument [117]. The failure rate increases along with inappropriate handling, repeated cleaning, sterilization, and over-frequent high-voltage current use [108]. The incidence of insulation defects differs not significantly between hospitals that routinely apply hospital-based detection programs and those not doing so (19% vs. 33%) [110]. The fact that the incidence of insulation-related complications is much less than the incidence of insulation defects is thank to "active electrode monitoring" (AEM) technology, which prevents stray current burns from insulation failure and capacitive coupling [104, 108, 110]. Nevertheless, laparoscopic surgeon is primarily responsible for the recognition of instrument defects.

### Capacitive coupling

Capacitor is defined as two conductors separated by a nonconducting medium (insulator). When electric current travels through a conductor, an electromagnetic field is generated around the conductor. This field can generate a secondary current in nearby conductors; they can be metal or plastic trocars, and also any other adjacent conductive material, for example, bowel or adhesions [104, 105, 110]. Capacitive coupling may transfer a percentage of the energy—"stored" in the intact insulator—to surrounding tissues or adjacent instruments without touching them with the active electrode. In this way capacitive coupling can cause significant visceral injuries away from visible surgical field. The percentage of energy coupled depends on the size of the capacitor, the activation mode, and the voltage of the waveform [104]. The use of hybrid trocars (metal cannula surrounded by plastic collar) can potentiate the capacitator effect and increase the risk of injury. According to Odell [110], capacitive coupling can occur when:

1. An active electrode's insulated shaft is placed against non-targeted organ or tissue such as the bowel and/or adhesion
2. An active electrode is placed inside a metal suction/irrigation tube
3. An active electrode is inserted through an operative laparoscope
4. An active electrode is placed through a metal trocar cannula
5. Single port access is used and cross capacitive coupling induces current into adjacent tissue and conductive devices
6. Two metal ring handle instruments are held by the surgeon and cross capacitive coupling induces current into the cold instrument

Similar to insulation failure, the use of AEM is the most effective prevention of mishaps due to stray currents caused by insulation failure and capacitive coupling. The surgeon can reduce the risk by avoiding hybrid trocars, shortening or interrupting the activation time as well as reducing the voltage setting of the active electrode [104, 108, 110, 117].

### Patient electrode burn

In monopolar electrosurgery, the current travels from the active electrode through the patient body via the path of least resistance to the dispersive (return) electrode. The return electrode has normally a large surface, decreasing the electron density and therefore local heat development. However, if the return electrode has been improperly attached to patients skin, the contact is diminished by hair, subcutaneous tumor, unintended detachment or adhesive pad failure, severe burns may happen within the consecutively smaller contact area to the skin. It is essential to attach the electrode to a clean, dry and healthy part of the body, which is in pelvic surgery usually the lateral part of the thigh. However, since introduction of return electrode monitoring (REM) technology this type of no adverse effects has become seldom [104, 108, 110].

### Electrosurgery and implantable devices

Monopolar electrosurgery can interfere with cardiac implantable electronic devices such as permanent pacemakers or implantable cardioverter defibrillators, as well as other neurologic stimulators. Such interference can damage or inhibit the electronic device, burn the myocardium or cause arrhythmias and asystole [108]. Similarly, in patients with conductive protheses (e.g. hip joints) an alternative circuit can occur including the metal prothesis. For this reason, bipolar and ultrasonic devices should be preferred in those patients with intracorporal implants. If monopolar electrosurgery is not avoidable, the return electrode pad should be placed as possibly far away from conductive implants, to keep them out of the electrical circuit between active and dispersive electrode. Device specification and cardiologist's opinion should be known prior to surgery [104, 108].

## Instrument-related complications: morcellators

The minimal invasive approach to includes the minimal invasive evacuation of surgical specimen through port-site incisions. The possible evacuation routes are: power morcellation via port-site incisions, and manual morcellation via minilaparotomy or transvaginally. In all this cases, the evacuation of a bulky specimens presumes its fragmentation called morcellation. The market offers about a dozen of disposable or re-usable morcellators [95, 118]. The most of them use mechanical forces, usually a rotating blade, for cutting or peeling the bulky specimen. Alternatively, the active part of the morcellator is an integrated electrosurgical cutting device [95, 118]. Morcellation is essential part of myomectomy, LASH and total LH for large uteri [119, 120]. It can also be considered in macroscopically not suspicious ovarian fibroids.

The use of morcellators, however, harbors three types of risks:

- Direct injury of adjacent organs
- Intraperitoneal spread of a benign disease (peritoneal myoma, adenomyoma or endometriosis)
- Intraperitoneal spread of a malignant tumor [119–122]

Considering the individual morcellation-related risk should be part of any patient-centered therapeutic concept, since the decision toward or against morcellation determines the whole surgical approach in the individual patient.

### Direct injury

The morcellators blade rotates with 500–1000 revolutions per minute, resulting in a possible spread of tissue fragments into all parts of peritoneal cavity [95, 118, 120, 121]. As it is designed for removing large portions of tissue within seconds, morcellator-related injuries are often severe, affect in 20% of cases more than one organ, and are associated with high (10%) mortality [95]. In the analysis of Milad and Milad [95], the injuries involved in 47% of the intestine (with the large bowel being mostly affected), and vascular system (41%), followed by kidney, ureter, bladder, and diaphragm lacerations. In every third case, the complication was not recognized intraoperatively. In the majority of cases the "lack of experience, lack of training, lack of control," and less frequent "poor visualization" or "device malfunction" were the best identified contributing factors [95]. For this reason, direct morcellator-related organ injuries are easily preventable. The morcellation should always be performed under continuous vision by applying the lateral pealing technique. The tip of the morcellator shaft should stay in midline of the lower abdomen, in a safe distance from intestine or to blood vessels [119].

### Secondary nonmalignant morcellation-related conditions

The current discussion about morcellation side effects has been largely determined by the risk of malignant tumor spread. However, since the latter can have gravest consequences, one should be aware about much more realistic de novo development of morcellation-related benign conditions. LH or myomectomy with unconfined morcellation is associated with the risk of iatrogenic endometriosis at 1.4%, adenomyosis at 0.57%, parasitic myoma at 0.9%, and disseminated peritoneal leiomyomatosis at 0.1% [120]. The iatrogenic secondary condition and the necessary secondary surgery can be more extensive than the primary disease (**Figure 4.2**).

Parasitic myomas and adenomyomas can develop at unexpected localizations, like colon, diaphragm, omentum or umbilicus, and reach a diameter > 10 cm [121]. The median time to presentation is 5 years and the risk is significantly increased in women before menopause [120]. The risk of nonmalignant sequelae of laparoscopic morcellation is hard to eliminate, but should be minimized by thorough removal of all tissue fragments and meticulous peritoneal lavage after morcellation. The efficacy of in-bag morcellation for minimizing the risk of peritoneal leiomyomatosis is under discussion but still not supported by firm evidence [120, 121, 123].

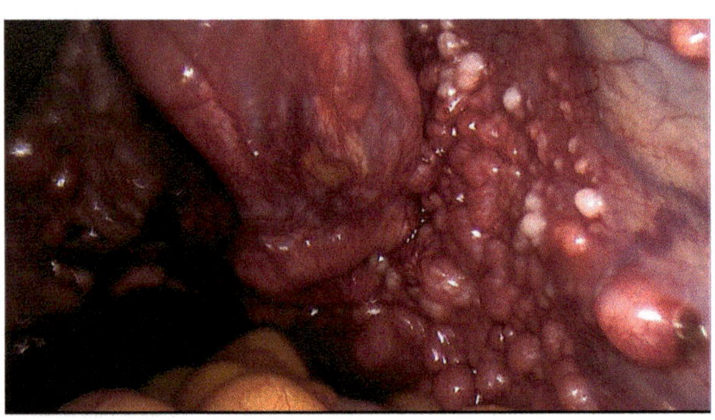

**FIGURE 4.2** Disseminated peritoneal leiomyomatosis: ten years after laparoscopic myomectomy.

### Inadvertent morcellation of a malignant tumor

The fragmentation of a malignant tumor usually significantly worsens its prognosis. This effect is most evident uterine leiomyosarcoma (LMS) [124]. Morcellation increases the overall (62% vs. 39%; OR: 3.16) and intra-abdominal (39% vs. 9%; OR: 4.11) recurrence rates as well as mortality rate (48% vs. 29%; OR: 2.42) in patients affected by unexpected LMS [125], while no differences in survival outcomes were observed for patients with, for example, low-grade endometrial stromal sarcomas [126]. Unlike open surgery, the morcellation of the uterus or myomas is a indivisible part of laparoscopic myomectomy or supracervical hysterectomy. For this reason, after the worldwide discussed case of the iatrogenic LMS morcellation in the U.S. patient Amy Reed, the U.S. Food and Drug Administration (FDA) released in 2014 a warning, followed by a statement advising against the use of power morcellators in myomectomy and hysterectomy. The reaction to this statement were numerous studies and position papers of leading laparoscopic societies, for example, the European Society of Gynecological Surgery and the American Association of Gynaecological Laparoscopists [119, 127]. In a nutshell, almost all publications supported the continuation of laparoscopic approach to presumed leiomyomas. A careful identification of high-risk cases should help to tailor the therapeutic approach.

The rates of any occult malignancy encountered in morcellated uterine specimens are reported between 0.25% (1 in 400) and 0.43% (1 in 230) [122, 128]. The lower rate was reported from a cohort in which 88% of patients were preoperatively screened using Pap-smear and transvaginal ultrasound or dilatation and curettage prior to LASH [122]. When limited to the LMS, the most reliable numbers range from 0.05% (1 in 2000) [127] to 0.14% (1 in 700) [119]. The LMS risk reported after myomectomy—0.08% (1 in 1,306)—is lower than after hysterectomy—0.15% (1 in 650) [119].

Careful patient and surgical approach selection are the cornerstones for reducing the risk to morcellate an unexpected malignancy during laparoscopic surgery for presumed benign indication. The preoperative decision making and informed consent should include individual attitudes of the patient toward risks and benefits of the minimal-invasive approach. The risk of LMS increases in patients older than 40 years. The presence of a rapidly growing, "large (≥8 cm), solitary, highly vascularized (peripheral and central) and irregular, heterogeneous myometrial tumor with central necrosis/degenerative cystic changes and absence of calcifications must raise the suspicion of a LMS" [119]. In those patients, a magnetic resonance imaging with contrast enhancement may help to differentiating between LMS and fibroid [119]. Furthermore, total LDH and LDH isozyme type 3 are often elevated in LMS, and the combination of MRI and LDH assay has been proven in a small study to have a 100% diagnostic accuracy in detection of uterine sarcoma [129]. In patients with abnormal uterine bleeding, an endometrial sampling prior to the operation is recommended, as it allows for the detection of uterine malignancy in 84% of cases [130]. The benefit of "in-bag" morcellation, however, according to the latest Cochrane Review, still remains unclear [123].

## Other procedure-related complications

### Intra-abdominal spillage of adnexal tumors

Intraoperative spillage accompanies 55%–65% (15%–100%) of laparoscopic removals of presumably benign ovarian cysts [131–133]. The relative risk compared to laparotomy is 5.55 (95%CI 1.88–16.33) [133]. However, the short- and long-term consequences of spillage of benign cells is not clear. The often threatened chemical peritonitis after contamination with dermoid cyst contain is observed rarely [131–132]. The use of an endoscopic retrieval bag for controlled volume reduction and evacuation of ovarian cysts is recommended. Alternatively, laparoscopically guided mini-laparotomy can prevent the intraoperative spillage without significant increase in patient short- and long-term discomfort [133].

## Trocar-site hernias

Trocar-site hernias complicate 0.5%–1% (0.6%–1.8%) of gynecological laparoscopic procedures. This is a low rate when compared to incisional hernia rates at 2%–6% after laparotomy for gynecologic indications, and 5%–20% performed by general surgeons [134, 135]. The risk for developing trocar-site hernia increases with the trocar diameter. Only 3% of reported trocar-site hernias are diagnosed at incision sites <8 mm, whereas 11% of them at sites 8–10 mm, and the majority (86%) at sites >10 mm [136]. In gynecology, umbilical defects are more common than lateral port-site defects [135, 137, 138], but remain in 16%–56% of cases asymptomatic [138]. Surgery-related risk factors are use of pyramidal trocars, 12-mm trocars and long operative times, whereas high parity, older age and a higher body mass index are reported as patient-related risk factors [138, 139]. A manifestation of an early herniation can be intestinal or omental strangulation developing within first few days after surgery. A late manifestation can be observed several months later as bulging of the abdominal wall [137, 139]. Closing the fascia trocar-sites ≥ 10 mm is a widely recommended prophylactic measure [5, 139], although in 90% of reported trocar site hernias after gynecologic laparoscopies, the surgeons declared they had sutured the fascia [136, 137]. These discrepancy can relate to improper suturing technique, so a full-thickness closure instead of facia-only closure has been recommended [139]. Additionally, the use of trocars with smallest possible diameter and preferring cone-shaped or blunt trocars instead of cutting ones seem to be a simple and effective measure to reduce the incidence of trocar-site herniations.

## Port-site metastases

Implantation or metastasis at trocar-site is a rare complication after laparoscopic removal of benign (dermoid cysts, fibroids) or malignant tumors (borderline ovarian tumors, ovarian carcinomas, uterine cancers, leiomyosarcoma, etc.) [140–143]. Port-site metastases are reported in 1.2%–2% of patients who underwent laparoscopic procedures for a malignant intra-abdominal condition, predominantly tubo-ovarian malignancies [140–141]. Half of the recurrences occur in the tissue-manipulating port [144]. The median time from the laparoscopic procedure to the diagnosis of port-site recurrence is 5–7 months, despite of underlying disease, when the average abdominal tumor diameter reaches about 2 cm [140, 144]. The clinical relevance of port-site metastases depend on the remaining extent of the disease. The overall survival of ovarian cancer patients with FIGO IV stage due to isolated abdominal wall metastases was with 58 months significantly longer than that of other FIGO IV patients (25 months), and non-significantly longer compared to FIGO IIIC (37 months) [145]. For this reason, a local excision and re-staging are mandatory in any patient with suspected port-site metastasis. Several hypotheses attempt to explain the pathogenesis of port-site metastases. The aerosolization of viable tumor cells and the implantation into the transabdominal trocar tunnels due to gas efflux has been proposed as "the chimney effect." Another studies suggested the role of carbon dioxide, showing that compared to gasless laparoscopy, carbon dioxide pneumoperitoneum resulted in increased tumor growth and a higher incidence of port-site and abdominal-wall metastases. Further concepts focus on the role of the—otherwise advantageous—lower local inflammatory activation by laparoscopy than by laparotomy, as well as on the surgical technique, since repeated removal and reintroduction of trocars during a laparoscopic procedure may contribute to the contamination of the trocar site with exfoliated tumor cells [141]. Prevention of port-site metastasis is feasible. Van Dam et al. achieved a reduction of port-site metastases in patients with ovarian cancer receiving diagnostic laparoscopy from 58% to 2% when additional to the skin suture also the rectus sheath and the peritoneum were closed separately. The bias of the study is the patients with all-layer closure were approached by open laparoscopy, while those with skin incision only with a closed technique [146]. Schneider et al. [147] investigated the efficacy of preventive maneuvers in pigs, in which laparoscopy was performed after intraperitoneal inoculation of "HeLa" tumor cells. In the study group, trocar fixation, prevention of gas leaks, rinsing of instruments with povidone-iodine, minilaparotomy protection, rinsing of trocars before removal, peritoneal closure, and rinsing of all wounds with povidone-iodine were applied. The reduction of port-site metastases in the intervention group dropped to 14%, compared to 64% in the control group.

## Vaginal cuff dehiscence

Earlier studies reported vaginal cuff dehiscence (VCD) rates after LH as high as 4.9%, which was a significantly higher rate in comparison to vaginal (0.29%) or abdominal (0.12%) hysterectomy [148]. Most recent studies report much lower incidences after LH (0.11%–0.75%), and slightly reduced or unchanged rates after vaginal (0.05%–0.13%) and open (0.02%–0.38%) hysterectomy, respectively [149–152]. Following risk factors for developing VCD after LH have been confirmed: premenopausal status, extensive use of electrosurgical technique, smoking habit, preexistent endometriosis, use of single instead of continuous stiches, postoperative infection and supravaginal hematoma [149, 151–154]. The use of barbed vs. conventional sutures, or single-versus double-layered closure did not impact the incidence of VCD [155–156]. In a large randomized controlled trial, the transvaginal route of vaginal vault closure was associated with a significant higher risk for VCD (2.7% vs. 1%), any cuff complication (9.8% vs. 4.7%), vaginal bleeding, vaginal cuff hematoma, postoperative infection, need for vaginal resuture, and reintervention of vaginal dehiscence as compared to laparoscopic closure [152]. Since sexual intercourse before the complete healing of the vaginal cuff is the main trigger event or VCD [149], sexual abstinence should be recommended for 8 weeks after LH.

## Retained surgical items

In laparoscopy, the most frequently retained surgical instruments are needles – lost or broken up. The diagnosis is usually made intraoperatively, but due to limited vision and restricted instrument flexibility, finding of a lost surgical needle (or a part of it) can be more demanding than in open surgery. A thorough inspection of the surgical field, trocar and abdominal port site examination, revision of the suction device, eventually intraoperative radiography should be carried out [157]. A laparoscopic magnet—provided its availability—was recommended as the "safest and most efficient way of retrieving lost needles during laparoscopy" [158]. When all those attempts fail or a prolonged operating time is contraindicated, a laparotomy should be performed.

## Retained specimen

An underreported category of forgotten "items" are retained surgical specimens [159, 160]. They can be overseen or "get lost" within abdominal cavity. Specimens (e.g., multiple myomas) or often intraoperatively collected in peritoneal pouches (Douglas, paracolic space) for being evacuated at the end of surgery. It is mandatory to thoroughly count all specimens and document their number both during and after surgery. A real mishap can be, for example, a small fibroid (2–3 cm) which "disappeared" between intestinal loops or is protruded into the subdiaphragmatic region. Some maneuvers should be tried before decision to a rescue laparotomy: lavage the abdominal cavity with 1.5–2 L saline, supine table position with head up tilt (reverse Trendelenburg), transient reduction of intra-abdominal pressure, inspection of trocars and abdominal insertion sites, and intraoperative transabdominal ultrasound.

## Pneumoperitoneum-related complications

Adverse events attributed to use of carbon dioxide for creating pneumoperitoneum are: subcutaneous emphysema, hypercarbia, and pneumothorax/pneumomediastinum. Additionally, pneumoperitoneum contributes both chemically and mechanically to the development of postlaparoscopic shoulder pain (PLSP).

### Subcutaneous emphysema, pneumothorax, and hypercarbia

Small, clinically not detectable amounts of carbon dioxide accumulate in the subfascial plane and subcutaneous tissue during the most laparoscopies. Rarely, in presence of congenital diaphragma micro-openings, insufflated gas can trespass from the peritoneal to pleural cavities causing pneumothorax. Hypercarbia and acidosis occur as consequence of $CO_2$ passage through large peritoneal surfaces; they can persist into postoperative period in presence of subcutaneous $CO_2$ reservoirs in cases of extensive emphysema [161]. By means of computed tomography residual pneumoperitoneum can be detected in 70%, and subcutaneous emphysema in 56% of patients 24 h after laparoscopy [162]. In an analysis of 968 laparoscopic procedures, grossly detectable subcutaneous emphysema was reported in 2.3%, pneumothorax/pneumomediastinum in 1.9%, and hypercarbia in 5.5% of cases [163].

Intraoperatively, hypercarbia is measured as end-tidal $CO_2 \geq$ 50 mmHg. The consequence can be elevated heart rate, increased systemic and central venous blood pressure, higher cardiac output, as well as decreased peripheral vascular resistance. Indicative for SE and pneumothorax/pneumomediastinum can be intraoperative insufflation problems (flow and pressure) and change in lung compliance. This immediate effects can be alleviated by anesthesiologist with increased ventilation rate and tidal volume, oxygen supply and by surgeon by—if possible—reduction of intra-abdominal pressure and gas insufflation flow [161, 163].

In the postoperative period, the pathognomonic clinical sign of SE is subcutaneous crepitus. This sensation is mostly limited to the abdominal wall and disappears spontaneously within 2–3 postoperative days following absorption of the $CO_2$ into blood. In extreme cases, SE can extend to vulva, limbs, chest, neck, and head [164]. Risk factors leading to subcutaneous emphysema are multiple attempts at abdominal entry, preperitoneal insufflation, use of more than 5 ports, to large incisions/loose fascial entry points, trocars acting as fulcrums, high gas volume and flow rates, and valveless trocar systems [161]. A common risk factor for development of hypercarbia (OR 2.02), subcutaneous emphysema (OR 5.27), and pneumothorax and/or pneumomediastinum (OR 20.49) are operative times greater than 200 minutes [163].

### Postlaparoscopic shoulder pain

PLSP is reported by 50%–80% of patients undergoing laparoscopic interventions. PLSP usually lasts 1–3 (sometimes up to 7) days and causes sometimes more discomfort as the surgical-site or trocar-incision pain [165]. The PLSP is a referred pain, caused by chemical irritation of the phrenic nerve during laparoscopy by $CO_2$ (converted to carbonic acid) and—additionally—by mechanical distention of liver capsule and parietal peritoneum. The nocioceptive signals forwarded from the viscera by the phrenic nerve (originating from C3-C5 spinal nerves) are referred to the C3–C5 dermatome and converge centrally with neck and shoulder pain, because the latter are sensory innervated by cervical nerves 3–5 [165, 166]. The pulmonary recruitment maneuver (PRM) has been shown as the most effective intervention reducing the incidence and severity of PLSP [167–169]. This maneuver consists of at least five manual pulmonary inspirations performed with a pressure of 22–45 mmHg (30–60 cm $H_2O$). Independent from or additional to PRM an intraperitoneal instillation of saline (15–20 mL/kg) [170, 171], intra-abdominal application or intradiaphragmaic injection of anesthetic agents [172] showed positive effects on PLSP. One randomized study observed a significant effect of perioperative intravenous application of vitamin C (1 g/day) [173]. Conflicting data exist in regard to applying low pressure pneumoperitoneum: while some studies confirm its ameliorating effect on PLSP [174], others underline longer surgical times and increased hemorrhage risk, which cannot be outweigh against lower PLSP risk [175]. In contrast, the use of drains, showed no efficacy in reducing PLSP [176]. The simplicity and effectivity of PRM with additional intra-abdominal saline installation makes this combination to the currently best available prevention of PLSP [167–171, 177].

## Surgeon-related complications

### Indication for surgery

A surgical complications occurs only when surgery is performed. It means that the decision to treat a condition surgically must presume a certain risk of surgical complications. In the most cases, this risk is significantly lower that the benefit of operation. "The right surgery offered to the right patient" is a banal, but though the right postulate. The rightness of the indication is primarily the responsibility of surgeon. This presumes that the physician by recommending the appropriate treatment is focused solely on the patient: her health and her personal autonomy. Notwithstanding this, 40% of requested German physicians admit that the indications for surgery are sometimes influenced by non-medical reasons [178]. Some striking differences between frequency of routine procedures between neighbor countries [179], or patients with different health insurance status [178, 180], raise questions about avoidable under- or overtreatments. Concerns about over numerous or sometimes unnecessary treatments performed in patients with private health insurance are repeatedly expressed [179–181]. In the study of Corona, unsupportive pathology was identified after 18.3% of hysterectomies [182]. A premature indication can roll back as subject of a lawsuit due to wrong indication [24]. So, during the decision making and informed consent process, reasonable conservative treatments should be discussed and evaluated, especially in cases of asymptomatic ovarian cysts or bleeding disorders without apparent uterine pathology [24, 181–183].

### Surgical volume

The occurrence of surgical complications is strongly related to individual surgical skills, and to less extent to institutional surgical volume. Numerous studies confirmed that the rate of surgical complications increases when patients are operated by an unexperienced ("low-volume") surgeon [184–186]. This fact explains why a large proportion of reported and litigated complications occur during basic or minor laparoscopies, often performed by less experienced doctors [6, 23]. Although firm evidence from around the world consequently indicates that surgeries performed by, or with participation of, high-volume surgeons result in better outcomes and less complications, several non-medical reasons lead to the fact that the majority of surgeries is performed by less skilled surgeons. The probability than they are faced with a serious complication is higher and that that they will recognize it and properly manage intraoperatively—lower. For instance, the overall complication rate of LH has been reported at is 2% for low-volume surgeons, and at 4.2% for high-volume surgeons [184]. In the United States, only 25% of laparoscopic hysterectomies are conducted by high-volume surgeons, and 68% of all surgeons performing a hysterectomy are low or very low-volume surgeons (less than 10 or 5 cases annually, respectively) [184, 185]. As compared to colleagues performing ≥21 hysterectomies per year, the complication rate of those surgeons is 60%–70% higher [185]. A meta-analysis from 2016 including 7,41,760 different gynecologic surgeries showed that patients operated by low-volume surgeons had an increased rate of intraoperative (OR 1.6) and postoperative complications (OR 1.4), and the mortality of oncologic patients almost doubled [186]. For this purpose, the French College of Obstetrics and Gynecology recommends that hysterectomy should be performed by surgeons removing at least 10 uteri per year [66]. Patients undergoing surgical procedures have right to be informed about the case volume of their surgeons and institutions.

### Psychological factors

Psychological factors—personality, burnout, chronic distress, or sleep deprivation—contributing to surgical performance and patient's safety are underestimated. For instance, surgical trainees with higher grade of impulsiveness are more likely to cause surgical errors [187], whereas introverted surgeons tend to have better surgical outcomes [188]. Kadzielski et al. [189] reported that macho attitude levels predicted 19% of the variation in surgeons' readmissions and reoperations rates. While practically, surgeons' personalities cannot be changed, several factors potentially impairing surgeons' work and patient safety are modifiable: anomalous workloads and sleep deficit, workplace-related distress and burnout; accumulating work-family conflicts, etc. In Germany, among 23 medical specialties gynecology is on the second place according to the burnout prevalence, on the fourth place regarding job distress, but only on the 16th place according to the job satisfaction [190]. A study including almost 8000 U.S. surgeons revealed that burnout and depression were the strongest factors associated with reporting a recent major medical error (the study design did not allow to determine whether distress caused errors or errors caused distress) [191]. Within the same cohort, a clear relationship between burnout, depression prevalence, working hours and nights on call per week was confirmed [192]. The prevalence of burnout ranged from 30% for surgeons working <60 hours/week to 50% for those working >80 hours/week. Importantly, those who worked >80 hours/week reported a significantly higher rates of medical errors compared with those who worked <60 hours/week (10.7% vs. 6.9). Additionally, depression, burnout, and work-home conflicts could be gradually predicted by hours and nights spent on call [192]. Gynecologists, especially those in low or medium-volume hospitals, often have to combine their surgical activity with obstetrical tasks and on-call duties, resulting in chronic sleep deprivation. As known from other high-risk industries "even minimal sleep disruption affect cognitive functioning (e.g., processing speed, visual-motor coordination, and reaction time), increasing the likelihood of poor work performance or injury" [193]. Forced wakefulness and mental fatigue increase attentional failure, risk taking, and decision-making bias [194]. Surgical performance, alertness, concentration, eye-hand coordination, mood, and self-assessed ability to perform measured in postcall surgeons are at comparable or worse levels as after ethanol intake resulting in its blood concentration of 0.6 g/L [195]. Moreover, gynecologic surgeons with a blood alcohol concentration 0.8 g/L perform basic and medium laparoscopic tasks faster and with a similar error rate as after acute sleep deprivation [196]. The immediate effects of acute sleep deprivation can be transient mitigated by cognitive mechanisms, experience, fatigue management [197], caffeine and taurine intake [198] and the fact that the postcall fatigue is greatest not directly on the "day after," but on the second postcall day [199]. However, if becoming chronic, surgeon's sleep deprivation arises to one of the factors most significantly influencing his performance. A most recent systematic review (as of 2020) addressing sleep deprivation and technical skills confirmed that sleepy surgeons have—depending on assessment instrument—12%–32% more reduced skill proficiency [197].

Unfortunately, the paramount role of psychological factors in complication prevention is faced with the fact that "hospitals become severely dysfunctional, which leads to an unhealthy culture, and this can exacerbate a surgeons' sense of mental fatigue" [200]. Workplace culture accepting duty hours devastating surgeon's health and impairing patient safety, violation of working hour laws and ignorance of human physiology are dangerous relicts, which should be eliminated from healthcare institutions.

## Adverse effects of laparoscopy on the surgeon

The numerous advantages of laparoscopy to the patient are paralleled by its sometimes devastating effects to the surgeon. Laparoscopy has been identified as "the most offensive procedure to the surgeon" performed in a "hostile ergonomic environment" [201]. Fixed trocar positions, repetitive motions, two-dimensional images while working in a three-dimensional space, continuous gaze fixation on the monitor and compromised tactile information are causes for a surgeon's fixed head and neck position, shoulder strain, prolonged wrist supination, performing precise manual maneuvers while standing on one leg and activating foot switches with the other, etc. [201, 202]. These challenges result in physical and mental strain, pain, numbness, and fatigue which are significantly higher in laparoscopic as in open surgery.

Minimally invasive surgeons experience significantly more often fatigue (OR 8.1), numbness (OR 6.8), pain in the neck (OR 2.77), arm or shoulder (OR 4.59), hands (OR 2.99), and legs (OR 12.34) compared with surgeons performing open surgery [203].

Studies focusing on gynecological laparoscopists revealed that the vast majority of them (88%) experienced pain and physical discomfort related to performing minimally invasive procedures. Body areas most affected were lower back (75.6%), neck (72.9%), shoulder (66.6%), upper back (61.6%), and wrist/hand (60.9%). Increased pain symptoms were associated with surgeon's female gender, age, height, and glove size, as well as patient's body mass index [202, 204]. Work-related risk factors were: >25 h spent on surgeries per week, working in standing position >4 h per day, surgeries lasting >3 h, long surgical experience (>10 years) and experiencing work-family conflict [205]. Although every second of them reported persistent pain, only 29% sought treatment and 16% had received ergonomic training [202, 204]. To decrease pain, surgeons changed positions (78%), limited the number of cases per day (14%), or total number of cases (3%), or spread cases throughout the week (6%) [204]. The chronic biomechanical and mental strains associated with performing laparoscopy make interventions improving surgical ergonomics (surgeon's posture, positioning of instruments), implementing of short breaks into surgical flow, as well changes in the medico-institutional culture indispensable.

## References

1. Chen R, Su Z, Yang L, Xin L, Yuan X, Wang Y. The effects and costs of laparoscopic versus abdominal myomectomy in patients with uterine fibroids: a systematic review and meta-analysis. BMC Surg. 2020;20:55. doi: 10.1186/s12893-020-00703-0.
2. Baggish MS. Major laparoscopic complications: a review in two parts. J Gynecol Surg. 2012; 28:315–332. doi: 10.1089/gyn.2012.0088.
3. Pulcinelli FM, Schimberni M, Marci R, Bellati F, Caserta D. Laparoscopic versus laparotomic surgery for adnexal masses: role in elderly. World J Surg Oncol. 2016;14:105. doi: 10.1186/s12957-016-0861-1.
4. Capozzi VA, Sozzi G, Gambino G, et al. Laparoscopy versus laparotomy for surgical treatment of obese women with endometrial cancer: a cost-benefit comparative analysis. Mol Clin Oncol. 2019;11:335–342. doi: 10.3892/mco.2019.1901.
5. Magrina JF. Complications of laparoscopic surgery. Clin Obstet Gynecol. 2002;45:469–480. doi: 10.1097/00003081-200206000-00018.
6. Fuentes MN, Rodríguez-Oliver A, Naveiro Rilo JC, Paredes AG, Aguilar Romero MT, Parra JF. Complications of laparoscopic gynecologic surgery. JSLS. 2014;18:e2014.00058. doi: 10.4293/JSLS.2014.00058.
7. Chapron C, Fauconnier A, Goffinet F, Bréart G, Dubuisson JB. Laparoscopic surgery is not inherently dangerous for patients presenting with benign gynaecologic pathology. Results of a meta-analysis. Hum Reprod. 2002;17:1334–1342.
8. Ates S, Tulandi T. Malpractice claims and avoidance of complications in endoscopic surgery. Best Pract Res Clin Obstet Gynaecol. 2013;27:349–361. doi: 10.1016/j.bpobgyn.2012.12.007.
9. Molloy D, Kaloo PD, Cooper M, Nguyen TV. Laparoscopic entry: a literature review and analysis of techniques and complications of primary port entry. Aust N Z J Obstet Gynaecol. 2002;42:246–254. doi: 10.1111/j.0004-8666.2002.00246.x.
10. Champault G, Cazacu F, Taffinder N. Serious trocar accidents in laparoscopic surgery: a French survey of 103,852 operations. Surg Laparosc Endosc. 1996;6:367–370.
11. Vilos GA. Litigation of laparoscopic major vessel injuries in Canada. J Am Assoc Gynecol Laparosc. 2000;7:503–509.
12. Sandadi S, Johannigman JA, Wong VL, Blebea J, Altose MD, Hurd WW. Recognition and management of major vessel injury during laparoscopy. J Minim Invasive Gynecol. 2010;17:692–702. doi: 10.1016/j.jmig.2010.06.005.
13. Baggish MS. Analysis of 31 cases of major vessel injury associated with gynecologic laparoscopy operations. J Gynecol Surg. 2003; 19:63–73. doi: 10.1089/104240603322145201.
14. Baggish MS. Sixty-four cases of major vessel injury associated with laparoscopic surgery. J Gynecol Surg. 2016; 32:73–78. 10.1089/gyn.2015.29001.bag
15. Llarena NC, Shah AB, Milad MP. Bowel injury in gynecologic laparoscopy: a systematic review. Obstet Gynecol. 2015;125:1407–1417. doi: 10.1097/AOG.0000000000000855.
16. Adelman MR, Bardsley TR, Sharp HT. Urinary tract injuries in laparoscopic hysterectomy: a systematic review. J Minim Invasive Gynecol 2014;21:558–566. doi: 10.1016/j.jmig.2014.01.006.
17. Behbehani S, Suarez-Salvador E, Buras M, Magtibay P, Magrina J. Mortality rates in benign laparoscopic and robotic gynecologic surgery: a systematic review and meta-analysis. J Minim Invasive Gynecol. 2020;27:603–612.e1. doi: 10.1016/j.jmig.2019.10.005.
18. Peterson HB, Greenspan JR, Ory HW. Death following puncture of the aorta during laparoscopic sterilization. Obstet Gynecol. 1982;59:133–134.
19. Gawande AA, Thomas EJ, Zinner MJ, Brennan TA. The incidence and nature of surgical adverse events in Colorado and Utah in 1992. Surgery 1999;126:66–75.
20. Wu AW. Medical error: the second victim. The doctor who makes the mistake needs help too. BMJ. 2000;320:726–727. doi: 10.1136/bmj.320.7237.726.
21. Jena AB, Seabury S, Lakdawalla D, Chandra A. Malpractice risk according to physician specialty. N Engl J Med. 2011;365:629–636. doi: 10.1056/NEJMsa1012370.
22. Glaser LM, Alvi FA, Milad MP. Trends in malpractice claims for obstetric and gynecologic procedures, 2005 through 2014. Am J Obstet Gynecol. 2017;217:340.e1–340.e6. doi: 10.1016/j.ajog.2017.05.037.
23. Sandberg EM, Bordewijk EM, Klemann D, Driessen SRC, Twijnstra ARH, Jansen FW. Medical malpractice claims in laparoscopic gynecologic surgery: a Dutch overview of 20 years. Surg Endosc. 2017;31:5418–5426. doi: 10.1007/s00464-017-5624-8.
24. Vilos GA, Ternamian A, Vilos AG, Abu-Rafea B, Zhu C. Direct laparoscopic trocar insertion: lessons learned from nine litigated cases. J Minim Invasive Gynecol. 2017;24:960–970. doi: 10.1016/j.jmig.2017.05.014.
25. Chapron C, Pierre F, Harchaoui Y, et al. Gastrointestinal injuries during gynaecological laparoscopy. Hum Reprod. 1999;14:333–337. doi: 10.1093/humrep/14.2.333. PMID: 10099974.
26. Baggish MS. One hundred and thirty small-and-large-bowel injuries associated with gynecologic laparoscopic operations. J Gynecol Surg 2007;23:83–95. doi: 10.1089/gyn.2007.B-02287.
27. Clavien PA, Sanabria JR, Strasberg SM. Proposed classification of complications of surgery with examples of utility in cholecystectomy. Surgery. 1992;111:518–526.
28. Dindo D, Demartines N, Clavien PA. Classification of surgical complications: a new proposal with evaluation in a cohort of 6336 patients and results of a survey. Ann Surg. 2004;240:205–213. doi: 10.1097/01.sla.0000133083.54934.ae.
29. Sokol DK, Wilson J. What is a surgical complication? World J Surg. 2008;32:942–944. doi: 10.1007/s00268-008-9471-6.
30. Biyani CS, Pecanka J, Rouprêt M, Jensen JB, Mitropoulos D. Intraoperative Adverse Incident Classification (EAUiaiC) by the European Association of Urology ad hoc Complications Guidelines Panel. Eur Urol. 2020;77:601–610. doi: 10.1016/j.eururo.2019.11.015.
31. Strasberg SM, Linehan DC, Hawkins WG. The accordion severity grading system of surgical complications. Ann Surg. 2009;250:177–186. doi: 10.1097/SLA.0b013e3181afde41.
32. Chapron C, Querleu D, Bruhat MA, et al. Surgical complications of diagnostic and operative gynaecological laparoscopy: a series of 29,966 cases. Hum Reprod. 1998;13:867–872. doi:10.1093/humrep/13.4.867.
33. Radosa MP, Meyberg-Solomayer G, Radosa J, et al. Standardised registration of surgical complications in laparoscopic-gynaecological therapeutic procedures using the Clavien-Dindo classification. Geburtshilfe Frauenheilkd. 2014;74:752–758. doi: 10.1055/s-0034-1382925.
34. Arbeitsgemeinschaft Gynäkologische Endoskopie. MIC-Qualifikation: erforderliche Fallzahlen/Eingriffstypen. https://www.ag-endoskopie.de/sites/age/files/media/fallzahlen_und_eingriffstypen_1-2019_0.pdf. Accessed 21 April 2020.
35. Bolliger M, Kroehnert JA, Molineus F, Kandioler D, Schindl M, Riss P. Experiences with the standardized classification of surgical complications (Clavien-Dindo) in general surgery patients. Eur Surg. 2018;50:256–261. doi: 10.1007/s10353-018-0551-z.
36. Szabó I, László A. Veres needle: in memoriam of the 100th birthday anniversary of Dr János Veres, the inventor. Am J Obstet Gynecol. 2004;191:352–353. doi: 10.1016/j.ajog.2004.01.030.
37. Yoong W, Saxena S, Mittal M, Stavroulis A, Ogbodo E, Damodaram M. The pressure profile test is more sensitive and specific than Palmer's test in predicting correct placement of the Veress needle. Eur J Obstet Gynecol Reprod Biol. 2010;152:210–213. doi: 10.1016/j.ejogrb.2010.06.007.

38. Teoh B, Sen R, Abbott J. An evaluation of four tests used to ascertain Veres needle placement at closed laparoscopy. J Minim Invasive Gynecol. 2005;12:153–158. doi: 10.1016/j.jmig.2005.01.011.
39. Azevedo OC, Azevedo JL, Sorbello AA, Miguel GP, Wilson Junior JL, Godoy AC. Evaluation of tests performed to confirm the position of the Veres needle for creation of pneumoperitoneum in selected patients: a prospective clinical trial. Acta Cir Bras 2006;21:385–391. doi: 10.1590/s0102-86502006000600006.
40. Alkatout I. Complications of laparoscopy in connection with entry techniques. J Gynecol Surg. 2017;33:81–91. doi: 10.1089/gyn.2016.0111.
41. Pickett SD, Rodewald KJ, Billow MR, Giannios NM, Hurd WW. Avoiding major vessel injury during laparoscopic instrument insertion. Obstet Gynecol Clin North Am. 2010;37:387–397. doi: 10.1016/j.ogc.2010.05.002.
42. Shields J, Kho K, Majewicz A. Laparoscopic trocar insertion: a comparison of insertional and rotational forces between expert and novice surgeons. J Minim Invasive Gynecol 2018: 25; S75. doi: 10.1016/j.jmig.2018.09.194.
43. Alkatout I, Mettler L, Maass N, Noé GK, Elessawy M. Abdominal anatomy in the context of port placement and trocars. J Turk Ger Gynecol Assoc. 2015;16:241–251. doi: 10.5152/jtgga.2015.0148.
44. Hurd WW, Amesse LS, Gruber JS, Horowitz GM, Cha GM, Hurteau JA. Visualization of the epigastric vessels and bladder before laparoscopic trocar placement. Fertil Steril. 2003;80:209–212.
45. Baggish M. How to avoid major vessel injury during gynecologic laparoscopy. OBG Manag. 2012;24:20–28.
46. Ahmad G, Baker J, Finnerty J, Phillips K, Watson A. Laparoscopic entry techniques. Cochrane Database Syst Rev. 2019;1:CD006583. doi: 10.1002/14651858.CD006583.pub5.
47. Cuss A, Bhatt M, Abbott J. Coming to terms with the fact that the evidence for laparoscopic entry is as good as it gets. J Minim Invasive Gynecol. 2015;22:332–341. doi: 10.1016/j.jmig.2014.10.023.
48. Rohrich RJ, Sorokin ES, Brown SA, Gibby DL. Is the umbilicus truly midline? Clinical and medicolegal implications. Plast Reconstr Surg. 2003;112:259–263. doi: 10.1097/01.PRS.0000066367.41067.C2.
49. Ambardar S, Cabot J, Cekic V, et al. Abdominal wall dimensions and umbilical position vary widely with BMI and should be taken into account when choosing port locations. Surg Endosc. 2009;23:1995–2000. doi: 10.1007/s00464-008-9965-1.
50. Mulayim B, Gurses C, Karadag B, Sozel YK. The relationship between the umbilicus and the aortic bifurcation in Turkish women: implications for laparoscopic entry. Arch Gynecol Obstet. 2017;296:1175–1180. doi: 10.1007/s00404-017-4552-0.
51. Hurd W, Bude RO, DeLancey JO, Gauvin JM, Aisen AM. Abdominal wall characterization with magnetic resonance imaging and computed tomography. The effect of obesity on the laparoscopic approach. J Reprod Med. 1991;36:473–476.
52. Polyzos D, Papadopoulos N, Chapman L, et al. Where is the aorta? Is it worth palpating the aorta prior to laparoscopy? Acta Obstet Gynecol Scand. 2007;86:235–239. doi: 10.1080/00016340601090147.
53. Nezhat F, Brill AI, Nezhat CH, Nezhat A, Seidman DS, Nezhat C. Laparoscopic appraisal of the anatomic relationship of the umbilicus to the aortic bifurcation. J Am Assoc Gynecol Laparosc. 1998;5:135–140. doi: 10.1016/s1074-3804(98)80079-0.
54. Audebert AJ, Gomel V. Role of microlaparoscopy in the diagnosis of peritoneal and visceral adhesions and in the prevention of bowel injury associated with blind trocar insertion. Fertil Steril. 2000;73:631–635. doi: 10.1016/s0015-0282(99)00555-5.
55. Levrant SG, Bieber EJ, Barnes RB. Anterior abdominal wall adhesions after laparotomy or laparoscopy. J Am Assoc Gynecol Laparosc. 1997;4:353–356. doi: 10.1016/s1074-3804(05)80227-0.
56. Nezhat CH, Dun EC, Katz A, Wieser FA. Office visceral slide test compared with two perioperative tests for predicting periumbilical adhesions. Obstet Gynecol. 2014;123:1049–1056. doi: 10.1097/AOG.0000000000000239.
57. Lee M, Kim HS, Chung HH, Kim JW, Park NH, Song YS. Prediction of intra-abdominal adhesions using the visceral slide test: A prospective observational study. Eur J Obstet Gynecol Reprod Biol. 2017;213:22–25. doi: 10.1016/j.ejogrb.2017.04.011.
58. Gerner-Rasmussen J, Donatsky AM, Bjerrum F. The role of non-invasive imaging techniques in detecting intra-abdominal adhesions: a systematic review. Langenbecks Arch Surg. 2019;404:653–661. doi: 10.1007/s00423-018-1732-8.
59. Palmer R. Safety in laparoscopy. J Reprod Med. 1974 Jul;13(1):1–5.
60. Lee CL, Huang KG, Jain S, Wang CJ, Yen CF, Soong YK. A new portal for gynecologic laparoscopy. J Am Assoc Gynecol Laparosc. 2001;8:147–150. doi: 10.1016/s1074-3804(05)60565-8.
61. Jain N, Sareen S, Kanawa S, Jain V, Gupta S, Mann S. Jain point: a new safe portal for laparoscopic entry in previous surgery cases. J Hum Reprod Sci. 2016;9:9–17. doi: 10.4103/0974-1208.178637.
62. Deffieux X, Ballester M, Collinet P, Fauconnier A, Pierre F; French National College of Gynaecologists and Obstetricians. Risks associated with laparoscopic entry: guidelines for clinical practice from the French College of Gynaecologists and Obstetricians. Eur J Obstet Gynecol Reprod Biol. 2011;158:159–166. doi: 10.1016/j.ejogrb.2011.04.047.
63. Aust TR, Kayani SI, Rowlands DJ. Direct optical entry through Palmer's point: a new technique for those at risk of entry-related trauma at laparoscopy. Gynecol Surg. 2010; 7:315–317. doi: 10.1007/s10397-009-0500-8.
64. Watrowski R. Unifying local hemostasis and adhesion prevention during gynaecologic laparoscopies: experiences with a novel, plant-based agent. J Obstet Gynaecol. 2020;40:586–588. doi: 10.1080/01443615.2019.1636779.
65. Vilos GA, Ternamian A, Dempster J, Laberge PY; Laparoscopic entry: a review of techniques, technologies, and complications. J Obstet Gynaecol Can. 2007;29:433–447. doi: 10.1016/S1701-2163(16)35496-2.
66. Pasic R, Levine RL, Wolf WM Jr. Laparoscopy in morbidly obese patients. J Am Assoc Gynecol Laparosc. 1999;6:307–312.
67. Peters A, Rindos NB. Dermatologic manifestations of laparoscopic port site vascular injuries. J Minim Invasive Gynecol. 2019; 26:16–17. doi:10.1016/j.jmig.2018.03.004.
68. Asfour V, Smythe E, Attia R. Vascular injury at laparoscopy: a guide to management. J Obstet Gynaecol. 2018;38:598–606. doi: 10.1080/01443615.2017.1410120.
69. Fuller J, Ashar BS, Carey-Corrado J. Trocar-associated injuries and fatalities: an analysis of 1399 reports to the FDA. J Minim Invasive Gynecol. 2005;12:302–307. doi: 10.1016/j.jmig.2005.05.008.
70. Paśnik B, Modrzejewski A. Major vascular injury during laparoscopy. Pol Przegl Chir. 2018;91:36–40. doi: 10.5604/01.3001.0012.6659.
71. Lam A, Kaufman Y, Khong SY, Liew A, Ford S, Condous G. Dealing with complications in laparoscopy. Best Pract Res Clin Obstet Gynaecol. 2009;23:631–646. doi: 10.1016/j.bpobgyn.2009.03.004.
72. Kyung MS, Choi JS, Lee JH, Jung US, Lee KW. Laparoscopic management of complications in gynecologic laparoscopic surgery: a 5-year experience in a single center. J Minim Invasive Gynecol. 2008;15:689–694. doi: 10.1016/j.jmig.2008.07.006.
73. Chiantera V, Erdemoglu E, Vercellino G, Straube M, Schneider A. Laparoscopic management of external iliac artery injury using yasargil clamps and intracorporeal suture. J Minim Invasive Gynecol. 2011;18:516–519. doi: 10.1016/j.jmig.2011.03.005.
74. Watrowski R, Jäger C, Forster J. Improvement of perioperative outcomes in major gynecological and gynecologic-oncological surgery with hemostatic gelatin-thrombin matrix. In Vivo. 2017;31:251–258. doi: 10.21873/invivo.11053.
75. Lewis KM, Ikeme S, Olubunmi T, Kuntze CE. Clinical effectiveness and versatility of a sealing hemostatic patch (HEMOPATCH) in multiple surgical specialties. Expert Rev Med Devices. 2018;15:367–376. doi:10.1080/17434440.2018.1464909.
76. Kim CS, Kim JY, Kwon JY, et al. Venous air embolism during total laparoscopic hysterectomy: comparison to total abdominal hysterectomy. Anesthesiology. 2009;111:50–54. doi: 10.1097/ALN.0b013e3181a05ac7.
77. van der Voort M, Heijnsdijk EA, Gouma DJ. Bowel injury as a complication of laparoscopy. Br J Surg. 2004;91:1253–1258.
78. Baggish M. How to avoid intestinal and urinary tract injuries during gynecologic laparoscopy. OBG Manag. 2012;24:34–44.

79. Teeluckdharry B, Gilmour D, Flowerdew G. Urinary tract injury at benign gynecologic surgery and the role of cystoscopy: a systematic review and meta-analysis. Obstet Gynecol 2015;126:1161–1169. doi: 10.1097/AOG.0000000000001096.
80. Burks FN, Santucci RA. Management of iatrogenic ureteral injury. Ther Adv Urol. 2014;6:115–124. doi: 10.1177/1756287214526767.
81. Chan JK, Morrow J, Manetta A. Prevention of ureteral injuries in gynecologic surgery. Am J Obstet Gynecol. 2003 May;188:1273–1277.
82. Wong JMK, Bortoletto P, Tolentino J, Jung MJ, Milad MP. Urinary tract injury in gynecologic laparoscopy for benign indication: a systematic review. Obstet Gynecol. 2018;131:100–108. doi: 10.1097/AOG.0000000000002414.
83. Hwang JH, Kim BW. Laparoscopic radical hysterectomy has higher risk of perioperative urologic complication than abdominal radical hysterectomy: a meta-analysis of 38 studies. Surg Endosc. 2020;34:1509–1521. doi: 10.1007/s00464-020-07366-1.
84. Baggish MS. Urinary tract injuries secondary to gynecologic laparoscopic surgery: analysis of seventy-five cases. J Gynecol Surg. 2010;26:79–92. doi: 10.1089/gyn.2010.0019.
85. Tan-Kim J, Menefee SA, Reinsch CS, et al. Laparoscopic hysterectomy and urinary tract injury: experience in a health maintenance organization. J Minim Invasive Gynecol. 2015;22:1278–1286. doi: 10.1016/j.jmig.2015.07.016.
86. Dassel MW, Adelman MR, Sharp HT. Recognition and management of urologic injuries with laparoscopic hysterectomy. Clin Obstet Gynecol. 2015;58:805–811. doi: 10.1097/GRF.0000000000000159.
87. Watrowski R, Babbel B, Fisch D. Renal calyceal rupture following ureteral injury after total laparoscopic hysterectomy. Gynecol Minim Invasive Ther 2020;9(3):166–169. doi: 10.4103/GMIT.GMIT_28_19.
88. Barber EL, Polan RM, Strohl AE, Siedhoff MT, Clarke-Pearson DL. Cystoscopy at the time of hysterectomy for benign indications and delayed lower genitourinary tract injury. Obstet Gynecol. 2019;133:888–895. doi: 10.1097/AOG.0000000000003192.
89. Sharp HT, Adelman MR. Prevention, recognition, and management of urologic injuries during gynecologic surgery. Obstet Gynecol. 2016;127:1085–1096. doi: 10.1097/AOG.0000000000001425.
90. Hurd WW, Chee SS, Gallagher KL, Ohl DA, Hurteau JA. Location of the ureters in relation to the uterine cervix by computed tomography. Am J Obstet Gynecol 2001;184:336–339. doi:10.1067/mob.2001.110296.
91. Odegard SE, Abernethy MG, Mueller ER. Does side make a difference? Anatomical differences between the left and right ureter. Female Pelvic Med Reconstr Surg 2015;21:249–251. doi: 10.1097/SPV.0000000000000185.
92. Mandovra P, Kalikar V, Patankar RV. Real-time visualization of ureters using indocyanine green during laparoscopic surgeries: can we make surgery safer? Surg Innov. 2019;26:464–468. doi: 10.1177/1553350619827152.
93. Chou MT, Wang CJ, Lien RC. Prophylactic ureteral catheterization in gynecologic surgery: a 12-year randomized trial in a community hospital. Int Urogynecol J Pelvic Floor Dysfunct. 2009;20:689–693. doi: 10.1007/s00192-008-0788-3.
94. Dallas KB, Rogo-Gupta L, Elliott CS. Urologic injury and fistula after hysterectomy for benign indications. Obstet Gynecol. 2019;134:241–249. doi: 10.1097/AOG.0000000000003353.
95. Milad MP, Milad EA. Laparoscopic morcellator-related complications. J Minim Invasive Gynecol. 2014;21:486–491. doi: 10.1016/j.jmig.2013.12.003.
96. Abdalmageed OS, Bedaiwy MA, Falcone T. Nerve injuries in gynecologic laparoscopy. J Minim Invasive Gynecol. 2017;24:16–27. doi: 10.1016/j.jmig.2016.09.004.
97. Kuponiyi O, Alleemudder DI, Latunde-Dada A, Eedarapalli P. Nerve injuries associated with gynaecological surgery. Obstetrician Gynaecologist 2014;16:29–36. doi: 10.1111/tog.12064.
98. Bradshaw AD, Advincula AP. Postoperative neuropathy in gynecologic surgery. Obstet Gynecol Clin North Am. 2010;37:451–459. doi: 10.1016/j.ogc.2010.05.008.
99. Arnold A, Abbott J. Complications of laparoscopic surgery. Obstet Gynaecol Reprod Med 2014; 24; 250–253. doi: 10.1016/j.ogrm.2014.05.003.
100. Ha A, Richards C, Criman E, Piaggione J, Yheulon C, Lim R. The safe use of surgical energy devices by surgeons may be overestimated. Surg Endosc. 2018;32:3861–3867. doi: 10.1007/s00464-018-6116-1.
101. Mayooran Z, Pearce S, Tsaltas J, et al. Ignorance of electrosurgery among obstetricians and gynaecologists. BJOG. 2004;111:1413–1418. doi: 10.1111/j.1471-0528.2004.00334.x.
102. Watanabe Y, Kurashima Y, Madani A, et al. Surgeons have knowledge gaps in the safe use of energy devices: a multicenter cross-sectional study. Surg Endosc. 2016;30:588–592. doi: 10.1007/s00464-015-4243-5.
103. Feldman LS, Fuchshuber P, Jones DB, Mischna J, Schwaitzberg SD; FUSE Task Force. Surgeons don't know what they don't know about the safe use of energy in surgery. Surg Endosc. 2012;26:2735–2739. doi: 10.1007/s00464-012-2263-y.
104. Alkatout I, Schollmeyer T, Hawaldar NA, Sharma N, Mettler L. Principles and safety measures of electrosurgery in laparoscopy. JSLS. 2012;16:130–139. doi: 10.4293/108680812X13291597716348.
105. Ferreira H, Ferreira C. Principle and use of electrosurgery in laparoscopy. In: Agarwal M, Mettler L, Alkatout I. A Manual of Minimally Invasive Gynaecology. Jaypee Brothers Medical Publishers Ltd. 2015. pp. 69–77.
106. Vilos GA, Rajakumar C. Electrosurgical generators and monopolar and bipolar electrosurgery. J Minim Invasive Gynecol. 2013;20:279–287. doi: 10.1016/j.jmig.2013.02.013.
107. Massarweh NN, Cosgriff N, Slakey DP. Electrosurgery: history, principles, and current and future uses. J Am Coll Surg. 2006;202(3):520–530. PubMed PMID: 16500257.
108. El-Sayed M, Mohamed S, Saridogan E. Safe use of electrosurgery in gynaecological laparoscopic surgery. Obstetrician Gynaecologist 2020;22:9–20. doi: 10.1111/tog.12620.
109. Jaiswal A, Huang KG. Energy devices in gynecological laparoscopy - Archaic to modern era. Gynecol Minim Invasive Ther. 2017;6:147–151. doi: 10.1016/j.gmit.2017.08.002.
110. Odell RC. Surgical complications specific to monopolar electrosurgical energy: engineering changes that have made electrosurgery safer. J Minim Invasive Gynecol. 2013;20:288–298. doi: 10.1016/j.jmig.2013.01.015.
111. Tulikangas PK, Smith T, Falcone T, Boparai N, Walters MD. Gross and histologic characteristics of laparoscopic injuries with four different energy sources. Fertil Steril. 2001;75:806–810.
112. Choi C, Do IG, Song T. Ultrasonic versus monopolar energy-based surgical devices in terms of surgical smoke and lateral thermal damage (ULMOST): a randomized controlled trial. Surg Endosc. 2018;32:4415–4421. doi: 10.1007/s00464-018-6183-3.
113. Hefermehl LJ, Largo RA, Hermanns T, Poyet C, Sulser T, Eberli D. Lateral temperature spread of monopolar, bipolar and ultrasonic instruments for robot-assisted laparoscopic surgery. BJU Int. 2014;114:245–252. doi: 10.1111/bju.12498.
114. Družijanić N, Pogorelić Z, Perko Z, Mrklić I, Tomić S. Comparison of lateral thermal damage of the human peritoneum using monopolar diathermy, harmonic scalpel and LigaSure. Can J Surg. 2012;55:317–321.
115. Seehofer D, Mogl M, Boas-Knoop S, et al. Safety and efficacy of new integrated bipolar and ultrasonic scissors compared to conventional laparoscopic 5-mm sealing and cutting instruments. Surg Endosc. 2012;26:2541–2549. doi: 10.1007/s00464-012-2229-0.
116. Çaltekin MD, Aydoğmuş S, Yalçin SE, et al. Comparison of three different new bipolar energy modalities and classic bipolar in vivo for tissue thermal spread. Turk Patoloji Derg. 2017;33:144–149. doi: 10.5146/tjpath.2016.01377.
117. Montero PN, Robinson TN, Weaver JS, Stiegmann GV. Insulation failure in laparoscopic instruments. Surg Endosc. 2010;24:462–465. doi:10.1007/s00464-009-0601-5.
118. Driessen SR, Arkenbout EA, Thurkow AL, Jansen FW. Electromechanical morcellators in minimally invasive gynecologic surgery: an update. J Minim Invasive Gynecol. 2014;21:377–383. doi:10.1016/j.jmig.2013.12.121.

119. Brölmann H, Tanos V, Grimbizis G, et al. Options on fibroid morcellation: a literature review. Gynecol Surg. 2015;12:3–15. doi:10.1007/s10397-015-0878-4.
120. Tulandi T, Leung A, Jan N. Nonmalignant sequelae of unconfined morcellation at laparoscopic hysterectomy or myomectomy. J Minim Invasive Gynecol. 2016;23:331–337. doi: 10.1016/j.jmig.2016.01.017.
121. Darii N, Anton E, Doroftei B, et al. Latrogenic parasitic myoma and iatrogenic adenomyoma after laparoscopic morcellation: a mini-review. J Adv Res. 2019;20:1–8. doi: 10.1016/j.jare.2019.04.004.
122. Theben JU, Schellong AR, Altgassen C, Kelling K, Schneider S, Große-Drieling D. Unexpected malignancies after laparoscopic-assisted supracervical hysterectomies (LASH): an analysis of 1,584 LASH cases. Arch Gynecol Obstet. 2013;287:455–462. doi:10.1007/s00404-012-2559-0.
123. Zullo F, Venturella R, Raffone A, Saccone G. In-bag manual versus uncontained power morcellation for laparoscopic myomectomy. Cochrane Database Syst Rev. 2020;5:CD013352. doi: 10.1002/14651858.CD013352.pub2.
124. Xu X, Lin H, Wright JD, et al. Association between power morcellation and mortality in women with unexpected uterine cancer undergoing hysterectomy or myomectomy. J Clin Oncol. 2019;37:3412–3424. doi:10.1200/JCO.19.00562.
125. Bogani G, Cliby WA, Aletti GD. Impact of morcellation on survival outcomes of patients with unexpected uterine leiomyosarcoma: a systematic review and meta-analysis. Gynecol Oncol. 2015;137:167–172. doi:10.1016/j.ygyno.2014.11.011.
126. Raspagliesi F, Maltese G, Bogani G, et al. Morcellation worsens survival outcomes in patients with undiagnosed uterine leiomyosarcomas: A retrospective MITO group study. Gynecol Oncol. 2017;144:90–95. doi: 10.1016/j.ygyno.2016.11.002.
127. Pritts EA, Vanness DJ, Berek JS, et al. The prevalence of occult leiomyosarcoma at surgery for presumed uterine fibroids: a meta-analysis. Gynecol Surg. 2015;12:165–177. doi:10.1007/s10397-015-0894-4.
128. Wright JD, Tergas AI, Cui R, et al. Use of electric power morcellation and prevalence of underlying cancer in women who undergo myomectomy. JAMA Oncol. 2015;1:69–77. doi:10.1001/jamaoncol.2014.206.
129. Goto A, Takeuchi S, Sugimura K, Maruo T. Usefulness of Gd-DTPA contrast-enhanced dynamic MRI and serum determination of LDH and its isozymes in the differential diagnosis of leiomyosarcoma from degenerated leiomyoma of the uterus. Int J Gynecol Cancer. 2002;12:354–361. doi:10.1046/j.1525-1438.2002.01086.x.
130. Bansal N, Herzog TJ, Burke W, Cohen CJ, Wright JD. The utility of preoperative endometrial sampling for the detection of uterine sarcomas. Gynecol Oncol. 2008;110(1):43–48. doi:10.1016/j.ygyno.2008.02.026.
131. Shawki O, Ramadan A, Askalany A, Bahnassi A. Laparoscopic management of ovarian dermoid cysts: potential fear of dermoid spill, myths and facts. Gynecol Surg 2007; 4: 255–260. doi: 10.1007/s10397-007-0295-4.
132. Hizkiyahu R, Yahav L, Yakovi S, Davidesko S, Abecassis A, Weintraub AY. Short- and long-term outcomes of intraoperative spillage during laparoscopic removal of benign ovarian cysts. Surg Endosc. 2019;34(9):3883–3887. doi: 10.1007/s00464-019-07154-6.
133. Panici PB, Palaia I, Bellati F, Pernice M, Angioli R, Muzii L. Laparoscopy compared with laparoscopically guided minilaparotomy for large adnexal masses: a randomized controlled trial. Obstet Gynecol. 2007;110(2 Pt 1):241–248. doi: 10.1097/01.AOG.0000275265.99653.64.
134. Bewö K, Österberg J, Löfgren M, Sandblom G. Incisional hernias following open gynecological surgery: a population-based study. Arch Gynecol Obstet. 2019;299:1313–1319. doi: 10.1007/s00404-019-05069-0.
135. Schiavone MB, Bielen MS, Gardner GJ, et al. Herniation formation in women undergoing robotically assisted laparoscopy or laparotomy for endometrial cancer. Gynecol Oncol. 2016;140:383–386. doi: 10.1016/j.ygyno.2016.01.010.
136. Montz FJ, Holschneider CH, Munro MG. Incisional hernia following laparoscopy: a survey of the American Association of Gynecologic Laparoscopists. Obstet Gynecol. 1994;84:881–884.
137. Wells A, Germanos GJ, Salemi JL, Mikhail E. Laparoscopic surgeons' perspectives on risk factors for and prophylaxis of trocar site hernias: a multispecialty national survey. JSLS. 2019;23:e2019.00013. doi: 10.4293/JSLS.2019.00013.
138. Pereira N, Hutchinson AP, Irani M, et al. 5-millimeter trocar-site hernias after laparoscopy requiring surgical repair. J Minim Invasive Gynecol. 2016;23:505–511. doi: 10.1016/j.jmig.2016.03.001.
139. Swank HA, Mulder IM, la Chapelle CF, Reitsma JB, Lange JF, Bemelman WA. Systematic review of trocar-site hernia. Br J Surg. 2012;99:315–323. doi: 10.1002/bjs.7836.
140. Zivanovic O, Sonoda Y, Diaz JP, et al. The rate of port-site metastases after 2251 laparoscopic procedures in women with underlying malignant disease. Gynecol Oncol. 2008;111:431–437. doi: 10.1016/j.ygyno.2008.08.024.
141. Ramirez PT, Wolf JK, Levenback C. Laparoscopic port-site metastases: etiology and prevention. Gynecol Oncol. 2003;91:179–189. doi: 10.1016/s0090-8258(03)00507-9.
142. Ota T, Huang KG, Sicam RV, Ueng SH, Lee CL. Unusual trocar site metastasis in a uterine leiomyosarcoma after laparoscopic hysterectomy. J Minim Invasive Gynecol. 2012;19:252–254. doi: 10.1016/j.jmig.2011.10.012.
143. Shin YJ, Lee HJ, Kim KR, Nam JH, Park JY. Port-site recurrence 6 years after laparoscopic surgery for early stage ovarian borderline malignancy. J Obstet Gynaecol. 2018;38(2):291–292. doi: 10.1080/01443615.2017.1340437.
144. Ramirez PT, Frumovitz M, Wolf JK, Levenback C. Laparoscopic port-site metastases in patients with gynecological malignancies. Int J Gynecol Cancer. 2004;14:1070–1077. doi: 10.1111/j.1048-891X.2004.14604.x.
145. Ataseven B, du Bois A, Harter P, et al. Impact of abdominal wall metastases on prognosis in epithelial ovarian cancer. Int J Gynecol Cancer. 2016;26:1594–1600. doi: 10.1097/IGC.0000000000000826.
146. van Dam PA, DeCloedt J, Tjalma WA, Buytaert P, Becquart D, Vergote IB. Trocar implantation metastasis after laparoscopy in patients with advanced ovarian cancer: can the risk be reduced? Am J Obstet Gynecol. 1999;181:536–541. doi: 10.1016/s0002-9378(99)70489-8.
147. Schneider C, Jung A, Reymond MA, et al. Efficacy of surgical measures in preventing port-site recurrences in a porcine model. Surg Endosc. 2001;15:121–125. doi: 10.1007/s004640010069.
148. Hur HC, Guido RS, Mansuria SM, Hacker MR, Sanfilippo JS, Lee TT. Incidence and patient characteristics of vaginal cuff dehiscence after different modes of hysterectomies. J Minim Invasive Gynecol. 2007;14:311–317.
149. Ceccaroni M, Berretta R, Malzoni M, et al. Vaginal cuff dehiscence after hysterectomy: a multicenter retrospective study. Eur J Obstet Gynecol Reprod Biol. 2011;158:308–313. doi: 10.1016/j.ejogrb.2011.05.013.
150. Hur HC, Donnellan N, Mansuria S, Barber RE, Guido R, Lee T. Vaginal cuff dehiscence after different modes of hysterectomy. Obstet Gynecol. 2011;118:794–801. doi: 10.1097/AOG.0b013e31822f1c92.
151. Ala-Nissilä S, Laurikainen E, Mäkinen J, Jokimaa V. Vaginal cuff dehiscence is observed in a higher rate after total laparoscopic hysterectomy compared with other types of hysterectomy. Acta Obstet Gynecol Scand. 2019;98(1):44–50. doi: 10.1111/aogs.13459.
152. Uccella S, Malzoni M, Cromi A, et al. Laparoscopic vs. transvaginal cuff closure after total laparoscopic hysterectomy: a randomized trial by the Italian Society of Gynecologic Endoscopy. Am J Obstet Gynecol. 2018;218:500.e1–500.e13. doi: 10.1016/j.ajog.2018.01.029.
153. Fuchs Weizman N, Einarsson JI, Wang KC, Vitonis AF, Cohen SL. Vaginal cuff dehiscence: risk factors and associated morbidities. JSLS. 2015;19:e2013.00351. doi:10.4293/JSLS.2013.00351.
154. Boersen Z, Aalders CIM, Klinkert ER, Maas JWM, Nap AW. Vaginal cuff dehiscence after endometriosis surgery. JSLS. 2019;23. pii: e2019.00018. doi: 10.4293/JSLS.2019.00018.

155. Kim JH, Byun SW, Song JY, Kim YH, Lee HJ, Park TC, Lee KH, Hur SY, Park JS, Lee SJ. Barbed versus conventional 2-layer continuous running sutures for laparoscopic vaginal cuff closure. Medicine (Baltimore). 2016;95(39):e4981. doi: 10.1097/MD.0000000000004981.
156. Yildirim D, Ozyurek SE, Kiyak H, et al. Single-layer versus double-layer closure of the vaginal cuff with barbed sutures in laparoscopic hysterectomy. Ginekol Pol. 2018;89:229–234. doi: 10.5603/GP.a2018.0040. PubMed PMID: 30084473.
157. Medina LG, Martin O, Cacciamani GE, Ahmadi N, Castro JC, Sotelo R. Needle lost in minimally invasive surgery: management proposal and literature review. J Robot Surg. 2018;12(3):391–395. doi: 10.1007/s11701-018-0802-9.
158. Barto W, Yazbek C, Bell S. Finding a lost needle in laparoscopic surgery. Surg Laparosc Endosc Percutan Tech. 2011;21(4):e163–e165. doi: 10.1097/SLE.0b013e3182203b49.
159. Lieng M, Istre O, Busund B, Qvigstad E. Severe complications caused by retained tissue in laparoscopic supracervical hysterectomy. J Minim Invasive Gynecol. 2006;13(3):231–233. doi: 10.1016/j.jmig.2006.01.006.
160. Smith CD. The retained surgical specimen, an unappreciated retained foreign object. J Laparoendosc Adv Surg Tech A. 2011;21(8):737–739. doi: 10.1089/lap.2011.0368.
161. Ott DE. Subcutaneous emphysema–beyond the pneumoperitoneum. JSLS. 2014;18:1–7. doi: 10.4293/108680813X13693422520882. PMID: 24680136.
162. McAllister JD, D'Altorio RA, Snyder A. CT findings after uncomplicated percutaneous laparoscopic cholecystectomy. J Comput Assist Tomogr. 1991;15:770–772.
163. Murdock CM, Wolff AJ, Van Geem T. Risk factors for hypercarbia, subcutaneous emphysema, pneumothorax, and pneumomediastinum during laparoscopy. Obstet Gynecol. 2000;95(5):704–709. doi: 10.1016/s0029-7844(00)00781-x.
164. Asano R, Suzuki Y, Saito S, Kamiya N, Aoki M, Miyagi E. Massive subcutaneous emphysema extending to the face during total laparoscopic hysterectomy. J Minim Invasive Gynecol. 2019;26:589–590. doi: 10.1016/j.jmig.2018.09.004.
165. Lee DH, Song T, Kim KH, Lee KW. Incidence, natural course, and characteristics of postlaparoscopic shoulder pain. Surg Endosc. 2018;32:160–165. doi: 10.1007/s00464-017-5651-5.
166. Struller F, Weinreich FJ, Horvath P, et al. Peritoneal innervation: embryology and functional anatomy. Pleura Peritoneum. 2017;2(4):153–161. doi: 10.1515/pp-2017-0024.
167. Phelps P, Cakmakkaya OS, Apfel CC, Radke OC. A simple clinical maneuver to reduce laparoscopy-induced shoulder pain: a randomized controlled trial. Obstet Gynecol. 2008;111(5):1155–1160. doi:10.1097/AOG.0b013e31816e34b4.
168. Pergialiotis V, Vlachos DE, Kontzoglou K, Perrea D, Vlachos GD. Pulmonary recruitment maneuver to reduce pain after laparoscopy: a meta-analysis of randomized controlled trials. Surg Endosc. 2015;29(8):2101–2108. doi:10.1007/s00464-014-3934-7.
169. Lee J, Park C, Kim J, Ki Y, Cha SH, Kim JY. Effect of low-pressure pulmonary recruitment maneuver on postlaparoscopic shoulder pain: randomized controlled trial. J Minim Invasive Gynecol. 2020;27:173–177. doi: 10.1016/j.jmig.2019.03.020.
170. Tsai HW, Wang PH, Yen MS, Chao KC, Hsu TF, Chen YJ. Prevention of postlaparoscopic shoulder and upper abdominal pain: a randomized controlled trial. Obstet Gynecol. 2013;121:526–531. doi: 10.1097/AOG.0b013e318283fcca.
171. Ryu KH, Lee SH, Cho EA, Kim JA, Lim GE, Song T. Comparison of impacts of intraperitoneal saline instillation with and without pulmonary recruitment maneuver on post-laparoscopic shoulder pain prevention: a randomized controlled trial. Surg Endosc. 2019;33:870–878. doi: 10.1007/s00464-018-6354-2.
172. Mostafa RH, Mekki YM. Comparative evaluation of intraperitoneal bupivacaine and bupivacaine ketamine combined with lung recruitment for reducing postoperative shoulder pain in laparoscopic cholecystectomy. Egypt J Anaesth 2018;34:159–164. doi: 10.1016/j.egja.2018.10.001.
173. Moon S, Lim SH, Cho K, Kim M-H, Lee W, Cho YH. The efficacy of vitamin C on postlaparoscopic shoulder pain: a double-blind randomized controlled trial. Anesth Pain Med 2019;14:202–207. doi: 10.17085/apm.2019.14.2.202.
174. Özdemir-van Brunschot DM, van Laarhoven KC, Scheffer GJ, Pouwels S, Wever KE, Warlé MC. What is the evidence for the use of low-pressure pneumoperitoneum? A systematic review. Surg Endosc. 2016;30(5):2049–2065. doi: 10.1007/s00464-015-4454-9.
175. Topçu HO, Cavkaytar S, Kokanalı K, Guzel AI, Islimye M, Doganay M. A prospective randomized trial of postoperative pain following different insufflation pressures during gynecologic laparoscopy. Eur J Obstet Gynecol Reprod Biol. 2014;182:81–85. doi: 10.1016/j.ejogrb.2014.09.003.
176. Craciunas L, Stirbu L, Tsampras N. The use of a peritoneal gas drain following gynecological laparoscopy: a systematic review. Eur J Obstet Gynecol Reprod Biol. 2014;179:224–228. doi: 10.1016/j.ejogrb.2014.04.012.
177. Donatsky AM, Bjerrum F, Gögenur I. Surgical techniques to minimize shoulder pain after laparoscopic cholecystectomy. A systematic review. Surg Endosc. 2013;27:2275–2282. doi:10.1007/s00464-012-2759-5.
178. Wehkamp KH, Naegler H. The commercialization of patient-related decision making in hospitals. Dtsch Arztebl Int. 2017;114:797–804. doi:10.3238/arztebl.2017.0797.
179. Sawicki PT. [Quality of healthcare in Germany. A six-country comparison]. Med Klin (Munich). 2005;100:755–768. doi:10.1007/s00063-005-1105-2.
180. Fourquet J, Zavala DE, Missmer S, Bracero N, Romaguera J, Flores I. Disparities in healthcare services in women with endometriosis with public vs private health insurance. Am J Obstet Gynecol. 2019;221(6):623.e1–623.e11. doi: 10.1016/j.ajog.2019.06.020.
181. Broder MS, Kanouse DE, Mittman BS, Bernstein SJ. The appropriateness of recommendations for hysterectomy. Obstet Gynecol. 2000;95(2):199–205. doi:10.1016/s0029-7844(99)00519-0.
182. Corona LE, Swenson CW, Sheetz KH, et al. Use of other treatments before hysterectomy for benign conditions in a statewide hospital collaborative. Am J Obstet Gynecol. 2015;212:304.e1–7. doi: 10.1016/j.ajog.2014.11.031.
183. Parazzini F, Frattaruolo MP, Chiaffarino F, Dridi D, Roncella E, Vercellini P. The limited oncogenic potential of unilocular adnexal cysts: A systematic review and meta-analysis. Eur J Obstet Gynecol Reprod Biol. 2018;225:101–109. doi:10.1016/j.ejogrb.2018.04.019.
184. Wallenstein MR, Ananth CV, Kim JH, et al. Effect of surgical volume on outcomes for laparoscopic hysterectomy for benign indications. Obstet Gynecol. 2012;119(4):709–716. doi:10.1097/AOG.0b013e318248f7a8.
185. Mehta A, Xu T, Hutfless S, et al. Patient, surgeon, and hospital disparities associated with benign hysterectomy approach and perioperative complications. Am J Obstet Gynecol. 2017;216:497.e1–497.e10. doi: 10.1016/j.ajog.2016.12.020.
186. Mowat A, Maher C, Ballard E. Surgical outcomes for low-volume vs high-volume surgeons in gynecology surgery: a systematic review and meta-analysis. Am J Obstet Gynecol. 2016;215:21–33. doi:10.1016/j.ajog.2016.02.048.
187. Kengen B, IJgosse WM, van Goor H, Luursema JM. Fast or safe? The role of impulsiveness in laparoscopic simulator performance. Am J Surg. 2020;S0002-9610(20)30137–30139. doi:10.1016/j.amjsurg.2020.02.056.
188. Lovejoy C, Nashef SA. Surgeons' personalities and surgical outcomes. The Bull Royal College Surg Eng. 2018;100:259–263. doi: 10.1308/rcsbull.2018.259.
189. Kadzielski J, McCormick F, Herndon JH, Rubash H, Ring D. Surgeons' attitudes are associated with reoperation and readmission rates. Clin Orthop Relat Res. 2015;473:1544–1551. doi:10.1007/s11999-014-3687-6.
190. Bauer J, Groneberg DA. [Working conditions of physicians in hospitals–A comparison of specialties in German hospitals (iCept-Study)]. Dtsch Med Wochenschr. 2015;140:e150–e158. doi:10.1055/s-0041-103165.

191. Shanafelt TD, Balch CM, Bechamps G, et al. Burnout and medical errors among American surgeons. Ann Surg. 2010;251:995–1000. doi: 10.1097/SLA.0b013e3181bfdab3.
192. Balch CM, Shanafelt TD, Dyrbye L, et al. Surgeon distress as calibrated by hours worked and nights on call. J Am Coll Surg. 2010;211(5):609–619. doi: 10.1016/j.jamcollsurg.2010.06.393.
193. Stout JW, Beidel DC, Brush D, Bowers C. Sleep disturbance and cognitive functioning among firefighters. J Health Psychol. 2020:1359105320909861. doi: 10.1177/1359105320909861.
194. Sugden C, Athanasiou T, Darzi A. What are the effects of sleep deprivation and fatigue in surgical practice? Semin Thorac Cardiovasc Surg. 2012 Autumn;24(3):166–175. doi: 10.1053/j.semtcvs.2012.06.005.
195. Huizinga CRH, de Kam ML, Stockmann HBAC, van Gerven JMA, Cohen AF, van der Bogt KEA. Evaluating fitness to perform in surgical residents after night shifts and alcohol intoxication: the development of a "Fit-to-Perform" test. J Surg Educ. 2018;75:968–977. doi: 10.1016/j.jsurg.2018.01.010.
196. Mohtashami F, Thiele A, Karreman E, Thiel J. Comparing technical dexterity of sleep-deprived versus intoxicated surgeons. JSLS. 2014;18(4):e2014.00142. doi:10.4293/JSLS.2014.00142.
197. Whelehan DF, McCarrick CA, Ridgway PF. A systematic review of sleep deprivation and technical skill in surgery. Surgeon. 2020;18(6):375–384. doi:10.1016/j.surge.2020.01.004.
198. Aggarwal R, Mishra A, Crochet P, Sirimanna P, Darzi A. Effect of caffeine and taurine on simulated laparoscopy performed following sleep deprivation. Br J Surg. 2011;98:1666–1672. doi:10.1002/bjs.7600.
199. Coleman JJ, Robinson CK, Zarzaur BL, Timsina L, Rozycki GS, Feliciano DV. To sleep, perchance to dream: acute and chronic sleep deprivation in acute care surgeons. J Am Coll Surg. 2019;229:166–174. doi: 10.1016/j.jamcollsurg.2019.03.019.
200. Campbell DA Jr. Physician wellness and patient safety. Ann Surg. 2010;251(6):1001–1002. doi: 10.1097/SLA.0b013e3181e06fea.
201. Gofrit ON, Mikahail AA, Zorn KC, Zagaja GP, Steinberg GD, Shalhav AL. Surgeons' perceptions and injuries during and after urologic laparoscopic surgery. Urology. 2008;71:404–407. doi: 10.1016/j.urology.2007.07.077.
202. Adams SR, Hacker MR, McKinney JL, Elkadry EA, Rosenblatt PL. Musculoskeletal pain in gynecologic surgeons. J Minim Invasive Gynecol. 2013;20:656–660. doi: 10.1016/j.jmig.2013.04.013.
203. Stucky CH, Cromwell KD, Voss RK, et al. Surgeon symptoms, strain, and selections: systematic review and meta-analysis of surgical ergonomics. Ann Med Surg (Lond). 2018;27:1–8. doi:10.1016/j.amsu.2017.12.013.
204. Franasiak J, Ko EM, Kidd J, et al. Physical strain and urgent need for ergonomic training among gynecologic oncologists who perform minimally invasive surgery. Gynecol Oncol. 2012;126:437–442. doi: 10.1016/j.ygyno.2012.05.016.
205. Dianat I, Bazazan A, Souraki Azad MA, Salimi SS. Work-related physical, psychosocial and individual factors associated with musculoskeletal symptoms among surgeons: implications for ergonomic interventions. Appl Ergon. 2018;67:115–124. doi:10.1016/j.apergo.2017.09.011.

# 5

# OVARIAN ENDOMETRIOMA SURGERY

**Liselotte Mettler, Ibrahim Alkatout, and Ivo Meinhold-Heerlein**

## Introduction

The ovarian localization of endometriosis is most frequently called endometrioma. Endometriomas are found in 17%–44% of endometriosis patients [1]. They can grow up to 15 cm in size; up to 50% of ovarian endometrioses appear bilaterally [2].

While endometriosis patients can also suffer from simple or functional cysts filled with hematoma, endometriosis cysts are characterized, and classified, by a distinct histopathological pattern. This includes a broad range of stroma, endometrioid cells, and collagenous fibers. The diagnosis requires the detection of pigment macrophages, so-called pseudoxanthoma cells retaining lipofuscin and haemofuscin. The inner side presents a cubic or cylindric epithelial layer; older cysts often show collagenous fibers only. Like the endometrial tissue, the cyst epithelial layers can show metaplastic changes [2]. In fact, the new "WHO classification of ovarian, fallopian tube, and primary peritoneal cancer" distinguishes between endometriosis cyst, endometrioid cystadenoma, and endometrioid cystadenofibroma and puts endometriomas in a context with some type of ovarian cancer [3, 4]. This connection is based on the fact that ovarian cancer, especially endometrioid and clear cell ovarian cancer, can be associated with so-called atypical ovarian endometriosis characterized by specific mutations (e.g., ARID 1a mutations) which can be found in both ovarian endometriosis and ovarian cancer of the same patient [2]. Altogether, endometriosis patients have a 50% greater risk of developing ovarian cancer [5].

Apart from the latter findings, the origin and pathogenesis of endometriomas remains mainly unclear. As far as we know there are three theories. Hughesdon suggested that an invagination of the ovarian cortex results in a pseudocyst collecting menstrual debris from endometrial implants [6]. Brosens and co-authors shared the theory of invagination but assumed that active implants have to be located at the site of invagination [7]. Donnez and co-authors suggested that the coelomic epithelial layer of the ovarian surface undergoes a metaplasia [8, 9]. Finally, Nezhat and co-authors assumed that endometrial implants within functional ovarian cysts may form endometriomas [10].

Since endometriomas barely respond to systemic treatment, surgical excision is still the most frequent way of treating them. The indications for treatment may include symptoms (mostly pain), infertility, sonographic suspicion of malignancy or a premalignant lesion such as a borderline tumor. If continued study confirms an association between atypical endometriosis and ovarian cancer, it may lead to the conclusion that removal is indicated for oncological reasons (reviewed in Refs. [2, 11]).

## Indications for surgery

Surgical removal of endometriomas – in case of symptoms or in case of infertility – is one of the standard procedures for the treatment of ovarian endometriosis recommended in national and international guidelines such as Dunselman et al. [12]. The most frequent indications for surgery are cyst-related symptoms, mainly pain. Despite a lack of profound data from prospective randomized trials, there is clear evidence that surgical removal or even ablation of an endometriosis cyst leads to pain reduction [13, 14]. In addition, it has been shown that complete removal of endometriosis, including the ovarian endometriosis, can lead to an increase in the fertility rate within a period of up to 12 months after surgery. By contrast a recent Cochrane analysis comparing aspiration, cyst enucleation, and expectant management did not show a significant difference in the pregnancy rate when these different procedures were followed by artificial reproductive technology (ART) [15].

Although the sensitivity and specificity of (transvaginal) ultrasound or tumor markers analysis are both insufficient to distinguish among a benign, a premalignant, or even a malignant ovarian tumor, nonetheless there are morphological aspects that support the decision to surgically remove it in order to obtain a histopathological certainty and not overlook a malignant lesion.

Finally, ovarian as well as other forms of deep-infiltrating endometriosis are associated with a 50% increase in the development of ovarian cancer. Thus, it may become important to reduce the cancer risk by removing the endometriosis at a later time [16–20].

However, a recurrence risk always remains, even after a second-line complete cyst enucleation; such risk increases over time, up to one third (37%) or 5 years after surgery [21].

## Discussion about endometrioma enucleation

There are serious arguments for and against surgical removal of endometriomas. Removal of an endometrioma may not only reduce pain but may also impair the integrity of primordial and antral follicles. It has been shown that in the neighborhood of an endometrioma primordial follicles are lost and the density of cells decreases [22–24]. Some authors blame this on increased oxidative stress in the surroundings and free iron inside the cyst [22, 24, 25]. In addition, a focal inflammation may lead to fibrosis of cortex-specific stroma. Oxidative stress and inflammation together may lead to enhanced follicular recruitment and atresia of follicles [26]: ovulation may be impaired [27] and the response to stimulation reduced. In fact, Barri and co-authors detected a contrast between a pregnancy rate after spontaneous conception of 12% with endometrioma in situ and a pregnancy rate of 54% after surgical removal [28]. For sure, the risk of adnexal torsion, cyst growth and rupture, and malignant progression may favor a surgical removal [29].

One further important aspect is "relapsed endometriosis." Neither of the two surgical methods – the stripping technique or ablation (i.e., opening and coagulation of the endometriosis cyst without removing it) – leads to a significantly different relapse rate. In fact, in a study by Muzii and co-workers comparing the two techniques in 51 patients with bilateral endometriomas, the recurrence rate was 6% after stripping and 2% after coagulation. Thus, even if the available data conflict among studies, it may be preferable to perform an ablation in patients desiring children

[13, 30]. However, when it comes to a relapse, a secondary surgery seems to impair the ovarian reserve and worsen the reproductive performance; then the pregnancy outcome might be even better after direct ART as shown by Park and co-workers [31].

Major obstacles for endometriosis patients trying to conceive are the parameters "ovarian reserve" and the quality of germ cells. While the germ cells undergo a more rapid process of ageing as compared to those in women without endometriosis, the ovarian reserve is reduced even further due to the above-mentioned effects of endometrioma. The so-called ovarian reserve can be measured – indirectly – as antral follicle count or as the level of anti-Mueller hormone (AMH). These different aspects (reduced ovarian reserve in endometriosis patients in general, further impairment with occurrence of endometrioma and damage due to any surgical procedure such as stripping or coagulation) have to be taken into account when counseling a patient about surgery of ovarian endometriosis [32].

Even although the results of many studies are conflicting, many studies have shown that surgical excision can decrease the ovarian reserve. One reason for the decrease may be the removal of healthy ovarian tissue, any damage due to coagulation, or local inflammation after surgery. In fact it has been shown that removal of an endometrioma leads more often to removal of ovarian tissue than does removal of another benign cyst, such as a dermoid or a functional cyst [33]. This applies in particular to repeated operations. Hormonal stimulation of an ovary seems to be more difficult after surgery. However, neither the pregnancy rate of IVF alone nor the sequence of surgery and IVF leads to a statistically significant difference [11].

## Decision on surgical removal of endometrioma or conservative management in view of fertility

In counseling a patient about surgery, it is mandatory to consider the motivation for surgery. We recommend a differentiated strategy:

- For pain or other endometriosis-related symptoms, surgical removal of cyst (stripping or coagulation)
- For infertility, surgical removal before or after fertility treatment; in case of unilateral endometrioma and first operation, surgery; in case of relapsing endometrioma, direct fertility treatment without surgery
- For ovarian cancer risk (atypical endometriosis), surgical removal of cyst

## Laparoscopic surgical technique

*Trocar placement and intra-operative setting:* For enucleation of an ovarian cyst, two working trocars are usually sufficient. However, in case of advanced surgery, for example, dense adhesions, obesity, bowel involvement it may be helpful to insert a third working trocar for assistance. In addition, it may be useful to antevert the uterus using a uterine manipulator. The placement of trocars depends on the surgeon's preference. We put the two standard working trocars in the lower abdomen lateral to the inferior epigastric artery (e.g., lateral umbilical ligament).

For the third working trocar, we prefer the paraumbilical site (medioclavicular line) or, alternatively, the median position cranial to the symphysis is frequently used.

*Salpingoovariolysis*: Endometriosis leads to dense adhesions of the ovary to the environment such that it may be adherent to the pelvic side wall, the uterus, the bowel, and – depending on size and bilaterality – the contralateral ovary. To remove any cyst, it is important to free the ovary completely without damaging either the ovary or adjacent structures. If the bowel is adherent, one should pull with gentle traction on to the bowel so that the plane of dissection between bowel and ovary is visible. The adhesions should be cut with scissors rather than with an energy device to prevent any thermic injury to the tissues. In case of "frozen pelvis," it may be useful to open the retroperitoneal space at the level of the sacral promontory so that the ureter can be identified. Then, the ureter is followed and the bowel, ureter, and ovary are separated from each other. The next step may be to detach the ovary from the uterus. It may be necessary to apply traction to the ovary using a grasper. Then, the adhesion can be identified and cut with scissors or with an energized dissection device (i.e., based on mono- or bipolar current or ultrasound). The last step is to separate the ovary from the pelvic side wall. The ovary is held ventrally with a grasper, either in one of the surgeon's hands or one of the assistant's. It is now possible to bluntly dissect with the suction/irrigation device, carefully detaching the ovary from the endometriosis-affected peritoneal tissue of the pelvic side wall. The device is swiped in parallel fashion – not perpendicular – between ovary and pelvic wall. Often the cyst ruptures at this stage of surgery, and the chocolate cyst is confirmed. The fluid is evacuated and the preparation continued in the same fashion until the ovary is completely freed. Bipolar current may be used carefully to coagulate any bleeding. Usually the anatomical structures of the ovarian ligament, infundibulopelvic ligament, fallopian tube, ovary, and pelvic wall can be identified. Do not coagulate the pelvic wall before identifying the ureter, because the latter is *always* close and is susceptible to thermic injury.

*Cyst enucleation*: Most endometriomas rupture during the ovariolysis. If that happens, the ruptured site of the ovary can serve as the starting point for cyst enucleation. The opening should be enlarged along the axis of the ovary or equatorially so that the ovary is divided into two equal parts.

It is now important to identify the proper plane of preparation. This may be difficult because endometriomas are stuck to the ovarian tissue, especially in a case of *fibroblastic* rather than *fibrocystic* histological pattern. Any preparation has to be performed very carefully and slowly so that the normal ovarian tissue is damaged as little as possible. If at one location one fails to separate the layers, another one should be tried. Always first perform the preparation where it succeeds easily and leave the most difficult part until the end. The graspers should always be close to each other, for otherwise if the surgeon ends up pulling a long peace of tissue, the normal tissue may tear, or even the cyst may tear, and this makes the preparation more difficult. One should try to avoid a forced coagulation so that safe germ cells are saved; most bleeders will stop by themselves. Only the heavier bleeders should be coagulated selectively. If the endometrioma measures 5 cm or less, the ovary shrinks after cyst enucleation of the cyst and this renders reconstruction with sutures unnecessary. If the defect approximates the ovarian ligament, an (intracorporeal) suture may be used, taking care to avoid stitching the vessels (**Figures 5.1–5.7**).

*Ovariopexy*: In almost all cases of ovarian endometriosis, the ovary is involved with peritoneal endometriosis of the pelvic wall. Therefore, a removal of the peritoneal and deep-infiltrating endometriosis of the adjacent tissues (i.e., peritoneal tissue of ovarian fossa and uterosacral ligament) is indicated. To expose the field for this operating step, an ovariopexy is recommended. There are many ways to fix the ovary temporarily. We prefer an extracorporeal suture introduced inside the abdominal cavity under vision lateral to the lower working port with a straight needle. The needle

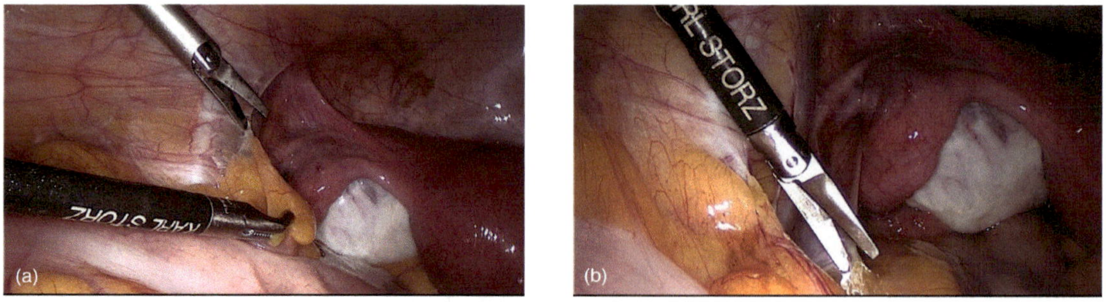


**FIGURE 5.1** Adhesiolysis. (a) Gentle traction on the mesosigma exposes an avascular plane which is cut with scissors. (b) The adhesion is cut such that the sigmoid colon is freed completely.

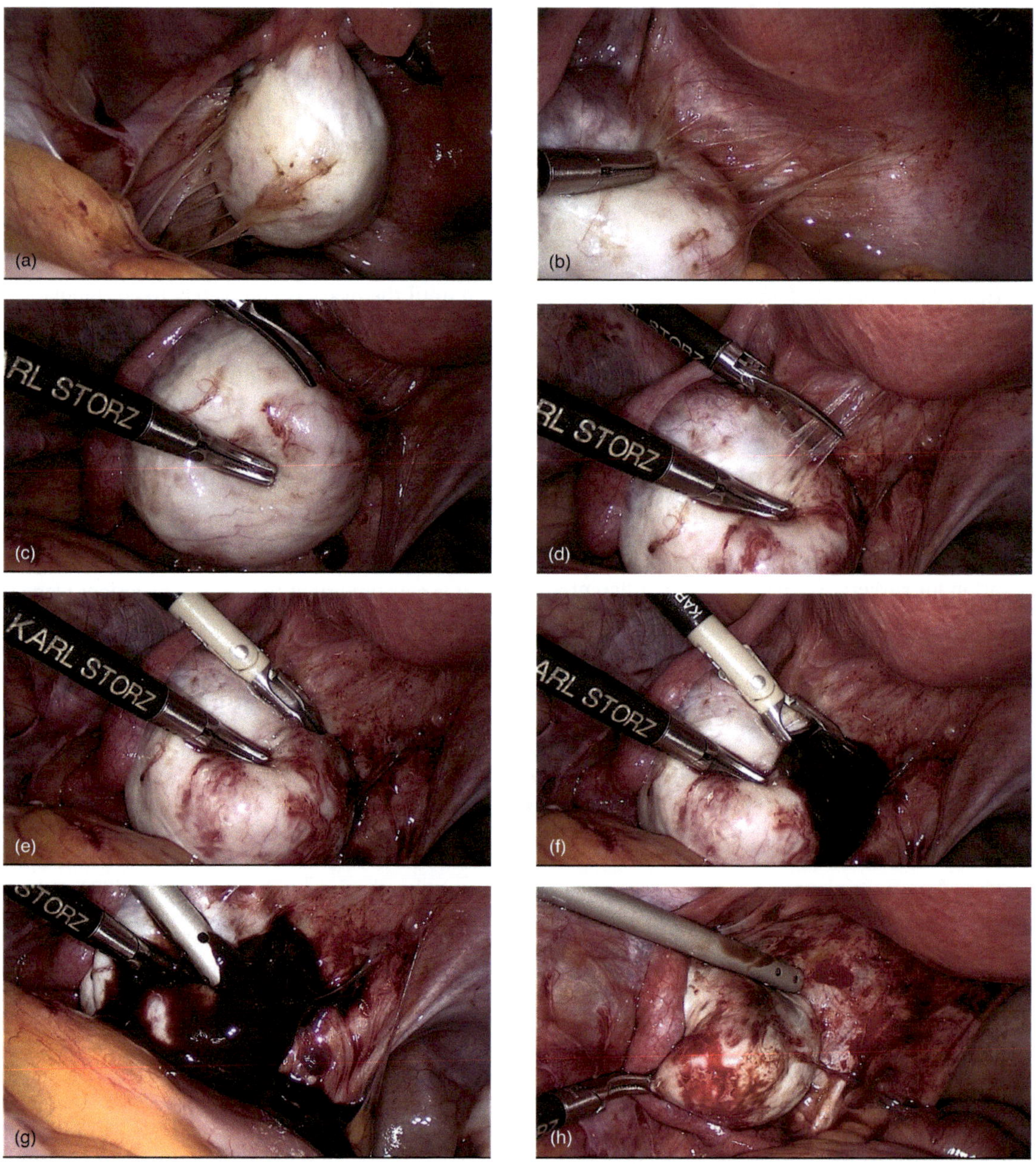


**FIGURE 5.2** Ovariolysis. (a) The uterus is anteverted and the adhesions between ovary and pelvic wall are exposed. (b) Between ovary and uterus, a blunt dissection may free the ovary. (c) and (d) Impression of the ovary exposes the flimsy adhesions between ovary and uterus close to the ovarian ligament. (e) Ovary and uterus are gently forced apart using the bipolar Maryland grasper but without current. (f) During dissection, the cyst often ruptures and a chocolate-like fluid is seen. (g) The fluid is evacuated. (h) A blunt dissection parallel to the dissection line between ovary and adjacent tissue of the pelvic wall is performed using the rinsing/suction device.

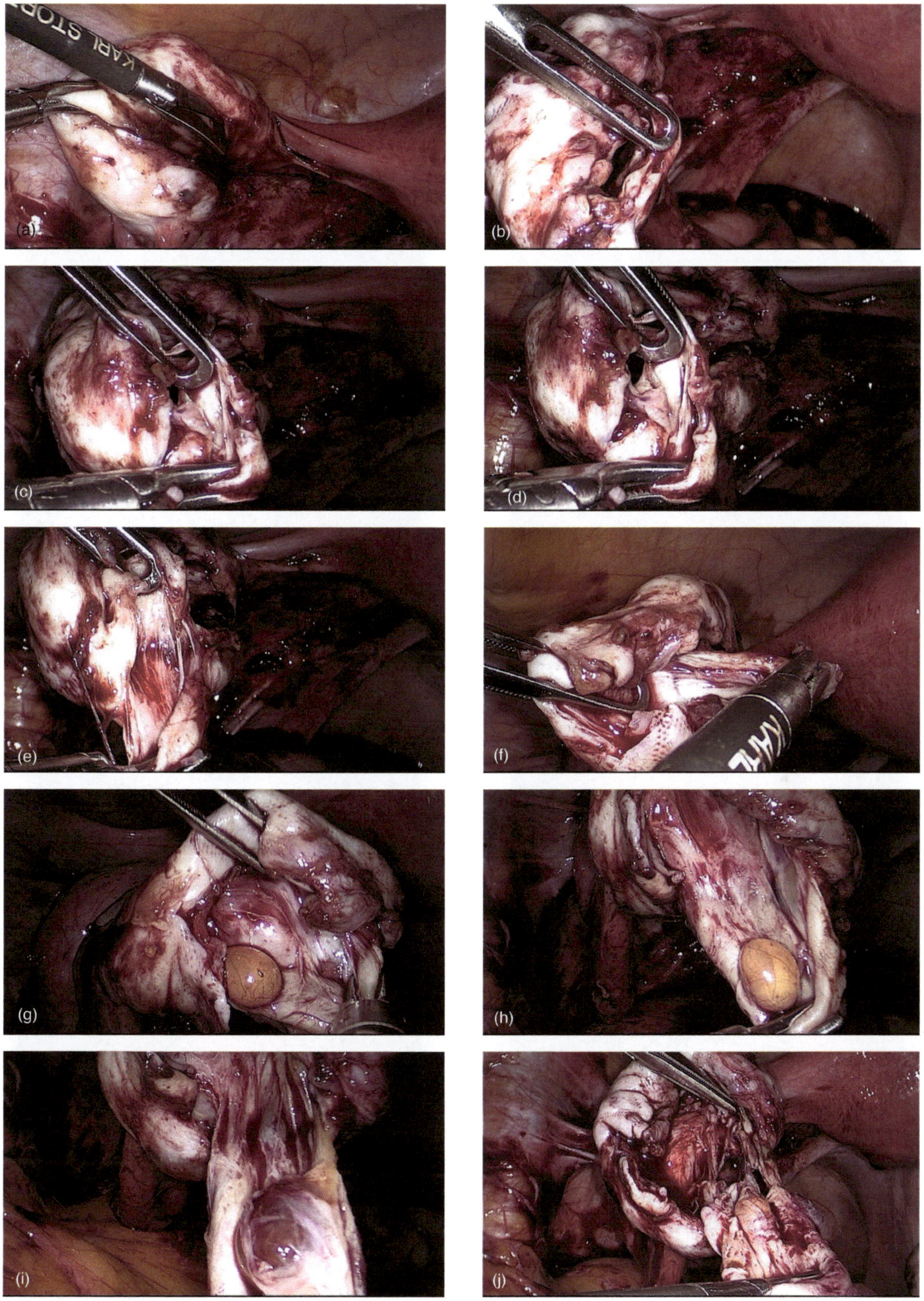

**FIGURE 5.3** Cyst enucleation ("stripping"). (a) The ovary is pulled ventro-laterally. The rupture site is exposed and enlarged utilizing scissors. (b–d) Normal ovary and cyst are identified and grasped separately. (e) The line (plane) between ovary and cyst is visualized, and pulling gently and slowly in a perpendicular fashion, the cyst is gradually separated from the normal ovarian tissue. If performed on the correct plane, little or no bleeding occurs. While stripping the cyst, the two graspers should not be too far apart. (g–j) Even if the preparation is performed very carefully, normal tissue (i.e., little functional cyst) is removed with the endometrioma. After removing the endometriosis cyst, bleeding vessels are coagulated sparingly.

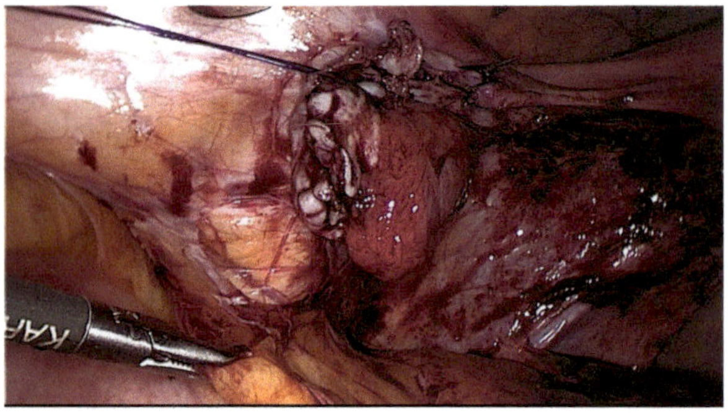

**FIGURE 5.4** Ovariopexy. An ovariopexy helps to expose the ovarian fossa.

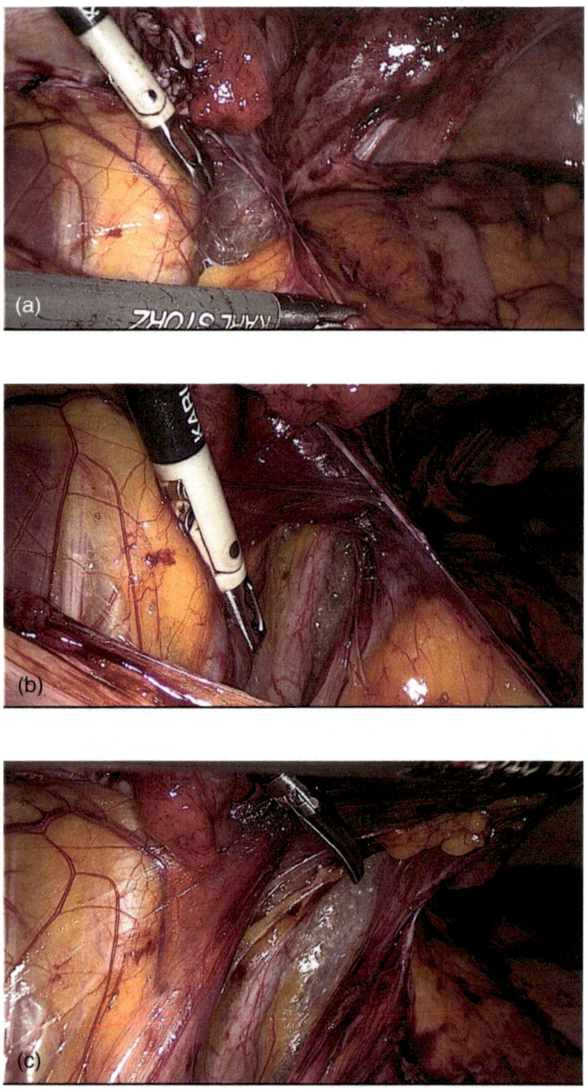

**FIGURE 5.5** Ureterolysis. (a–b) The sigmoid colon is gently pulled. The Maryland grasper is used for blunt dissection, identifying and exposing the ureter. (c) Scissors are used to cut avascular fibers of connective tissue.

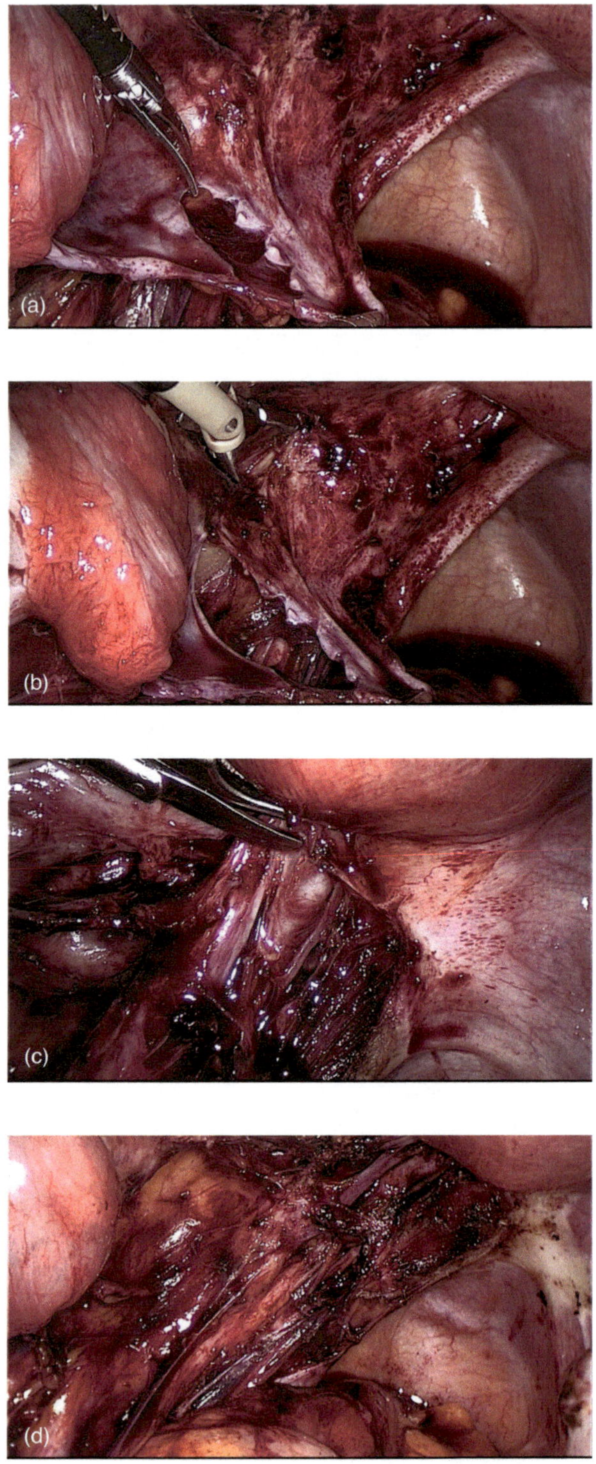

**FIGURE 5.6** Deperitonealization of ovarian fossa. (a) The peritoneum is pulled and the endometriosis-affected peritoneal tissue is excised with scissors. (b) The Maryland grasper may help to force apart healthy and affected peritoneal tissue. (c) The peritoneum is excised with scissors close the uterus. (d) Final view after deperitonealization of ovarian fossa.

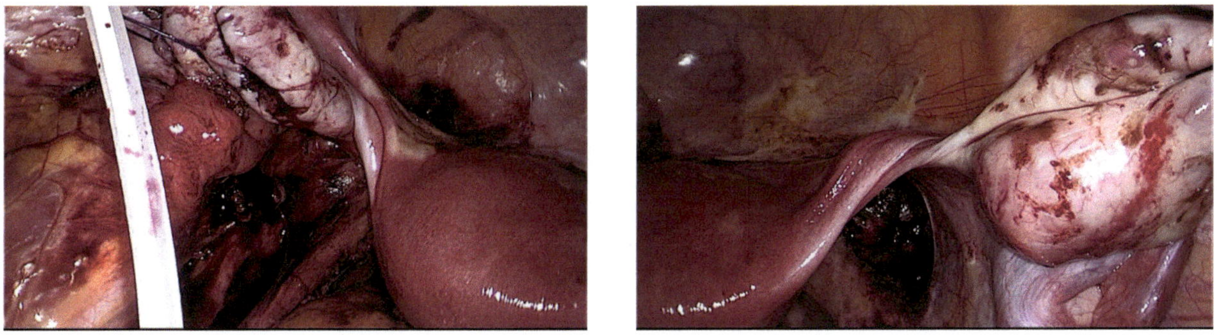

**FIGURE 5.7** Final view at the end of surgery (left, right). The ovariopexy remains in place for 2 days. The drain remains until the ichor decreases.

is then stitched through the ovary and returned through the abdominal wall. The suture is knotted outside the abdomen. It is possible to keep the ovary in that position even postoperatively for 1–2 days to prevent immediate postoperative adhesions between ovary and, respectively, the pelvic wall or bowel. Alternatively, an assistant can lift up the ovary with a grasper to expose the field for deperitonealization and ureterolysis, respectively.

*Deperitonealization of ovarian fossa and ureterolysis*: The peritoneum adjacent to the ureter is often involved with endometriosis. Since deep-infiltrating endometriosis can cause hydroureter and hydronephrosis, and because complete excision represents the best prevention of recurrence and leads to the best pregnancy rate after complete resection, deperitonealization of ovarian fossa and, perhaps, of uterosacral ligament are recommended. Thus to save the ureter, the ureter needs to be identified and ureterolysis performed, carefully preserving the vessels and nerve fibers accompanying the ureter.

The ureter is to be visualized where it crosses the iliac vessels, approximately at the level of the sacral promontory. The retroperitoneal space is then opened parallel to the ureter. This can occur bluntly by dissection with a Maryland grasper. One should look for unaffected peritoneum to start the preparation. The ureter is followed caudally until the uterine artery is seen thereby crossing the ureter to medially reach the uterus. It may be necessary to dissect the ureter even further until the parametrial tissue is reached. The peritoneum is stripped so that all endometriosis-affected tissue is removed.

The following imperative tips may help free the ureter safely:

- Dissect parallel
- Do not apply traction to the ureter
- Carefully use bipolar
- Thin out peritoneum
- Keep the ureter in his web
- Expect endometriosis at the crossover of ureter and uterine artery
- Use DJ stents, if necessary
- Internalize the fact that if you operate an endometriosis as radically as you would a cancer, you can expect the same side effects

*Adhesion prophylaxis*: To prevent adhesions, surgeons may prefer any barrier method (such as oxidized regenerated cellulose (Interceed®), expanded polytetrafluoroethylene (Gore-Tex®) and sodium hyaluronate with carboxymethylcellulose (Seprafilm®) as prophylaxis against adhesions. However, there is no clear evidence that any barrier method may prevent adhesion formation or lead to an improvement of the pregnancy rate (Ahmad, Cochrane 2015).

*Drain*: Since one should avoid coagulating the ovary extensively, the cyst bed may still ooze at the end of the surgery. It is recommended instead to introduce a drain until the drained fluid amounts to less than 100 cc in 24 hours.

## Statistical analysis of surgery for endometrioma

### Material and methods

At the Department of Obstetrics and Gynecology, University Clinics of Schleswig-Holstein, Kiel, Germany, we analyzed retrospectively 3057 patient medical records and surgical reports. From these records and reports, we histologically verified 550 patients with ovarian endometriotic cysts undergoing conservative excision via laparoscopy or laparotomy. Data regarding general patient characteristics, endometrioma symptoms, and diagnostic and surgical findings were collected from clinical records and reviewed (**Figure 5.8**). Patient characteristics are summarized in **Table 5.1**. Letters were sent to the patients asking them to fill in and return a questionnaire. With a final return rate of 52.5%, there were 289 patients in the follow-up study. The questionnaire inquired about patients' postoperative occurrence of another endometriosis cyst, temporal occurrence, and dignity, as well as reoperation rate, operation type, and recurrent pain symptoms (pain lasting > 1 week, dysmenorrhea, and dyspareunia). Patients were surveyed about their preoperative and postoperative fertility, whether a planned spontaneous pregnancy with or without complications had occurred, and, in cases of infertility followed by and pregnancy, whether artificial insemination had been successful. The recurrence of ovarian endometrioma was defined as a positive response to the presence of an endometriosis cyst as reported by the patient on the questionnaire. The average follow-up period was 12.9 years with a minimal time of 7.0 years and a maximum time of 16.9 years between operation and follow-up.

Data for analysis were recorded using Microsoft (Redmond, Washington) Access software. Statistical analysis was performed using Microsoft Excel and SPSS (IBM Corporation, Armonk, New York) programs. Patient identification numbers were assigned to ensure data protection. The percentages are based primarily on the total number; but in the absence of information, the corrected probability is given. $\chi^2$ was used in the analysis of categorical values. The statistical significance level was set at 5% ($P < 0.05$). The recurrence-free interval probabilities were estimated according to the Kaplan–Meier method. The log-rank

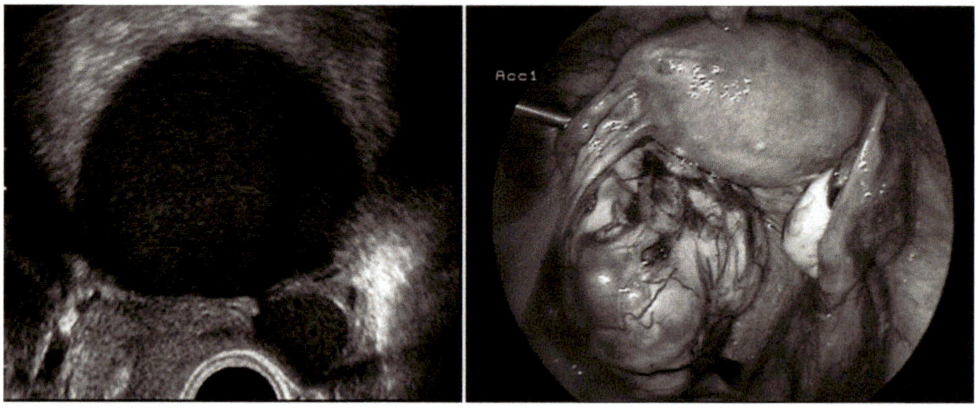


**FIGURE 5.8** Transvaginal ultrasonogram of a 6-cm (diameter), left ovarian endometrioma and its corresponding laparoscopic image.

test (Mantel–Cox) was used to compare the survival time of two groups with each other. Postmenopausal women were not considered in the postoperative analysis of dysmenorrhea [34].

### *Results*

At the time of surgery, the mean age of all endometrioma patients was 37.2 (±9.0) years; at follow-up, it was 50.5 (±9.3) years (**Table 5.1**). Preoperatively younger age, nulliparity, and previous laparoscopic surgery for ovarian endometrioma positively predicted the presence of pain and dysmenorrhea. Larger cyst size (>8 cm) was also associated with occurrence of pain, while primary or secondary sterility was associated with a higher rate of dysmenorrhea.

Factors associated with recurrence of dysmenorrhea were younger age ($P < 0.01$), nulliparity ($P < 0.05$), and larger cyst size

**TABLE 5.1: Patient Characteristics ($n = 550$)**

| Factors | | Number of Cases (%) |
|---|---|---|
| **Age** (years) | | 37.2 ± 9.0[a] |
| **BMI** (kg/m$^2$) | < 19 | 43 (7.8) |
| | 19–24 | 344 (62.5) |
| | 25–30 | 123 (22.4) |
| | > 30 | 40 (7.3) |
| **Sterility** | primary | 261 (47.5) |
| | secondary | 52 (9.5) |
| **Parity** | ≥ 1 | 194 (35.3) |
| **Abortion or miscarriage** | ≥ 1 | 72 (13.1) |
| **Pain** | | 338 (61.5) |
| **Dysmenorrhea** | | 214 (38.9) |
| **Recurrence of previous endometrioma** | | 153 (27.8) |
| **Previous laparoscopic surgery of endometrioma** | | 226 (41.1) |
| **Presence of uterine myoma** | | 105 (19.1) |
| **CA-125**[b] (U/mL) | increased (> 35 U/ml) | 147 (47.6) |
| **Cyst size** (cm) | 2–4 | 316 (57.5) |
| | 5–8 | 209 (38.0) |
| | > 8 | 25 (4.5) |
| **Cyst rupture** | preoperative | 23 (4.2) |
| | intra-operative | 281 (51.1) |
| **Follow-up patient characteristics ($n = 289$)** | | |
| **Age** (years) | | 50.5 ± 9,3[a] |
| **Postoperative medical treatment** | | 162 (56.1) |
| **Postoperative pain** | | 96 (33.2) |
| **Postoperative dysmenorrhea**[b] | | 93 (34.8) |
| **Recurrence of first diagnosed ovarian endometrioma**[b] | | 47 (23.9) |
| **Re-operation rate of first diagnosed ovarian endometrioma**[b] | | 32 (68.1) |
| **Postoperative pregnancy desire** | | 111 (38.4) |
| **Postoperative pregnancy**[b] | | 60 (54.1) |

[a] Mean ± SD.
[b] The sum does not add up to the total because of missing values or because of a new subtotal.

TABLE 5.2: Analysis of Factors Related to the Occurrence and Recurrence of Pain and Dysmenorrhea

| | Preoperative | Postoperative | Preoperative | Postoperative |
|---|---|---|---|---|
| | Pain | | Dysmenorrhea | |
| Factors | *P-value* (*n* = 550) | *P-value* (*n* = 289) | *P-value* (*n* = 550) | *P-value* (*n* = 267) |
| Younger age (years) | < 0.01 | NS | < 0.01 | < 0.01 |
| BMI (kg/m²) | NS | NS | NS | NS |
| Sterility | NS | NS | < 0.01 | NS |
| Nulliparity | < 0.05 | NS | < 0.05 | < 0.05 |
| Abortion/Miscarriage | NS | NS | NS | NS |
| Previous laparoscopy of endometrioma | < 0.01 | < 0.05 | < 0.05 | NS |
| Larger cyst size (>8 cm) | < 0.05 | NS | NS | < 0.05 |
| Cyst rupture | NS | NS | NS | NS |

NS = not significant.
*Source:* Courtesy of Maul L.V., et al. JSLS. 2014;18(3) [34]. With permission.

($P < 0.05$). Previous laparoscopic surgery for ovarian endometrioma ($P < 0.05$) was the only significant risk factor to be found for recurrence of pain (**Table 5.2**).

One hundred ninety-seven patients were initially diagnosed with endometriomas at the time of surgery; of these, 47 patients showed recurrent ovarian endometrioma (23.9%) in the follow-up period. 68.1% of the same set of patients (32 of 47) had undergone a reoperation in the follow-up period (**Table 5.1**). Of those 32 patients, 17 (53.1%) had needed 1 reoperation; 9 patients (28.1%) had needed 2 reoperations; and 6 patients (18.8%) had required ≥ 3 reoperations due to new endometriosis cysts. The probability of a recurrent-free interval was 76.1% for all primarily diagnosed endometriomas over our study period.

Patients with preoperative pain showed a significantly higher recurrence rate (log-rank test $P = 0.013$). The Kaplan–Meier graph demonstrates that patients without preoperative pain had a significantly higher recurrence-free interval of 84.7% when compared with patients who had a history of preoperative pain. The latter group were only 69.4% recurrence-free by the end of the follow-up period (**Figure 5.9**). Another statistically significant risk factor for endometrioma recurrence was preoperative dysmenorrhea (log-rank test $P = 0.013$). The Kaplan–Meier curve (**Figure 5.10**) illustrates that women without preoperative dysmenorrhea have a recurrence-free interval of 81.4% compared with a recurrence-free interval of only 66.2% in women with preoperative dysmenorrhea.

Other risk factors that were not significant but showed an association with higher rate of recurrence were larger cyst size (>8 cm; rate of recurrence was 33.3% [5 of 15] versus 16.3% [15 of 92] in cyst size 5–8 cm and 16.8% [24 of 143] in cyst size <5 cm), younger age at surgery (<25 years: 6.4% [3 of 47] in the recurrence cohort versus 2.8% [8 of 289] in the follow-up cohort), and preoperative cyst rupture (with a rate of recurrence of 28.6% [2 of 7] versus 20.5%

As to the effectiveness of endometrioma surgery, laparoscopy exhibited the best results in terms of freedom from symptoms in the postoperative period: after laparoscopic surgery, 49.0% of the patients were symptom-free, while after laparotomy only 33.3%

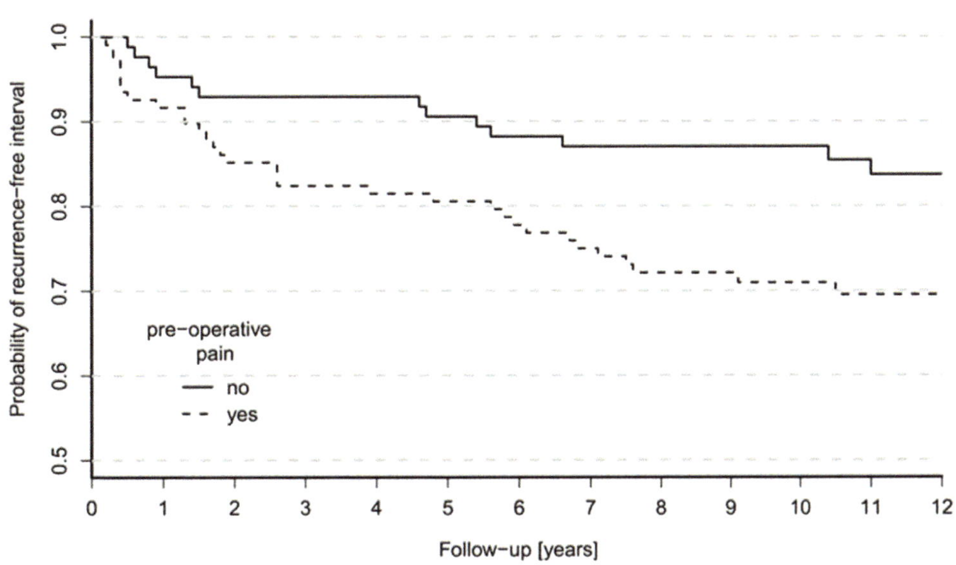


FIGURE 5.9 Probability of recurrence-free interval within the follow-up period in patients with and without preoperative pain. (Courtesy of Maul L.V., et al. JSLS. 2014;18(3) [34]. With permission.)

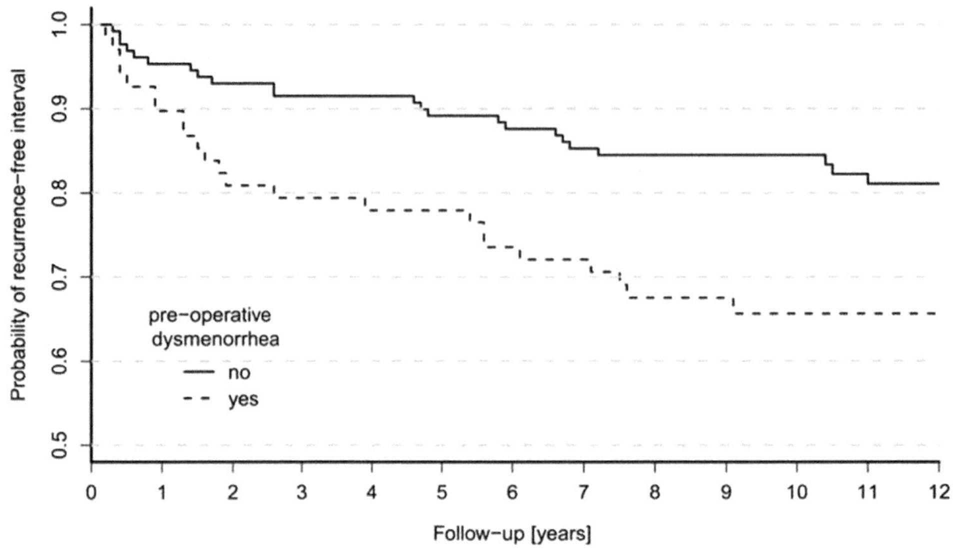


**FIGURE 5.10** Probability of recurrence-free interval within the follow-up period in patients with and without preoperative dysmenorrhea. (Courtesy of Maul L.V., et al. JSLS. 2014;18(3) [34]. With permission.)

remained free of symptoms. By transition from laparoscopy to laparotomy, only 43.7% were asymptomatic.

Postoperative medical treatment was given in 56.1% of the cases (162 of 289). Additional postoperative hormone therapy (gonadotropin-releasing hormone agonist, oral contraceptive, medroxyprogesterone acetate, or danazol) led to a higher recurrence of endometrioma, with a recurrence-free interval rate of only 70.5% versus 82.6% in patients who did not receive hormonal therapy (log-rank test $P = 0.050$) (**Figure 5.11**). The recurrence rates in both groups increased constantly with time from diagnostic surgery. Comparing combined surgical and hormonal treatment with exclusive surgical therapy, the following differences were shown: postoperative pain in 36.4% versus 29.1%, dysmenorrhea in 37.8% versus 26.0%, and dyspareunia in 19.1% versus 18.1%.

111 of 289 patients expressed a desire to become pregnant in the postoperative period (38.4%). Combined surgical and hormonal treatment was given to 61 of 111 patients (55.0%), whereas surgery alone was performed in 50 of 111 patients (45.0%). Among these patients, the postoperative spontaneous pregnancy rate was 54.1% (60 of 111). Of the 60 patients who had become pregnant, 46 of 111 (41.4%) had surgical treatment combined with medical treatment, and 14 of 111 (12.6%) had had surgery alone. A statistically significant difference ($P < .001$) was observed between combined surgical and hormonal therapy and exclusive surgery.

### *Discussion*

Our retrospective cohort study looked at risk factors, the effectiveness of endometrioma surgery comparing laparoscopy versus

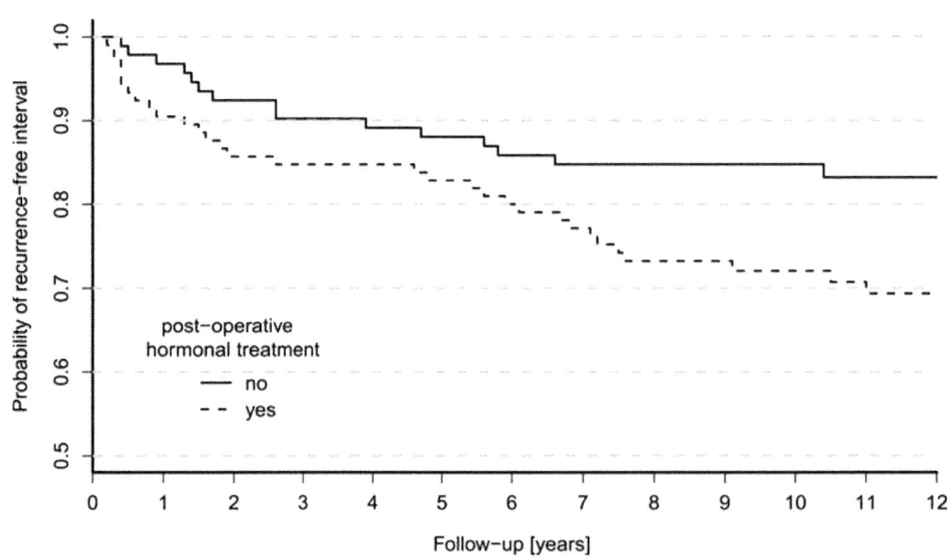


**FIGURE 5.11** Probability of recurrence-free interval within the follow-up period in patients with and without postoperative hormonal treatment. (Courtesy of Maul L.V., et al. JSLS. 2014;18(3) [34]. With permission.)

laparotomy, and the effect of additional medical treatment on recurrence of endometrioma and on pregnancy rates.

The preoperative risk factors observed as having significant predictive value for the presence of pain and dysmenorrhea were younger age, previous laparoscopic surgery of ovarian endometrioma, and nulliparity. Occurrence of pain seemed to be significantly associated with larger cyst size (> 8 cm), while primary or secondary sterility was associated with a higher rate of dysmenorrhea. As for recurrent symptoms, younger age, nulliparity, and larger cyst diameter significantly influenced the recurrence of dysmenorrhea, while only previous laparoscopic surgery of ovarian endometrioma could be determined to be a significant risk factor for the recurrence of pain as reported by Busacca et al. and Porpora et al. [34–36]. In accordance with Vercellini et al., a lower incidence of dysmenorrhea in older age is found to be justifiable due to the postmenopausal changes [37]. Other studies have also suggested that adhesions are causally important in pain associated with endometriosis, but on the other hand the cyst diameter produces no significant correlation between cyst size and pain symptoms [38, 39].

As with earlier studies that have indicated that pregnancy is a protective factor against pain associated with endometriosis, the present study also attributes a predictive value for pain symptoms to nulliparity [36, 40].

Many studies have analyzed the recurrence rate of endometriomas after laparoscopic surgery and found a recurrence rate between 11.0% and 30.4% after ≥ 2 years of observation [37, 40]. As recurrence is among the most significant challenges of endometriosis, reoperation is often regarded as the best treatment option at present, though the extent and duration of the effect of the second-line operation remains unclear [41]. In the present follow-up, a reoperation rate of 68.1% was observed in 32 of 47 patients with recurrent endometrioma who had ovarian endometriomas initially diagnosed at surgery. These observations agree with those made by Cheong et al. but not with the lower rate of required reoperation in other observations [41–43].

A history of preoperative pain or preoperative dysmenorrhea was shown to be a significant factor associated with higher recurrence rates, which agrees with a study by Renner et al. [44]. Our study observed significantly lower recurrence-free intervals for such preoperative complaints. In the present study larger cyst size, as also reported by Kikuchi et al. and Koga et al., younger age at surgery, and preoperative cyst rupture seemed to increase the risk of recurrence of ovarian endometrioma [40, 45].

Laparoscopy produced the best results regarding effectiveness of endometrioma surgery. This was in terms of a symptom-free postoperative course and pain reduction. In fact, because of its good tolerance, low morbidity, and low total cost of treatment, laparoscopy with sampling for histological investigation is the gold standard for diagnosis of endometriosis in the evaluation of persistent complaints [36, 46].

The impact of postoperative hormone therapy on ovarian endometriosis remains unclear at present. To determine the effect of additional postoperative medical treatment in the present follow-up, patients with hormone therapy (56.1%) were compared with those without (43.9%). Our study was in line with previous observations that patients do not significantly benefit from additional postoperative hormone therapy (gonadotropin-releasing hormone agonist, oral contraceptive, medroxyprogesterone acetate, or danazol) in terms of reduced risk of disease and recurrence of pain [36, 41, 47–49]. We observed even lower probabilities for a recurrence-free interval by reference to an average follow-up of 12.9 years in patients receiving hormone therapy versus in those who exclusively received surgical therapy. A retrospective study indicated that previous medical treatment of endometriosis was a significant risk factor ($P = .009$) for higher recurrence [40]. Yap et al. indicated that there was a significant improvement in the recurrence rate after postoperative hormone intake, and there were no recorded beneficial effects on pain and pregnancy rate in addition to surgery alone [50].

Among the 111 patients who had wished to conceive, the postoperative spontaneous pregnancy rate was 54.1%, which correlates with fertility rates observed by Vercellini et al. and Jones and Sutton [37, 51]. As the present study analyzes only the surgical outcome of total endometrioma excision, we were unable to draw comparisons with other surgical techniques such as fenestration or ablation [14, 52]. The present study indicates that additional medical treatment positively impacts the postoperative spontaneous pregnancy rate, which is in line with previous observations [53, 54]. Other studies by contrast have failed to observe a hormonal impact on the fertility rate after surgery [55–57]. Further studies are necessary to determine the most effective treatment of ovarian endometrioma.

A limitation of this study is that its study model, a retrospective cohort study, provides worse evidence and validity than would a prospective randomized controlled study. The definition of recurrence varies in the literature. Some studies define recurrence as a typical morphological change represented in a vaginal ultrasonogram; others define it as a recurrence or worsening subjective perception of pain. Although the general definition of a recurrent endometriosis remains to be determined, our definition represents a limitation because it is based on a questionnaire.

Biases in this study include the varying surgeon's experience, the low return rate of questionnaires, and developments in the field of hormonal treatment over the period of data collection and observation (e.g., danazol, in spite of its interesting immunosuppressive effects, is no longer commonly applied as drugs with fewer side effects, such as GnRh analogues and pure "gestagen preparations," have become more common.

Among the strengths of the study are the long follow-up period, large sample size, and the fact that all patients were operated upon at the same hospital.

Our study identifies risk factors for recurrent ovarian endometrioma in our patient population as preoperative pain, preoperative dysmenorrhea, and larger cyst size.

The present study also indicates that patients with ovarian endometriomas who wish to conceive seem to benefit from additional postoperative medical treatment. For patients whose family planning is fulfilled, the indications for additional postoperative medical treatment must be thoroughly evaluated according to the patient's preferences.

## *Summary*

Endometriosis cysts of the ovary occur in up to 44% of all endometriosis patients. Again, half of these patients suffer from bilateral endometrioma. Surgical treatment, in particular surgeries to enucleate ("stripping") or coagulate the cyst, represent the most frequent treatment modality because it has been shown that complete removal of endometriosis leads to the most effective reduction of symptoms and a significant increase in the pregnancy rate [57]. Apart from endometriosis-related symptoms, endometriosis cysts may impair fertility. However, there is controversial debate whether any endometriosis cysts should be removed as other studies have indicated that any kind of manipulation may worsen the outcome of fertility treatment by affecting the ovarian reserve. Translational research has detected that endometriosis is associated with endometrioid, clear cell, and low-grade serous ovarian cancer. However, ovarian endometriosis is frequently removed upon identification of symptoms together with unwanted childlessness. This chapter provides an introduction to the controversial debate and specifies the indications and describes the technique of surgical treatment.

## References


1. Alborzi, S., et al., *The impact of laparoscopic cystectomy on ovarian reserve in patients with unilateral and bilateral endometriomas.* Fertil Steril, 2014. **101**(2): p. 427–34.
2. Schmidt, D. and U. Ulrich, *[Endometriosis-related ovarian tumors].* Pathologe, 2014. **35**(4): p. 348–54.
3. Meinhold-Heerlein, I., et al., *Statement by the Kommission Ovar of the AGO: The New FIGO and WHO Classifications of Ovarian, Fallopian Tube and Primary Peritoneal Cancer.* Geburtshilfe Frauenheilkd, 2015. **75**(10): p. 1021–27.
4. Kurman, R.J., et al., *WHO classification of tumours of female reproductive irgans,* in WHO Classification of Tumours. 2014, WHO Press: Lyon.
5. Vercellini, P., et al., *Endometriosis: pathogenesis and treatment.* Nat Rev Endocrinol, 2014. **10**(5): p. 261–75.
6. Hughesdon, P.E., *The structure of endometrial cysts of the ovary.* J Obstet Gynaecol Br Emp, 1957. **64**(4): p. 481–7.
7. Brosens, I.A., P.J. Puttemans, and J. Deprest, *The endoscopic localization of endometrial implants in the ovarian chocolate cyst.* Fertil Steril, 1994. **61**(6): p. 1034–8.
8. Donnez, J., et al., *Large ovarian endometriomas.* Hum Reprod, 1996. **11**(3): p. 641–6.
9. Nisolle, M. and J. Donnez, *Peritoneal endometriosis, ovarian endometriosis, and adenomyotic nodules of the rectovaginal septum are three different entities.* Fertil Steril, 1997. **68**(4): p. 585–96.
10. Nezhat, F., et al., *Clinical and histologic classification of endometriomas. Implications for a mechanism of pathogenesis.* J Reprod Med, 1992. **37**(9): p. 771–6.
11. Keyhan, S., et al., *An update on surgical versus expectant management of ovarian endometriomas in infertile women.* Biomed Res Int, 2015. **2015**: p. 204792.
12. Dunselman, G.A., et al., *ESHRE guideline: management of women with endometriosis.* Hum Reprod, 2014. **29**(3): p. 400–12.
13. Brown, J. and C. Farquhar, *Endometriosis: an overview of Cochrane Reviews.* Cochrane Database Syst Rev, 2014. **3**: p. CD009590.
14. Hart, R.J., et al., *Excisional surgery versus ablative surgery for ovarian endometriomata.* Cochrane Database Syst Rev, 2008. 2: p. CD004992.
15. Benschop, L., et al., *Interventions for women with endometrioma prior to assisted reproductive technology.* Cochrane Database Syst Rev, 2010. 11: p. CD008571.
16. Pavone, M.E. and B.M. Lyttle, *Endometriosis and ovarian cancer: links, risks, and challenges faced.* Int J Womens Health, 2015. 7: p. 663–72.
17. Brinton, L.A., et al., *Relationship of benign gynecologic diseases to subsequent risk of ovarian and uterine tumors.* Cancer Epidemiol Biomarkers Prev, 2005. **14**(12): p. 2929–35.
18. Rossing, M.A., et al., *Risk of epithelial ovarian cancer in relation to benign ovarian conditions and ovarian surgery.* Cancer Causes Control, 2008. **19**(10): p. 1357–64.
19. Sainz de la Cuesta, R., et al., *Histologic transformation of benign endometriosis to early epithelial ovarian cancer.* Gynecol Oncol, 1996. **60**(2): p. 238–44.
20. Forte, A., M. Cipollaro, and U. Galderisi, *Genetic, epigenetic and stem cell alterations in endometriosis: new insights and potential therapeutic perspectives.* Clin Sci (Lond), 2014. **126**(2): p. 123–38.
21. Kim, M.L., et al., *Recurrence of ovarian endometrioma after second-line, conservative, laparoscopic cyst enucleation.* Am J Obstet Gynecol, 2014. **210**(3): p. 216 e1-6.
22. Sanchez, A.M., et al., *Iron availability is increased in individual human ovarian follicles in close proximity to an endometrioma compared with distal ones.* Hum Reprod, 2014. **29**(3): p. 577–83.
23. Maneschi, F., et al., *Ovarian cortex surrounding benign neoplasms: a histologic study.* Am J Obstet Gynecol, 1993. **169**(2 Pt 1): p. 388–93.
24. Sanchez, A.M., et al., *The distinguishing cellular and molecular features of the endometriotic ovarian cyst: from pathophysiology to the potential endometrioma-mediated damage to the ovary.* Hum Reprod Update, 2014. **20**(2): p. 217–30.
25. Matsuzaki, S., et al., *Analysis of risk factors for the removal of normal ovarian tissue during laparoscopic cystectomy for ovarian endometriosis.* Hum Reprod, 2009. **24**(6): p. 1402–6.
26. Kitajima, M., et al., *Enhanced follicular recruitment and atresia in cortex derived from ovaries with endometriomas.* Fertil Steril, 2014. **101**(4): p. 1031–7.
27. Benaglia, L., et al., *Endometriotic ovarian cysts negatively affect the rate of spontaneous ovulation.* Hum Reprod, 2009. **24**(9): p. 2183–6.
28. Barri, P.N., et al., *Endometriosis-associated infertility: surgery and IVF, a comprehensive therapeutic approach.* Reprod Biomed Online, 2010. **21**(2): p. 179–85.
29. Pearce, C.L., et al., *Association between endometriosis and risk of histological subtypes of ovarian cancer: a pooled analysis of case-control studies.* Lancet Oncol, 2012. **13**(4): p. 385–94.
30. Muzii, L., et al., *Comparison between the stripping technique and the combined excisional/ablative technique for the treatment of bilateral ovarian endometriomas: a multicentre RCT.* Hum Reprod, 2016. **31**(2): p. 339–44.
31. Park, H., et al., *Effect of second-line surgery on in vitro fertilization outcome in infertile women with ovarian endometrioma recurrence after primary conservative surgery for moderate to severe endometriosis.* Obstet Gynecol Sci, 2015. **58**(6): p. 481–6.
32. Seyhan, A., B. Ata, and G. Uncu, *The impact of endometriosis and its treatment on ovarian reserve.* Semin Reprod Med, 2015. **33**(6): p. 422–8.
33. Perlman, S. and J.J. Kjer, *Ovarian damage due to cyst removal. A comparison of endometriomas and dermoid cysts.* Acta Obstet Gynecol Scand, Nordic Federation of Societies of Obstetrics and Gynecology, Acta Obstetricia et Gynecologica Scandinavica 95(2016) 285–290.
34. Maul, L.V., Morrision J.E., Schollmeyer T., et al., *Surgical therapy of ovarian endometrioma: recurrence and pregnancy rates.* JSLS, 2014. **18**(3).
35. Busacca, M., et al., *Recurrence of ovarian endometrioma after laparoscopic excision.* Am J Obstet Gynecol, 1999. **180**(3 Pt 1): p. 519–23.
36. Porpora, M.G., et al., *Pain and ovarian endometrioma recurrence after laparoscopic treatment of endometriosis: a long-term prospective study.* Fertil Steril, 2010. **93**(3): p. 716–21.
37. Vercellini, P., et al., *Reproductive performance, pain recurrence and disease relapse after conservative surgical treatment for endometriosis: the predictive value of the current classification system.* Hum Reprod, 2006. **21**(10): p. 2679–85.
38. Fauconnier, A., et al., *Relation between pain symptoms and the anatomic location of deep-infiltrating endometriosis.* Fertil Steril, 2002. **78**(4): p. 719–26.
39. Kaya, H., et al., *Does the diameter of an endometrioma predict the extent of pelvic adhesions associated with endometriosis?* J Reprod Med, 2005. **50**(3): p. 198–202.
40. Koga, K., et al., *Recurrence of ovarian endometrioma after laparoscopic excision.* Hum Reprod, 2006. **21**(8): p. 2171–4.
41. Vercellini, P., et al., *Repetitive surgery for recurrent symptomatic endometriosis: what to do?* Eur J Obstet Gynecol Reprod Biol, 2009. **146**(1): p. 15–21.
42. Cheong, Y., et al., *Laparoscopic surgery for endometriosis: How often do we need to re-operate?* J Obstet Gynaecol, 2008. **28**(1): p. 82–5.
43. Abbott, J.A., et al., *The effects and effectiveness of laparoscopic excision of endometriosis: a prospective study with 2-5 year follow-up.* Hum Reprod, 2003. **18**(9): p. 1922–7.
44. Renner, S.P., et al., *Preoperative pain and recurrence risk in patients with peritoneal endometriosis.* Gynecol Endocrinol, 2010. **26**(3): p. 230–5.

45. Kikuchi, I., et al., *Recurrence rate of endometriomas following a laparoscopic cystectomy.* Acta Obstet Gynecol Scand, 2006. **85**(9): p. 1120–4.
46. Mettler, L., et al., *Accuracy of laparoscopic diagnosis of endometriosis.* JSLS, 2003. 7(1): p. 15–8.
47. Sesti, F., et al., *Recurrence rate of endometrioma after laparoscopic cystectomy: a comparative randomized trial between postoperative hormonal suppression treatment or dietary therapy vs. placebo.* Eur J Obstet Gynecol Reprod Biol, 2009. **147**(1): p. 72–7.
48. Bianchi, S., et al., *Effects of 3 month therapy with danazol after laparoscopic surgery for stage III/IV endometriosis: a randomized study.* Hum Reprod, 1999. **14**(5): p. 1335–7.
49. Tsai, Y.L., et al., *Short-term postoperative GnRH analogue or danazol treatment after conservative surgery for stage III or IV endometriosis before ovarian stimulation: a prospective, randomized study.* J Reprod Med, 2004. **49**(12): p. 955–9.
50. Yap, C., S. Furness, and C. Farquhar, *Pre and post operative medical therapy for endometriosis surgery.* Cochrane Database Syst Rev, 2004(3): p. CD003678.
51. Jones, K.D. and C.J. Sutton, *Pregnancy rates following ablative laparoscopic surgery for endometriomas.* Hum Reprod, 2002. **17**(3): p. 782–5.
52. Alborzi, S., et al., *A prospective, randomized study comparing laparoscopic ovarian cystectomy versus fenestration and coagulation in patients with endometriomas.* Fertil Steril, 2004. **82**(6): p. 1633–7.
53. Alkatout, I., et al., *Combined surgical and hormone therapy for endometriosis is the most effective treatment: prospective, randomized, controlled trial.* J Minim Invasive Gynecol, 2013. **20**(4): p. 473–81.
54. Mettler, L., *Pathogenesis, diagnosis and treatment of genital endometriosis.* Acta Obstet Gynecol Scand Suppl, 1989. **150**: p. 31–7.
55. Loverro, G., et al., *A randomized study comparing triptorelin or expectant management following conservative laparoscopic surgery for symptomatic stage III-IV endometriosis.* Eur J Obstet Gynecol Reprod Biol, 2008. **136**(2): p. 194–8.
56. Busacca, M., et al., *Postoperative GnRH analogue treatment after conservative surgery for symptomatic endometriosis stage III-IV: a randomized controlled trial.* Hum Reprod, 2001. **16**(11): p. 2399–402.
57. Mettler, L., Alkatout, I., Keckstein, J., Meinhold-Heerlein, I. Endometriosis. A concise practical guide to current diagnosis and treatment. Endo Press, 2017: p. 1–478.

# 6

## MANAGEMENT OF MYOMETRIAL CYSTIC ADENOMYOSIS

**Huda Afaneh, Mohammed R. Said, and Mostafa I. Abuzeid**

### Introduction

Adenomyosis is defined by the presence of endometrial stroma and glands within the myometrium of the uterus [1]. This is further characterized as focally present in an area of myometrium, or present throughout the myometrium in a diffuse form. The pathophysiology of adenomyosis is incompletely understood at this time. One hypothesis involves the inciting aspect of uterine surgery or pregnancy; however, even uteri that do not possess these risk factors can be affected by adenomyosis, although they are not the majority [1]. In these foci of endometrial implants, cyclic bleeding is minimal due to the lack of proliferation and secretory phases that occur during the menstrual cycle [1]. This chapter will focus on a rare entity of focal adenomyosis, namely the type with large cystic lesions occurring within a focal area of adenomyosis or cystic adenomyosis. The cystic part of the nomenclature refers to a distinct cavity that forms within the myometrium and contains evidence of hemorrhage and bleeding that is comparable to the "chocolate-like" material of an endometrioma. However, it is important to note that the nomenclature does vary among different reviews of the literature depending on, the type of classification used, the individual cases presented, as well as the proposed etiology of the lesion [2–4]. This makes establishing universal terminology challenging. Cystic adenomyosis can be classified into two types depending on patient's age into adult and juvenile forms. Juvenile cystic adenomyoma (JCA) represents a focal form of adenomyosis present in women of younger reproductive age [5]. The chronic nature of progression of this pathology when it occurs in older age groups may explain why many women diagnosed with adult cystic adenomyosis (ACA) appear to be in the end of the reproductive years.

### Incidence

Cystic lesions in the literature were reported as early as 1908 [2, 6, 7]. One of the earliest cases of JCA defined in the literature was by Tamura et al. in 1996 [8]. In this case report, cystic lesions as isolated entities within the uterus, were reported as rare, and less than 1%. The incidence of JCA is currently unclear and is possibly difficult to be determined accurately [2]. In comparison with older reproductive age groups, younger reproductive age groups such as adolescents are rarely reported to be affected by adenomyosis [1, 2]. There is speculation that misdiagnoses of other syndromes that present similarly may also contribute to the lack of representation of JCA in the literature. For example, unicornuate uteri with non-communicating rudimentary horns with hematometra displaying a collection of hemorrhage within a capsule may be misdiagnosed as a focal area of cystic adenomyosis [9]. Another hypothesis for the development of JCA may be a defect in the embryological process of the gubernaculums [10]. The adult form of cystic adenomyosis is less reported in the literature compared to the lesions affecting the younger age demographic [2].

### Pathogenesis

The exact mechanism of adenomyosis is largely unknown and based on theoretical pathological processes. There are proposed hypotheses of invasion of the stratum basalis of the endometrium into the myometrial tissue [1, 11]. Any type of process which potentially creates an extension from the endometrium to the myometrium can in theory cause adenomyosis. Such processes include pregnancy, curettage, or other uterine surgery, cesarean delivery or even endometrial ablation. There are of course hormonal influences during the reproductive years and pregnancy. The pathogenesis of a cystic collection with hemorrhage is not thoroughly understood but can be related to hormonal receptors present on adenomyotic implants [12]. Interestingly, other authors propose an alternative etiology. Acién et al. (2010) [9] discussed the possibility of juvenile cystic adenomyoma as a variation or alternative Müllerian anomaly, one that involves a rudimentary or accessory horn of the uterine corpus [9]. They proposed that the accessory uterine cavity as well as cystic adenomyoma are of the same pathologic entity [9]. The discussion of the possibility of a new Müllerian anomaly associated with a defect in the gubernaculum development of the broad and/or round ligament during embryologic development is also explored [10]. These findings have been discussed in a few case reports involving older reproductive age women [2]. Takeuchi et al. (2010) [13] disputed this as the uterine corpus itself remains relatively normal, while the cystic lesion of the juvenile cystic adenomyoma functions independently [13]. There are unresolved definitions in the literature regarding the etiology of these cysts and their pathophysiology at this time. These inferences allow us to develop differential diagnosis when evaluating a patient who presents with secondary dysmenorrhea, abnormal uterine bleeding, and abnormal pelvic findings on imaging.

### Classification

The focal form of adenomyosis is much less common than the diffuse form [11–14]. As mentioned earlier, cystic adenomyosis can be classified into two types depending on patient's age, adult and juvenile forms. Takeuchi et al. (2010) [13] reviewed the literature and created their own diagnostic criteria for juvenile cystic adenomyoma including (1) age less than 30 years, (2) the presence of a lesion measuring greater than 1 cm in diameter and surrounded by myometrial tissue and (3) clinical symptoms of dysmenorrhea [13]. Alternatively, the adult form refers to women older than 30 years of age and a cystic lesion that can be confined anywhere in the uterus, which follows the pathogenesis of adenomyosis as its etiology. The cysts also tend to be larger, contain clear fluid and presence of ciliated epithelium [2].

### Diagnosis

The diagnosis of JCA should be considered in a patient younger than age 30 [13]. Some authors cite individuals of 13–20 years

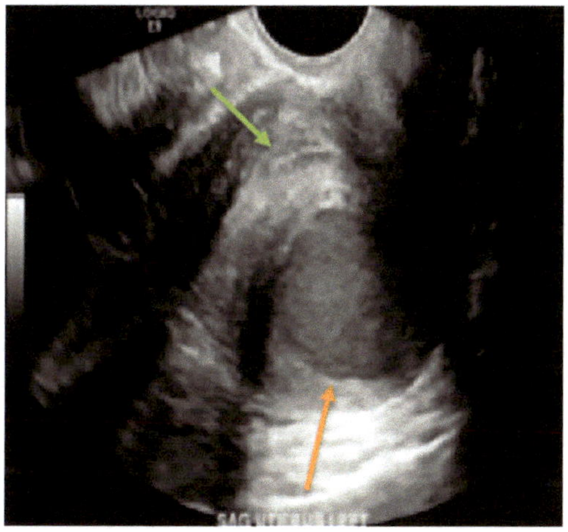

**FIGURE 6.1** TV 2D US of a juvenile cystic adenomyoma in the posterior wall of the uterus (orange arrow), showing the endometrial strip separate from the cyst (green arrow).

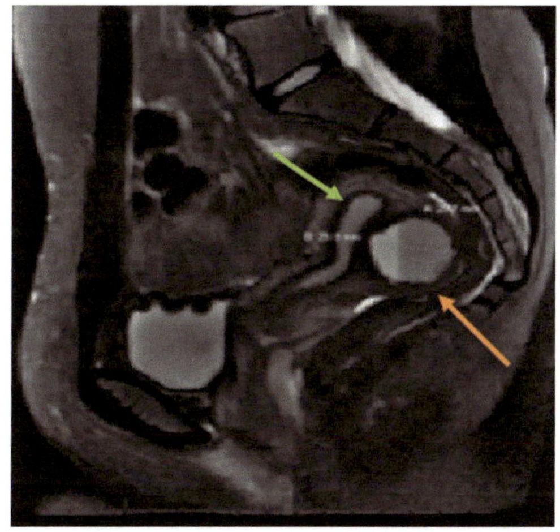

**FIGURE 6.2** MRI of a juvenile cystic adenomyoma in the posterior wall of the uterus (orange arrow) of the same patient in **Figure 6.1**, showing the endometrial strip separate from the cyst (green arrow).

age, who present with severe dysmenorrhea refractory to conventional first-line therapy with nonsteroidal anti-inflammatory drugs or hormonal treatment [15]. Other nonspecific symptoms also include abnormal uterine bleeding, pelvic pain, and/or infertility [16]. Pelvic examination may or may not display uterine enlargement. On the other end of the spectrum, women with ACA can be asymptomatic, but these cases are likely to be underreported [17]. Although histopathology of cyst specimens confirms the diagnosis, imaging modalities such as magnetic resonance imaging (MRI) and pelvic ultrasonography have been used more frequently to identify the signs of adenomyosis on imaging preoperatively [18]. Imaging with pelvic transvaginal 2D &3D ultrasonography (TV 2D and 3D US) or MRI is essential to narrowing the diagnosis when there are findings of a focal, cystic lesion within the myometrium of the uterus [14]. The pelvic sonogram is the cornerstone to any initial gynecologic pathology work-up. However, it may have limitations in delineating specific changes in the pelvic anatomy. TV 2D US can suggest adenomyosis characteristics in the uterus of the diffuse or focal type, when evaluating the entire shape of the uterus or myometrial thickness [1]. In addition, TV 2D US can detect a cystic structure in the myometrium (**Figure 6.1**). MRI provides more detail regarding any cystic lesions or presence of hematometra to help determine the diagnosis (**Figure 6.2**) [1]. Hysterosalpingogram can be used when considering congenital anomaly as a primary diagnosis, but MRI will likely be a follow-up study [14, 16]. Surgical evaluation with hysteroscopy is a more invasive approach and will only help with intracavitary lesions, or when visualizing absent tubal ostia in patients with unicornuate uterus.

## Differential diagnosis

Much of the literature debates the presence of cystic forms of adenomyosis as a subset of adenomyosis or as a form of congenital anomaly. Some authors reported cases where the preoperative diagnosis was a non-communicating horn of a unicornuate uterus with hematometra, and later were diagnosed as a juvenile cystic adenomyoma [11, 14]. The specific uterine malformations on the differential diagnosis include unicornuate uterus with non-communicating rudimentary horn (Class IIb of AFS classification) and complete septate uterus (Class Va of AFS classification) with non-communicating hemi-cavity [19, 20]. However, when a cystic lesion is visualized on imaging and the patient's pain is refractory to medical treatment, other diagnoses should also be explored. These include possible leiomyoma undergoing degeneration, ovarian masses benign or neoplastic, cervical retention cysts and intra-myometrial endosalpingiosis [21]. Green et al. (2019) [22] reported a case series of eleven patients from their institution with symptoms mostly consisting of persistent pelvic pain and abnormal uterine bleeding [22]. Seven out of the eleven patients had a diagnosis of cystic adenomyosis based on imaging and/or histologic findings [22]. The patient's age ranged between 28 and 54 years of age, with the majority being older than 30 years of age [22]. Other findings included cystic leiomyoma (cyst with smooth muscle lining without an epithelial lining), Müllerian cysts (cyst with smooth muscle wall lining with columnar epithelium), adenomatoid tumors, and intra-myometrial hydrosalpinx. The most common diagnosis was cystic adenomyosis [22]. In addition, endosalpingiosis can act as a subset of endometriosis and can also present with uterine cysts [17].

## Medical management

Conservative therapy with medical management should be thoroughly explored and does depend on the patients' goals of treatment. Medical treatment can include nonsteroidal anti-inflammatory drugs (NSAIDs) and other over-the-counter analgesics. GnRH-a agonist and continuous oral contraceptive pills are also reported to be effective [5]. A focal adenomyotic lesion can be approached similarly to the conservative medical therapy appropriate for endometriosis, such as using a 12-month course of GnRH-a agonist therapy, aromatase inhibitors or oral contraceptives in conjunction with acetaminophen and NSAIDs [23, 24]. The risks of surgery, especially with a young patient should be considered against debilitating pain that may severely affect daily or weekly functioning of a patient during her menses.

Few reports supported the use of medical treatment as the first line with successful outcome [5, 25]. Fisseha et al. (2006) [25] started a 13-year-old girl with JCA associated with pelvic pain and vaginal bleeding for 10 months on continuous oral contraceptive pills and reported significant relief of her pelvic pain, vaginal bleeding as well as decrease in cyst size. Follow-up ultrasounds at 6 months, 1 year, and 2 years showed a decrease in cyst size from 2 cm to less than 1 cm. The patient remained asymptomatic on oral contraceptive pills throughout her follow-up [25]. Branquinho et al. (2012) [5] used continuous oral contraceptive pills to manage a 17-year-old patient with severe dysmenorrhea associated with JCA unresponsive to NSAIDs. They also reported a significant relief of her pelvic pain, in addition to a significant decrease in mass size from 3.5 cm to less than 2.5 on ultrasound and MRI after 6 months, and less than 1.5 cm after 1 year. The patient remained asymptomatic throughout her follow-up [5].

On the other hand, there are several reports in the literature of failed medical treatment or a combined sclerotherapy and medical treatment. Akar et al. (2010) [26] described a case of robot-assisted laparoscopic removal of a JCA in a 15-year-old girl with intermittent episodic right-sided periumbilical pain and severe dysmenorrhea unresponsive to medical suppression with aromatase inhibitors, progestins, oral contraceptives, or GnRH-a agonist for 2 years [26]. Pontrelli et al. (2015) [27] reported a hysteroscopic management of a giant 8 cm cystic adenomyoma in a 27-year-old nulliparous patient that presented with worsening dysmenorrhea, chronic pelvic pain, and abnormal uterine bleeding unresponsive to continuous oral contraceptive therapy for 5 years [27]. Deblaere et al. (2019) [28] managed a 16-year-old girl with JCA presenting with pelvic pain and progressing dysmenorrhea with transabdominal ultrasound-guided cyst aspiration followed by injection of 3.5 mL ethanol in the cystic cavity and aspiration of this ethanol after 5 minutes [28]. They reported symptomatic relief for 2 months, followed by recurrence of the symptoms unresponsive to daily oral progestins, with worsening of her symptoms [28]. A laparoscopic excision of the cyst was performed followed by 6 months of continuous contraceptive pills. They reported full relief from the pelvic pain and major improvement in the patient's dysmenorrheal [28].

Other examples of failed medical treatment requiring definitive surgical treatments were reported by Ball et al. (2009), Akar et al. (2010), Kamio et al. (2007), Ho et al. (2009), Nabeshima et al. (2008), and Takeda et al. (2007) [15, 26, 29–32]. Nabeshima et al. (2008) [31] reported failure of medical treatment for 4 years using NSAIDs, GnRH-a agonist therapy, and oral contraceptives [31]. Overall, although there are a couple of reports of successful medical treatment of JCA, the majority of the limited published data suggest a high failure rate of medical treatment. Based on this, the authors of this chapter believe that an attempt at medical treatment should be tried first, but if it fails to achieve adequate relief, a definitive surgical treatment with laparoscopic resection should be performed by an experienced reproductive surgeon.

## Surgical treatment of JCA

There are various approaches when considering surgical management for patients affected by JCA. The benefit of minimally invasive therapy and fertility conservation should be employed when possible.

## Laparoscopic excision of JCA

Depending on surgeon expertise and comfort, laparoscopy is an excellent minimally invasive approach to JCA. Nabeshima et al. (2008) [31] reported the first total laparoscopic resection in the literature of a cystic adenomyoma in a 27-year-old woman after unsuccessful laparotomy [31]. The patient was diagnosed with a cystic adenomyoma, medical treatment was ineffective and surgical laparotomy failed because the uterine surface was visually normal and there was no imaging guidance available to locate the cystic lesion [31]. The patient underwent medical therapy using NSAIDs, GnRH-a agonist, oral contraceptives for 4 years without any improvement [31]. Laparoscopic resection of the cystic region with ultrasonographic guidance was done because the location of the cystic adenomyoma could not be detected precisely [31]. Transtrocar ultrasonography was performed using an intra-operative phased-array sector probe with an endfire laparoscopic microconvex probe that was compatible with a 12-mm port [31]. Diluted Vasopressin with physiologic saline was injected into the myometrium, and the cyst was excised followed by double-layer uterine closure [31]. Postoperatively the cyst completely disappeared on follow-up ultrasonography and the patient was asymptomatic up to 1-year after the surgery [31]. Ball et al. (2009) [15] described a case of JCA in a 19-year-old patient who had failed medical treatment. She underwent hysteroscopy as well as operative laparoscopy. There were 4 ports used including a 10-mm umbilical port [15]. The 2 cm lesion was located on the left aspect of the uterus caudal to the round ligament [15]. Vasopressin (1U in 50 mL of normal saline) was injected for hemostasis [15]. A Harmonic Ace scalpel (Ethicon, Johnson & Johnson Health Care Systems Inc., USA) was then used to make the initial transverse incision over the cystic lesion [15]. The chocolate-like contents were drained [15]. Bipolar diathermy was used for hemostasis during removal of the cyst [15]. The remaining defect was closed using 2-0 PDS suture on a CT1 needle and the serosal and muscularis layers were closed using 3-0 PDS [15]. The surgical time was 90 minutes, and estimated blood loss was less than 20 mL [15]. They reported successful postoperative outcome [15]. Histopathology confirmed the diagnosis of cystic adenomyoma [15]. Takeuchi et al. (2010) [13] described laparoscopic resection of JCA in 9 cases with significant improvement of symptoms within 6 months following the surgery [13]. Their laparoscopic technique was performed through an 11 mm primary port, two 5 mm accessory ports bilaterally inserted, and a 12 mm trocar that was inserted into the left upper abdomen on the anterior axillary line on the surgeon's side [13]. Diluted Vasopressin was injected into the myometrium surrounding the cyst [13]. The serosa over the cyst was incised horizontally using a monopolar probe followed by cyst wall extraction using a 0-Polysorb Z suture in the cyst parenchyma after separation of cyst from the overlying serosa [13]. The myometrium was closed in two or three layers using a 0-Polysorb in a continuous technique. Thereafter, the serosa was closed by a continuous mattress or baseball suture using 0-Polysorb [13]. Tissue samples were collected from the pouch of Douglas using an 11 mm trocar inserted via the posterior vaginal fornix that was closed laparoscopically with a continuous 2-0 Polysorb suture [13]. No lesion recurrence was reported during the postoperative period in all cases [13]. In addition, pregnancy was reported in two of three patients who wished to become pregnant. Tubal patency was also established in all the five patients who underwent tubal patency testing postoperatively [13]. Similarly, Grimbizis et al. (2008) [33], discuss six cases at their institution that were successfully managed with laparoscopic treatment of focal cystic adenomyoma [33]. They treated nonpregnant women of reproductive age with ages ranging from 29 to 38 years old [33]. Their symptoms included dysmenorrhea, menorrhagia, and pregnancy loss [33]. They utilized a longitudinal incision along the cystic lesion and dissected using monopolar and bipolar diathermy [33]. The uterine seromuscular wall was reapproximated in two layers using absorbable suture [33]. All their surgeries were uncomplicated with an unremarkable postoperative course [33]. The histology confirmed adenomyosis in all the cases [33]. Follow up after 13 months revealed complete regression of all their patients' symptoms [33]. Kriplani et al. (2011) [14] described performing laparoscopy and hysteroscopy for four cases of JCA. Hysteroscopy was done to rule out any Müllerian anomalies or submucous component of the lesion [14]. Laparoscopy was performed through an 11 mm primary port and three 5 mm accessory ports followed by diluted Vasopressin injection into the lesion [14]. Thereafter, the myometrium overlying the cystic lesion was dissected using both monopolar and bipolar electrocautery and it was separated from the lesion [14]. Chocolate-colored fluid was subsequently drained from the cyst cavity, then, myometrium closure was performed using 2-0 polyglactin sutures, with complete obliteration of dead space [14]. All cases showed significant improvement at 3 months follow up visits; however, no pregnant cases were recorded [14]. Takeda et al. (2007) [32] published laparoscopic resection of JCA in 2 cases [32]. The first case was a 20-year-old female with severe dysmenorrhea unresponsive to NSAIDs. Her symptoms improved on a 6 months course of GnRH-a agonist [32]. However, her symptoms reoccurred once the medication was discontinued [32]. Gasless laparoscopic surgery was performed by the subcutaneous abdominal wall-lift method and a 5-mm laparoscope (Olympus, Tokyo, Japan) was placed through a 5-mm Optiview port (Ethicon, Tokyo, Japan) that was placed at the superior edge of the umbilicus, and an additional 5 mm port that was placed on the left side at the level of the umbilicus, and another two 12 mm ports were placed [32]. Diluted vasopressin was then injected into the nodule and then it was incised at the midline portion by Harmonic scalpel (Ethicon, Tokyo, Japan) [32]. After reaching the cystic cavity, the dark-brown content was drained. The upper half of the cyst was grasped by claw forceps and pulled through the suprapubic port using a claw forceps [32]. The cyst base was then excised by Harmonic scalpel. Single-layer closure of the myometrium was done and then covered by Interceed (Johnson & Johnson, Tokyo, Japan) to prevent adhesion [32]. A 2 months GnRH-a agonist treatment was given. Complete disappearance of dysmenorrhea was achieved with the first menstrual cycle after the surgery [32]. The second case was also a 20-year-old patient with similar presentation and laparoscopic resection was done in a similar technique to the first case; however, a three-dimensional transvaginal ultrasonography (Voluson 730 System, GE Yokogawa Medical Systems, Tokyo, Japan) was performed due to inability to locate the nodule using the laparoscopy alone [32]. Postoperatively, the patient also reported complete disappearance of her symptoms [32]. Deblaere et al. (2019) [28] described a laparoscopic excision of JCA followed by 6 months of continuous contraceptive pills in a 16-year-old girl after failed medical treatment and ultrasound guided alcohol sclerotherapy [28]. The authors located the cyst by using a laparoscopic ultrasound probe [28]. The serosa overlying the cyst was opened with a 4 cm incision and the brown viscous fluid was then drained from the cyst cavity [28]. Monopolar scissor and bipolar forceps were used to dissect the cyst from the surrounding myometrium [28]. Afterward the myometrial defect was closed in two layers with interrupted resorbable Vicryl 2-0 sutures (Ethicon, Johnson & Johnson, USA) [28]. This was followed by placement of Hyalobarrier gel on the suture line (Nordic Pharma Group, Paris, France) in an attempt to prevent adhesion formation [28]. They reported full relief from the pelvic pain and major improvement in the patient's dysmenorrheal [28]. Few other reports were published describing laparoscopic excision of JCA [11, 34, 35]. In addition, there are 3 case reports in the literature of laparoscopic excision of a cystic mass from a unique location, namely the broad ligament [16, 36, 37]. Interestingly, two of these reports named the cystic lesions endometrioma instead of JCA [36, 37].

The authors of this chapter managed three patients with JCA (2016–2019). They aged 16–30 years and they all presented with chronic pelvic pain (CPP). Hormonal treatment was attempted in two cases but it failed. Cystic lesions in the myometrium ($n$ = 2), and the broad ligament ($n$ = 1) was detected on TV 2D US and/or MRI (**Figures 6.1** and **6.2**, respectively). The cyst was separated from the endometrial cavity in all the cases. The cysts were within the myometrium of the posterior wall of the uterus (**Figure 6.3a–d**), within the cornual region of the myometrium (**Figure 6.4a–i**), and within the broad ligament near the cornual region (**Figure 6.5a–f**) in the three cases, respectively. The cystic lesions were confirmed on laparoscopy, and laparoscopic excision of the cysts with adequate repair of the myometrial beds were performed in all cases with fertility preservation (**Figure 6.3a–d**), (**Figure 6.4a–i**), (**Figure 6.5a–f**). Robotic assistance was chosen in one case, with the cyst in the broad ligament for better visualization (unpublished data), [**Figure 6.5a–f**]. The endometrial cavity was entered in one case (0.5 cm), [**Figure 6.4a–i**]. Pathology report confirmed the diagnosis of JCA is all cases. All three patients reported relief of their symptoms up to 6–8 months after surgery. No recurrence of the JCA was reported using TV 2D US in all cases (**Figure 6.6**). Two of these cases were published, one as a manuscript [Afaneh et al. (2020)] and the other case as an abstract [Zaghmout et al. (2017)] [38, 39]. It is worth of note that in the case published by Afaneh et al. (2020) [38], the dissection of the cystic lesion was difficult (**Figure 6.3a–d**) [38]. Although, the dissection of the cyst wall was done in piece meal, it was complete at the conclusion of the procedure (**Figure 6.3a–d**) [38]. The authors believe that in this case they were dealing with the typical JCA present in a focal area of adenomyosis [38]. On the other hand, in the case published by Zaghmout et al. (2016) [39], the dissection of the cyst wall was done easily from the myometrial bed and it was done in one piece, very similar to the dissection of a typical endometrioma from the ovarian bed (**Figure 6.4a–i**) [39]. Therefore, the authors named this lesion an endometrioma of the myometrium, especially that the pathology report revealed endometrial tissue in the cyst wall [39].

The presence of typical endometrioma outside the ovary is very rare. There are 4 reports of such endometrioma in the literature, all of them were found in the broad ligament. The first was reported by Whitehouse (1926) [40]. The second was reported by Rizzuto and Odejinmi (2009) [41]. More recently two other reports of endometrioma of the broad ligament were published [36, 37]. Trehan et al. (2014) [36] and Chauhan et al. (2017) [37] in their reports acknowledged that endometriomas can rarely be present within the broad ligament [36, 37]. These authors indicated that endometrioma within the broad ligament suggest that the etiology of endometriomas can (at least in some cases) be explained by methods other than retrograde menstruation [36, 37]. Chauhan et al. (2017) [37] suggested the possibility of Müllerian remnant etiology of the abnormal cystic lesion [37]. The authors indicated that laparoscopic excision of such lesions appear to be safe and effective in experienced hands [36, 37].

## Robotic-assisted laparoscopic excision of JCA

Another option for laparoscopic approach is utilizing the robotic system [26]. Akar et al. (2010) [26] described the first case of robotic-assisted laparoscopic excision in a case of JCA. The cyst was dissected with a higher degree of visualization and precise motion. The defect was closed in four layers [26]. The data

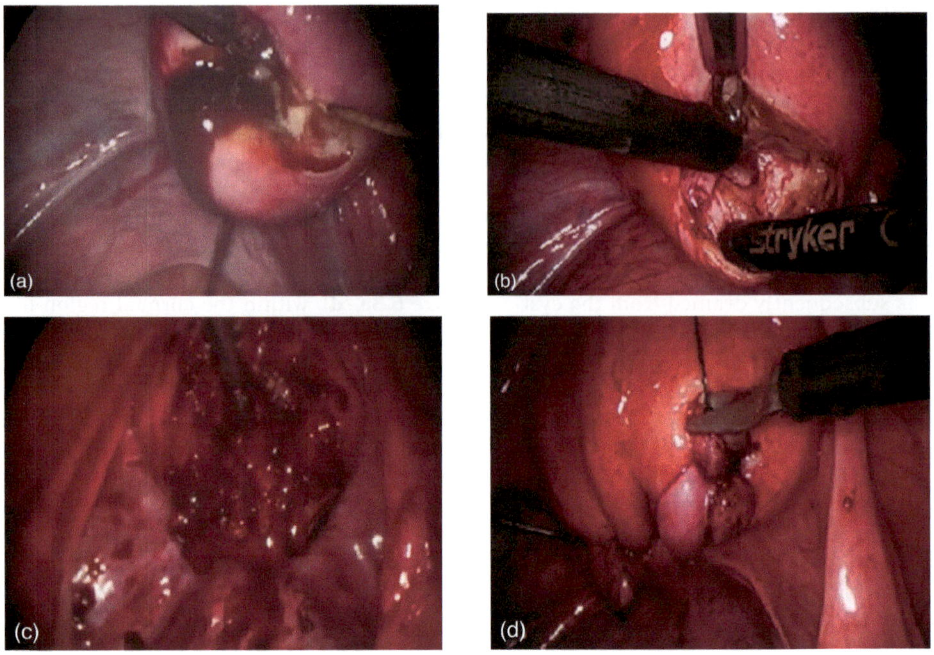


**FIGURE 6.3** Stages of laparoscopic excision of juvenile cystic adenomyoma in the patient in **Figures 6.1** and **6.2**. (a) Chocolate-like material exiting from the adenomyoma cyst on the posterior aspect of uterus. (b) Removal of the cyst wall bit by bit. (c) Adenomyoma cyst bed, following excision, with no evidence of entry of the endometrial cavity. (d) End result after two-layer repair of the adenomyoma cyst bed was carried out with a continuous 2-0 V-lock suture. (From Afaneh H, et al. Obstet Gynecol Cases Rev. 2020;7:162 [38]. With permission.)

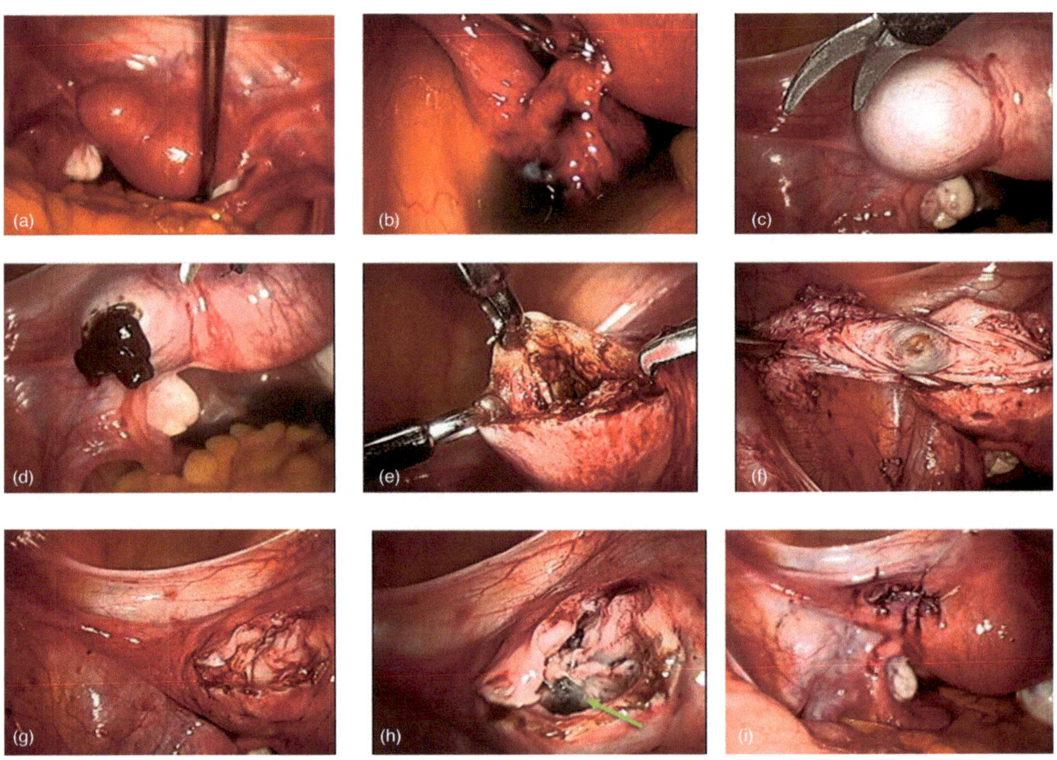


**FIGURE 6.4** Top row: (a,b) Cystic mass within the myometrium of the anterior wall of the uterus near the left cornual region in close proximity of the left fallopian tube which was patent. (c) Mass after injecting diluted vasopressin. Middle row: (d) Chocolate-like material exiting from the cystic mass after a transverse incision was made along the myometrium covering the cyst. (e) Cyst wall appears similar to that of endometrioma in the ovaries. (f) Final step of stripping the cyst wall from the myometrium in one piece. Bottom row: (g,h) Myometrial bed, after the cyst was excised, to be hemostatic, with the endometrial cavity entered in a small area (5 mm) with diluted indigo carmin dye seen (green arrow). (i) End result after the myometrial bed was repaired in three layers using interrupted figure of eight 2-0 Vicryl sutures.

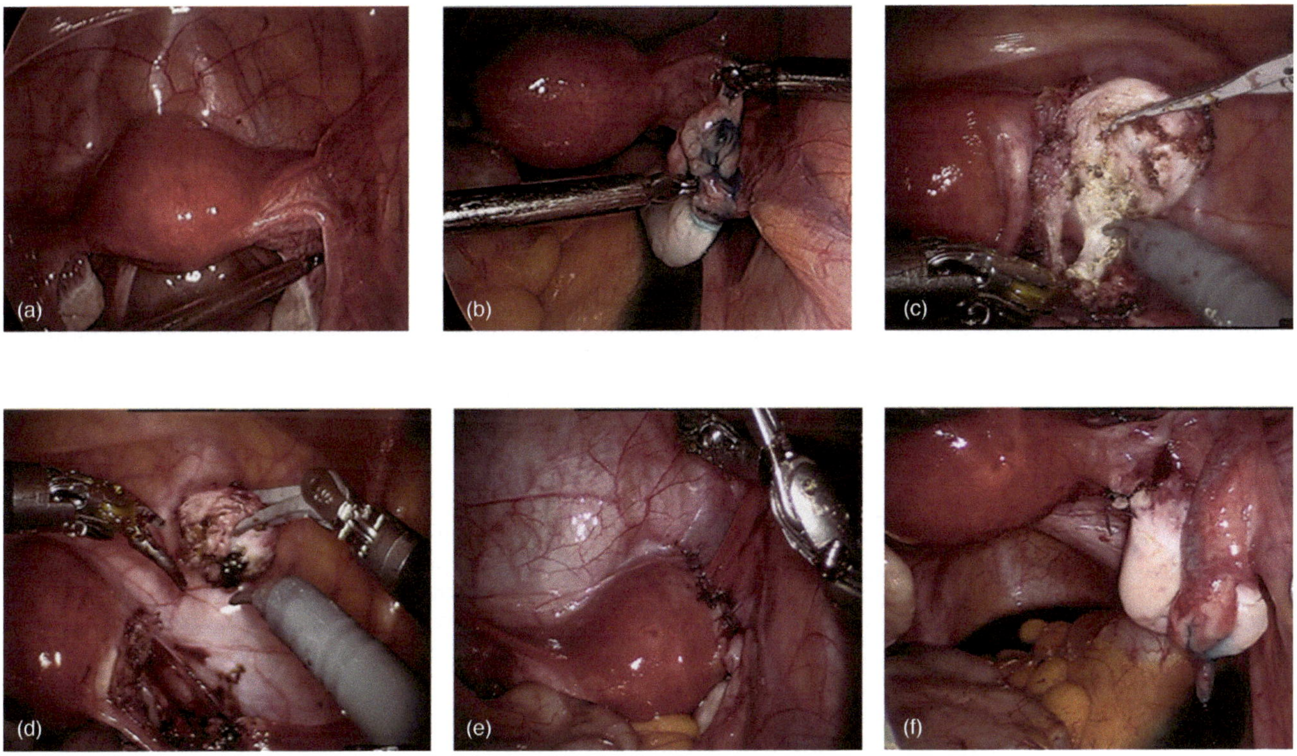


**FIGURE 6.5** Top row: (a,b) 2 cm juvenile cystic adenomyoma mass in the right broad ligament which appeared to be continuous with the myometrium near the right cornual region and in close proximity of the isthmic portion of the right fallopian tube which was patent. (c) Robotic-assisted laparoscopic excision of the cystic mass. Bottom row: (d) Robotic-assisted laparoscopic excision of the cystic mass. (e) End results of the surgery after suturing the broad ligament. (f) Tubal patency at the conclusion of the procedure.

on the risks of uterine rupture during pregnancy is limited. In theory, there may be an increased risk of such complication [42]. Akar et al. (2010) [26] suggested that the robotic-assisted approach would be not only more efficient but also safer for patients who conceive in the future [26].

The authors of this chapter performed a robotic-assisted laparoscopic excision in a case of JCA (unpublished data), (**Figure 6.5a–f**). The patient was a 27-year-old, gravida 0, with a history of chronic pelvic pain refractory to medical treatment with continuous oral contraceptive pills and 6 months of GnRH-a agonist. A diagnostic laparoscopy was performed by her gynecologist 1 year earlier and a 2 cm mass was found in broad ligament. The mass was not removed due to proximity to the isthmic portion of the right fallopian tube and the increased vascularity surrounding the mass from the right uterine artery. The mass was left in place and the patient was advised to have excision of the mass together with right salpingectomy at a later date. TV 2D and 3D US at our unit revealed a 3 cm cystic mass in the right broad ligament which appeared to be continuous with the myometrium near the right cornual region. The cystic mass was removed with preservation of the right fallopian tube via robotic-assisted operative laparoscopy. An area of healed endometriosis was present on left uterosacral ligaments and in the pouch of Douglas inferior to the right uterosacral ligament. The patient had uneventful recovery. The pathology report confirmed the presence of an endometrioma. Therefore, the diagnosis of juvenile cystic adenomyoma was made. The patient did have relief of her pain. Three months later, histosalpingogram (HSG) revealed patent tubes. She had a follow-up appointment 8 months following her surgery, and she continued to have relief of her previous symptoms.

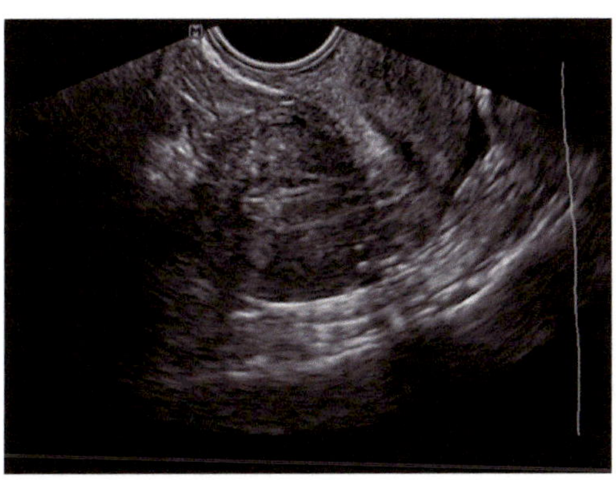

**FIGURE 6.6** Transvaginal 2D US performed 8 weeks after laparoscopic excision of the juvenile cystic adenomyoma in the patient in **Figures 6.1** and **6.2**, illustrating normal appearing uterus with no evidence of recurrence of the cyst.

## Laparotomy excision of JCA

Tamura et al. (1996) [8] described the first case of JCA in the literature which was successfully excised via laparotomy [8]. Kamio et al. (2007) [29] reported a successful excision of a 3 cm

JCA in a 23-year-old, nulliparous patient who was suffering from heavy menstrual bleeding and dysmenorrheal. Medical treatment failed after using different medications including, danazol, GnRH-a agonist and oral contraceptive therapy. The cyst was excised via laparotomy and there was no communication between the cyst and the endometrial cavity [29]. The authors reported complete disappearance of the patient's symptoms postoperatively [29]. Wang et al. (2007) [43] described a case of JCA that occurred after dilatation and curettage for cornual ectopic pregnancy. The cyst was excised successfully via laparotomy [43]. Few other reports of successful surgical treatment of JCA via laparotomy were published [17, 30, 44]. In addition, Nabeshima et al. 2007 [31] attempted to excise a JCA via laparotomy but they failed to localize the cyst [31]. Subsequently, these authors were successful to excise the cyst laparoscopically under ultrasound guidance intra-operatively as detailed above [31].

## Hysteroscopy resection of JCA

Alternatively, hysteroscopy can be considered with lesions that are more easily accessible through the endometrial cavity. Pontrelli et al. (2015) [27] encountered a cystic mass measuring 8 cm with locations along the posterior wall of the uterine cavity in a 27-year-old nulliparous patient [27]. The initial diagnosis was cornual hematometra within a bicornuate uterus on preoperative pelvic ultrasound scan and MRI. The thickness of the uterine wall below was very thin (4 mm) [27]. They decided to proceed with a diagnostic hysteroscopy to rule out bicornuate uterus. They encountered difficulty in distending the endometrial cavity due to a large cystic mass on the posterior wall of the uterus not communicating with the endometrial cavity. The decision was to proceed with operative hysteroscopy. A standard 26-Fr irrigating resectoscope (Karl Storz, GmbH, Germany) was used [27]. The distending medium used was sorbitol-mannitol solution [27]. A 2 cm incision was made into the posterior uterine wall using a monopolar resectoscope loop [27]. The cyst was exposed, and chocolate-like material drained [27]. The ability to irrigate, and suction with the resectoscope was essential for the success of this surgery [27]. Next, a right angled monopolar resectoscope loop was used to completely resect the cyst capsule from the anterior and lateral walls in small 3 mm chips [27]. In view of proximity of the posterior cyst wall to the serosal layer, they only coagulated that portion to avoid uterine perforation [27]. The procedure was uneventful. The pathology report confirmed the diagnosis of JCA. Patient's symptoms improved postoperatively [27]. At the conclusion of the operative hysteroscopy, the endometrial cavity appeared normal with a pouch in the posterior wall at the site of the previously removed lesion [27]. Subsequent pelvic ultrasound scans and hysteroscopies revealed a gradual decrease in the size of the posterior wall pouch and its complete disappearance, and normal appearance of the posterior wall 18 months postoperatively [27]. This unique method of surgical management requires further consideration by only very experienced reproductive surgeon and longtime evaluation of safety and efficacy especially during pregnancy and delivery.

## Surgical management of ACA

In ACA, the surgical treatment discussed in the literature includes both conservative minimally invasive surgery and hysterectomy. Chung et al. (1997) [45] described a deeply embedded lesion in the right broad ligament in a 41-year-old patient following tamoxifen therapy for 3 years due to breast cancer [45]. The mass was cystic in nature, located in the right broad ligament with a fibrous band connecting it to the uterus. Total abdominal hysterectomy with bilateral salpingo-oophorectomy was performed [45]. The pathology report confirmed adenomyosis with cyst formation and an unusual thick capsule, suggesting ACA [45]. Similarly, Isik et al. (2015) [46] performed a hysterectomy with bilateral salpingo-oophorectomy in a 47-year-old perimenopausal patient with ACA in the cervix [46]. Koga et al. (2006) [47] performed a hysterectomy in a 37-year-old patient for a giant ACA, 17 × 11 × 8 cm after a lack of response to GnRH-a agonist [47]. The patient's past history included two myomectomies and two dilation and curettage for a hydatidiform mole [47]. Two years prior to hysterectomy, she underwent transvaginal ultrasound guided aspiration of chocolate-like fluid cystic mass in the uterine wall and injection of ethanol, minocycline, and danazol [47]. After pregnancy and delivery by cesarean section, her symptoms worsened. The cyst contained 1150 mL of serous non-colored clear fluid [47]. The pathology report revealed the cyst was lined by stratified squamous cells, and partially lined by endometrial like epithelia with squamous metaplasia, suggesting the diagnosis of cystic adenomyosis with epithelial metaplasia [47].

Laparoscopic excision of ACA was reported in the literature. Calagna et al. (2015) [48] described a unique case of a pedunculated ACA that spread to a myoma in the uterus in a 39-year-old patient [48]. The cyst was successfully excised laparoscopically [48]. Shen et al. (2017) [49] reported a successful laparoscopic excision of a cystic adenomyoma that was preoperatively diagnosed as an adnexa chocolate cyst in a 37-year-old woman. At the time of laparoscopy, the patient was found to have stage IV endometriosis and extensive pelvic adhesions [49]. Postoperative patient's symptoms of dysmenorrhea and dyschezia were improved significantly [49]. Patient was also placed on oral progestogen to prevent recurrence and the authors reported no recurrence 6 months after the surgery [49].

ACA is considered benign lesions. However, Mori et al. (2015) [50] reported a case of a 67-year-old asymptomatic patient who was evaluated for a cystic lesion in the pelvis. Total abdominal hysterectomy with bilateral salpingo-oophorectomy was performed [50]. The patient was found to have an endometrioid adenocarcinoma arising from cystic adenomyosis [50]. The authors suggested that cystic adenomyoma possesses the risk of malignant transformation. They stressed the importance of long-term follow-up with imaging examination [50].

## Conclusion

Cystic adenomyoma are represented infrequently in the literature but present a clinical and surgical challenge to the gynecologist. The exact pathogenesis is incompletely understood but it is acknowledged that there is possible difference in the pathogenesis depending on dealing with adult vs juvenile type. The symptoms of dysmenorrhea, pelvic pain and dyspareunia can be remarkably debilitating. The approach to therapy depends highly on a patient's desire for future fertility. Medical treatment can be attempted in patients with JCA, but if it fails one should proceed with surgical treatment. For women wishing to preserve their fertility potential and require surgery, we encourage the minimally invasive approach. Laparoscopic surgery is a safe and effective option in experienced hands. Robotic-assisted laparoscopic surgery may have a role in certain cases. However, laparotomy and hysterectomy are options for select patients.

## References

1. Hoffman B, Schorge J, Bradshaw K, Halvorson L, Schaffer J, Corton M. *Williams Gynecology*. New York, McGraw-Hill Education 2016:213.
2. Brosens I. Uterine cystic adenomyosis: A disease of younger women. *J Pediatr Adol Gynec*. 2015;28(6):420–426. https://doi:10.1016/j.jpag.2014.05.008
3. Habiba M, Benagiano G, Brosens I. *Uterine Adenomyosis*. Marwan Habiba and Giuseppe Benagiano Editors, Springer International Publishing Switzerland 2016;2015:163–167. https://doi.10.1007/978-3-319-13012-5
4. Gordts S, Grimbizis G, Campo R. Symptoms and classification of uterine adenomyosis, including the place of hysteroscopy in diagnosis. *Fert Steril*. 2018;109(3):380–388.e1. https://doi.org/10.1016/j.fertnstert.2018.01.006
5. Branquinho MM, Marques AL, Leite HB, Silva IS. Juvenile cystic adenomyoma. *Case Reports*. 2012;2012:bcr2012007006. https://doi:10.1136/bcr-2012-007006
6. Cullen TS. Adenomyoma of the uterus. *Am J Med Sci*. 1909; 137(1):121–122.
7. Garcia L and Isaacson K. Adenomyosis: Review of the Literature. *J Minimal Invasive Gynecol*. 2011;18(4):428–437. https://doi.org/10.1016/j.jmig.2011.04.004
8. Tamura M, Fukaya T, Takaya R, Ip CW, Yajima A. Juvenile adenomyotic cyst of the corpus uteri with dysmenorrhea. *Tohoku J Exp Med*. 1996;178(3):339–344. https://doi.org/10.1620/tjem.178.339
9. Acién P, Acién M, Fernández F, Mayol MJ, Aranda I. The cavitated accessory uterine mass. *Obstet Gynecol*. 2010;116(5):1101–1109. https://doi:10.1097/aog.0b013e3181f7e735
10. Acién P, del Campo FS, Mayol MJ, Acién M. The female gubernaculum: role in the embryology and development of the genital tract and in the possible genesis of malformations. *Eur J Obstet Gyn RB*. 2011;159(2):426–432.
11. Dadhwal V, Sharma A, Khoiwal K. Juvenile cystic adenomyoma mimicking a uterine anomaly: a report of two cases. *Eurasian J Med*. 2017;49(1):59–61. https://doi:10.5152/eurasianjmed.2017.17028
12. Troiano RN, Flynn SD, and McCarthy S. Cystic adenomyosis of the uterus: MRI. J Magn Reson Imaging. 1998;8(6):1198–1202. https://doi:10.1002/jmri.1880080603
13. Takeuchi H, Kitade M, Kikuchi I, Kumakiri J, Kuroda K, Jinushi M. Diagnosis, laparoscopic management, and histopathologic findings of juvenile cystic adenomyoma: a review of nine cases. *Fertil Steril*. 2010;94(3):862–868. https://doi.org/10.1016/j.fertnstert.2009.05.010
14. Kriplani A, Mahey R, Agarwal N, Bhatla N, Yadav R, Singh MK. Laparoscopic management of juvenile cystic adenomyoma: four cases. *J Minimal Invasive Gynecol*. 2011;18(3):343–348. https://doi:10.1016/j.jmig.2011.02.001
15. Ball E, Ganji M, Janik G, Koh C. Laparoscopic resection of cystic adenomyosis in a teenager with arcurate uterus. *Gynecol Surg*. 2009;6(4):367–370. https://doi:10.1007/s10397-009-0505-3
16. Shah N, Paranjpe SH, Puri J. Juvenile cystic adenomyoma managed laparoscopically. http://www.jpgo.org/2018/08/juvenile-cystic-adenomyoma-managed.html.
17. Dogan E, Gode F, Saatli B, Seçil M. Juvenile cystic adenomyosis mimicking uterine malformation: a case report. *Arch Gynecol Obstet*. 2008;278(6):593–595. https://doi:10.1007/s00404-008-0618-3
18. Krentel H, Cezar C, Becker S, Di Spiezio S, Tanos V, Wallwiener M, De Wilde RL. From clinical symptoms to MR imaging: diagnostic steps in adenomyosis. *Biomed Res Int*. 2017;2017:1514029. https://doi:10.1155/2017/1514029
19. The American Fertility Society classifications of adnexal adhesions, distal tubal occlusion, tubal occlusion secondary to tubal ligation, tubal pregnancies, Müllerian anomalies and intrauterine adhesions. *Fertil Steril*. 1988;49(6):944–955.
20. Santiago I, Cavalheiro F, Coelho P, Noruégas MJ, Sanches MC. Juvenile cystic adenomyosis. *Eurorad*. 2011 https://doi10.1594/EURORAD/CASE.9066
21. Kataoka ML, Togashi K, Konishi I, et al. MRI of adenomyotic cyst of the uterus. *J Comput Assist Tomogr*. 1998;22(4):555–559. https://doi:10.1097/00004728-199807000-00010
22. Green LJ, Sokhi T, Balogun M, Ganesan R. Myometrial cysts: a case series. *Case Rep Women Health*. 2019;24:e00155. https://doi.org/10.1016/j.crwh.2019.e00155
23. Ho M, Raptis C, Hulett R, McAlister W, Moran K, Bhalla S. Adenomyotic cyst of the uterus in an adolescent. *Pediatr Radiol*. 2008;38(11):1239–1242. https://doi:10.1007/s00247-008-0948-0
24. American College of Obstetricians and Gynecologists. Practice Bulletin No. 114: Management of endometriosis. *Obstet Gynecol*. 2010; 116(1):223–36. https://doi10.1097/AOG.0b013e3181e8b073
25. Fisseha S, Smith YR, Kumetz LM, Mueller GC, Hussain H, Quint EH. Cystic myometrial lesion in the uterus of an adolescent girl. *Fertil Steril*. 2006;86(3):716–718. https://doi:10.1016/j.fertnstert.2006.03.019
26. Akar ME, Leezer KH, Yalcinkaya TM. Robot-assisted laparoscopic management of a case with juvenile cystic adenomyoma. *Fertil Steril*. 2010;94(3):e55–e56. https://doi:10.1016/j.fertnstert.2010.06.001
27. Pontrelli G, Bounous VE, Scarperi S, Minelli L, Di Spiezio Sardo A, Florio P. Rare case of giant cystic adenomyoma mimicking a uterine malformation, diagnosed and treated by hysteroscopy. *J Obstet Gyn Res*. 2015;41(8):1300–1304.
28. Deblaere L, Froyman W, Van den Bosch T, van Rompuy AS, Kaijser J, Deprest J, Timmerman D. Juvenile cystic adenomyosis: a case report and review of the literature. *Australasian J Ultrasound Med*. 2019;22(4):295–300. https://doi:10.1002/ajum.12171
29. Kamio M, Taguchi S, Oki T, Tsuji T, Iwamoto I, Yoshinaga M, Douchi T. Isolated adenomyotic cyst associated with severe dysmenorrhea. *J Obstet Gynecol Res*. 2007;33(3):388–391. https://doi:10.1111/j.1447-0756.2007.00543.x
30. Ho ML, Ratts V, Merritt D. Adenomyotic cyst in an adolescent girl. *J Pediatr Adolesc Gynecol*. 2009;22:e33–e38.
31. Nabeshima H, Murakami T, Nishimoto M, Sugawara N, Sato N. Successful total laparoscopic cystic adenomyomectomy after unsuccessful open surgery using transtrocar ultrasonographic guiding. *J Minimal Invasive Gynecol*. 2008;15(2):227–230. https://doi:10.1016/j.jmig.2007.10.007
32. Grimbizis GF, Mikos T, Zepiridis L, Theodoridis T, Miliaras D, Tarlatzis BC, Bontis JN. Laparoscopic excision of uterine adenomyomas. *Fertil Steril*. 2008;89:953–961.
33. Takeda A, Sakai K, Mitsui T, Nakamura H. Laparoscopic management of juvenile cystic adenomyoma of the uterus: Report of two cases and review of the literature. *J Minimal Invasive Gynecol*. 2007;14(3):370–374. https://doi:10.1016/j.jmig.2007.01.005
34. Jain N, Goel S. Cystic adenomyoma simulates uterine malformation: a diagnostic dilemma: case report of two unusual cases. *J Hum Reprod Sci*. 2012;5(2):285–288. https://doi.10.4103/0974-1208.106342
35. Strelec M, Banovic M, Banovic V, Sirovec A. Juvenile cystic adenomyoma mimicking a Müllerian uterine anomaly successfully treated by laparoscopic excision. *Int J Gyecol Obstet*. 2019;142(2):265–266. https://doi.10.1002/ijgo.12864
36. Trehan A, Trehan AK. Endometrioma contained within the broad ligament. *BMJ Case Rep*. 2014;2014:bcr2013203441. https://doi.10.1136/bcr-2013-203441
37. Chauhan R, Dadhich R, Sahu B, Sahni S. Endometriosis in broad ligament: a rare case. *Int J Reprod Contracept Obstet Gynecol*. 2017; 6:2676.
38. Afaneh H, Moses K, Young O, Abuzeid M Surgical management of a juvenile cystic adenomyoma: a unique presentation of adenomyosis. *Obstet Gynecol Cases Rev*. 2020;7:162. https://doi.org/10.23937/2377-9004/1410162
39. Zaghmout OA, Abuzeid O, Heber J, Abuzeid M. Endometrioma embedded within the myometrium. *Am J Obstet Gynecol*. 2017; S629:34.
40. Whitehouse HB. Endometrioma between the layers of the broad ligament. *Proc R Soc Med, Obstet_Gynaecol*. 1926;19:16.

41. Rizzuto MI, Odejinmi F. Laparoscopic 'day case' management of an 'endometrioma' within the broad ligament. *J Obstet Gynaecol.* 2009;29(6):561–562.
42. Koo YJ, Im KS, Kwon YS. Conservative surgical treatment combined with GnRH agonist in symptomatic uterine adenomyosis. Pak J Med Sci 2011;27(2):365–370.
43. Wang JH, Wu RJ, Xu KH, Lin J. Single large cystic adenomyoma of the uterus after cornual pregnancy and curettage. *Fertil Steril.* 2007;88(4):965–967.
44. Manta L, Suciu N, Constantin A, Toader O, Popa F. Focal adenomyosis (intramural endometriotic cyst) in a very young patient - differential diagnosis with uterine fibromatosis. *J Med Life.*2016;9(2):180–182.
45. Chung YP, Lin HH, Sheu BC, Mao TL, Chang DY, Huang SC. Adenomyosis in the broad ligament and tamoxifen: report of a case. *J Obstet Gynecol Res.* 1997;23(1):69–73.
46. Isik Y, Dag ZO, Celik H. A giant adenomyotic cyst originating from the cervix. *International J Gynecol Obstet.* 2015;131:205–208.
47. Koga K, Osuga Y, Hiroi H, et al. A case of giant cystic adenomyosis. *Fertil Steril.* 2006;85(3):748–749.
48. Calagna G, Cucinella G, Tonni G, et al. Cystic adenomyosis spreading into subserosal-peduncolated myoma: How to explain it? *Int J Surg Case Rep.* 2015;8:29–31.
49. Shen J, Masuda K, Onoue M, et al. A case of difficult to diagnose cystic adenomyoma treated with laparoscopic surgery. *Clin Obstet Gynecol Reprod Med.* 2017;3(6). https://doi:10.15761/cogrm.1000199
50. Mori M, Furusawa A, Kino N, Uno M, Ozaki Y, Yasugi T. Rare case of endometrioid adenocarcinoma arising from cystic adenomyosis. *J Obstet Gynecol Res.* 2015;41(2):324–328. https://doi.101111/jog.12513

# 7

## DEEP-INFILTRATING ENDOMETRIOSIS

**Nupur Tamhane and Emad Mikhail**

### Definition and epidemiology

Endometriosis is an inflammatory condition defined by the presence of endometrium like tissue outside the uterus, predominantly but not exclusively in the pelvic compartment. Its prevalence is estimated to be 10% of reproductive aged females [1, 2].

Deep-infiltrating endometriosis (DIE) is a phenotype of endometriosis characterized by infiltration depth > 5 mm in the peritoneum with the presence of endometrial implants, fibrosis, and muscular hyperplasia [3, 4]. DIE is broadly subdivided into the anterior compartment disease involving the bladder and the posterior compartment involving the vagina, uterosacral ligaments (USL), rectum, rectovaginal septum (RVS), and the ureters. The prevalence of deep pelvic endometriosis is estimated to be 15%–30% of the women suffering from endometriosis [5–7]. The order of involvement of DIE from highest to lowest occurrence is uterosacral ligament, rectosigmoid colon (**Figure 7.1**), vagina (**Figure 7.2**), and the bladder (**Figure 7.3**) [8].

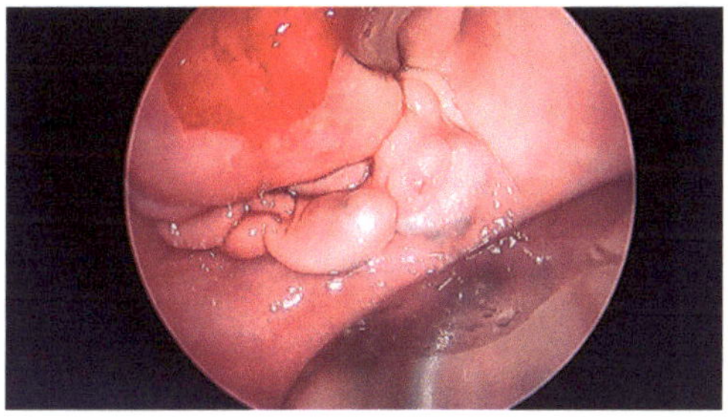

FIGURE 7.2 Posterior Fornix DIE.

### Clinical presentation

The clinical presentation of patients with endometriosis varies with a wide spectrum of symptoms ranging from being asymptomatic to experiencing severe pain. Endometriosis usually presents with chronic pelvic pain lasting > 6 months and is associated with dysmenorrhea, dyspareunia, deep pelvic pain, and lower abdominal pain with or without back pain [9]. Dysmenorrhea (80%) and deep dyspareunia (30%) are considered the most frequent symptoms of endometriosis [10, 11]. Other less frequent symptoms are dyschezia, dysuria, and inter-menstrual pelvic pain and are often associated with anatomic location of lesions or ovulation [12]. Characteristic of pain may vary and eventually worsen over time. Moreover, DIE is associated with more severe pain and infertility [12]. Hyperalgesia described as excruciating pain with nonpainful stimuli is observed in some women especially with deep endometriosis. It is a result of invasion of sensory nerve fibers by endometriotic stromal cells in turn engaging a vicious inflammatory cascade [13, 14]. However, no symptoms are specific to endometriosis and the estimated prevalence of endometriosis in symptomatic population is 35%–50% [9].

Correlation is observed between anatomic location and type of endometriotic pain [15]. This is demonstrated by conspicuous association of deep dyspareunia with deep-infiltrating lesions of the uterosacral and cardinal ligaments, pouch of Douglas, posterior vaginal fornix, and anterior rectal wall [10, 12, 15, 16]. Bladder and bowel associated symptoms such as nausea, distension, early satiety, constipation, urinary urgency, dysuria appear cyclically in some patients [17].

Despite the correlation of symptoms and anatomic location of DIE, clinical examination has reduced value for assessing the extent of the disease and majority of DIE nodules are not diagnosed on clinical examination [18]. However, certain positive signs on clinical examination can alarm the clinician to suspect DIE. Fixed uterine retroversion or painful uterine mobilization are frequently observed due to USL infiltration or Pouch of Douglas (POD) adhesions indicating DIE [19]. Digital vaginal or rectal examination may reveal a hard, tender nodule on posterior vaginal fornix or rectal wall indicating bowel involvement [20].

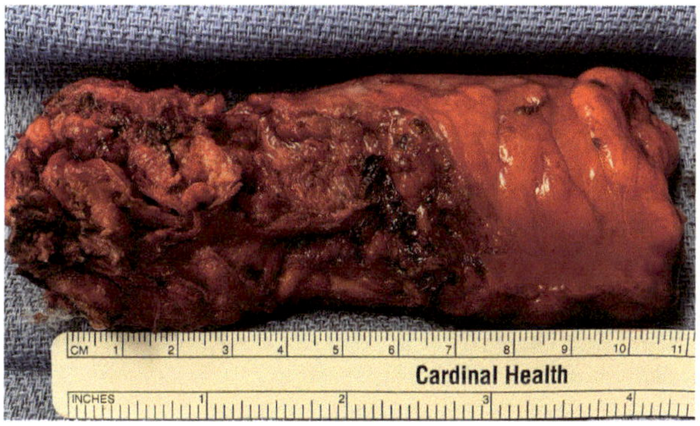



FIGURE 7.1 Surgical specimen of DIE of the rectum post low anterior resection.

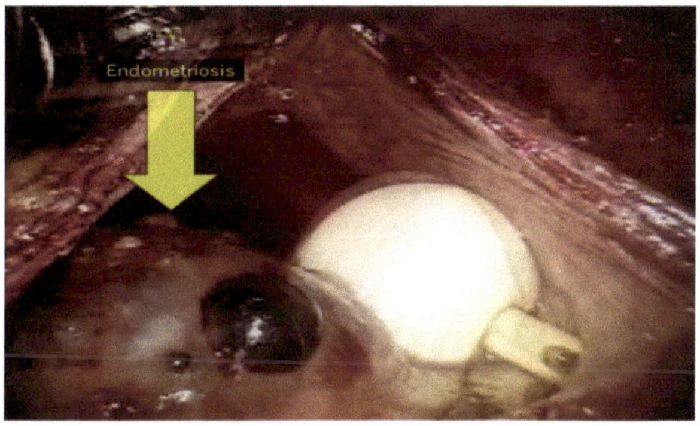



FIGURE 7.3 Large DIE nodule of the bladder.

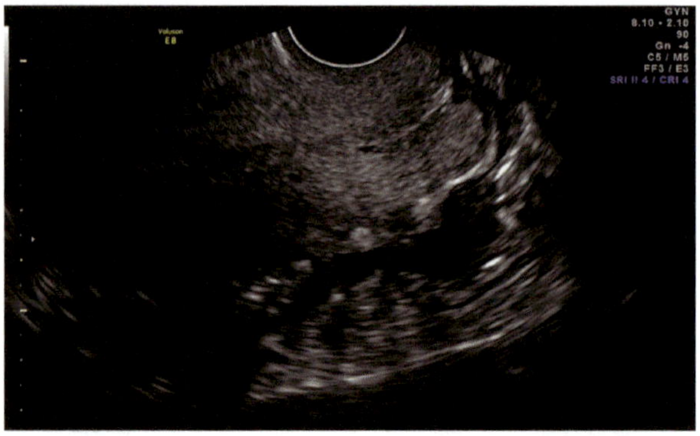

**FIGURE 7.4** 2D TV US image of DIE of the rectovaginal septum.

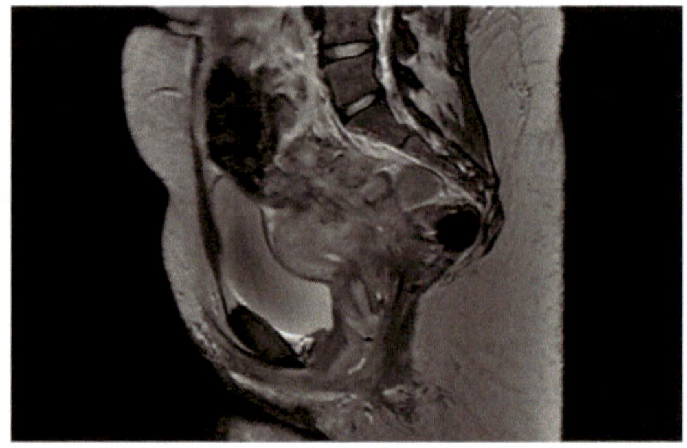

**FIGURE 7.6** T2 sagittal MRI image showing DIE of the rectovaginal septum.

## Diagnosis

In the event of clinical suspicion of DIE, it can be further evaluated by diagnostic tests such as transvaginal ultrasonography (TV US), rectosigmoid endoscopy sonography (RES), and MRI. TV US is considered first line diagnostic tool as it is cheaper than MRI but it is operator dependent.

TVUS in hands of an experienced operator and in consultation with a clinician or surgeon is a useful tool [18]. The sensitivity, specificity, and positive and negative predictive values of TV US for the diagnosis of deep pelvic endometriosis are found to be 78.5%, 95.2%, 95.4%, and 77.9%, respectively (**Figure 7.4**) [21]. A recent IDEA (International Deep Endometriosis Analysis Group) study formulated few fundamental steps to improve diagnosis of DIE on TV US; routine examination of uterus and adnexa for presence or absence of disease, evaluation of TV US soft markers like specific tenderness and ovarian mobility, POD assessment, and evaluation of DIE nodules in anterior and posterior compartment (**Figure 7.5**) [22]. Nevertheless, a positive ultrasonographic diagnosis of endometriosis in absence of symptoms should not be considered as an indication of surgery [18].

MRI is another extremely effective diagnostic tool to confirm clinical suspicion of endometriosis as it is not operator dependent and can provide details about lesions even at the level of sigmoid colon [4, 23, 24]. It is also a valuable tool for surgical planning and incorporation of multidisciplinary team approach if indicated (**Figure 7.6**).

Rectal endoscopy sonography (RES) is a diagnostic procedure that involves use of endoscopic sonography through the rectum with the lesions of DIE identified as hypoechoic nodules or mass. Diagnostic accuracy of RES for rectosigmoid endometriosis is only slightly higher than MRI [pooled sensitivity was 0.84 (95% CI 0.79–0.88) for MRI, and 0.91 (95% CI 0.87–0.94) for RES]. Additionally, RES has limited value as compared to MRI for diagnosis of DIE in locations other than intestinal endometriosis [25].

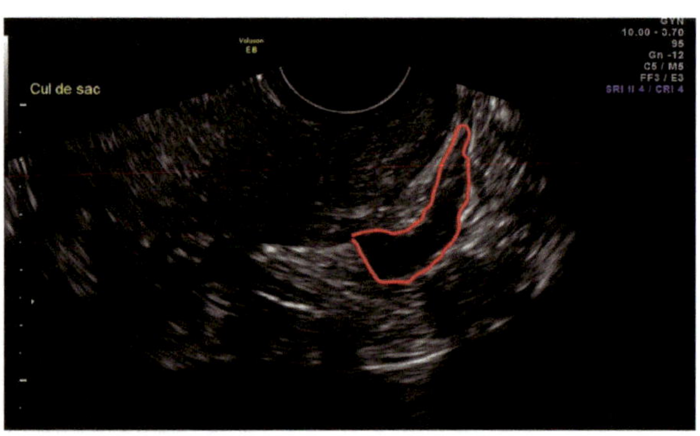


**FIGURE 7.5** 2D TV US images with DIE nodule of the anterior rectal wall marked.

Initially, it was observed that TV US did not prove to be very helpful in diagnosis of sigmoid endometriosis [26] and studies also demonstrated that MRI had a higher sensitivity for diagnosis of uterosacral ligament (84.4%) and vaginal endometriosis ((80%) [4]. However, a recent meta-analysis concluded that TV US is not inferior to MRI in diagnosis of DIE of uterosacral ligament, rectovaginal septum, and rectosigmoid [27]. Hence to summarize, TVUS should be considered primary approach for DIE diagnosis as it is less invasive than RES and less expensive than MRI [27]. MRI should be reserved for centers where highly skilled sonographers are not available.

The requirement for noninvasive diagnostic test cannot be emphasized enough and hence numerous blood biomarkers for diagnosis of endometriosis such as CA-125, CA-19.9, IL-6 (to name a few) have also been studied. However, none have proved clinically accurate for diagnosing endometriosis [28].

Nevertheless laparoscopic surgical evaluation and histopathological examination remains the gold standard for diagnosis of endometriosis [19]. The major factor influencing the decision for surgery is clinical evaluation as compared to radiographic evaluation. MRI and TV US provide invaluable information preoperatively in terms of size estimation, location, lateral extensions of the lesions, etc. [29].

## Surgical management

Laparoscopy due to its advantages of lesser complications and faster recovery time is the preferred technique to evaluate and treat benign conditions in the pelvis and the abdomen [30]. It also provides a better visualization of the peritoneal cavity due to its magnified view and is the only acceptable method till date to determine the extent and severity of the disease [28]. Despite various classification systems for endometriosis, the extensively used and internationally accepted rASRM (revised American Society for Reproductive Medicine) classification system uses characteristics visualized during laparoscopy such as appearance, size, depth of implants, adhesions [31].

The ESHRE guidelines (European Society of Human Reproduction and Embryology Special Interest Group for Endometriosis) also reinstated the fact that for most forms of endometriosis, symptomatic women cannot obtain a definitive diagnosis without laparoscopic inspection of the pelvis [32]. Nonetheless only a third of women undergoing a laparoscopic procedure receive a diagnosis of endometriosis and therefore many disease-free women are unnecessarily exposed to surgical risk [33]. The validity of laparoscopy as a diagnostic test for endometriosis is highly dependent on the skills of the surgeon and should preferably be performed by an experienced surgeon [28].

Additionally, laparoscopy provides opportunity to excise the entire diseases portion including adhesions, peritoneal lesions, endometriomas, and deep-infiltrating lesion. DIE should be managed by only expert surgeons and preferably at specialized centers with multidisciplinary team including colorectal surgeon or urologist or both [19].

Surgical technique for management of endometriosis depends on age of the patient, severity of symptoms, extent and location of disease, and her desire for future fertility.

## Urologic endometriosis

Urologic involvement is seen in 1.2%–3.9% of women with endometriosis [34]. Bladder (84%) is most common location of urinary tract endometriosis and the retro-trigone and dome of bladder are frequently affected sites [35]. Sixty percent of these patients initially present with cyclic micturition syndrome [35, 36]. Bladder endometriosis can be confirmed by cystoscopic biopsy in certain cases. Other common locations of urinary endometriosis are ureter (15%), kidney (4%), and urethra (2%) [37]. It has also been observed by Knabben et al. that patients with endometriosis of bladder are frequently symptomatic as compared to those with ureteric involvement [38].

Ureteral involvement is commonly extrinsic and leads to compression and fibrosis of ureters while the intrinsic lesions are less frequent, originating from lymphatic or venous drainage and leading to obstruction or cyclic hematuria [39]. Intrinsic ureteral endometriosis can be evaluated effectively with excretory urography [40]. Ureteral endometriosis affects kidney function in <30% of cases. Notably 50% of ureteral endometriosis patients are asymptomatic [41]. Hence, preoperative diagnosis of hydronephrosis is essential as it is associated with 18% intra-operative ureteral lesions and necessitates preoperative ureteral stenting [42]. This diagnosis can be accomplished by ultrasound, contrast MRI, and CT scans.

MRI has increased specificity in diagnosing urinary endometriosis and differentiating from other benign and malignant urinary pathology [43]. A noteworthy correlation was observed by Knabben et al. between the ureteral involvement and size of rectovaginal nodule, nodule > 30 mm had four-fold risk of ureteral endometriosis [38].

Surgery is treatment of choice for urinary tract endometriosis [35] and the choice of surgery depends on location, extent of involvement of the urinary tract and experience of the surgeon [44]. Laparoscopic conservative management for bladder and ureteral endometriosis has consistently proved to be feasible and safe choice [44–47].

Ureterolysis is generally performed for minimal, intrinsic, and non-obstructive ureteral endometriosis while segmental ureteral resection is reserved for more severe and infiltrative cases. Ureterocystoneotomy restores the urinary tract axis in patients undergoing ureteric resection. Double J stents are usually used for few weeks postoperatively.

Surgery of choice for bladder endometriosis is partial cystectomy with complete excision of all bladder lesions [37, 45, 47, 48]. Special attention to the ureteral orifices is needed during resection and repair. Sieracchioli et al. have demonstrated that these approaches in management of urinary tract endometriosis also significantly reduce preoperative symptoms without relapse at long-term follow-up [48]. Bladder surgeries can typically be performed by an expert gynecologic laparoscopic surgeon, however ureteral resection and reconstruction is a complex surgery requiring involvement of urologists with expertise [19].

## Colorectal endometriosis

Gastrointestinal tract is the most common extra genital pelvic location of endometriotic lesions [49, 50]. The prevalence of bowel endometriosis is estimated to be 3.8%–37% of all the patients with endometriosis [51]. The most frequent anatomic location of colorectal endometriosis is sigmoid colon (>65% cases), followed by rectum, ileum, appendix and cecum [52]. Other sites are appendiceal endometriosis, observed in 5%–20% patients [53–55], small intestinal lesions comprise 5%–16%, and mostly affect the terminal ileum [56, 57] and few extremely rare locations are the gallbladder, Meckel diverticulum, stomach, and endometriotic cyst of pancreas and liver [58]. Majority of GI lesions affect the serosal surface and they are categorized as deep endometriosis only after the muscularis layer is invaded [59, 60]. Multifocality is commonly observed in intestinal deep endometriosis. Multifocal lesions are deep lesions found within 2 cm of main area and are encountered in 62% cases while multicentric lesions are satellite nodule found > 2 cm from main lesion and observed in 38% cases [61]. Laparoscopy remains gold standard for diagnosis and GI endometriosis may be accidentally encountered during surgery due to its nonspecific preoperative signs [62].

Several studies have demonstrated that removal of endometriotic lesions is beneficial leading to improvement in GI symptoms and quality of life [63–65]. The decision to choose a technique for rectal and sigmoid endometriosis is determined by clinical factors, imaging characteristics, recurrence rate and impact on quality of life [60].

Superficial bowel lesions affecting the serosal surface are removed by a process called shaving that involves lifting the lesion with grasping forceps and simultaneously excising it with sharp or blunt dissection [66]. Diathermy excision advocates caution due to thermal damage to bowel. Additionally, any defect in the bowel wall should be repaired by interrupted sutures [67]. However, care should be taken that the direction of the suture needle is parallel to the long axis of the bowel to prevent postoperative stenosis of the lumen.

Another technique used for bowel endometriosis repair is full thickness disc excision. It is reserved for cases where submucosal fibrosis is present and luminal entry is inevitable [68]. In this technique, two stay sutures are applied on either side of bowel defect that aid in transforming it into transverse defect and the bowel lumen is then closed intracorporeally [69]. This technique can be modified for low rectal lesions and for disease involving less than one-third circumference of rectum by using a circular stapler. The entire defect is enclosed in the stapler and removed through the anus after firing the stapler [70] (**Figure 7.7**).

Laparoscopic segmental resection and anastomosis is a technique that is proven to be safe and feasible and performed in cases of single lesion ≥3 cm in diameter, single lesion infiltrating ≥50% of the bowel wall, and if more than 3 lesions infiltrating the muscular layer are present [63]. Bowel resection is preferred to other conservative methods as it has lower recurrence rate however it comes at a cost of increased complications [71]. Postoperative

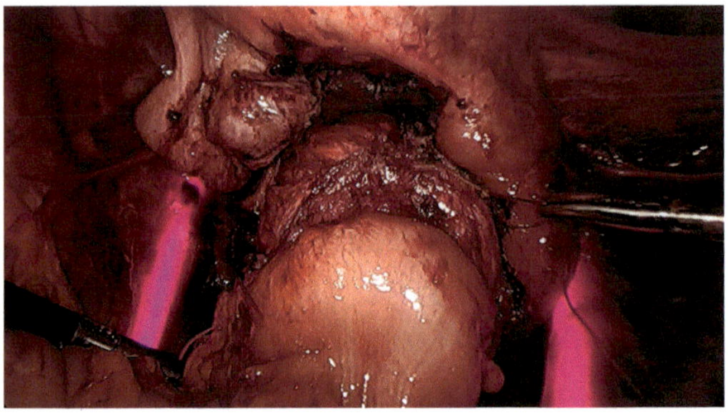

**FIGURE 7.7** Laparoscopic view for discoid excision using transanal stapler.

complications commonly observed are rectovaginal fistula, anastomotic leak and pelvic abscesses. The major risk factors for complications are opening of the vagina at the time of the bowel surgical procedure [72]; excessive use of electrocoagulation increasing the risk of rectovaginal fistulae and abscesses; and surgical treatment of low rectal lesions (5–8 cm from the anal verge) which increases the risk of anastomotic leaks [73, 74]. Hence, it is important to consider all factors before deciding the technique to excise deep endometriotic lesion of the bowel (**Figure 7.8**).

A large retrospective cohort study of 371 consecutive patients with deep endometriosis of rectosigmoid was conducted. It was observed that rate of complications was 11.8% and two-third of the cases were treated by bowel resection ($p < 0.001$) [75]. It was also observed that the surgical groups were not similar in characteristics, with more severe and extensive disease present in resection group. Hence, they concluded that a strategy to prioritize shaving should be employed whenever possible to decrease complication rate but also the advantages of resection for extensive disease should be assessed against the complications which could very well be due to the severity of the disease.

The results of a recent RCT conducted by Roman et al. suggested that there was no long-term difference in surgical outcomes between discoid excision and bowel resection. The 5 year-recurrence rate for discoid excision was 3.7% compared to 0% for resection ($P = 1$), and 55.6% versus 53.6% of patients subjectively reported normal bowel movements ($P = 1$) [76].

Data has also consistently shown that shaving is feasible even in advanced disease. The recurrence of pain for the patients undergone shaving is <10% [77, 78] with 4% at 3-year follow-up [78] and 8.7% after 5-year follow-up [79]. The risk of immediate complications after conservative approach is lower than after colorectal resection, allowing for better functional outcomes. The alleged higher risk of recurrence of disease after shaving has also not been demonstrated. Hence, Roman et al. concluded that surgeons should consider rectal shaving as a first-line surgical treatment of rectovaginal DE, regardless of nodule size or association with other digestive localizations, disc excision should be performed with unsatisfactory shaving and ultimately segmental resection should be reserved for advanced lesions causing major stenosis or cases with multiple nodules infiltrating the rectosigmoid junction or sigmoid colon [80].

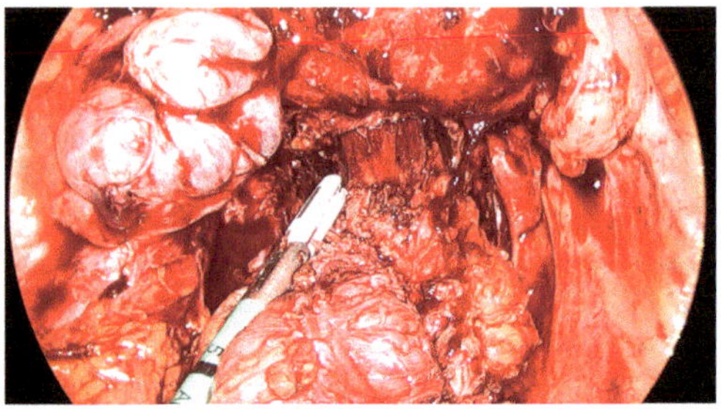

**FIGURE 7.8** Laparoscopic view of DIE nodule of the rectum.

## Latest advances for intra-operative visualization

### ICG dye

Indocyanine green (ICG) is a sterile, anionic, water-soluble but relatively hydrophobic tricarbocyanine fluorophore dye that can be used under near infrared (NIR) fluorescence to assess perfusion and highlight the desired anatomy. ICG due to its non-toxic and non-ionizing property has a good safety profile. The high signal to noise ratio of ICG allows illumination of the target more than the background thus producing good contrast [81]. ICG fluoresces green in NIR spectrum at wavelengths equal to or longer than 820 nm [82]. In recent years ICG has been incorporated in laparoscopic surgery to improve the view and highlight the anatomical details during surgery [83, 84].

Identification of endometriotic lesions is essential as incomplete resection during primary surgery results in postoperative recurrence [85, 86]. Appearance of peritoneal endometriosis varies greatly ranging from non-pigmented subtle lesions to hypervascularized areas described as powder burns [87, 88]. Application of ICG fluorescence in endometriosis involves detecting the hyper-vascularization of occult endometriotic lesions due to angiogenesis as a result of chronic inflammation [89]. This principle was used by Cosentino et al. in their pilot study for patients undergoing laparoscopic procedures for endometriosis by injecting 0.25 mg/kg ICG dye intravenously. They removed a total of 116 lesion by NIR imaging, 100 of which were already detected by white light and found a PPV of 97.8%, NPV of 82.3%, sensitivity of 82%, and specificity of 97.9% [90]. Levey et al. have described similar procedure in their case report where they used a 5 mg bolus of ICG intravenously and the endometriotic lesions suspected on conventional laparoscopic mode fluoresced green in NIR imaging mode of the robotic system. An additional area that appeared normal on conventional mode was detected by fluorescence only and later confirmed positive on histological examination [91]. Neef et al. in their preliminary study found that ICG in dose of 0.25 mg/kg was beneficial in delineating deep-infiltrating endometriotic lesions of the rectovaginal septum from the healthy rectal tissues during laparoscopic procedures and achieved complete macroscopic resection without rectal perforation [92].

### Lighted stents

Iatrogenic ureteral injury is a serious complication that can arise during abdominal or pelvic procedures. More than 50% cases are encountered in gynecologic surgery [93]. The incidence of ureteral injury in colorectal surgery is 0.7%–10% whereas in gynecologic surgery it is 0.2%–2.5% [94]. Ureteral injury can be primarily prevented by accurate identification of the ureter [95]. In the event of ureteral injury, immediate intra-operative identification and prompt treatment improves the clinical outcomes [93, 95, 96] (**Figure 7.9**).

Ureteral stents are open ended catheters that are preoperatively placed under cystoscopic guidance, for protection of the ureter. Lighted ureteral stents are a variant of these stents illuminated by an external power source. The glow of the ureters cautions the

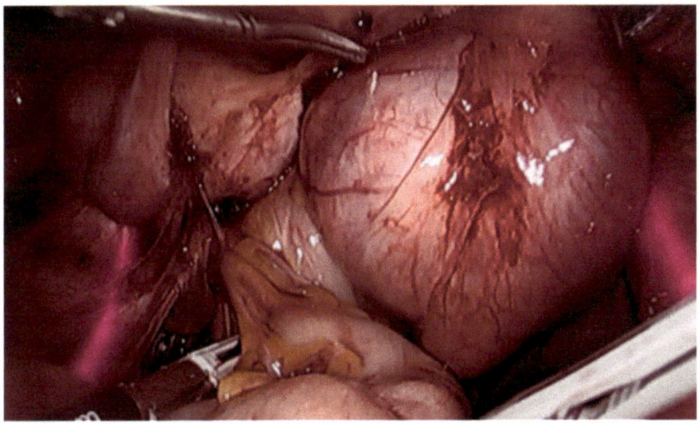

**FIGURE 7.9** Laparoscopic view showing utilization of lighted stents in stage IV endometriosis.

surgeon about its proximity thus preventing potential damage [97]. In an advent of injury, the stent is directly visible through the exposed ureteral lumen facilitating early identification and repair.

A retrospective study of a cohort of 151 patients who underwent procedures such as laparoscopic hysterectomy, colectomy, and pelvic adhesiolysis revealed absence of ureteral injury in the presence of ureteric stent placement. Additionally, the operative time was shortened by 0–45 min as the stents allowed rapid identification of the ureters [98]. Lighted ureteral stent are also found beneficial for ureterovaginal fistula repair as it requires dissection and precise transection of the ureters in distorted anatomy [99]. Lighted ureteral stents have a clear potential in minimally invasive surgery to improve operative efficiency. Its ability to delineate the location of ureter allows for confident dissection in complex pelvic procedures with distorted anatomy such as in deep endometriosis.

## Postoperative care

DIE surgery is a major surgery and is associated with postoperative complications including urinary retention or bladder dysfunction and more frequently seen when nodules are bigger, extending laterally deep into the pararectal space [100, 101]. This is due to the fact that parasympathetic nerves infiltrate endometriotic nodule and dissection turns out to be difficult either leaving endometriosis in place or damaging nerve fibers. Urinary retention usually resolves within a few weeks. As seen earlier deep endometriosis requires ureteral and bowel surgery and is prone to complications, postoperative care should therefore be meticulous requiring expertise. The most severe complications during the first week are late bowel perforations and late ureteral perforations and other complications are rectovaginal, ureterovaginal, and vesicovaginal fistulae [18].

## References


1. Johnson NP, Hummelshoj L, World Endometriosis Society Montpellier C: Consensus on current management of endometriosis. *Hum Reprod* 2013, 28(6):1552–1568.
2. Vigano P, Parazzini F, Somigliana E, Vercellini P: Endometriosis: epidemiology and aetiological factors. *Best Pract Res Clin Obstet Gynaecol* 2004, 18(2):177–200.
3. Cornillie FJ, Oosterlynck D, Lauweryns JM, Koninckx PR: Deeply infiltrating pelvic endometriosis: histology and clinical significance. *Fertil Steril* 1990, 53(6):978–983.
4. Bazot M, Lafont C, Rouzier R, Roseau G, Thomassin-Naggara I, Darai E: Diagnostic accuracy of physical examination, transvaginal sonography, rectal endoscopic sonography, and magnetic resonance imaging to diagnose deep-infiltrating endometriosis. *Fertil Steril* 2009, 92(6):1825–1833.
5. Noventa M, Saccardi C, Litta P, Vitagliano A, D'Antona D, Abdulrahim B, Duncan A, Alexander-Sefre F, Aldrich CJ, Quaranta M, et al: Ultrasound techniques in the diagnosis of deep pelvic endometriosis: algorithm based on a systematic review and meta-analysis. *Fertil Steril* 2015, 104(2):366–383 e362.
6. Bazot M, Darai E: Diagnosis of deep endometriosis: clinical examination, ultrasonography, magnetic resonance imaging, and other techniques. *Fertil Steril* 2017, 108(6):886–894.
7. Nnoaham KE, Hummelshoj L, Webster P, d'Hooghe T, de Cicco Nardone F, de Cicco Nardone C, Jenkinson C, Kennedy SH, Zondervan KT, World Endometriosis Research Foundation Global Study of Women's Health: Impact of endometriosis on quality of life and work productivity: a multicenter study across ten countries. *Fertil Steril* 2011, 96(2):366–373 e368.
8. Jenkins S, Olive DL, Haney AF: Endometriosis: pathogenetic implications of the anatomic distribution. *Obstet Gynecol* 1986, 67(3):335–338.
9. Giudice LC, Kao LC: Endometriosis. *Lancet* 2004, 364(9447): 1789–1799.
10. Vercellini P, Fedele L, Aimi G, Pietropaolo G, Consonni D, Crosignani PG: Association between endometriosis stage, lesion type, patient characteristics and severity of pelvic pain symptoms: a multivariate analysis of over 1000 patients. *Hum Reprod* 2007, 22(1):266–271.
11. Ballard KD, Seaman HE, de Vries CS, Wright JT: Can symptomatology help in the diagnosis of endometriosis? Findings from a national case-control study–Part 1. *BJOG* 2008, 115(11):1382–1391.
12. Fauconnier A, Chapron C: Endometriosis and pelvic pain: epidemiological evidence of the relationship and implications. *Hum Reprod Update* 2005, 11(6):595–606.
13. Anaf V, Simon P, El Nakadi I, Fayt I, Buxant F, Simonart T, Peny MO, Noel JC: Relationship between endometriotic foci and nerves in rectovaginal endometriotic nodules. *Hum Reprod* 2000, 15(8): 1744–1750.
14. Anaf V, Simon P, El Nakadi I, Fayt I, Simonart T, Buxant F, Noel JC: Hyperalgesia, nerve infiltration and nerve growth factor expression in deep adenomyotic nodules, peritoneal and ovarian endometriosis. *Hum Reprod* 2002, 17(7):1895–1900.
15. Fauconnier A, Chapron C, Dubuisson JB, Vieira M, Dousset B, Breart G: Relation between pain symptoms and the anatomic location of deep-infiltrating endometriosis. *Fertil Steril* 2002, 78(4): 719–726.
16. Ferrero S, Esposito F, Abbamonte LH, Anserini P, Remorgida V, Ragni N: Quality of sex life in women with endometriosis and deep dyspareunia. *Fertil Steril* 2005, 83(3):573–579.
17. Bulletins–Gynecology ACoP: ACOG Practice Bulletin No. 51. Chronic pelvic pain. *Obstet Gynecol* 2004, 103(3):589–605.
18. Koninckx PR, Ussia A, Adamyan L, Wattiez A, Donnez J: Deep endometriosis: definition, diagnosis, and treatment. *Fertil Steril* 2012, 98(3):564–571.
19. Rolla E: Endometriosis: advances and controversies in classification, pathogenesis, diagnosis, and treatment. *F1000Res* 2019, 8.
20. Cameron IC, Rogers S, Collins MC, Reed MW: Intestinal endometriosis: presentation, investigation, and surgical management. *Int J Colorectal Dis* 1995, 10(2):83–86.
21. Bazot M, Thomassin I, Hourani R, Cortez A, Darai E: Diagnostic accuracy of transvaginal sonography for deep pelvic endometriosis. *Ultrasound Obstet Gynecol* 2004, 24(2):180–185.
22. Guerriero S, Condous G, van den Bosch T, Valentin L, Leone FP, Van Schoubroeck D, Exacoustos C, Installe AJ, Martins WP, Abrao MS, et al.: Systematic approach to sonographic evaluation of the pelvis in women with suspected endometriosis, including terms, definitions and measurements: a consensus opinion from the International Deep Endometriosis Analysis (IDEA) group. *Ultrasound Obstet Gynecol* 2016, 48(3):318–332.

23. Saba L, Guerriero S, Sulcis R, Pilloni M, Ajossa S, Melis G, Mallarini G: MRI and "tenderness guided" transvaginal ultrasonography in the diagnosis of recto-sigmoid endometriosis. *J Magn Reson Imaging* 2012, 35(2):352–360.
24. Bazot M, Gasner A, Lafont C, Ballester M, Darai E: Deep pelvic endometriosis: limited additional diagnostic value of postcontrast in comparison with conventional MR images. *Eur J Radiol* 2011, 80(3):e331–339.
25. Bazot M, Detchev R, Cortez A, Amouyal P, Uzan S, Darai E: Transvaginal sonography and rectal endoscopic sonography for the assessment of pelvic endometriosis: a preliminary comparison. *Hum Reprod* 2003, 18(8):1686–1692.
26. Hudelist G, English J, Thomas AE, Tinelli A, Singer CF, Keckstein J: Diagnostic accuracy of transvaginal ultrasound for non-invasive diagnosis of bowel endometriosis: systematic review and meta-analysis. *Ultrasound Obstet Gynecol* 2011, 37(3):257–263.
27. Noventa M, Scioscia M, Schincariol M, Cavallin F, Pontrelli G, Virgilio B, Vitale SG, Lagana AS, Dessole F, Cosmi E, et al.: Imaging modalities for diagnosis of deep pelvic endometriosis: comparison between transvaginal sonography, rectal endoscopy sonography and magnetic resonance imaging. A head-to-head meta-analysis. *Diagnostics (Basel)* 2019, 9(4).
28. Nisenblat V, Bossuyt PM, Shaikh R, Farquhar C, Jordan V, Scheffers CS, Mol BW, Johnson N, Hull ML: Blood biomarkers for the non-invasive diagnosis of endometriosis. *Cochrane Database Syst Rev* 2016(5):CD012179.
29. Ballester M, Santulli P, Bazot M, Coutant C, Rouzier R, Darai E: Preoperative evaluation of posterior deep-infiltrating endometriosis demonstrates a relationship with urinary dysfunction and parametrial involvement. *J Minim Invasive Gynecol* 2011, 18(1):36–42.
30. Medeiros LR, Rosa DD, Bozzetti MC, Fachel JM, Furness S, Garry R, Rosa MI, Stein AT: Laparoscopy versus laparotomy for benign ovarian tumour. *Cochrane Database Syst Rev* 2009(2):CD004751.
31. Revised American Society for Reproductive Medicine classification of endometriosis: 1996. *Fertil Steril* 1997, 67(5):817–821.
32. Kennedy S, Bergqvist A, Chapron C, D'Hooghe T, Dunselman G, Greb R, Hummelshoj L, Prentice A, Saridogan E, Endometriosis ESIGf, et al.: ESHRE guideline for the diagnosis and treatment of endometriosis. *Hum Reprod* 2005, 20(10):2698–2704.
33. Frishman GN, Salak JR: Conservative surgical management of endometriosis in women with pelvic pain. *J Minim Invasive Gynecol* 2006, 13(6):546–558.
34. Ball TL, Platt MA: Urologic complications of endometriosis. *Am J Obstet Gynecol* 1962, **84**:1516–1521.
35. Perez-Utrilla Perez M, Aguilera Bazan A, Alonso Dorrego JM, Hernandez A, de Francisco MG, Martin Hernandez M, de Santiago J, de la P, Barthel J: Urinary tract endometriosis: clinical, diagnostic, and therapeutic aspects. *Urology* 2009, 73(1):47–51.
36. Vercellini P, Meschia M, De Giorgi O, Panazza S, Cortesi I, Crosignani PG: Bladder detrusor endometriosis: clinical and pathogenetic implications. *J Urol* 1996, 155(1):84–86.
37. Donnez J, Spada F, Squifflet J, Nisolle M: Bladder endometriosis must be considered as bladder adenomyosis. *Fertil Steril* 2000, 74(6): 1175–1181.
38. Knabben L, Imboden S, Fellmann B, Nirgianakis K, Kuhn A, Mueller MD: Urinary tract endometriosis in patients with deep-infiltrating endometriosis: prevalence, symptoms, management, and proposal for a new clinical classification. *Fertil Steril* 2015, 103(1):147–152.
39. Fujita K: Endometriosis of the ureter. *J Urol* 1976, 116(5):664.
40. Yohannes P: Ureteral endometriosis. *J Urol* 2003, 170(1):20–25.
41. Comiter CV: Endometriosis of the urinary tract. *Urol Clin North Am* 2002, 29(3):625–635.
42. De Cicco C, Schonman R, Craessaerts M, Van Cleynenbreugel B, Ussia A, Koninckx PR: Laparoscopic management of ureteral lesions in gynecology. *Fertil Steril* 2009, 92(4):1424–1427.
43. Togashi K, Nishimura K, Kimura I, Tsuda Y, Yamashita K, Shibata T, Nakano Y, Konishi J, Konishi I, Mori T: Endometrial cysts: diagnosis with MR imaging. *Radiology* 1991, 180(1):73–78.
44. Villa G, Mabrouk M, Guerrini M, Mignemi G, Montanari G, Fabbri E, Venturoli S, Seracchioli R: Relationship between site and size of bladder endometriotic nodules and severity of dysuria. *J Minim Invasive Gynecol* 2007, 14(5):628–632.
45. Gustilo-Ashby AM, Paraiso MF: Treatment of urinary tract endometriosis. *J Minim Invasive Gynecol* 2006, 13(6):559–565.
46. Antonelli A, Simeone C, Zani D, Sacconi T, Minini G, Canossi E, Cunico SC: Clinical aspects and surgical treatment of urinary tract endometriosis: our experience with 31 cases. *Eur Urol* 2006, 49(6):1093–1097; discussion 1097–1098.
47. Chapron C, Dubuisson JB, Jacob S, Fauconnier A, Da Costa Vieira M: [Laparoscopy and bladder endometriosis]. *Gynecol Obstet Fertil* 2000, 28(3):232–237.
48. Seracchioli R, Mabrouk M, Montanari G, Manuzzi L, Concetti S, Venturoli S: Conservative laparoscopic management of urinary tract endometriosis (UTE): surgical outcome and long-term follow-up. *Fertil Steril* 2010, 94(3):856–861.
49. Bergqvist A: Different types of extragenital endometriosis: a review. *Gynecol Endocrinol* 1993, 7(3):207–221.
50. Forsgren H, Lindhagen J, Melander S, Wagermark J: Colorectal endometriosis. *Acta Chir Scand* 1983, 149(4):431–435.
51. Remorgida V, Ferrero S, Fulcheri E, Ragni N, Martin DC: Bowel endometriosis: presentation, diagnosis, and treatment. *Obstet Gynecol Surv* 2007, 62(7):461–470.
52. Keckstein J, Ulrich U, Kandolf O, Wiesinger H, Wustlich M: [Laparoscopic therapy of intestinal endometriosis and the ranking of drug treatment]. *Zentralbl Gynakol* 2003, 125(7-8):259–266.
53. Schipper E, Nezhat C: Video-assisted laparoscopy for the detection and diagnosis of endometriosis: safety, reliability, and invasiveness. *Int J Womens Health* 2012, 4:383–393.
54. Pittaway DE: Appendectomy in the surgical treatment of endometriosis. *Obstet Gynecol* 1983, 61(4):421–424.
55. Tumay V, Ozturk E, Ozturk H, Yilmazlar T: Appendiceal endometriosis mimicking acute appendicitis. *Acta Chir Belg* 2006, **106**(6):712–713.
56. Teunen A, Ooms EC, Tytgat GN: Endometriosis of the small and large bowel. Study of 18 patients and survey of the literature. *Neth J Med* 1982, 25(5):142–150.
57. Rio FW, Edwards DL, Regan JF, Schmutzer KJ: Endometriosis of the small bowel. *Arch Surg* 1970, 101(3):403–405.
58. Charatsi D, Koukoura O, Ntavela IG, Chintziou F, Gkorila G, Tsagkoulis M, Mikos T, Pistofidis G, Hajiioannou J, Daponte A: Gastrointestinal and urinary tract endometriosis: a review on the commonest locations of extrapelvic endometriosis. *Adv Med* 2018, 2018:3461209.
59. Chapron C, Fauconnier A, Vieira M, Barakat H, Dousset B, Pansini V, Vacher-Lavenu MC, Dubuisson JB: Anatomical distribution of deeply infiltrating endometriosis: surgical implications and proposition for a classification. *Hum Reprod* 2003, 18(1):157–161.
60. Abrao MS, Petraglia F, Falcone T, Keckstein J, Osuga Y, Chapron C: Deep endometriosis infiltrating the recto-sigmoid: critical factors to consider before management. *Hum Reprod Update* 2015, 21(3):329–339.
61. Kavallaris A, Kohler C, Kuhne-Heid R, Schneider A: Histopathological extent of rectal invasion by rectovaginal endometriosis. *Hum Reprod* 2003, 18(6):1323–1327.
62. Zhang C, Sun Y, Zhang D, Sun Y: Letter to the editor: recurrent symptoms of gastrointestinal tract caused by isolated endometriosis in a middle-aged female. *Int J Colorectal Dis* 2016, 31(8): 1511–1513.
63. Remorgida V, Ragni N, Ferrero S, Anserini P, Torelli P, Fulcheri E: The involvement of the interstitial Cajal cells and the enteric nervous system in bowel endometriosis. *Hum Reprod* 2005, 20(1): 264–271.
64. Thomassin I, Bazot M, Detchev R, Barranger E, Cortez A, Darai E: Symptoms before and after surgical removal of colorectal endometriosis that are assessed by magnetic resonance imaging and rectal endoscopic sonography. *Am J Obstet Gynecol* 2004, 190(5): 1264–1271.

65. Ribeiro PA, Rodrigues FC, Kehdi IP, Rossini L, Abdalla HS, Donadio N, Aoki T: Laparoscopic resection of intestinal endometriosis: a 5-year experience. *J Minim Invasive Gynecol* 2006, 13(5):442–446.
66. Roman H, Vassilieff M, Gourcerol G, Savoye G, Leroi AM, Marpeau L, Michot F, Tuech JJ: Surgical management of deep-infiltrating endometriosis of the rectum: pleading for a symptom-guided approach. *Hum Reprod* 2011, 26(2):274–281.
67. Keckstein J, Wiesinger H: Deep endometriosis, including intestinal involvement–the interdisciplinary approach. *Minim Invasive Ther Allied Technol* 2005, 14(3):160–166.
68. Nezhat C, Nezhat F, Pennington E, Nezhat CH, Ambroze W: Laparoscopic disk excision and primary repair of the anterior rectal wall for the treatment of full-thickness bowel endometriosis. *Surg Endosc* 1994, 8(6):682–685.
69. Roman H, Tuech JJ: New disc excision procedure for low and mid rectal endometriosis nodules using combined transanal and laparoscopic approach. *Colorectal Dis* 2014, 16(7):O253–256.
70. Woods RJ, Heriot AG, Chen FC: Anterior rectal wall excision for endometriosis using the circular stapler. *ANZ J Surg* 2003, 73(8):647–648.
71. Fanfani F, Fagotti A, Gagliardi ML, Ruffo G, Ceccaroni M, Scambia G, Minelli L: Discoid or segmental rectosigmoid resection for deep-infiltrating endometriosis: a case-control study. *Fertil Steril* 2010, 94(2):444–449.
72. Meuleman C, Tomassetti C, D'Hoore A, Van Cleynenbreugel B, Penninckx F, Vergote I, D'Hooghe T: Surgical treatment of deeply infiltrating endometriosis with colorectal involvement. *Hum Reprod Update* 2011, 17(3):311–326.
73. Ruffo G, Scopelliti F, Scioscia M, Ceccaroni M, Mainardi P, Minelli L: Laparoscopic colorectal resection for deep-infiltrating endometriosis: analysis of 436 cases. *Surg Endosc* 2010, 24(1):63–67.
74. Trencheva K, Morrissey KP, Wells M, Mancuso CA, Lee SW, Sonoda T, Michelassi F, Charlson ME, Milsom JW: Identifying important predictors for anastomotic leak after colon and rectal resection: prospective study on 616 patients. *Ann Surg* 2013, 257(1):108–113.
75. Abo C, Moatassim S, Marty N, Saint Ghislain M, Huet E, Bridoux V, Tuech JJ, Roman H: Postoperative complications after bowel endometriosis surgery by shaving, disc excision, or segmental resection: a three-arm comparative analysis of 364 consecutive cases. *Fertil Steril* 2018, 109(1):172–178 e171.
76. Roman H, Tuech JJ, Huet E, Bridoux V, Khalil H, Hennetier C, Bubenheim M, Branduse LA: Excision versus colorectal resection in deep endometriosis infiltrating the rectum: 5-year follow-up of patients enrolled in a randomized controlled trial. *Hum Reprod* 2019, 34(12):2362–2371.
77. Reich H, McGlynn F, Salvat J: Laparoscopic treatment of cul-de-sac obliteration secondary to retrocervical deep fibrotic endometriosis. *J Reprod Med* 1991, 36(7):516–522.
78. Roman H, Moatassim-Drissa S, Marty N, Milles M, Vallee A, Desnyder E, Stochino Loi E, Abo C: Rectal shaving for deep endometriosis infiltrating the rectum: a 5-year continuous retrospective series. *Fertil Steril* 2016, **106**(6):1438–1445 e1432.
79. Roman H, Milles M, Vassilieff M, Resch B, Tuech JJ, Huet E, Darwish B, Abo C: Long-term functional outcomes following colorectal resection versus shaving for rectal endometriosis. *Am J Obstet Gynecol* 2016, 215(6):762 e761–762 e769.
80. Donnez O, Roman H: Choosing the right surgical technique for deep endometriosis: shaving, disc excision, or bowel resection? *Fertil Steril* 2017, 108(6):931–942.
81. Alander JT, Kaartinen I, Laakso A, Patila T, Spillmann T, Tuchin VV, Venermo M, Valisuo P: A review of indocyanine green fluorescent imaging in surgery. *Int J Biomed Imaging* 2012, 2012:940585.
82. Luo S, Zhang E, Su Y, Cheng T, Shi C: A review of NIR dyes in cancer targeting and imaging. *Biomaterials* 2011, 32(29):7127–7138.
83. Schaafsma BE, Mieog JS, Hutteman M, van der Vorst JR, Kuppen PJ, Lowik CW, Frangioni JV, van de Velde CJ, Vahrmeijer AL: The clinical use of indocyanine green as a near-infrared fluorescent contrast agent for image-guided oncologic surgery. *J Surg Oncol* 2011, 104(3):323–332.
84. Verbeek FP, Schaafsma BE, Tummers QR, van der Vorst JR, van der Made WJ, Baeten CI, Bonsing BA, Frangioni JV, van de Velde CJ, Vahrmeijer AL, et al.: Optimization of near-infrared fluorescence cholangiography for open and laparoscopic surgery. *Surg Endosc* 2014, 28(4):1076–1082.
85. Taylor E, Williams C: Surgical treatment of endometriosis: location and patterns of disease at reoperation. *Fertil Steril* 2010, 93(1): 57–61.
86. Vignali M, Bianchi S, Candiani M, Spadaccini G, Oggioni G, Busacca M: Surgical treatment of deep endometriosis and risk of recurrence. *J Minim Invasive Gynecol* 2005, 12(6):508–513.
87. Stegmann BJ, Sinaii N, Liu S, Segars J, Merino M, Nieman LK, Stratton P: Using location, color, size, and depth to characterize and identify endometriosis lesions in a cohort of 133 women. *Fertil Steril* 2008, 89(6):1632–1636.
88. Laufer MR: Identification of clear vesicular lesions of atypical endometriosis: a new technique. *Fertil Steril* 1997, 68(4):739–740.
89. Asante A, Taylor RN: Endometriosis: the role of neuroangiogenesis. *Annu Rev Physiol* 2011, 73:163–182.
90. Cosentino F, Vizzielli G, Turco LC, Fagotti A, Cianci S, Vargiu V, Zannoni GF, Ferrandina G, Scambia G: Near-infrared imaging with indocyanine green for detection of endometriosis lesions (Gre-Endo trial): a pilot study. *J Minim Invasive Gynecol* 2018, 25(7):1249–1254.
91. Levey KA: Use of fluorescence imaging technology to identify peritoneal endometriosis: a case report of new technology. *Surg Laparosc Endosc Percutan Tech* 2014, 24(2):e63–65.
92. De Neef A, Cadiere GB, Bourgeois P, Barbieux R, Dapri G, Fastrez M: Fluorescence of deep-infiltrating endometriosis during laparoscopic surgery: a preliminary report on 6 cases. *Surg Innov* 2018, 25(5):450–454.
93. Schimpf MO, Gottenger EE, Wagner JR: Universal ureteral stent placement at hysterectomy to identify ureteral injury: a decision analysis. *BJOG* 2008, 115(9):1151–1158.
94. Pokala N, Delaney CP, Kiran RP, Bast J, Angermeier K, Fazio VW: A randomized controlled trial comparing simultaneous intra-operative vs. sequential prophylactic ureteric catheter insertion in re-operative and complicated colorectal surgery. *Int J Colorectal Dis* 2007, 22(6):683–687.
95. Neuman M, Eidelman A, Langer R, Golan A, Bukovsky I, Caspi E: Iatrogenic injuries to the ureter during gynecologic and obstetric operations. *Surg Gynecol Obstet* 1991, 173(4):268–272.
96. Pettit PD, Petrou SP: The value of cystoscopy in major vaginal surgery. *Obstet Gynecol* 1994, 84(2):318–320.
97. Lee Z, Kaplan J, Giusto L, Eun D: Prevention of iatrogenic ureteral injuries during robotic gynecologic surgery: a review. *Am J Obstet Gynecol* 2016, 214(5):566–571.
98. Redan JA, McCarus SD: Protect the ureters. *JSLS* 2009, 13(2):139–141.
99. Siddighi S, Carr KR: Lighted stents facilitate robotic-assisted laparoscopic ureterovaginal fistula repair. *Int Urogynecol J* 2013, 24(3): 515–517.
100. Ballester M, Chereau E, Dubernard G, Coutant C, Bazot M, Darai E: Urinary dysfunction after colorectal resection for endometriosis: results of a prospective randomized trial comparing laparoscopy to open surgery. *Am J Obstet Gynecol* 2011, 204(4):303 e301–306.
101. Gabriel B, Nassif J, Trompoukis P, Lima AM, Barata S, Lang-Averous G, Wattiez A: Prevalence and outcome of urinary retention after laparoscopic surgery for severe endometriosis–does histology provide answers? *Int Urogynecol J* 2012, 23(1):111–116.

# 8

# ROBOTIC TECHNIQUES FOR ENDOMETRIOSIS

**Sara Rahman, Jordan S. Klebanoff, and Gaby N. Moawad**

## Introduction

Surgical treatment of endometriosis has continued to play an essential role in its diagnosis and therapy, despite the efforts to find non-invasive diagnostic tests and other medical treatments. The goal of surgical therapy is two-fold: one, for definitive confirmation or exclusion of endometriosis, and two, to re-establish normal anatomy as best possible by removing all visible endometriotic lesions and adhesions; repairing trauma to affected sites and improving quality of life [1].

Surgical treatment may not cure endometriosis, but it plays a crucial role in the management of the disease, including relieving pain and improving fertility [2–7]. Laparoscopy is the standard approach for diagnosis and removal of endometriotic lesions, reserving laparotomy for specific circumstances only. Surgery for pain related to endometriosis has been shown to significantly reduce pain scores at both 6 and 12 months postoperatively compared to diagnostic laparoscopy alone [8]. The goal of this chapter is to discuss the decision-making process of surgical treatment of endometriosis and how robotic surgery plays an integral role in its management.

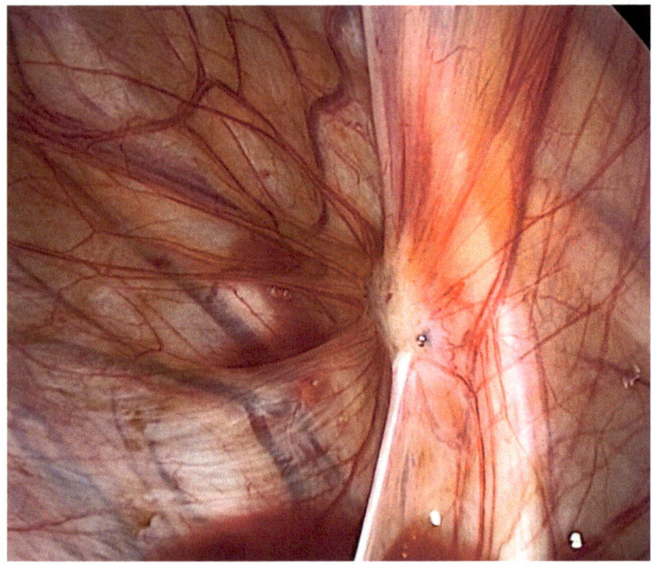

**FIGURE 8.1** Visible lesions.

## Surgical management of endometriosis

There are multiple indications for surgical management of endometriosis. Some include failure or intolerance of medical therapy, diagnosis, immediate treatment, and infertility [9]. When considering surgical management of endometriosis, the surgeon must discuss the patient's goals and understanding of the options so that the patient may adequately plan for surgery.

### Conservative vs definitive surgery

In regard to conservative versus definitive surgery, the most important issue is the reproductive plans of the patient. For patients desiring future fertility, a conservative approach is best. This involves only removal or destruction of visible lesions (**Figure 8.1**), which may help the patient's dysmenorrhea or pain, and/or improve fertility for the [10].

If, however, patients have completed childbearing or do not desire fertility, hysterectomy with or without ovarian conservation should be offered. Additionally, definitive surgery is a better option for those who have severe pain refractory to medical management and/or have had previous conservative surgery for endometriosis [1]. Both types of surgery, conservative and definitive, have shown to alleviate dysmenorrhea postoperatively, however, there is a high rate of reoperation for endometriosis if either the uterus and/or the ovaries are not removed [8, 11].

### Concurrent oophorectomy

Prior research has shown that patient who undergo conservative surgery have the highest rates of reoperation, in contrast to the low rates of reoperation in patients who have undergone a hysterectomy and concurrent oophorectomy [11]. Namnoum et al. found that a majority of patients (60%) with ovarian conservation for endometriosis had a reoccurrence of symptoms (**Figure 8.2**). In fact, 30% of those women required repeat surgery. This is a stark contrast to the 3.7% of women who required repeat surgery that did not have ovarian tissue preserved in their initial surgery [12].

Counseling and discussion play a pivotal role in the decision for oophorectomy at the time of hysterectomy. Patients must comprehend that although concurrent oophorectomy leads to better long-term suppression of pain, surgical menopause has

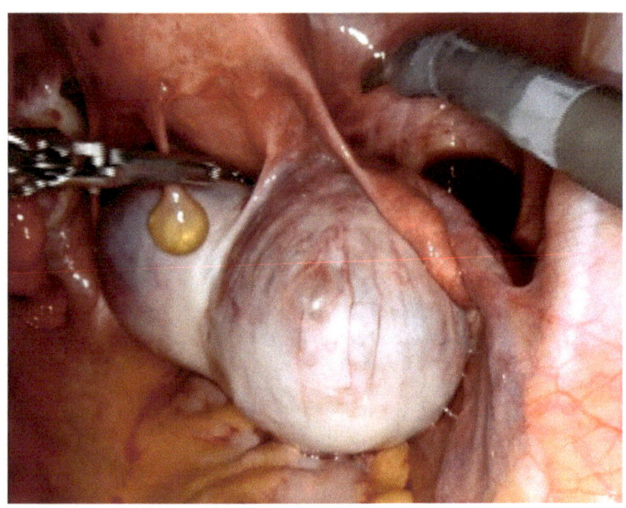

**FIGURE 8.2** Recurrent symptoms.

consequences [1]. Early menopause, whether surgically induced or natural progression, affects women's bone mineral density and cardiovascular health, and it causes significant side effects [13]. Some women may require hormone replacement therapy. Additionally, it is important that patients understand that, as common with the disease of endometriosis in particular, removal of all ovarian tissues does not guarantee complete symptom resolution [14].

### Supracervical hysterectomy

Some have looked into the role of supracervical hysterectomy in endometriosis; supporters hypothesize that this type of hysterectomy reduces the risk of surgical damage to ureters, bladder, nerves, and may even allow women a better sex life for long term [15, 16]. However, research does not support this claim; there is no evidence exists that suggest that supracervical hysterectomies provide any benefits over total hysterectomies. Often, patients require future trachelectomy due to persistent pain [17, 18].

## Minimally invasive surgery versus laparotomy in the surgical management of endometriosis

Surgical management of endometriosis is performed via laparoscopy or laparotomy. Laparoscopy can be further sub-divided into robotic-assisted laparoscopy or traditional laparoscopy ("key hole" or "straight stick"). Non-randomized studies comparing laparoscopy and laparotomy have shown that both surgical methods are effective at long-term pain reduction for endometriosis [19–23].

Although studies show no difference with regard to long-term pain reduction between the two surgical approaches, there are several other outcomes that clearly demonstrate laparoscopy as the superior method. Several studies have shown that laparoscopic treatment of endometriosis has decreased postoperative recovery time, lower cost, decreased immediate post-surgical pain and less analgesic use, and decreased infection rates compared to laparotomy [24–27]. Additionally, laparoscopic surgery decreases the incidence of adhesion formation compared to laparotomy [28].

For endometriosis-related surgical treatment for fertility, laparoscopy is associated with a higher spontaneous pregnancy rate [29, 30]. Several factors can explain this positive effect of the minimally invasive surgical approach for endometriosis. As mentioned previously, the amount of adhesion formation is lower after laparoscopy when compared to open, which likely has an effect on tubal and ovarian functions [28]. Additionally, the shorter recovery time after laparoscopy means that intercourse can be resumed earlier [31].

Although laparoscopy is the preferred method, sometimes conversion to laparotomy still needs to be performed in cases of difficult visualization with extensive disease and the need for multiple complex procedures involving other organ structures [32]. The rate of conversion to open surgery has varied in the literature and depends on the difficulties of the case, but overall, is low in the hands of a skilled minimally invasive surgeon [33].

## Robotics in gynecologic surgery: History, current, and advantages

### A historical perspective

Research in medical technology allows for novel breakthroughs, an effect seen with the establishment and rapid advancement of robotic surgery in the field of gynecologic surgery [34, 35]. Robotic surgery was initially developed for use in military battle zones. The goal was to allow surgeons in a remote location to perform procedures with similar skill, technique, and outcomes as if done in a regular operating room [36, 37]. These earlier military models paved the way for the advanced systems in use today.

The first robotic system available commercially was used in orthopedic hip prosthesis surgery, allowing accurate incisions in the femur bone for implant insertion [37]. The only robotic surgical system used today is the da Vinci Surgery system by Intuit. This system's first successful surgery was a cholecystectomy done in 1997 in Belgium [38]. Shortly afterward, in 2000, the da Vinci became the first robotic system approved by the United States Food and Drug Administration (FDA) for general laparoscopic surgery. This was the first time the FDA approved an all-encompassing system of surgical instruments and camera utensils. In 2005, the da Vinci surgical system was cleared by the FDA for use in gynecologic procedures, and it also has full regulatory clearance with the coveted Conformité Européenne (CE) mark in Europe [39].

### The da Vinci robotic system

The current da Vinci consists of three components: a surgeon console, a patient side cart, and a vision cart. The surgeon sits at the console and has a three-dimensional (3D) view of the surgical field. The da Vinci surgical system's 3D vision system is produced from two endoscopes, allowing the surgeon to view the operative area with high-resolution clarity (**Figure 8.3**).

The patient side cart consists of four robotic arms. One arm is used for the camera, and the other three arms are interactive operative arms. The side cart can be docked between the patients' legs or to either side of the patient. The side-docking technique gives improved access to the uterine manipulator and is becoming increasingly popular in benign gynecologic surgery. The da Vinci's one-centimeter diameter surgical arms represent a significant advancement in robotic surgery from the earlier large-armed systems. With such miniaturized operating arms, the da Vinci robot removes the need to leverage the sides of the incision walls. This advancement allows for less contact between exposed interior tissue and the surgical device, greatly reducing the risk of infection.

The surgeon controls the camera and operative robotic arms through the surgeon console. Robotic arms should be thought of as an extension of the surgeon's arms. The Endowrist system

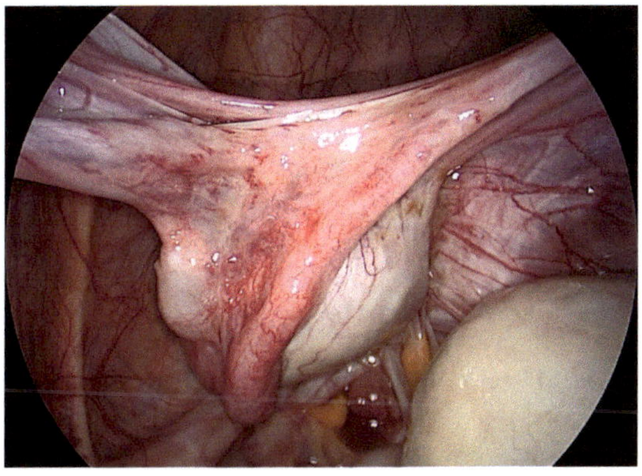

**FIGURE 8.3** Two endoscopes allow the surgeon to view the operative area with high-resolution clarity.

gives seven degrees of motion, which mimics the dexterity of the human hand. This feature of the operating arms replicate the skilled movements of the surgeon and improved accuracy in small operating spaces. The instruments can be rotated a full 360 degrees, allowing for a high degree of flexibility and precision.

The last component of the da Vinci system is the vision cart, which is the integration hub for the power generation, image processing, and information systems. It also includes a high-definition display, which allows others in the operating room to watch the procedure.

## Adoption of robotic surgery

The current debate surrounding robotic-assisted laparoscopy is the same skepticism that traditional laparoscopy met in the 1980s and 1990s [40, 41]. Robotic surgery has revolutionized gynecologic surgery, making minimally invasive technique a feasible and an appropriate option for many patients. Robotic surgery is used in a multitude of gynecologic procedures, including endometriosis, myomectomies, benign hysterectomies, urogynecology, and gynecological oncology with good success and low morbidity [42–44]. Other surgical fields, including colorectal, urology, and general surgery, have learned from gynecologic robotic surgeons and have successfully applied this technology to their own surgical fields [44]. The evidence shows that minimally invasive surgery is the preferred surgical approach over laparotomy for patient outcomes, pain, satisfaction, cost, and complications, and robotic surgery can make difficult laparoscopic procedures more feasible [45, 46].

## Benefits and advantages of robotic surgery

There is a large volume of literature that discusses the various benefits and advantages of robotic surgery [47]. The benefits can be broken down into various components, further described below:

1. *Field and depth of view*: The ability to see in a 3D, as mentioned earlier, is truly a remarkable feature. As an old adage of surgical techniques, the need for adequate exposure and visualization is vital. The robot has improved visual quality over the traditional laparoscopic technique, which has a limited two-dimensional view. The 3D stereoscopic vision allows depth perception not seen on a standard laparoscopic monitor. Additionally, robotic surgery enables increased magnification which adds ability for more precise fine microsurgery techniques. The robot also eliminates the counterintuitive motion of standard laparoscopy and aligns the eyes and hands over the area of interest with improved ergonomics.
2. *Precision*: The robotic surgical system improved precision due to different factors such as the EndoWrist, tremor reduction (explained below), and improved field of view. It allows an increased freedom of instrument movement by allowing wristed and finger movements that standard laparoscopic instruments do not have. This increases the degrees of freedom from four movements to seven, allowing more precision in the surgical field which more closely mimics open surgery.
3. *Control and motion dampening*: This technology reduces the tremors created naturally by the extension of the fingers or the resultant tension due to fatigue as operating times increase. It eliminates the fulcrum effect and motion scaling, minimizing instrument tremor from the console to the patient. The robot is also able to filter out unnecessary hand and finger motions which results in safer, more accurate intracorporeal movements.
4. *Dexterity*: The invention of the ergonomic wrist instruments allowed for more accurate replication of the movement at the wrist, including rotation. Surgeons can use very fine suture material with improved handling when compared to traditional laparoscopy.
5. *Decreased blood loss*: This can be seen as a direct result of the factors above, especially greater instrument control, viewing ability, and small entry sites.
6. *Decreased surgeon fatigue*: The surgeon operator console provided on the robotic surgical system is a great enhancement, especially in longer operations [48].
7. *Learning curve*: Studies have evaluated the required learning to be proficient in both laparoscopic and robotic techniques and have noted robotic surgical skills are less difficult to acquire. This is likely due to the ergonomic setup and more counter-intuitive hand movements needed compared to a laparoscopic style. Additionally, only 20 robotic procedures are needed for proficiency [49, 50]. Another important point is that operative times tend to decrease as the surgeon's experience increase.
8. *Teaching*: The robotic setup that includes a viewing station for the assistants and other staff in the room provides both a great interactive learning and teaching viewing option unique to this system. Additionally, the visual system can be expanded to remote location or telesurgery [51].

The advantages of robotics are not limited to above mentioned themes. Surgeons who have adopted minimally invasive techniques of robotic-assisted laparoscopy are embracing the other clinical benefits including shorter postoperative hospital stays, less analgesia, and improved cosmesis. Moreover, these surgeons are responding to the market pressure of patients' desire. With significant improvements from standard laparoscopy, the robot has enabled surgeons to perform procedures laparoscopically which were formerly performed by laparotomy, while giving patients the benefits of minimally invasive surgery.

## Limitations

The da Vinci robotic system is not without some limitations. The initial cost is around one to two million U.S. dollars, which does not include the fee for the recommended yearly maintenance. The system itself is large, with three components, which restricts its use to large operating rooms. Additionally, once the system is docked, the surgeon cannot change the position of the patient. If the patient needs to be moved, the robot has to be undocked and then re-docked after the position change is made, increasing the time in the operating room and overall cost.

Another limitation includes decreased tactile feedback. Lack of tactile feedback can lead to suture breakage from the use of excessive force during knot tying. The surgeon must learn to utilize visual cues over tactile cues, especially on tissue, to overcome the reduced tactile feedback during the procedure. Despite this limitation, the robotic platform is a reliable and durable way to be very precise in surgical dissection and reconstruction.

Currently, there are not any published guidelines on patient selection in regard to robotic surgery. Age, size, weight, disease type, and disease extent play a limited role in the decision to proceed with robotic surgery. However, one patient factor that plays a key role is the ability of the patient to tolerate steep Trendelenburg, which is necessary to complete the surgery. Nonetheless, patients with multiple comorbidities need not be

| Advantages | Drawbacks |
|---|---|
| • Higher degree of freedom in the robotic instrument | • Cost of implementation and maintenance |
| • Reduction in tremor interference | • Time required to dock and separate the robotic cart from the patient |
| • Three-dimensional vision | • Inability to move patient once robot is docked |
| • Ambidextrous capability | • Lack of tactile feedback |
| • Better ergonomics | |
| • Telesurgery | |

**FIGURE 8.4** Advantages and drawbacks of robotic-assisted laparoscopy for surgical treatment of endometriosis.

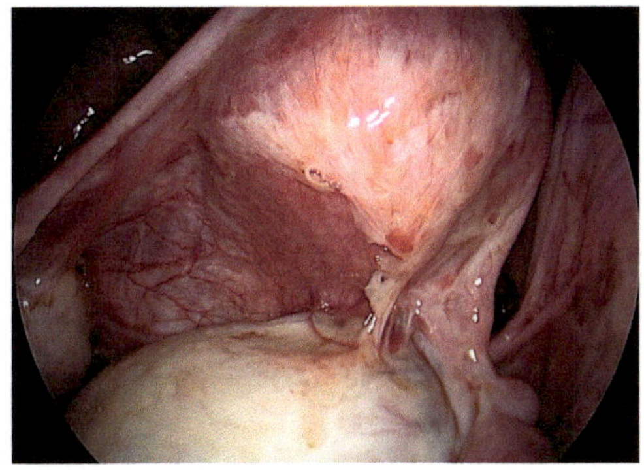

**FIGURE 8.5** Deep-infiltrating endometriosis.

excluded from a robotic surgical approach if they are appropriately counseled, have proper preoperative clearance, and have approval by the anesthesia team.

The initial and maintenance cost, lack of haptic feedback, and the bulky size of the equipment make can robotics less attractive to some surgeons and medical institutions. Despite these limitations, the da Vinci surgical system has achieved increasing popularity in gynecologic surgery due to immediate and long-term patient outcomes, especially when cases are able to be performed minimally invasively instead of via laparotomy which make it worthwhile (**Figure 8.4**).

## Role of robotic surgery compared to traditional laparoscopy in surgical endometriosis

As mentioned previously in this chapter, endometriosis can be treated by laparotomy, but a minimally invasive approach has been the preferred method since the initial reports of the application of laparoscopy for the diagnosis and treatment of endometriosis [52]. In terms of robotic-assisted laparoscopy, there is limited data describing the use of robotic surgery for endometriosis. Initial studies discussed robotic-assisted resection of endometriosis located in the bladder, ureter, or rectum, and reported favorable outcomes [53–57]. Some recent case series showed that using the robotic system for surgical management of deep-infiltrating endometriosis is feasible and that patients showed clinical improvement from their disease symptoms postoperatively [58, 59].

Few studies exist that compare robotic surgery with conventional laparoscopy for the treatment of endometriosis [60–62]. Both surgical approaches seem to have similar perioperative outcomes. Some report longer operative with the robotic approach (191 minutes robotically vs. 159 minutes conventionally). However, it is important to note that disease stage was not similar between the robotic and traditional laparoscopic groups in many of these studies. A different study reported a 16% shorter operating time for robotics as compared with laparoscopy for patients with deep-infiltrating endometriosis (stage III/IV) (**Figure 8.5**). They additionally found that this increase in operative time in traditional laparoscopic approach was an independent risk factor for postoperative complications and longer hospital stay [63].

One study found surgeon ergonomics were improved with the robot in comparison to traditional laparoscopy [61]. The loss of 3D, restricted degrees of movement, and presence of fulcrum effect in conventional laparoscopy likely affects surgeon fatigue [64].

It is important to recognize the aforementioned studies are retrospective, and long-term postoperative outcomes, such as quality of life and pain scores, were not been investigated. It is possible that the observed differences in these retrospective studies may be explained by patient selection or surgeon experience.

The LAROSE study is the first multicenter, randomized control trial comparing robotics with traditional laparoscopy for the treatment of endometriosis [65]. This trial brought to light several important points. First, no differences were noted in operative time between robotic and traditional laparoscopic groups. The similar operative times demonstrated in this trial stand in contrast to the retrospective studies that have been published to date [60–63]. Operatives times are important, as longer times implicate larger costs. Mean operative time and blood loss in the LAROSE study were within range of time and volumes in other studies, so the equivalent operative times between groups is unlikely due to patient selection and surgeon experience [65].

The LAROSE study also found no significant clinical differences observed over a 6-month follow-up period with regard to complications or quality of life. Notably, patients in each group improved in all aspects of quality of life scores; this attests to the value of surgical treatment of endometriosis [65]. Although equal in effectiveness in the intermediate term (up to 6 months postoperatively), more research needs to be conducted to see if robotic technology improves long-term results, especially over multiple years. Previous clinical trials with long-term follow-up of patients who had conventional laparoscopy for endometriosis found low recurrence of symptoms for the first 1–2 years, especially with medical postoperative suppressive therapy, but this has yet to be evaluated for robotic patients [11, 66].

To conclude, laparoscopy and robotic surgery for the treatment of endometriosis have comparable perioperative outcomes and significant improvement in quality of life after surgery. Other high-quality clinical trials evaluating clinical outcomes and intermediate- and long-term quality of life are needed. Robotic surgery for the treatment of endometriosis is a feasible option and is especially helpful in complex procedures.

## Robotic surgery techniques for endometriosis

The goal of surgical treatment of endometriosis is to restore normal anatomy by destroying or removing all visible endometriosis lesions (**Figure 8.6**) and repairing damaged organs and other sites [67]. Severe endometriosis involving the bowel, rectum, and/or bladder may require a different expertise and illicit a multidisciplinary team with gynecologists, general surgeons,

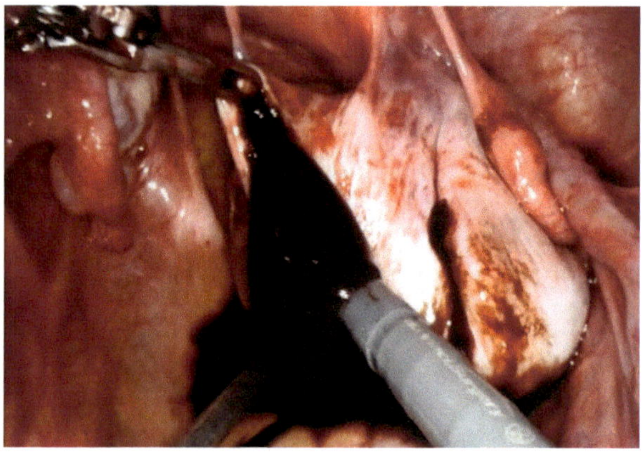

FIGURE 8.6 Removal of all visible endometriosis lesions.

and urologists. It is important to thoroughly consent and plan surgical approach for endometriosis patients, as surgery can have significant complications if important organs and structures are damaged [8].

### Excision and ablation

For patients undergoing conservative surgery for endometriosis, there are two mainstays of treating disease: excision or ablation of visible lesions. Only excision of disease can confirm the diagnosis of endometriosis with histologic analysis. Ablation of disease, while providing clinical benefit, precludes the ability for histologic confirmation. Confirmation histologically is an important consideration, as visual inspection alone has poor reliability for accurately diagnosing endometriosis [9].

Surgery, whether ablation or excision, reduces overall pain associated with endometriosis in the immediate postoperative period, at 6 months, and 12 months, when compared to diagnostic laparoscopy alone [3]. However, it is important to consider the impacts of both surgical approaches.

Ablation is limited to destruction of superficial lesions. For deeply infiltrative disease, ablation may not adequately eliminate the entire lesion [9]. Notably, ablation of lesions should not be attempted near certain intra-abdominal structures due to the potential for thermal spread and adjacent injury, such as the bowel, bladder, and ureters [9].

A meta-analysis reported that women who underwent excision had significantly greater reduction in symptoms in comparison to those who underwent ablation [68]. Additionally, patients treated with the excisional method had significantly greater improvement in symptoms 12 months postoperative compared to those treated with the ablation method [68].

### Lysis of adhesions

In some studies, laparoscopic adhesiolysis was utilized in addition to ablation and excision [69, 70]. The degree of reduction in overall pain is statistically significant at 6 months postoperatively when compared to those without lysis of adhesion in addition to ablation and excision [8].

### Deep-infiltrating endometriosis

Deep-infiltrating endometriosis (DIE) are endometriotic lesions infiltrating the retroperitoneum or the wall of the pelvic organs [71]. The prevalence of DIE is difficult to evaluate, as the diagnostic criteria in the literature vary widely [72–75]. It is estimated that DIE affects twenty percent of all endometriosis patients, and adequate management of this disease is an important challenge on a societal level because of its physical, social, and psychological consequences [76, 77]. The symptoms exhibited by patients, particularly urinary and digestive symptoms, often are correlated with the location and infiltration of the lesions—dysuria, tenesmus, diarrhea, dyschezia [78]. A multidisciplinary approach to its surgical management is necessary, as a one-time complete resection and if necessary, resection of involved organs, is the best approach for patients with DIE [21, 29].

DIE is one of the best indications for robotic-assisted laparoscopy. One multicenter international retrospective trial found no increases in surgical time, blood loss, or intra-operative or postoperative complications. Use of the robot also reduced the rates of conversion to laparotomy and of laparotomy itself [79]. Robotics has an established place in the surgical treatment of DIE, especially in the more aggressive stage IV disease [79].

### Bladder

Case reports have documented the feasibility of robotics for infiltrating bladder endometriosis. Liu et al. used the da Vinci system to resect the bladder lesions and then close the defect in two layers. The authors reported an estimated blood loss of 100 mL with a total operative time of 297 min. There were no complications to the procedure, and the patient was discharged home on postoperative day number two [55]. More research needs to be conducted on specific robotic techniques for bladder endometriosis, but the feasibility has been established.

### Colorectal

Bowel involvement is estimated to occur in 5.3%–12% of women with endometriosis, and the rectum and rectosigmoid junction together account for 70%–93% of all intestinal sites of endometriosis [71, 80–82]. Symptoms include dysmenorrhea, infertility, dyspareunia, dysuria, dyschezia, tenesmus, and pain on defecation [81, 83].

The management of intestinal endometriosis depends on the depth of the bowel wall invasion (superficial, partial, or full-thickness invasion). Preoperative diagnostic imaging confirms of rectosigmoid involvement with an accuracy of 99% (sensitivity of 98.1% and specificity of 100%) when transvaginal sonography with bowel preparation is used, allowing gynecologists to create a surgical team to include colorectal surgeons if needed [84].

Bowel endometriosis can be removed by either full-thickness disc or segmental resection [4, 85–87]. Endometriosis recurrence is higher if the bowel lesions are not excised [88–90]. One-third of patients with bowel endometriosis treated by full-thickness disc resection have persistent disease [91]. The best results in terms of recurrence rates and improvement of symptoms are achieved by intestinal resection. For lesions producing partial obstruction and/or in cases of extensive lesions, a bowel resection should be performed [71, 80, 88, 89]. Complete excision of deep endometriosis with bowel resection leads to a reliable and persistent relief of pain symptoms and improvement of quality of life [4, 30, 85, 86, 92–94].

Robotic-assisted laparoscopy is feasible tool for resection of endometriosis involving the bowel. Colorectal robotic-assisted laparoscopic bowel resection results in significant improvement in gynecologic and digestive symptoms, as well as the quality of life, and produced similar results as when using a laparoscopic approach [83, 93]. One study even found a 43% rate of natural pregnancy only 6 months after robotic resection [95]. In severe cases, robotic surgery was a successful tool to avoid conversions to laparotomy [54, 61].

The use of robotic assistance provides a very precise dissection of the pelvic area, allowing good visualization of the pelvic plexus nerves, thus providing resection without nerve injury. The stable camera and the freedom of movement allow a very delicate and accurate dissection, as well as identification and preservation of the superior hemorrhoidal artery, which provides good irrigation to the rectal stump and diminishes the incidence of rectal fistula. Robotic-assisted laparoscopic bowel resection surgery for the treatment of bowel endometriosis is feasible effective and safe.

### Endometriomas

Surgical management of endometriomas (**Figures 8.5** and **8.6**) is helpful to establish the diagnosis of an adnexal mass, to treat pain associated with the cyst, for subfertility and decreased ovarian reserve in affected ovaries, to prevent continued growth of existing cysts, and to relieve external compression of surrounding structures. It is important to counsel patients that any surgical intervention on the ovary can impact ovarian reserve. However, complete excision of an endometrioma cyst, as opposed to ablation of the cyst, is associated with a reduced rate of recurrence, a reduction in symptom recurrence, and increased pregnancy rates [96]. Unfortunately, both excision and ablation have an impact on ovarian reserve. Some data suggests a one-third decrease in antimüllerian hormone (AMH) levels removal of endometriomas [97]. Robotic surgery has been showed to be safe and effective when excising and ablating ovarian endometriomas [98].

## Conclusion

Currently, robotic technology systems represent the latest developments in minimally invasive surgery and have revolutionized conventional laparoscopy by offering improved ergonomics for the surgeon, three-dimensional visualization of the operating field, greater precision, and fine instrumentation, with six degrees of freedom allowing increased maneuverability of the instruments [99]. In addition, working of these systems is intuitive and the learning curve is rapid for surgeons who master conventional laparoscopy [100, 101]. The robotic system has shown feasibility in treatments of many locations and types of endometriosis and helps reduce the conversion to laparotomy. Robotic-assisted laparoscopy plays a crucial role in treatment of endometriosis.

## References


1. Howard FM. Surgical Treatment of Endometriosis. Vol. 38, Obstetrics and Gynecology Clinics of North America. Obstet Gynecol Clin North Am; 2011. p. 677–86.
2. Jacobson TZ, Duffy JMN, Barlow DH, Farquhar C, Koninckx PR, Olive D. Laparoscopic Surgery for Subfertility Associated with Endometriosis. Vol. 2014, Cochrane Database of Systematic Reviews. John Wiley and Sons Ltd; 2014.
3. Jacobson TZ, Duffy JMN, Barlow DH, Koninckx PR, Garry R. Laparoscopic Surgery for Pelvic Pain Associated with Endometriosis. Vol. 2014, Cochrane Database of Systematic Reviews. John Wiley and Sons Ltd; 2014.
4. Abbott JA. The effects and effectiveness of laparoscopic excision of endometriosis: a prospective study with 2-5 year follow-up. Hum Reprod. 2003:1922–7. Available from: https://academic.oup.com/humrep/article-lookup/doi/10.1093/humrep/deg275
5. Vercellini P, Somigliana E, Viganò P, Abbiati A, Barbara G, Crosignani PG. Surgery for Endometriosis-Associated Infertility: A Pragmatic Approach. Vol. 24, Human Reproduction. Oxford University Press; 2009; p. 254–69.
6. Vercellini P, Crosignani PG, Abbiati A, Somigliana E, Viganò P, Fedele L. The effect of surgery for symptomatic endometriosis: the other side of the story. Hum Reprod Update. 2009;15(2):177–88. Available from: https://academic.oup.com/humupd/article-lookup/doi/10.1093/humupd/dmn062
7. Vercellini P, Fedele L, Aimi G, De Giorgi O, Consonni D, Crosignani PG. Reproductive performance, pain recurrence and disease relapse after conservative surgical treatment for endometriosis: the predictive value of the current classification system. Hum Reprod. 2006;21(10):2679–85. Available from: https://academic.oup.com/humrep/article-lookup/doi/10.1093/humrep/del230
8. Duffy JMN, Arambage K, Correa FJS, Olive D, Farquhar C, Garry R, et al. Laparoscopic Surgery for Endometriosis. Cochrane Database of Systematic Reviews. 2014.
9. Falcone T, Flyckt-Rebecca R. Clinical management of endometriosis. Obstet Gynecol. 2018;
10. Howard FM. Laparoscopic evaluation and treatment of women with chronic pelvic pain. Am Assoc Gynecol Laparosc. 1994;1(4 part 1):325–31.
11. Shakiba K, Bena JF, McGill KM, Minger J, Falcone T. Surgical treatment of endometriosis: a 7-year follow-up on the requirement for further surgery. Obstet Gynecol. 2008;111(6):1285–92. Available from: http://www.ncbi.nlm.nih.gov/pubmed/18515510
12. Namnoum AB, Hickman TN, Goodman SB, Gehlbach DL, Rock JA. Incidence of symptom recurrence after hysterectomy for endometriosis. Fertil Steril. 1995;
13. Parker WH. Bilateral oophorectomy versus ovarian conservation: effects on long-term women's health. J Minim Invasive Gynecol. 2010;17(2):161–6.
14. Clayton RD, Hawe JA, Love JC, Wilkinson N, Garry R. Recurrent pain after hysterectomy and bilateral salpingo-oophorectomy for endometriosis: Evaluation of laparoscopic excision of residual endometriosis. BJOG An Int J Obstet Gynaecol. 1999;106(7):740–4.
15. Wilczyński M, Cieślak J, Malinowski A. Supracervical hysterectomy—The vaginal route. Wideochirurgia I Inne Tech Maloinwazyjne. 2014;9(2):207–12.
16. Zobbe V, Gimbel H, Andersen BM, Filtenborg T, Jakobsen K, Sørensen HC, et al. Sexuality after total vs. subtotal hysterectomy. Acta Obstet Gynecol Scand. 2004;83(2):191–6.
17. Tsafrir Z, Aoun J, Papalekas E, Taylor A, Schiff L, Theoharis E, et al. Risk factors for trachelectomy following supracervical hysterectomy. Acta Obstet Gynecol Scand. 2017;
18. Lieng M, Qvigstad E, Istre O, Langebrekke A, Ballard K. Long-term outcomes following laparoscopic supracervical hysterectomy. BJOG An Int J Obstet Gynaecol. 2008;115(13):1605–10.
19. Nezhat CH, Malik S, Nezhat F, Nezhat C. Laparoscopic ureteroneocystostomy and vesicopsoas hitch for infiltrative endometriosis. JSLS J Soc Laparoendosc Surg;8(1):3–7. Available from: http://www.ncbi.nlm.nih.gov/pubmed/14974654
20. Vercellini P, Pisacreta A, Pesole A, Vicentini S, Stellato G, Crosignani PG. Is ureteral endometriosis an asymmetric disease? BJOG. 2000;107(4):559–61. Available from: http://www.ncbi.nlm.nih.gov/pubmed/10759279
21. Abbott J, Hawe J, Hunter D, Holmes M, Finn P, Garry R. Laparoscopic excision of endometriosis: a randomized, placebo-controlled trial. Fertil Steril. 2004;82(4):878–84.
22. Donnez J, Nisolle M, Gillet N, Smets M, Bassil S, Casanas-Roux F. Large ovarian endometriomas. Hum Reprod. 1996;11(3):641–5.
23. Mais V, Ajossa S, Guerriero S, Piras B, Floris M, Palomba M, et al. Laparoscopic management of endometriomas: A randomized trial versus laparotomy. J Gynecol Surg. 1996;
24. Crosignani PG, Vercellini P, Biffignandi F, Costantini W, Cortesi I, Imparato E. Laparoscopy versus laparotomy in conservative surgical treatment for severe endometriosis. Fertil Steril. 1996;66(5):706–11.
25. Ahmad G, Baker J, Finnerty J, Phillips K, Watson A. Laparoscopic Entry Techniques. Vol. 2019, Cochrane Database of Systematic Reviews. John Wiley and Sons Ltd; 2019.
26. Somigliana E, Vigano P, Barbara G, Vercellini P. Treatment of endometriosis-related pain: options and outcomes. Front Biosci (Elite Ed). 2009;1:455–65. Available from: http://www.ncbi.nlm.nih.gov/pubmed/19482659
27. Schwenk W, Neudecker J, Haase O, Müller J. Short-Term Benefits for Laparoscopic Colorectal Resection. The Cochrane Database of Systematic Reviews. John Wiley & Sons; 2001.

28. Winkel CA. Evaluation and management of women with endometriosis. Obstet Gynecol. 2003;102(2):397–408. Available from: http://www.ncbi.nlm.nih.gov/pubmed/12907119
29. Daraï E, Dubernard G, Coutant C, Frey C, Rouzier R, Ballester M. Randomized trial of laparoscopically assisted versus open colorectal resection for endometriosis: Morbidity, symptoms, quality of life, and fertility. Ann Surg. 2010;251(6):1018–23.
30. Ferrero S, Anserini P, Abbamonte LH, Ragni N, Camerini G, Remorgida V. Fertility after bowel resection for endometriosis. Fertil Steril. 2009.
31. Pathogenesis, consequences, and control of peritoneal adhesions in gynecologic surgery: A committee opinion. Fertil Steril. 2013;
32. Zanelotti A, Decherney AH. Surgery and endometriosis. Clin Obstet Gynecol. 2017;60(3):477–84.
33. E. D, M. B, R. R, S. H, G. D. Outcome of laparoscopic colorectal resection for endometriosis. Current Opin Obstet Gynecol. 2007.
34. Robotic Surgery in Gynecology Committee on Gynecologic Practice Society of Gynecologic Surgeons.
35. Liu H, Lu D, Wang L, Shi G, Song H, Clarke J. Robotic surgery for benign gynaecological disease. Cochrane database Syst Rev. 2012;(2):CD008978. Available from: http://www.ncbi.nlm.nih.gov/pubmed/22336855
36. Satava RM. Robotic surgery: from past to future - a personal journey. Surg Clinics North Am. 2003;83:1491–500.
37. Bann S, Khan M, Hernandez J, Munz Y, Moorthy K, Datta V, et al. Robotics in surgery. J Am Coll Surg. 2003;196: 784–95.
38. Himpens J, Leman G, Cadiere GB. Telesurgical laparoscopic cholecystectomy. Surg Endoscopy. 1998;12:1091.
39. Reza M, Maeso S, Blasco JA, Andradas E. Meta-analysis of observational studies on the safety and effectiveness of robotic gynaecological surgery. Br J Surg. 2010;97(12):1772–83.
40. Nezhat C, Crowgey SR, Garrison CP. Surgical treatment of endometriosis via laser laparoscopy. Fertil Steril 1986;45(6):778–83. Available from: http://www.ncbi.nlm.nih.gov/pubmed/2940121
41. Kelley WE. The evolution of laparoscopy and the revolution in surgery in the decade of the 1990s. J Soc Laparoendosc Surg. 2008;12(4):351–7.
42. Nezhat C, Lavie O, Hsu S, Watson J, Barnett O, Lemyre M. Robotic-assisted laparoscopic myomectomy compared with standard laparoscopic myomectomy–a retrospective matched control study. Fertil Steril. 2009;91(2):556–9. Available from: http://www.ncbi.nlm.nih.gov/pubmed/18377901
43. Nezhat FR, Datta MS, Liu C, Chuang L, Zakashansky K. Robotic radical hysterectomy versus total laparoscopic radical hysterectomy with pelvic lymphadenectomy for treatment of early cervical cancer. J Soc Laparoendosc Surg. 2008;12(3):227–37.
44. Nezhat C, Saberi NS, Shahmohamady B, Nezhat F. Robotic-assisted laparoscopy in gynecological surgery. JSLS. 2006;10(3):317–20.
45. Frumovitz M, Escobar P, Ramirez PT. Minimally invasive surgical approaches for patients with endometrial cancer. Clin Obstet Gynecol. 2011;54(2):226–34.
46. Ayoubi JM, Carbonnel M, Pirtea P, Kvarnstr€ N, Dahm-K€Ahler P. Laparotomy or minimal invasive surgery in uterus transplantation: a comparison. [cited 2020 Feb 29]; Available from: https://doi.org/10.1016/j.fertnstert.2019.05.038
47. Company [Internet]. [cited 2020 Jan 19]. Available from: https://www.intuitive.com/en-us/about-us/company?gclid=Cj0KCQiAmZDxBRDIARIsABnkbYT4tv-CWS1IxW0xcjPKQRD4919wDu-3eNdw5l3K_y5oahpBgVrAhvNIaAnGtEALw_wcB
48. Fourman MM, Saber AA. Robotic bariatric surgery: a systematic review.Surg Obes Relat Dis. 2012;8:483–8.
49. Seamon LG, Fowler JM, Richardson DL, Carlson MJ, Valmadre S, Phillips GS, et al. A detailed analysis of the learning curve: Robotic hysterectomy and pelvic-aortic lymphadenectomy for endometrial cancer. Gynecol Oncol. 2009;114(2):162–7.
50. Fowler JM, Seamon LG, Cohn DE, Richardson DL, Valmadre S, Carlson MJ, et al. Robotic hysterectomy and pelvic-aortic lymphadenectomy for endometrial cancer. Obstet Gynecol. 2008;112(6):1207–13.
51. Hung AJ, Chen J, Shah A, Gill IS. Telementoring and telesurgery for minimally invasive procedures. J Urol. 2018;199:355–69.
52. Advancing Minimally Invasive Gynecology Worldwide A. AAGL Position Statement: Robotic-assisted laparoscopic surgery in benign gynecology. 2013 [cited 2020 Jan 25]; Available from: http://dx.doi.org/10.1016/j.jmig.2012.12.007
53. Chammas MF, Kim FJ, Barbarino A, Hubert N, Feuillu B, Coissard A, et al. Asymptomatic rectal and bladder endometriosis: a case for robotic-assisted surgery. Can J Urol. 2008;
54. Nezhat C, Hajhosseini B, King LP. Robotic-assisted laparoscopic treatment of bowel, bladder, and ureteral endometriosis. J Soc Laparoendosc Surg. 2011;
55. Liu C, Peresic D, Samadi D, Nezhat F. Robotic-assisted laparoscopic partial bladder resection for the treatment of infiltrating endometriosis. J Minim Invasive Gynecol. 2008;
56. Frick AC, Barakat EE, Stein RJ, Mora M, Falcone T. Robotic-assisted laparoscopic management of ureteral endometriosis. J Soc Laparoendosc Surg. 2011;15(3):396–9.
57. Averbach M, Popoutchi P, Marques OW, Abdalla RZ, Podgaec S, Abrão MS. Robotic rectosigmoidectomy - pioneer case report in Brazil. Current scene in colorectal robotic surgery. Arq Gastroenterol. 2010;
58. Ercoli A, Dasta M, Fagotti A, Fanfani F, Romano F, Baldazzi G, et al. Robotic treatment of colorectal endometriosis: technique, feasibility and short-term results. Hum Reprod. 2012;27(3):722–6.
59. Abo C, Roman H, Bridoux V, Huet E, Tuech J-J, Resch B, et al. Management of deep-infiltrating endometriosis by laparoscopic route with robotic assistance: 3-year experience. J Gynecol Obstet Hum Reprod. 2017;46(1):9–18.
60. Nezhat FR, Sirota I. Perioperative outcomes of robotic assisted laparoscopic surgery versus conventional laparoscopy surgery for Advanced-Stage endometriosis. J Soc Laparoendosc Surg. 2014;18(4):e2014.00094.
61. Nezhat C, Lewis M, Kotikela S, Veeraswamy A, Saadat L, Hajhosseini B, et al. Robotic versus standard laparoscopy for the treatment of endometriosis. Fertil Steril. 2010;94(7):2758–60.
62. Nezhat CR, Stevens A, Balassiano E, Soliemannjad R. Robotic-assisted laparoscopy vs conventional laparoscopy for the treatment of advanced stage endometriosis. J Minim Invasive Gynecol. 2015;22(1):40–4.
63. Magrina JF, Espada M, Kho RM, Cetta R, Chang YHH, Magtibay PM. Surgical Excision of Advanced Endometriosis: Perioperative Outcomes and Impacting Factors. J Minim Invasive Gynecol. 2015;22(6):944–50.
64. Chen CCG, Falcone T. Robotic gynecologic surgery: past, present, and future. Clin Obstet Gynecol. 2009;52(3):335–43.
65. Soto E, Luu TH, Liu X, Magrina JF, Wasson MN, Einarsson JI, et al. Laparoscopy vs. Robotic Surgery for Endometriosis (LAROSE): a multicenter, randomized, controlled trial. Fertil Steril. 2017:107(4):996–1002.
66. Touboul C, Ballester M, Dubernard G, Zilberman S, Thomin A, Daraï E. Long-term symptoms, quality of life, and fertility after colorectal resection for endometriosis: extended analysis of a randomized controlled trial comparing laparoscopically assisted to open surgery. Surg Endosc. 2015;29(7):1879–87.
67. Berlanda N, Vercellini P, Somigliana E, Frattaruolo MP, Buggio L, Gattei U. Role of surgery in endometriosis-associated subfertility. Semin Reprod Med. 2013;31(2):133–43.
68. Pundir J, Omanwa K, Kovoor E, Pundir V, Lancaster G, Barton-Smith P. Laparoscopic Excision Versus Ablation for Endometriosis-associated Pain: An Updated Systematic Review and Meta-analysis.J Minim Invasive Gynecol. 2017;24: 747–56.
69. Marcoux S, Maheux R, Bérubé S. Laparoscopic surgery in infertile women with minimal or mild endometriosis. Canadian Collaborative Group on Endometriosis. N Engl J Med. 1997;337(4):217–22.
70. Sutton CJG, Ewen SP, Whitelaw N, Haines P. Prospective, randomized, double-blind, controlled trial of laser laparoscopy in the treatment of pelvic pain associated with minimal, mild, and moderate endometriosis. Fertil Steril. 1994;62(4):696–700.
71. Chapron C, Dubuisson JB, Chopin N, Foulot H, Jacob S, Vieira M, et al. [Deep pelvic endometriosis: management and proposal for a "surgical classification"]. Gynecol Obstet Fertil. 2003.

72. Cramer DW, Missmer SA. The epidemiology of endometriosis. Ann New York Acad Sci. 2002.
73. Eskenazi B, Warner ML. Epidemiology of endometriosis. Obstet Gynecol Clin North Am. 1997.
74. Viganò P, Parazzini F, Somigliana E, Vercellini P. Endometriosis: Epidemiology and aetiological factors. Best Pract Res Clin Obstet Gynaecol. 2004;18(2):177–200.
75. Mahmood TA, Templeton A. Prevalence and genesis of endometriosis. Hum Reprod. 1991;6(4):544–9.
76. Birnbaum LS, Cummings AM. Dioxins and endometriosis: A plausible hypothesis. Environ Health Perspect. 2002;110(1):15–21.
77. Fauconnier A, Fritel X, Chapron C. [Endometriosis and pelvic pain: Epidemiological evidence of the relationship and implications] Gynecol Obstet Fertil. 2009;37(1):57–69.
78. Panel P, Renouvel F. Management of endometriosis: clinical and biological assessment. J Gynecol Obstet Biol Reprod (Paris). 2007;36(2):119–28.
79. Collinet P, Leguevaque P, Neme RM, Cela V, Barton-Smith P, Hébert T, et al. Robot-assisted laparoscopy for deep-infiltrating endometriosis: International multicentric retrospective study. Surg Endosc. 2014;28(8):2474–9.
80. Weed JC, Ray JE. Endornetriosis of the bowel. Obstet Gynecol. 1987.
81. Coronado C, Franklin RR, Lotze EC, Bailey HR, Valdes CT. Surgical treatment of symptomatic colorectal endometriosis. Fertil Steril. 1990;53(3):411–6.
82. Bailey HR, Ott MT, Hartendorp P. Aggressive surgical management for advanced colorectal endometriosis. Dis Colon Rectum. 1994;37(8):747–53.
83. Daraï E, Marpeau O, Thomassin I, Dubernard G, Barranger E, Bazot M. Fertility after laparoscopic colorectal resection for endometriosis: preliminary results. Fertil Steril. 2005;84(4):945–50.
84. Chamié LP, Pereira RMA, Zanatta A, Serafini PC. Transvaginal US after bowel preparation for deeply infiltrating endometriosis: Protocol, imaging appearances, and laparoscopic correlation. Radiographics. 2010;30(5):1235–49.
85. Redwine DB, Wright JT. Laparoscopic treatment of complete obliteration of the cul-de-sac associated with endometriosis: Long-term follow-up of en bloc resection. Fertil Steril. 2001;76(2):358–65.
86. Fleisch MC, Xafis D, Bruyne F De, Hucke J, Bender HG, Dall P. Radical resection of invasive endometriosis with bowel or bladder involvement - long-term results. Eur J Obstet Gynecol Reprod Biol. 2005;123(2):224–9.
87. Verspyck E, Lefranc JP, Guyard B, Blondon J. Treatment of bowel endometriosis: A report of six cases of colorectal endometriosis and a survey of the literature. Eur J Obstet Gynecol Reprod Biol. 1997;71(1):81–4.
88. Anaf V. Sigmoid endometriosis and ovarian stimulation. Hum Reprod. 2000;15(4):790–4.
89. Nezhat C, Hajhosseini B, King LP. Laparoscopic management of bowel endometriosis: Predictors of severe disease and recurrence. J Soc Laparoendosc Surg. 2011;15(4):431–8.
90. D'Hooghe T, Hummelshoj L. Multi-disciplinary centres/networks of excellence for endometriosis management and research: a proposal. Hum Reprod. 2006;21(11):2743–8.
91. Remorgida V, Ragni N, Ferrero S, Anserini P, Torelli P, Fulcheri E. The involvement of the interstitial Cajal cells and the enteric nervous system in bowel endometriosis. Hum Reprod. 2005;20(1):264–71.
92. Kumar D. Irritable bowel syndrome, chronic pelvic inflammatory disease and endometriosis. Eur J Gastroenterol Hepatol. 2004.16(12):1251–2.
93. Dubernard G, Piketty M, Rouzier R, Houry S, Bazot M, Darai E. Quality of life after laparoscopic colorectal resection for endometriosis. Hum Reprod. 2006;21(5):1243–7.
94. Landi S, Ceccaroni M, Perutelli A, Allodi C, Barbieri F, Fiaccavento A, et al. Laparoscopic nerve-sparing complete excision of deep endometriosis: Is it feasible? Hum Reprod. 2006;21(3):774–81.
95. Neme RM, Schraibman V, Okazaki S, Maccapani G, Chen WJ, Domit CD, et al. Deep-infiltrating colorectal endometriosis treated with robotic-assisted rectosigmoidectomy. J Soc Laparoendosc Surg. 2013;17(2):227–34.
96. Hart RJ, Hickey M, Maouris P, Buckett W. Excisional surgery versus ablative surgery for ovarian endometriomata. Cochrane Database of Systematic Reviews. 2008.
97. Uncu G, Kasapoglu I, Ozerkan K, Seyhan A, Oral Yilmaztepe A, Ata B. Prospective assessment of the impact of endometriomas and their removal on ovarian reserve and determinants of the rate of decline in ovarian reserve. Hum Reprod. 2013;28(8):2140–5.
98. Gargiulo AR, Feltmate C, Srouji SS. Robotic single-site excision of ovarian endometrioma. 2015 [cited 2020 Feb 29]; Available from: www.biomedcentral.com/submit
99. Monsarrat N, Collinet P, Narducci F, Leblanc E, Vinatier D. Robotic assistance in gynaecological surgery: State-of-the-art. Gynecol Obstet Fertil. 2009;37(5):415–24.
100. Falcone T, Goldberg JM. Robotics in gynecology. Surg Clin North Am. 2003.
101. Bokhari MB, Patel CB, Ramos-Valadez DI, Ragupathi M, Haas EM. Learning curve for robotic-assisted laparoscopic colorectal surgery. Surg Endosc. 2011;25(3):855–60.

# 9

## ENDOMETRIOSIS AND UTERINE ANOMALIES: DIAGNOSIS AND TREATMENT

**Damaris Freytag and Ibrahim Alkatout**

### Introduction

Endometriosis, defined as the presence of endometrial glands and stroma outside the internal epithelial lining of the uterine cavity, is regarded as the second most common benign female genital disease after uterine myoma. Endometriosis affects 6%–10% of women of reproductive age [1]. In terms of pathogenesis, the disease is attributed to various factors, including retrograde menstruation, coelomic metaplasia, metastasis, altered cellular immunity, and a multifactorial mode of inheritance with interactions between the environment and specific genes [2]. The patients experience chronic pelvic pain, dysmenorrhea, deep dyspareunia, cyclic bowel or bladder symptoms (such as dyschezia, bloating, constipation, rectal bleeding, diarrhea, or hematuria), subfertility, abnormal menstrual bleeding, chronic fatigue, and low back pain [3]. The percentage of women with confirmed endometriosis treated for infertility is 9%–50% [3]. Patients with endometriosis have a reduced quality and quantity of oocytes and embryos, low implantation and pregnancy rates, and high rates of spontaneous abortion [4].

Congenital uterine anomalies (CUA) are more common than previously assumed. Their clinical presentation depends on the anomalies and the woman's reproductive age. Some patients may be asymptomatic, with normal fertility and obstetric outcomes, while others may have primary amenorrhea, menstrual irregularities, endometriosis, and infertility. Some are subject to a high risk of recurrent implantation failure, recurrent spontaneous abortions, and adverse pregnancy outcomes. CUA are caused by abnormal development of the Müllerian ducts during embryogenesis. The two Müllerian ducts undergo descent, fusion, and resorption of the midline septum to form the uterus, tubes, cervix, and the upper part of the vagina [5]. Various prevalence rates have been reported for CUA, depending on the population and the diagnostic technique used. In the general population, CUA has been observed in 4.3%–6.7% of women. The prevalence of CUA is estimated to range between 3.4% and 8.0% in the infertile population, and between 12.6% and 18.2% in women with recurrent abortions [5].

The absence of a uniform classification system for CUA is a well-known problem. A correct diagnosis based on an accurate classification is essential in order to avoid inadequate or unnecessary surgery [6]. Four main systems have been suggested for the classification of congenital uterine anomalies: the American Society for Reproductive Medicine (ASRM) system, the embryological-clinical classification system of genitourinary malformations, the VCUAM, and the ESHRE/ESGE system [6–8].

The septate uterus is one of the most common structural uterine anomalies. It is associated with adverse reproductive outcomes, such as recurrent miscarriages or infertility. The surface of the septum differs from that of the endometrium or the uterine cavity. Lesser thickness and inadequate blood supply result in lower implantation rates. Lavergne et al. analyzed women with a septate uterus undergoing in vitro fertilization (IVF) treatment. Women with an untreated septate uterus had a poor outcome after IVF treatment compared to women who had undergone hysteroscopic dissection prior to IVF [9]. A close embryological relation exists between the development of the reproductive and urinary organs. Therefore, congenital renal defects may also be found in patients with Müllerian duct anomalies. Renal anomalies are present in 30%–50%. The distal part of the vagina, external genitals, and ovaries are spared because of their different embryological origin.

The association between endometriosis and CUA has been frequently mentioned in the published literature [10–14]. Especially obstructive Müllerian malformations may lead to severe retrograde menstruation and cause endometriosis. Data reported by Olive and Henderson support the concept of increased retrograde menstruation and the likelihood of endometriosis [14]. Ugur et al. [13] showed that obstructive anomalies were associated significantly more often with endometriosis than nonobstructive anomalies, but patients with nonobstructive anomalies did not have endometriosis more frequently than controls [13]. This was confirmed by Fedele et al. [12]. Yet other investigations have not consistently confirmed these data [15]. Recent studies have also reported a high rate of endometriosis among women with nonobstructive Müllerian duct anomalies. Nawroth et al. [10, 11], and recently LaMonica et al. described a high rate of endometriosis in women with a septate uterus [10, 11].

The etiology, classification, diagnosis, and management of Müllerian duct anomalies, especially the uterus subseptus, have been discussed for years [6–8, 16–18].

### Classification, definition, and diagnosis of CUA

The evaluation of women with a suspected anomaly should include a detailed medical history, with questions about previous miscarriages, adverse pregnancy outcomes, special obstetric features (such as breech presentation or placental complications), menstrual history (such as primary amenorrhea or menstrual irregularities), infertility, endometriosis, ureter, and kidney disease, as well as a physical examination and imaging investigations. Besides endometriosis, dysmenorrhea may be a sign of uterine malformations. Pelvic ultrasound is the first imaging procedure recommended for a patient with primary amenorrhea, dysmenorrhea, or cyclic pain. It may be difficult to detect an anomaly prior to puberty because of the small size of the uterus and the absence of endometrial stimulation [19]. Given the diversity of anomalies and clinical presentations, therapeutic approaches are equally variable. The treatment, when needed, is always surgery using simple procedures. However, the majority of anomalies do not require treatment. A correct diagnosis and an adequate classification are essential in order to avoid inadequate or unnecessary surgery [6]. Consultation with a gynecologist and a radiologist experienced in the diagnostic investigation of Müllerian duct anomalies may be helpful to establish the accurate diagnosis.

In general, these anomalies do not call for emergency surgery. However, in view of their complexity the anomalies are best managed by gynecologists who are familiar with their surgical management [19].

## Classification

The lack of a uniform classification system for uterine anomalies has been a well-known problem for many years. Several international societies, including the ASRM, ESHRE, and ESGE have published classification systems to describe and categorize uterine anomalies. Since the first descriptions of congenital anomalies and their classifications in the 19th century, more than 30 classifications and modifications have been mentioned in the published literature. The ASRM classification, published in 1988, is well known and seems to be most widely used by clinicians throughout the world. It consists of seven main groups: (i) agenesis and hypoplasias, (ii) unicornuate uteri, (iii) didelphys, (iv) bicornuate uteri, (v) septate uteri, (vi) arcuate uteri, and group (vii) malformations due to exposure to diethylstilbestrol (DES) [6, 8].

Despite its long-standing acceptance in the medical fraternity, the ASRM classification has some limitations. Other classifications have been suggested like the embryological-clinical classification system of genitourinary malformations and the VCUAM (Vagina, Cervix, Uterus, Adnex, and Associated Malformation) system based on the TNM principle in oncology – but they did not achieve widespread acceptance [6, 8]. In 2013, the European Society of Human Reproduction and Embryology (ESHRE) and the European Society for Gynaecological Endoscopy (ESGE) proposed a new classification system based on the anatomy of the female genital tract, including cervical and vaginal malformations [7, 20]. Anomalies are classified into six main categories: U0: normal uterus, U1: dysmorphic uterus, U2: septate uterus, U3: bicorporeal uterus, U4: hemiuterus, U5: aplastic uterus, and U6: unclassified cases. The main categories were divided into subclasses based on clinically significant anatomical variations. The independent subclasses of C and V have been suggested for cervical and vaginal anomalies [7].

## Diagnosis and imaging techniques

In the last few decades, several methods have been suggested for the diagnosis of uterine malformations, including two-dimensional transvaginal ultrasound, hysteroscopy and laparoscopy, hysterosalpingography (HSG), magnetic resonance imaging (MRI), and three-dimensional ultrasound (3D ultrasound). Laparoscopy is useful for the evaluation of the external contours of the uterus, while hysteroscopy permits the assessment of the uterine cavity. Hysteroscopy and laparoscopy as well as MRI have been considered the gold standard for the diagnosis of uterine malformations [21].

The first procedure is always a conventional two-dimensional ultrasound (2D ultrasound) investigation. It is easy, painless, economical, available nearly everywhere, and gynecologists are familiar with the technique. The endometrial line must be clearly visible for an accurate assessment of the uterine cavity. Timing the examination in the late proliferative or secretory phase of the menstrual cycle may enhance the contrast field and permit better visualization. Sagittal and transverse planes can be investigated. As shown in **Figure 9.1**, two separate endometrial echoes are the first sign of a septate uterus on 2D ultrasound. The latter provides additional information in cases of infertility due to potential intramural or intracavitary pathologies, such as myomas, adenomyosis, or polyps. When used as a screening test, the sensitivity of 2D ultrasound is about 70% [22], but the investigation does not permit the examiner to distinguish between the different types of anomalies. The technique does permit a limited assessment of the uterine cavity.

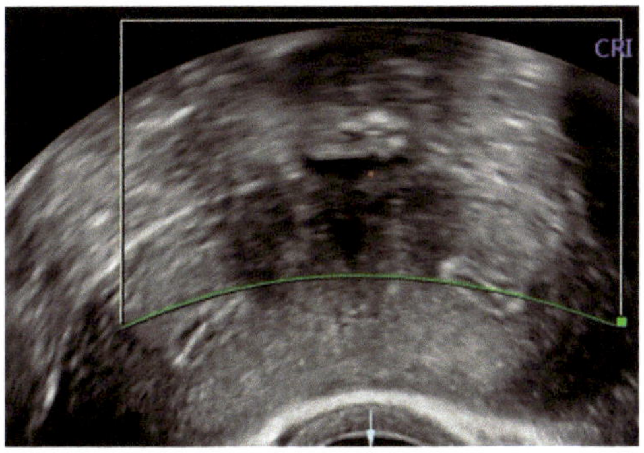


FIGURE 9.1 Imaging of the septate uterus. 2D ultrasound with two separate endometrial echoes in the transverse plane.

Compared with other techniques, three-dimensional ultrasound (3D ultrasound) and MRI provide information about the uterine cavity as well as the external contours of the uterus [23]. The advantage of 3D ultrasound is that the investigator is able to image the coronal plane and perform volumetric reconstruction, which provides a frontal view of the uterus and details of its anatomy. Thus, 3D ultrasound may well serve as a viable alternative to MRI [23]. Compared to other diagnostic procedures 3D ultrasound is non-invasive, safer, cheaper, and more tolerable. The technique has been recommended as the reference standard by the ESHRE [20]. As shown in **Figures 9.2a,b** and **9.3a,b**, 3D ultrasound permits an accurate and comprehensive diagnosis and classification of subtypes of uterine anomalies.

Saline contrast sonohysterography proved to be accurate, particularly when used in conjunction with 3D ultrasound, but is more invasive. Several studies have compared the sensitivity and specificity of 3D ultrasound and MRI for the detection of uterine anomalies. Using the ESHRE/ESGE classification system, Graupera et al. [23] compared the accuracy of 3D ultrasound with that of MRI for the diagnosis of uterine malformations. For the investigation of the normal uterus 3D ultrasound had a sensitivity of 83.3%, a specificity of 100%, PPV of 100%, NPV of 98.2%, and a kappa index of 0.900 compared to MRI. For septate uteri, the authors established a sensitivity of 100% and a specificity of 88.9%. The PPV was 95.5%, the NPV 100%, and kappa 0.918. For dysmorphic and hemi-uteri, the sensitivity, specificity, PPV and NPV of the procedure was 100%. For bicorporeal uteri the sensitivity was 83.3% and the specificity 100% [23].

Uterine malformations must be diagnosed accurately because they are associated with an adverse reproductive outcome. The accurate diagnosis is also needed in order to establish the prognosis of the reproductive procedure and devise an appropriate treatment strategy for the individual patient. 2D ultrasound only provides indirect information about the presence of uterine anomalies. Unlike 2D ultrasound, 3D ultrasound permits the diagnostician to distinguish between the different types of uterine malformations [23]. Salim et al. proved the intra- and interobserver reproducibility of 3D ultrasound for the diagnosis of uterine malformations [24].

The Thessaloniki ESHRE/ESGE consensus on the diagnosis of female genital anomalies was published in 2016 [20]. The distance between the interostial line and the external uterine profile at the mid-coronal plane was used to determine the thickness of the uterine wall. When the coronal plane is not available, an

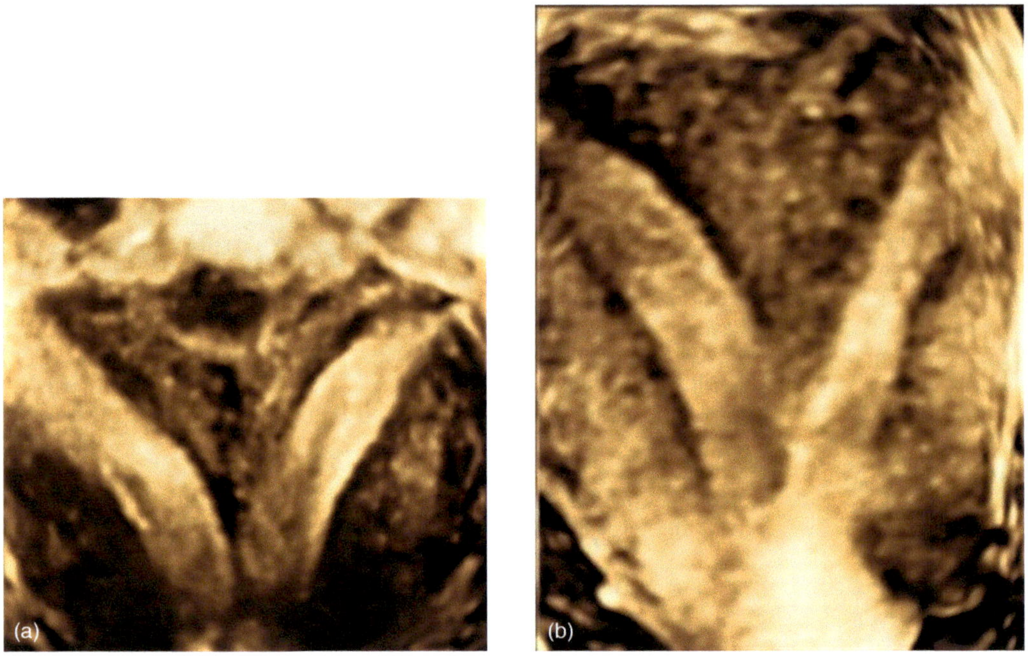

FIGURE 9.2 Image of (a) a septate uterus and (b) using transvaginal 3D ultrasonography.

alternative option is the mean anterior and posterior uterine wall thickness in 2D longitudinal planes. For the detection of anomalies, the ESHRE/ESGE consensus of 2016 recommends 2D ultrasound and a gynecological examination in cases of asymptomatic women, and 3D ultrasound for symptomatic women in high-risk groups. Furthermore, the consensus recommends 3D ultrasound in asymptomatic women whose routine investigations yield suspicion of a malformation. In ambiguous cases or in women with suspected complex anomalies, the consensus recommends MRI and endoscopy [20].

## Endometriosis

Causal treatment of endometriosis is rendered difficult by the fact that its pathogenesis is not clearly understood. Depending on its symptoms, the treatment options include expectant management, analgesia, hormonal therapy, surgery, and the combination of medical treatment before and/or after surgery. The treatment should be as radical as necessary and as minimal as possible. The recurrence rate among treated patients ranges between 5% and >60%, and is highly dependent on the existing management and surgical skills. Optimal treatment calls for intensive interdisciplinary cooperation for the purpose of diagnostic investigation as well as treatment. Both of these should be conducted at suitably equipped centers, especially in women with deep-infiltrating endometriosis [25–27].

**Figure 9.4** provides an overview of potential treatment options. Medical treatment with gonadotropin-releasing hormone (GnRH) analogs or progesterone (such as Visanne (Dienogest)) may be offered to patients with pain or other typical symptoms of endometriosis who do not wish to become pregnant. The GnRH agonist must be prescribed in combination with an add-back of estrogen in order to prevent the adverse effects of GnRH agonists, such as

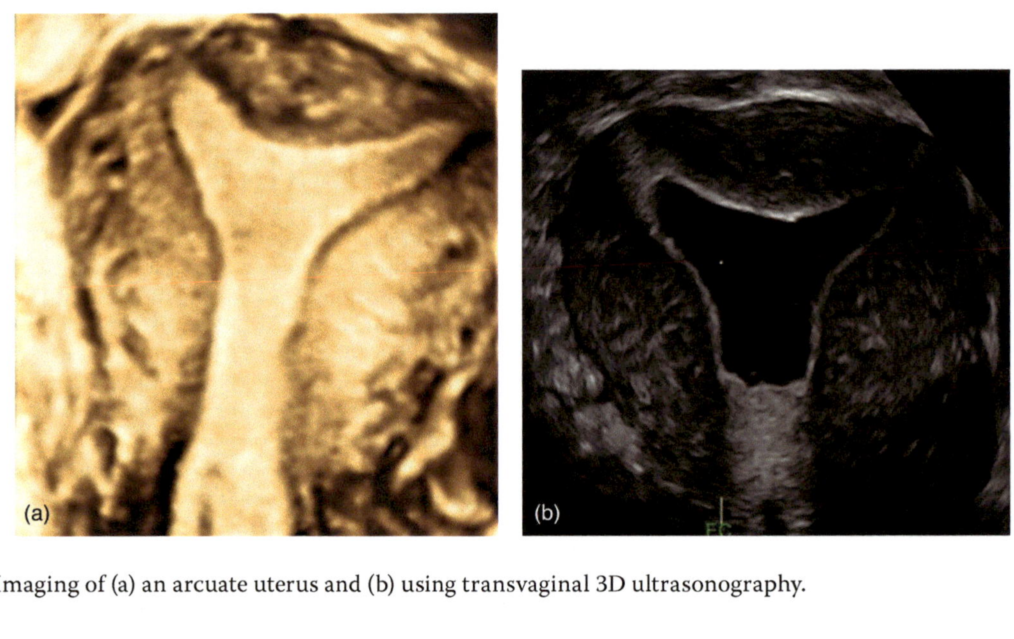

FIGURE 9.3 Imaging of (a) an arcuate uterus and (b) using transvaginal 3D ultrasonography.

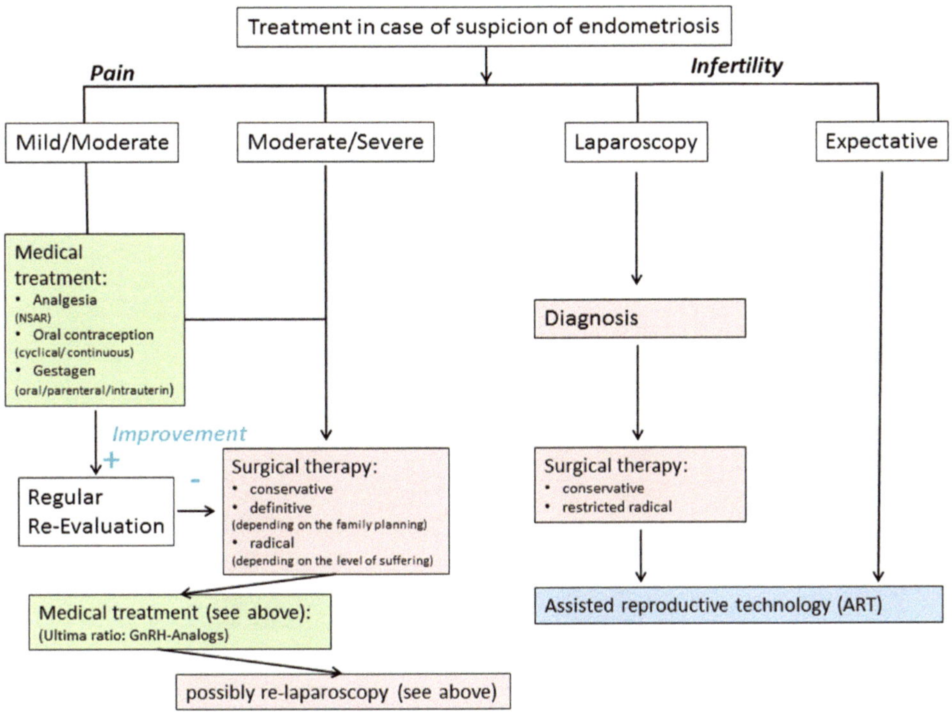


**FIGURE 9.4** Potential treatment options in women with endometriosis.

bone demineralization, vasomotor symptoms, and mood swings. A serum estradiol level of about 60 pg/mL is needed [3]. In cases of infertility, laparoscopy is the method of choice to detect and, if possible, eliminate endometriosis. The latter is a progressive disease that may destroy the anatomy of the reproductive organs. Therefore, surgery is of crucial importance [28, 29]. In advanced stages, pain and sterility are mainly caused by organ damage, fibrosis, and adhesions; these constitute a clear indication for surgery. Early laparoscopy can prevent any delay in diagnosing the disease and halt the progression of symptoms [30]. Most patients experience symptomatic relief after successful ablation/resection of endometriosis and adhesiolysis [31]. Combined treatment is a further option. It involves diagnostic laparoscopy, the removal of all visible endometriosis lesions, three to six months of endocrine therapy, and a subsequent second-look laparoscopy with resection of residual lesions, adhesiolysis, and reconstruction of organs [3].

In contrast to fibroids, polyps, and uterine septa, adenomyosis is difficult to treat and not accessible to surgery. Tremellen and Russell [32] reported four cases of recurrent implantation failure (RIF) in connection with adenomyosis; all patients were successfully treated with an ultra-long pituitary downregulation protocol [33].

## Endometriosis and Müllerian duct anomalies

The coexistence of endometriosis and Müllerian duct anomalies, which are frequently diagnosed during the exploration of infertility has been reported by many authors. The underlying pathological mechanism could be intensified retrograde menstruation. Several authors mention the association between endometriosis and obstructive Müllerian duct malformations, but not endometriosis and nonobstructive anomalies [12, 13]. Ugur et al. [13] showed that obstructive anomalies were associated significantly more often with endometriosis than nonobstructive anomalies. Endometriosis was as common in patients with nonobstructive anomalies as it was in controls [13]. This was confirmed by Fedele et al. [12], but not in other studies. Olive and Henderson support the concept of increased retrograde menstruation and the likelihood of endometriosis [14].

Since a septate uterus is the most common nonobstructive Müllerian anomaly, Nawroth and LaMonica recently addressed this anomaly alone; the authors compared the prevalence of a septum in women with and without endometriosis. Nawroth et al. registered a high rate of endometriosis in women with a septate uterus [10].

LaMonica [11] investigated whether the incidence of a septate uterus correlates with the severity of endometriosis. In 343 women of reproductive age undergoing hysteroscopy and laparoscopy for infertility, menorrhagia or pelvic pain, the authors found that the frequency of a septate uterus was significantly higher in women with endometriosis than in women without endometriosis (37% vs. 27%, $p = .046$), and was even higher in women with severe endometriosis (stage IV disease 41%, $p = .022$). The authors suggest that the presence of a uterine septum may predispose the patient to more advanced endometriosis. However, the conclusions of the study were limited by the heterogeneity of the groups (infertility, pain, and abnormal uterine bleeding) and different numbers of patients with endometriosis in stages I–IV [11].

## Diagnosis and management of common congenital anomalies and their association with endometriosis

**Figure 9.5** provides an overview of common uterine congenital malformations; the latter are described below in greater detail.

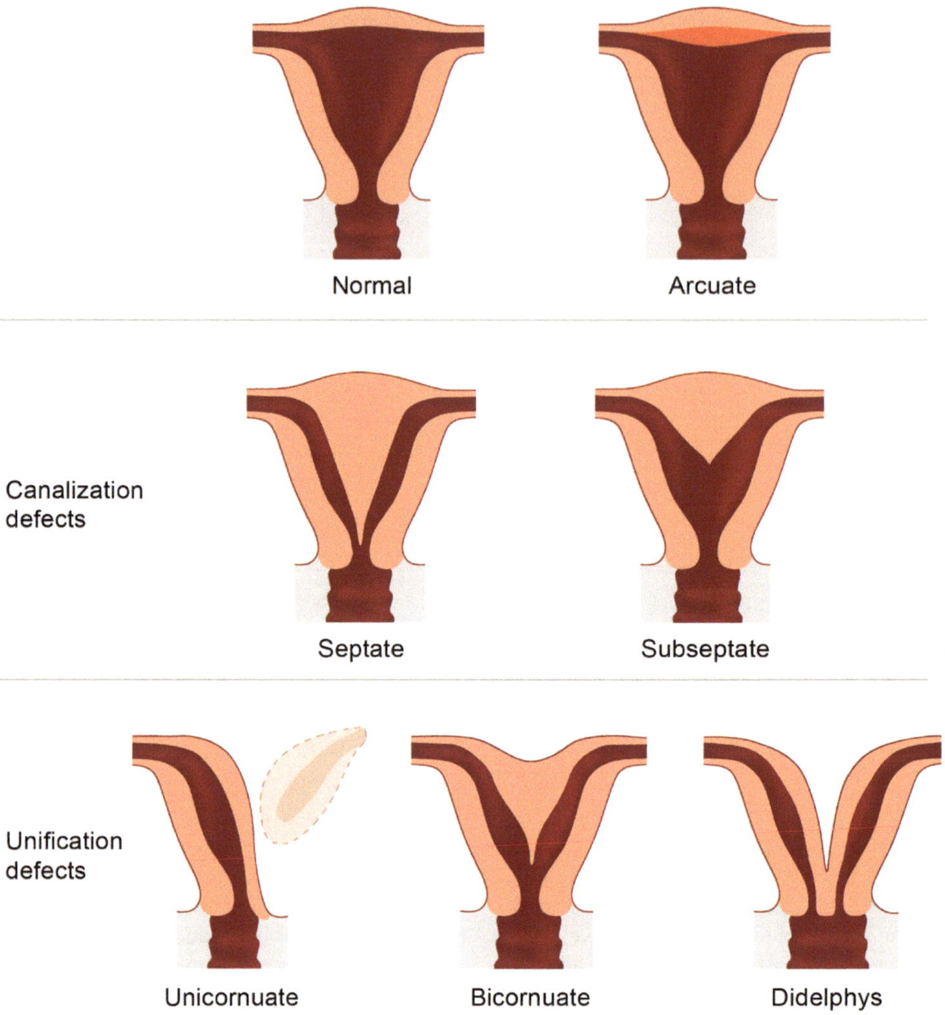


**FIGURE 9.5** Diagram of common uterine congenital malformations. The orange color marks the external uterine contour while red marks the uterine cavity.

## Septate uterus

The septate uterus (**Figure 9.5**, **Figure 9.1** and **Figure 9.2a,b**) is a controversial Müllerian duct anomaly. The controversy is attributed, on the one hand, to the ambiguous definition of the entity, and on the other hand to the dispute as to whether the clinical outcome is actually improved by surgery.

The septate uterus is the most common subtype of Müllerian duct anomalies, with a mean prevalence of 35% [5]. It results from the absence of resorption of the midline septum between the two Müllerian ducts. This anomaly has been associated with reduced fertility, a higher risk of preterm birth, malpresentation, miscarriage, and intrauterine growth retardation. The length, width, and vascularity of a septum may vary, ranging from an incomplete/partial septate to a complete septate uterus [17]. Definitions are not standardized and the majority of them have not been categorized systematically. The classifications of the European Society of Human Reproduction and Embryology, the European Society for Gynaecological Endoscopy (ESHRE/ESGE), and ASRM differ from each other. As shown in **Figure 9.6**, the criteria of the ESHRE/ESGE include a uterus with normal outlines and an internal indentation (septum) exceeding > 50% of the myometrial wall thickness. The criteria of the ASRM include an indentation angle <90° and an indentation depth >15 mm. The criteria for a normal/arcuate uterus include an indentation angle >90° and an indentation depth <10 mm [17] (**Figure 9.6**). The arcuate uterus is referred to as category VI in the ASRM classification. In the ESHRE/ESGE classification, arcuate uteri have not been defined as a separate category but assigned to "others" in class U1 (dysmorphic uteri). Class U1, in the ESHRE/ESGE classification, consists of the three subgroups U1a (T shaped), U1b (infantilis), and U1c (others).

As no uniform criteria exist for the diagnosis of a septate uterus, the various classifications may prompt clinicians to favor surgery more or less frequently to correct the anomaly. Some authors describe the risk of overdiagnosis and overtreatment of the septate uterus on the basis of the ESHRE/ESGE classification as compared to the ASRM classification [34]. Recently Ludwin et al. published a study evaluating the opinions of experts in distinguishing between the normal/arcuate and septate uterus [34]. They asked 15 experts (five clinicians, five surgeons, and five ultrasonographers) to state the diagnosis of a normal/arcuate or septate uterus after evaluating coronal 3D ultrasound images of the uteruses of 100 women with suspected fundal internal indentations. Two other observers performed the ultrasound investigations and measurements. The authors registered good agreement

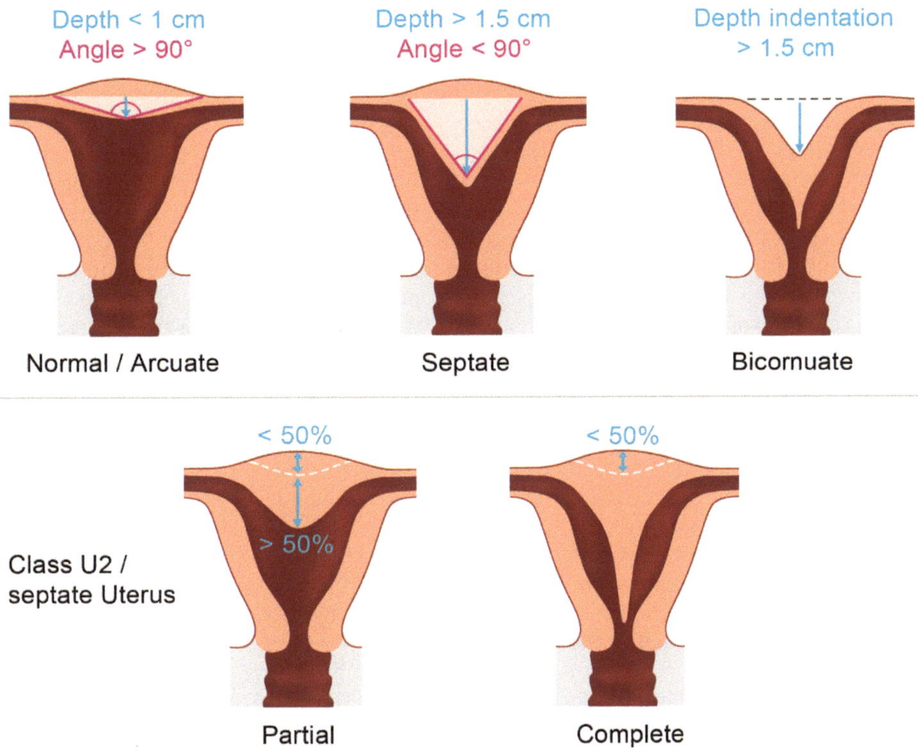


**FIGURE 9.6** Diagram of septate uteri. The upper illustrations show a normal/arcuate, septate, and bicornuate uterus according to the ASRM classification. Illustrated below is a septate uterus according to the ESHRE–ESGE classification.

between the evaluators, also known as CUME or Congenital Uterine Malformations Experts. The latter found 18 septate and 82 normal/arcuate uteri. According to the ESHRE/ESGE criteria, the experts found 80 septate and 20 normal/arcuate uteri, compared with 5 septate, 82 normal/arcuate, and 13 that could not be classified (gray zone) by the ASRM criteria. The agreement between CUME and ASRM was 87%, and that between CUME and ESHRE/ESGE 38%. The authors concluded that the prevalence of septate uteri was overestimated by the ESHRE/ESGE and underestimated by the ASRM classification. The following were established as the best cut-off values for a septate uterus: indentation angle <140°, indentation depth ≥10 mm and I:WT ratio >110% [34]. The experts recommend these measurements and consider them simple and reliable. Of these three, the simplest and most reliable measurement to distinguish between a normal/arcuate and a septate uterus is an internal indentation depth ≥10 mm. However, this classification was based on only one study that included 15 experts; further prospective studies will be needed to confirm these statements [18].

Surgical section of the uterine septum is considered a part of standard care in many countries, although evidence of the advantages of resection is limited and is mainly based on retrospective studies [35]. The pathophysiology underlying the negative impact of the septum on fertility and the outcome of pregnancy have not been clarified. The data suggest that the septum is a poor site for embryo implantation because of its assumed poor vascularization, and the fact that vascular endothelial growth factor (VEGF) receptors are altered in the endometrium of the septal region. Further reasons include uncoordinated contractility of the septum and reduced sensitivity to pre-ovulatory changes in the endometrium at this site [35].

The ASRM published its guidelines in 2016 [17], which include the following statements: there is insufficient evidence to conclude that a uterine septum is associated with infertility (Grade C), but some observational studies shows that hysteroscopic septum resection is associated with improved clinical pregnancy rates in women with infertility (Grade C). Furthermore, a uterine septum increases the risk of preterm birth and miscarriage (Grade B). According to the ASRM guidelines, some studies have shown that hysteroscopic septum resection reduces miscarriage rates and improves live birth rates in patients with a history of recurrent pregnancy loss (Grade C). Various technologies may be used for incision of the septum, including cold scissors, laser, unipolar, or bipolar cautery. The paucity of specific evidence does not permit recommendation of a specific method (Grade C). Furthermore, the guidelines state that there is insufficient evidence to recommend treatment for the prevention of adhesions after incision of the septum (Grade C) [17].

In 2017, a Cochrane Review was published by Rikken et al. [16] as an update of an earlier review of 2011 on the management of septum resection in women of reproductive age with a septate uterus. Since no RCTs have been published since 2011, the conclusions reported in 2011 remain valid. Accordingly, hysteroscopic septum resection is performed throughout the world in women of reproductive age with a septate uterus in order to improve the outcome of pregnancy. However, currently we have no evidence to support the surgical approach in these women. Randomized controlled trials are needed to address this aspect. Two trials are currently under way (The Randomized Uterine Septum Transsection Trial [TRUST] and the Pilot Randomized Controlled Trial of Hysteroscopic Septal Resection [ISRCTN28960271]), but the results have not been published yet [16]. The TRUST, a multicenter randomized controlled Dutch trial, includes women with a septate uterus, with reduced fertility or recurrent miscarriage. Patients will be randomized into expectant management and hysteroscopic septum resection. The primary outcome is live birth and the secondary outcomes include ongoing pregnancy, clinical pregnancy, complications after surgery, and miscarriage. The authors anticipate a better live birth rate after surgery [35].

Nawroth et al. [10] report a significantly higher rate of endometriosis in women with a septate uterus compared to controls without Müllerian malformations (25.8% vs. 15.2%, p = .006). In a retrospective study they evaluated 120 patients with a septate uterus. The control group consisted of 486 infertile women with a normal hysteroscopy and laparoscopy and without any Müllerian malformations. In all cases of a septate uterus, the authors performed a hysteroscopic septum dissection. The authors conclude that resection of the uterine septum cannot prevent endometriosis, because these are two different conditions. Their simultaneous presence may be a reason to perform an early laparoscopy/hysteroscopy in order to determine the presence and severity of endometriosis and decide about the resection of both, the endometriosis and the septum. The authors suggest that resection of endometriosis would enhance the likelihood of pregnancy in infertile women while resection of the septum would reduce abortion rates [10].

The first prospective study that showed a statistically significant association between a septate uterus and endometriosis was published in 2016 by LaMonica et al. [11]. In a group of 343 women of reproductive age undergoing hysteroscopy and laparoscopy for infertility, menorrhagia, or pelvic pain, the authors registered a uterine septum in 33%. The prevalence of a septate uterus was significantly higher in women with endometriosis than in those without (37% vs. 27%, p = .046), and was even higher in women with severe endometriosis (stage IV disease 41%, p = .022). The authors suggest that the presence of a uterine septum may predispose a woman to more advanced endometriosis disease [11]. This should be evaluated in larger prospective multicenter studies [11]. Several studies have shown that dissection of a septum improves the outcome of pregnancy. The authors suggest that further studies should also address the question as to whether resection of a septum will reduce the recurrence of endometriosis [11].

We believe that, in terms of normal anatomy, the uterine fundus should be flat or nearly flat. Any deviation from this condition should be investigated and, if abnormal, corrected in order to restore a normal uterine cavity. As suggested by Nawroth et al., this strategy would enhance the chances of pregnancy in infertile patients [10]. In view of the frequent coexistence of endometriosis and uterine malformations, precise imaging procedures should be used, and the decision in favor of or against surgery should be made early.

## Unicornuate uterus

The unicornuate uterus (**Figure 9.5**) results from the normal differentiation of only one Müllerian duct; it is found in 0.03%–0.1% of women. The unicornuate uterus accounts for 5%–20% of all Müllerian duct anomalies [8]. The four subgroups mentioned by the ASRM classification are the following: isolated unicornuate uterus, unicornuate uterus with a non-cavitary rudimentary horn, unicornuate uterus with a cavitary non-communicating rudimentary horn, and unicornuate uterus with a cavitary communicating rudimentary horn. The women typically experience symptoms such as dysmenorrhea, chronic pain, and hematometra after menarche. Women with this anomaly have higher frequencies of first- and second-trimester abortions, abnormal fetal presentations, and preterm labor. Women with communicating and non-communicating cavitary rudimentary horns are subject to a higher risk of endometriosis, adenomyosis, hematosalpinx, hematometra, and ectopic pregnancies in the rudimentary horn [36, 37]. Retrograde menstruation and metaplastic conversion of the omnipotential mesothelium into the functional endometrium have been mentioned as the cause of endometriosis [38]. Anomalies of the urinary tract are more commonly associated with this malformation than with other Müllerian duct anomalies. Renal agenesis contralateral to the main horn is the most common renal abnormality. Women with such agenesis are subject to a higher risk of pregnancy-induced hypertension. Imaging techniques for these women include hysterosalpingography, 3D ultrasound, and MRI if needed [38]. Surgical management has not been shown to improve pregnancy outcomes [39]. Removal of a functional rudimentary horn is recommended as the treatment for severe dysmenorrhea, dyspareunia, and chronic pelvic pain related to endometriosis. Surgery is also recommended to prevent conception in an obstructed horn [8].

## Bicornuate uterus

The bicornuate uterus (as shown in **Figure 9.5**) results from incomplete fusion of the two Müllerian ducts, occurs in 0.3% of women, and accounts for 10% of all Müllerian malformations. The ASRM classification mentions a complete or partial bicornuate uterus (class IV), while the ESHRE/ESGE classification mentions a partial, complete, and bicorporeal septate uterus (class U3) [7, 8]. The bicornuate uterus is characterized by two separate but communicating endometrial cavities and a single uterine cervix. In the ESHRE/ESGE classification system [7], class U3 is described as an external indentation at the fundal midline of > 50% of the thickness of the uterine wall and the uterine corpus may be partly or completely divided. Depending on the degree of deformity of the uterine corpus, this class is further divided into three subclasses (class U3a or a partial bicorporeal uterus, class U3b or complete bicorporeal uterus, and class U3c or bicorporeal septate uterus) [7]. A laparoscopy may not be necessary in this setting. A transvaginal 3D ultrasound, sonohysterography, and MRI may well be able to establish the differential diagnosis of a septate uterus. It is important to distinguish between a bicornuate and a septate uterus because the latter can be treated easily with hysteroscopic septal dissection.

In 1907, Paul Strassman was the first to describe surgical correction of this abnormality by performing an anterior colpotomy in a patient with recurrent pregnancy loss [40]. Currently metroplasty is performed by using various modifications of the Strassman technique, even by the laparoscopic procedure [41]. The majority of women with this abnormality need not undergo surgery. Currently the surgical approach is reserved for those patients who have repeated mid-trimester or preterm deliveries [8]. In a retrospective study, Mastrolia et al. studied maternal and fetal outcomes in the second and third trimester in women with a bicornuate uterus. The percentage of women with a bicornuate uterus in the study population was 0.15%. The authors report that women with a bicornuate uterus were of lower parity, had a higher rate of previous cesarean deliveries, were more susceptible to conception by assisted reproductive techniques, and had a significantly higher rate of recurrent abortions compared to controls. The authors conclude that this anomaly is an independent risk factor for cervical insufficiency [42].

## Uterus didelphys

A didelphys uterus (**Figure 9.5**) is a class III anomaly according to the ASRM classification and is characterized by complete failure of the Müllerian ducts to fuse, leading to separate uterine cavities, and two cervices. A partial or complete longitudinal vaginal septum may also be found. This anomaly is observed in 0.03%–0.1% of women and accounts for 5% of all Müllerian malformations [8]. The women are asymptomatic [43]. Of all major anomalies, the didelphys uterus has the best reproductive performance; it is associated with a spontaneous abortion rate of 21% and a fetal survival rate of 75%. The pregnancy is commonly located in the right uterus (76%) [43]. Imaging techniques include hysterosalpingography, transvaginal 2D and 3D ultrasound, and MRI. The ultrasound investigation reveals two completely separate and divergent uterine bodies with no communication between the endometrial cavities. Transvaginal 3D ultrasound in the coronal plane permits a distinction between this condition and a complete septate uterus. Two cervices must be proved either by clinical examination or ultrasound [8]. Published literature on this anomaly is very limited because of its rarity. Vaginal correction is indicated in cases of dyspareunia. General surgical management is not recommended unless the patient experiences repeated late-trimester losses or premature delivery has occurred without any other cause [43–45].

In 2010, Acién et al. published a retrospective study comprising 276 women with genitourinary malformations, in particular 60 cases with genital malformations and congenital unilateral renal agenesis, and 216 control cases with genital tract malformations and both kidneys present. The most commonly seen uterine anomalies in women with renal agenesis were unicornuate uteri, didelphys uteri, and uterus bicornis bicollis. The authors report that women with didelphys or bicornuate uteri and renal agenesis had more gynecological pathologies (such as endometriosis) than those with both kidneys present [46].

### Arcuate uterus

The arcuate anomaly (as shown in **Figure 9.5** and on 3D ultrasound in **Figure 9.3 a,b**) is regarded as a Müllerian duct malformation, but is often classified as a variation from the normal condition or a condition at the benign end of the spectrum of septate uteri [8]. The evaluation of reproductive outcomes in women with an arcuate uterus is hindered by the absence of a uniform definition for this malformation. The definition mentioned in the ASRM classification (category VI) includes a depth of fundal indentation <1 cm with an angle >90° (as shown in **Figure 9.6**). Arcuate uteri were not specifically mentioned in the ESHRE/ESGE classification and were summarized into a subcategory entitled "others" in the UI class (dysmorphic uteri). The latter class includes all cases with a normal outline of the uterus but an abnormal shape of the uterine cavity. The UI class is subdivided into three categories, namely class UIa or a T-shaped uterus, class UIb or uterus infantilis, and class UIc or others, which refers to an inner indentation < 50% of the thickness of the uterine wall at the fundal midline level [18]. The value of surgery for arcuate uteri has long been a subject of debate. The ASRM published its guidelines for the management of the uterine septum in 2016. They state that, in terms of development, the arcuate uterus is a type of resorption failure but should be regarded as a normal variation and differentiated from the septate uterus in terms of prognosis and surgical management [17, 34].

## Conclusion

The report of the published literature showed that the development of various classification systems for the management and diagnosis of CUA has culminated in a Tower of Babel. We need to find and speak a common language in order to define CUA, avoid inadequate or unnecessary surgery, eliminate conflicts between the different classification systems, and optimize the individual patient's treatment.

## References


1. Alkatout I, Egberts JH, Mettler L, et al. Interdisciplinary diagnosis and treatment of deep-infiltrating endometriosis. Zentralbl Chir. 2016;141:630–638.
2. Giudice LC, Kao LC. Endometriosis. Lancet 2004;364:1789–1799.
3. Alkatout I, Mettler L, Beteta C, et al. Combined surgical and hormone therapy for endometriosis is the most effective treatment: prospective, randomized, controlled trial. J Minim Invasive Gynecol. 2013;20:473–481.
4. Mate G, Bernstein LR, Torok AL. Endometriosis Is a cause of infertility. Does reactive oxygen damage to gametes and embryos play a key role in the pathogenesis of infertility caused by endometriosis? Front Endocrinol (Lausanne). 2018;9:725.
5. Grimbizis GF, Camus M, Tarlatzis BC, et al. Clinical implications of uterine malformations and hysteroscopic treatment results. Hum Reprod Update 2001;7:161–174.
6. Acién P, Acién MI. The history of female genital tract malformation classifications and proposal of an updated system. Hum Reprod Update 2011;17:693–705.
7. Grimbizis GF, Gordts S, Di Spiezio Sardo A, et al. The ESHRE-ESGE consensus on the classification of female genital tract congenital anomalies. Gynecol Surg. 2013;10:199–212.
8. Bhagavath B, Ellie G, Griffiths K, et al. Uterine malformations: An update of diagnosis, management, and outcomes. Obstet Gynecol Surv. 2017;72:377–392.
9. Lavergne N, Aristizabal J, Zarka V, et al. Uterine anomalies and in vitro fertilization: what are the results? Eur J Obstet Gynecol Reprod Biol. 1996;68:29–34.
10. Nawroth F, Rahimi G, Nawroth C, et al. Is there an association between septate uterus and endometriosis? Human Reprod. 2006; 21:542–544.
11. LaMonica R, Pinto J, Luciano D, et al. Incidence of septate uterus in reproductive-aged women with and without endometriosis. J Minim Invasive Gynecol. 2016; 23:610–613.
12. Fedele L, Bianchi S, Di Nola G, et al. Endometriosis and nonobstructive Müllerian anomalies. Obstet Gynecol. 1992;79:515–517.
13. Uğur M, Turan C, Mungan T, et al. Endometriosis in association with Müllerian anomalies. Gynecol Obstet Invest. 1995;40:261–264.
14. Olive DL, Henderson DY. Endometriosis and Müllerian anomalies. Obstet Gynecol. 1987;69:412–415.
15. Acién P: Endometriosis and genital anomalies: some histogenetic aspects of external endometriosis. Gynecol Obstet Invest. 1986;22:102–107.
16. Rikken JF, Kowalik CR, Emanuel MH, et al. Septum resection for women of reproductive age with a septate uterus. Cochrane Database Syst Rev. 2017;1:CD008576.
17. Practice Committee of the American Society for Reproductive Medicine. Uterine septum: a guideline. Fertil Steril. 2016; 106:530–540.
18. Corroenne R, Legendre G, May-Panloup P, et al. Surgical treatment of septate uterus in cases of primary infertility and before assisted reproductive technologies. J Gynecol Obstet Hum Reprod. 2018;47:413–418.
19. ACOG Committee Opinion Summary, Number 779. Management of acute obstructive uterovaginal anomalies. Obstet Gynecol. 2019; 133:1290–1291.
20. Grimbizis GF, Di Spiezio Sardo A, Saravelos SH, et al. The Thessaloniki ESHRE/ESGE consensus on diagnosis of female genital anomalies. Hum Reprod. 2016;31:2–7.
21. ACOG Committee Opinion, Number 779. Management of acute obstructive uterovaginal anomalies. Obstet Gynecol 2019; 133:e363–371.
22. Nicolini U, Bellotti M, Bonazzi B, et al. Can ultrasound be used to screen uterine malformations? Fertil Steril. 1987;47:89–93.

23. Graupera B, Pascual MA, Hereter L, et al. Accuracy of three-dimensional ultrasound compared with magnetic resonance imaging in diagnosis of Müllerian duct anomalies using ESHRE–ESGE consensus on the classification of congenital anomalies of the female genital tract. Ultrasound Obstet Gynecol 2015;46:616–622.
24. Salim R, Woelfer B, Backos M, et al. Reproducibility of three-dimensional ultrasound diagnosis of congenital uterine anomalies. Ultrasound Obstet Gynecol. 2003;21:578–582.
25. Alkatout I, Wedel T, Maass N. Combined treatment of endometriosis: radical yet gentle. Aktuelle Urol. 2018;49:60–72.
26. Alkatout I, Mettler L. Hysterectomy: a comprehensive surgical approach. J Turk Ger Gynecol Assoc. 2017;18:221–223.
27. Alkatout I, Mettler L, Maass N, et al. Robotic surgery in gynecology. J Turk Ger Gynecol Assoc. 2016;17:224–232.
28. Alkatout I, Meinhold-Heerlein I, Keckstein J, et al. Endometriosis: a concise practical guide to current diagnosis and treatment. J Turk Ger Gynecol Assoc. 2018;19:173–175.
29. Alkatout I. An atraumatic retractor for interdisciplinary use in conventional laparoscopy and robotic surgery. Minim Invasive Ther Allied Technol. 2018;27:265–271.
30. Mettler L, Ruprai R, Alkatout I. Impact of medical and surgical treatment of endometriosis on the cure of endometriosis and pain. Biomed Res Int. 2014;2014:264653.
31. Healey M, Ang WC, Cheng C. Surgical treatment of endometriosis: a prospective randomized double-blinded trial comparing excision and ablation. Fertil Steril. 2010;94:2536–2540.
32. Tremellen K, Russell P. Adenomyosis is a potential cause of recurrent implantation failure during IVF treatment. Aust N Z J Obstet Gynaecol. 2011. 51:280–283.
33. Coughlan C, Ledger W, Wang Q, Liu F, et al. Recurrent implantation failure: definition and management. Reprod Biomed Online 2014;28:14–38.
34. Ludwin A, Martins WP, Nastri CO, et al. Congenital Uterine Malformation by Experts (CUME): better criteria for distinguishing between normal/arcuate and septate uterus? Ultrasound Obstet Gynecol. 2018;51:101–109.
35. Rikken JFW, Kowalik CR, Emanuel MH, et al. The randomised uterine septum transsection trial (TRUST): design and protocol. BMC Womens Health. 2018;18:163.
36. Reichman D, Laufer MR, Robinson BK. Pregnancy outcomes in unicornuate uteri: a review. Fertil Steril. 2009;91:1886–1894.
37. Liu MM. Unicornuate uterus with rudimentary horn. Int J Gynaecol Obstet. 1994;44:149–153.
38. Khati NJ, Frazier AA, Brindle KA. The unicornuate uterus and its variants: clinical presentation, imaging findings, and associated complications. J Ultrasound Med. 2012;31:319–331.
39. Acién P, Acién M, Sánchez-Ferrer ML. Complex malformations of the female genital tract. New types and revision of classification. Hum Reprod 2004a;19:2377–2384.
40. Tomasz R, Marta M, Aleksandra B. Clinical effectiveness of Strassman operation in the treatment of bicornuate uterus. Ginekologia Polska. 2009;80:88–92.
41. Alborzi S, Asefjah H, Amini M, et al. Laparoscopic metroplasty in bicornuate and didelphic uteri: feasibility and outcome. Arch Gynecol Obstet. 2015;291:1167–1171.
42. Mastrolia SA, Baumfeld Y, Hershkovitz R, et al. Bicornuate uterus is an independent risk factor for cervical os insufficiency: A retrospective population based cohort study. J Matern Fetal Neonatal Med. 2017;30:2705–2710.
43. Kachhawa G, Kriplani A. Management of reproductive tract anomalies. J Obstet Gynaecol India. 2017;67(3):162–167.
44. Rackow BW, Arici A. Reproductive performance of women with Müllerian anomalies. Curr Opin Obstet Gynecol. 2007;19:229–237.
45. Taylor E, Gomel V. The uterus and fertility. Fertil Steril. 2008;89:1–16.
46. Acién P, Acién M. Unilateral renal agenesis and female genital tract pathologies. Acta Obstet Gynecol Scand. 2010;89:1424–1431.

# 10

## SURGICAL TREATMENT OF FIBROIDS

**Ibrahim Alkatout**

### Introduction

Fibroids (uterine leiomyomas) are benign tumors of the uterus and the most common pelvic tumor in women.

Usually, asymptomatic leiomyomas do not have to be treated as the histological diagnosis is not necessary in most cases. Treatment might be necessary for women with submucosal fibroids who are contemplating pregnancy (**Table 10.1**).

The treatment of fibroids usually depends on the symptoms they are causing, such as bleeding disorders, pain or displacement complaints. Bleeding disorders occur mostly in submucous or intramural placement. Here, the tumor borders on the endometrium and the uterine cavity is deformed, thereby increasing the endometrial bleeding surface [1–3]. Nevertheless, the type and time of any treatment should be individualized according to relevant factors, such as:

- Type of symptoms and subjective discomfort
- Number and size(s) of fibroid(s)
- Location of fibroid(s)
- Age of patient
- Family planning and/or obstetrical history

**TABLE 10.1: Indications for Treatment**

| | | | |
|---|---|---|---|
| Fibroid | Symptoms | yes | *Treatment* |
| | | no | *No measures if:*<br>*- no growths*<br>*- no desire for children* |
| | Growths | yes | *Control* |
| | | no | *No measures if:*<br>*- no symptoms*<br>*- no desire for children* |
| | Desire for Children | yes | *Treatment dependent on: size, localisation, number* |
| | | no | *No measures if:*<br>*- no symptoms*<br>*- no growths* |

In this review article, an overview of surgical treatment will be given in relation to other treatment options (**Table 10.2**). The surgical treatment of fibroids can be differentiated between less invasive and more invasive surgical techniques. Time and type of treatment have to be chosen individually and are dependent on the patient and the treating gynecologist.

### Expectant management

Wait-and-see is a possibility if patients are asymptomatic, decline medical or surgical treatment or have contraindications to any kind of treatment. However, existing data describe the possibility that fibroids can shrink substantially either by optimizing endocrinological disorders, such as hypothyroidism, or during the postpartum period [4, 5].

To pursue the idea of expectant management, the pelvic mass must definitely be classified as a fibroid and differentiated from an ovarian mass. The complete blood count should be regular, especially in patients with severe symptoms, such as menorrhagia or hypermenorrhea. The women must also be informed that the risk of miscarriage, premature labor and delivery, abnormal fetal position and placental abruption is increased [6].

### Medical therapy

The benefit of medical treatment in the management of women with symptomatic fibroids is still difficult to prove. Medical therapy can provide adequate symptom relief, especially in cases where hypermenorrhea is the leading problem. The benefit of symptom improvement decreases in long-term treatment periods so that more than 50% undergo surgery within two years [7].

Nevertheless, there has been a shift in traditional thinking that medical treatment of fibroids is solely based on the manipulation of steroid hormones. A deeper analysis and understanding of specific genes or pathways associated with leiomyomatosis may open new possibilities for prevention and medical treatment [8].

### Alternative treatment methods

If the patient does not want to undergo surgery or there are contraindications to surgery, there are alternative procedures:

Uterine artery embolization: This minimally invasive therapeutical option allows an occlusion of the specific arteries supplying blood to the fibroids. A catheter is introduced via the femoral artery under local anesthesia and particles are injected to block the blood flow to the fibroid. This can be an effective treatment option if the uterus should not be removed, surgery is contraindicated and family planning is completed. It results in myoma shrinkage of up to 46%. Nevertheless, there is still a significant rate of postinterventional complications [9, 10].

Magnetic resonance-guided focused ultrasound: This is a more recent treatment method for uterine fibroids in premenopausal

TABLE 10.2: Treatment Options for Uterine Fibroids

| Treatment Options for Uterine Fibroids | | | | | | | | |
|---|---|---|---|---|---|---|---|---|
| **Conservative** | **Alternative** | **Surgical** | | | | | | |
| **Expectant Treatment** | **Uterine Artery Embolization** | **Myomectomy** | | | | **Hysterectomy** | | |
| Medical therapy | High intensity focused ultrasound | Hysteroscopic | Laparoscopic | Abdominal | Robotic assisted | Vaginal | Laparoscopic | Abdominal |
| • Hormonal | Miscellaneous methods (myoma coagulation, myolysis) | | | | | | • Supracervical | |
| • GnRH agonist | | | | | | | • Total | |
| • Ulipristal acetate | | | | | | | | |

women. Again, the patients must have completed their family planning. In a noninvasive thermoablative technique multiple waves of ultrasound energy are converged on a small volume of tissue, resulting in maximal thermal destruction. The limiting factors are size, vascularity and access [11, 12].

## Surgical treatment of fibroids

### Indications

Surgical treatment of fibroids is still the main pillar in the treatment of leiomyomas. Hysterectomy is the only definitive solution and can be performed as supracervical or total hysterectomy. Myomectomy performed by hysteroscopy, laparoscopy, abdominal access or with robotic assistance is an alternative surgical method.

Indications for surgical therapy of uterine fibroids are (**Table 10.1**):

1. Abnormal uterine bleeding disorders (hypermenorrhea, dysmenorrhea, menorrhagia and metrorrhagia)
2. Bulk-related symptoms
3. Primary or secondary infertility and recurrent pregnancy loss

### Counseling and informed consent

Patients undergoing an operative procedure have to be informed of the risks and potential complications as well as alternative operating methods. Counseling before surgery should include discussion of the entry technique and the associated risks: injury of the bowel, urinary tract, blood vessels, omentum and other surrounding organs and, at a later date, wound infection, adhesion-associated pain and hernia formation.

Counseling needs to integrate the individual risk dependent on the body mass index of the patient. Depending on the medical history, it is important to consider anatomical malformations, number of vaginal births, midline abdominal incisions, a history of peritonitis or inflammatory bowel disease [13].

### *Myomectomy*

Myomectomy is a surgical treatment option for women who have not completed their family planning or who wish to retain their uterus for any other reasons. The enucleation of fibroids by any method is an effective therapy for bleeding disorders or displacement pressure in the pelvis. Nevertheless, the risk of recurrence remains after myomectomy. Furthermore, if any other pathologies might be causative or only co-causative for the symptoms (such as adenomyosis uteri), these problems will persist [14]. Enucleated myomas and pregnancy-related complications have been investigated extensively. All operating possibilities, especially laparoscopic versus laparotomic, but recently also laparoscopic versus robotic-assisted myomectomy have been evaluated. Uterine rupture or uterine dehiscence is rare and occurs in only 2%–4% of laparoscopic cases and even less seldom in robotic-assisted and laparotomic cases. Careful patient selection and secure preparation and suture techniques appear to be the most important variables for myomectomy in women of reproductive age [15, 16]. Uteri with multiple fibroids have an increased number of uterine arterioles and venules. Therefore, myomectomy can lead to a significant blood loss and corresponding arrangements should be made [17].

### Hysteroscopic myomectomy

Submucosal fibroids have their origin in myometrial cells underneath the endometrium and represent about 15%–20% of all fibroids. Before the establishment of hysteroscopy as a minimally invasive and effective treatment method, these myomas were removed by hysterotomy or even hysterectomy. Increased surgical training, improvement of technology and the widespread use of hysteroscopic myomectomy have made it a safe, fast, effective and cheap method of fibroid resection while preserving the uterus [18].

Patient selection concentrates on intracavitary submucous and some intramural fibroids. More than 50% of the fibroid circumference needs to be protruding into the uterine cavity. Deep myometrial leiomyomas require advanced operative skills and have an increased risk for perioperative complications and incomplete resection. The depth of myometrial penetration correlates with the volume of distension fluid absorbed [19, 20]. Few data are available on the size of myoma that prevents the use of the hysteroscopic approach. The European Society of Hysteroscopy suggests to limit the myoma size to 4 cm but the few existing data report a significant increase of complications in fibroids that are >3 cm. Surgical skills determine the size and number of myomas that can be resected [21].

Prior to hysteroscopy, knowledge of the patient's medical history is important, for example, history of cesarian section or any other reason to expect an anatomical disorder. A vaginal ultrasound scan must be performed to precisely determine the uterus location, size and all cervical and uterine pathologies [22]. If available and feasible, fluid hystero-sonography should be performed to better differentiate the relationship of leiomyoma to the endometrial cavity and the myometrium. No prophylactic antibiotic is required to prevent surgical site infection.

The first step is the dilation of the cervical channel with Hegar dilators up to Hegar 9. The most commonly used instrument for fibroid resection is the monopolar or bipolar wire loop. Using a monopolar device the fluid medium must be non-electrolytic, using a bipolar device the fluid medium is isotonic [23]. A continuous flow allows the clearance of blood out of the uterine cavity to improve visualization. Furthermore, the resected pieces can be retracted. Nevertheless, the surface of the myoma and the time needed for resection increase the risk of excessive fluid absorption [24].

The resectoscope is inserted through the cervix into the uterine cavity and after distension with fluid the uterine cavity is carefully inspected. The monopolar resectoscope requires a cutting current of 60 to 120 watts. Bipolar resectoscopes offer the possibility of simultaneous cut and coagulation. The wire loop passes easily through the tissue. The incision starts at the highest point of the myoma. Only in pedunculated fibroids might the incision cut the peduncle first. The loop is then moved toward the surgeon using the spring mechanism and simultaneously the entire resectoscope is gently pulled backwards. The wire loop must be in view of the surgeon during the whole procedure. This motion is repeated until the whole myoma has been resected and the surrounding myometrium (depth) and endometrium (side) can be differentiated. All resected specimen is sent to the pathologist. In cases of heavy bleeding and reduced vision the endometrium and the cutting surface have to be reinspected. These areas can be desiccated with the coagulating current.

The resected area will be recovered by the surrounding endometrium during the following weeks. The complication rate is low (0.8%–2.6%) [24, 25]. Complications that can occur, especially after extensive resection, are uterine perforation or excessive fluid absorption. Absorption of distension fluid might result in hyponatremia or volume overload [26]. The recurrence rate is about 20% in a follow-up period of more than 3 years [21].

## Laparoscopic myomectomy

With the improvement of laparoscopic techniques and skills, myomectomy can be performed laparoscopically in most women. The laparoscopic approach is usually used for intramural or subserosal fibroids. The main advantage compared to abdominal myomectomy is decreased morbidity and a shorter recovery period. Nevertheless, laparoscopic myomectomy is limited by surgical expertise and especially laparoscopic suturing skills [2, 27]. Selection criteria for laparoscopic myomectomy are location, size and number of fibroids. Nevertheless, these characteristics are variable in relation to the surgical expertise. Preoperative imaging is performed by vaginal ultrasound to assess the precise features of the leiomyomas [22, 28–30].

Laparoscopic myomectomy starts with the usual placement of ports and trocars. After placement of the initial port in the umbilicus, two ancillary trocars are placed in the lower abdomen about 2 cm medial of each iliac crest [30–32]. Myomectomy can lead to severe bleeding that will complicate the procedure due to reduced vision. Vessel bleeding is controlled by bipolar electrosurgical paddles. Intraoperative bleeding can be reduced using vasopressin or other vasoconstrictors. Vasopressin is diluted (e.g., 20 units in 100 mL of saline) and injected into the planned uterine incision site. Vasopressin constricts the smooth muscle in the walls of capillaries, small arterioles and venules. Nevertheless, due to side effects the surgeon should pull back the plunger of the syringe before insertion to check that the needle is not inserted intravascularly [33–35]. Alternatively, misoprostol can be administered vaginally about one hour before surgery to reduce blood loss [36].

The uterine incision is preferably made vertically as this allows a more ergonomic suturing of the defect. The incision is performed with a monopolar hook directly over the fibroid and carried through deeply until the entire myoma tissue has been reached. After exposure of the myoma, it is grasped with a tenaculum or sharp forceps and traction and countertraction are applied. The removal of the myoma can easily be performed with blunt and sharp dissecting devices. Capsular vessels should be coagulated before complete removal of the myoma as coagulation becomes more difficult if traction is unsuccessful and bipolar coagulation occurs in the remaining myometrium wall. Subsequent to removal, the myoma is morcellated with an electromechanical device under direct vision and at a safe distance to all structures, such as the small bowel, to avoid inadvertent injury. The myoma tissue is removed and sent for pathologic evaluation. The uterine defect is closed with delayed absorbable sutures in one or two layers, depending upon the depth of the myometrial defect. It is important that the suture starts at the deepest point to avoid any cavity that might lead to a weak uterine wall. Furthermore, we tie the knot extracorporally so that the knot can be pushed into the deep layers with full strength (**Figure 10.1**). Alternatively, barbed sutures, such as V-lock, can be used to tighten the tissue or a third ancillary trocar can be inserted to hold the suture tight. The security of the uterine closure has bearing on the risk of uterine rupture in subsequent pregnancy. Different kinds of adhesion prevention barriers can be applied [37–39]. Women should wait at least 4–6 month before attempting to conceive [40].

For an overview of laparoscopic myomectomy and uterus reconstruction, see **Figures 10.1–10.7**.

## Abdominal myomectomy

Abdominal or open myomectomy has its origin in the early 1900s as a uterus preserving procedure. Today, it is mostly performed for women with intramural or subserosal myomas and less frequently for submucosal localization. Since the introduction of endoscopic procedures, the indication for abdominal myomectomy has become rare. It becomes an option if hysteroscopic or laparoscopic myomectomy is not feasible or if a laparotomy is required for any other reason. The indication to exclude uterine sarcomas has to be taken very strictly; however, uterine sarcoma is a very rare malignancy and the rate of sarcoma after clinical diagnosis of myoma is very low. The risk of severe complications in association with open surgery is higher than with hysteroscopic or laparoscopic moymectomy. Prophylactic antibiotics should be given for any abdominal fibroid operation [41, 42]. After the Pfannenstiel incision either a vertical or transverse uterine incision is performed [43]. The myoma enucleation is performed by traction on the myometrial edges, for example, with Allis clamps. After exposure of the fibroid it can be extirpated. The pseudocapsule is typically dissected bluntly. The uterine defects are closed with sutures in in several layers to reapproximate the tissue and achieve hemostasis without excessive bipolar coagulation.

## Robotic myomectomy

Robot-assisted myomectomy is a relatively new approach. The advantages of robotic surgery are three-dimensional: imaging, mechanical improvement, including 7 degrees of freedom for each instrument, stabilization of the instruments within the surgical field and improved ergonomics for the surgeon. Technical difficulties are decreased as suturing is easier than during conventional laparoscopy; however, there are few data comparing robot-assisted with conventional laparoscopic myomectomy [44–46]. The advantages compared to abdominal myomectomy are decreased blood loss and shorter recovery time. Nevertheless, operation duration and operating costs are much higher than for conventional procedures. Furthermore, robotic devices are large and bulky. Robotic surgery is limited by the lack of tactile feedback and additional team training is necessary to minimize the

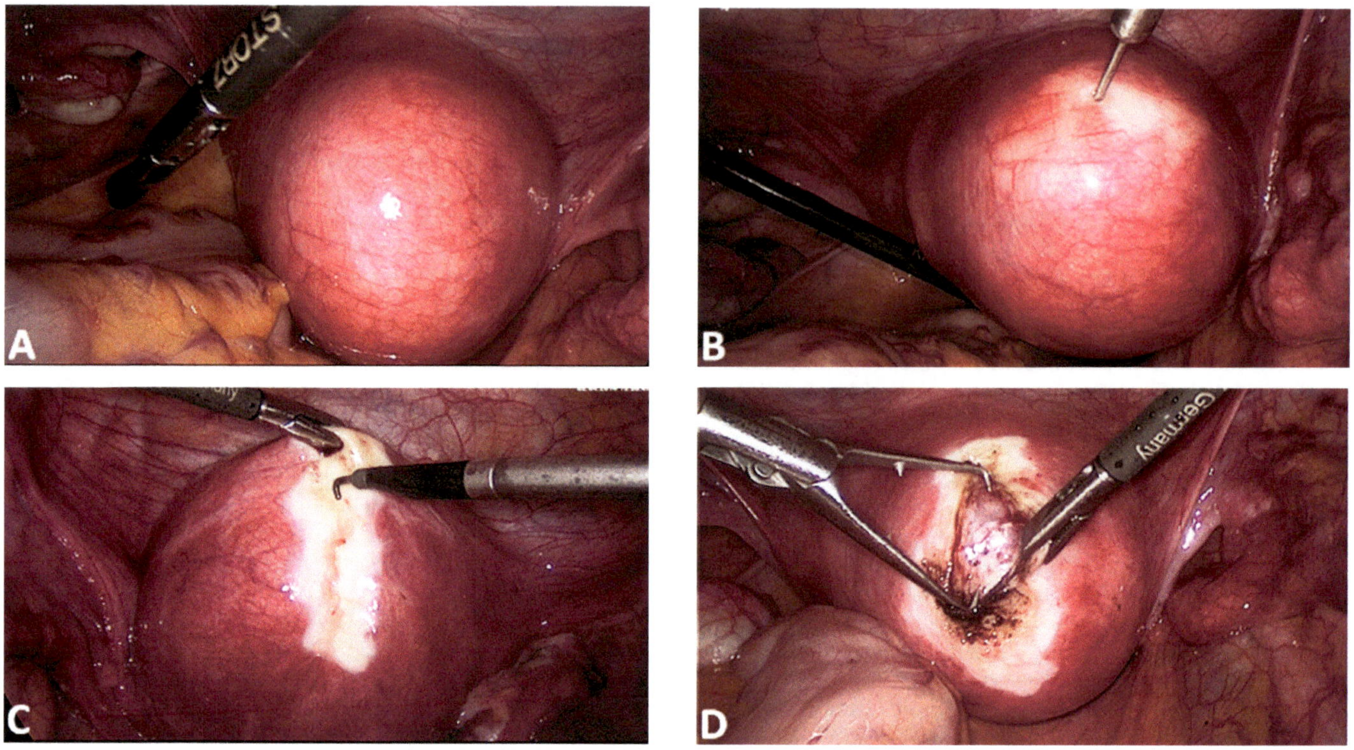

FIGURE 10.1 Performance of the extracorporeal "von Leffern" knot. (A) Pulling out the suture, removing the needle, half hitch. (B) Holding the knot with the left hand and reaching over with the right hand. (C) Grasping the short end from below and leading it back, exiting before the half hitch. (D) Turning back the knot. Holding the straight suture and tightening the knot.

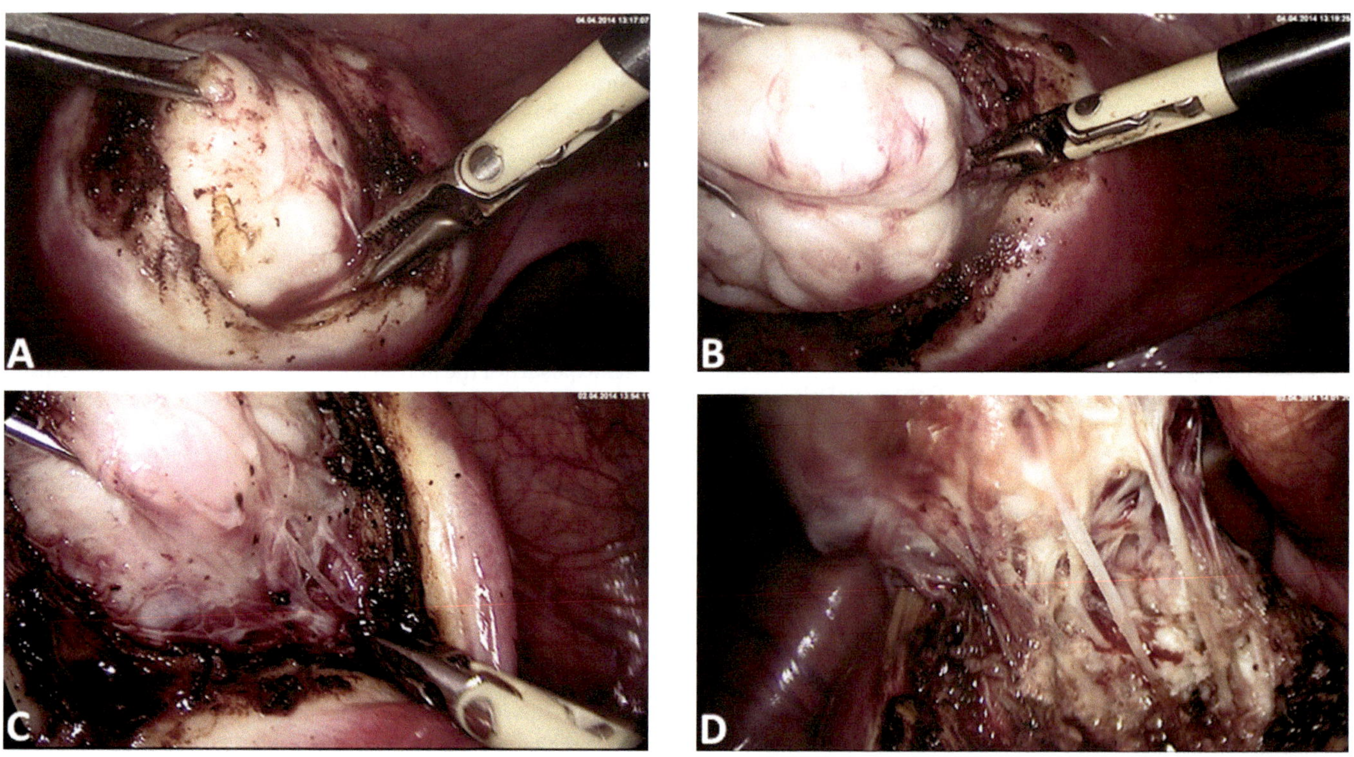

FIGURE 10.2 Laparoscopic myoma enucleation. (A) Situs of a fundal/anterior wall fibroid. (B) Prophylactic hemostasis with 1:100 diluted vasopressin solution (gylcilpressin) in separate wells. The injection intends to separate the pseudocapsule from the fibroid and reduces bleedings. (C) Bipolar superficial coagulation of the longitudinal incision strip and opening of the uterine wall with the monopolar hook or needle till the fibroid surface. (D) Grasping of the fibroid and beginning of the enucleation. The pseudocapsule remains within the uterine wall and is pushed off bluntly.

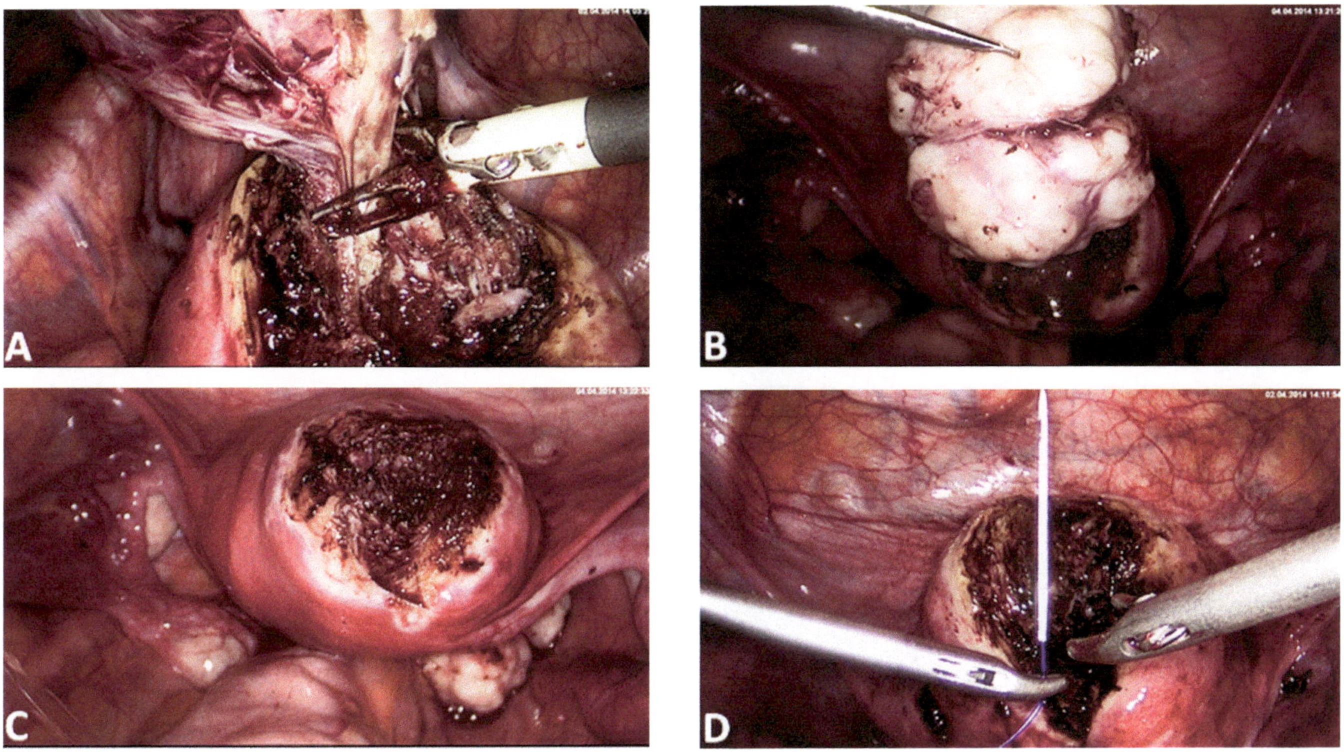

FIGURE 10.3 Laparoscopic myoma enucleation. (A) Traction of the fibroid with a tenaculum and blunt delineation from the capsule. (B) Focal bipolar coagulation of basic vessels. (C) Continuous enucleation of the fibroid under traction and specific coagulation of capsule fibers containing vessels. (D) Magnification of remaining capsule fibers to be coagulated and cut.

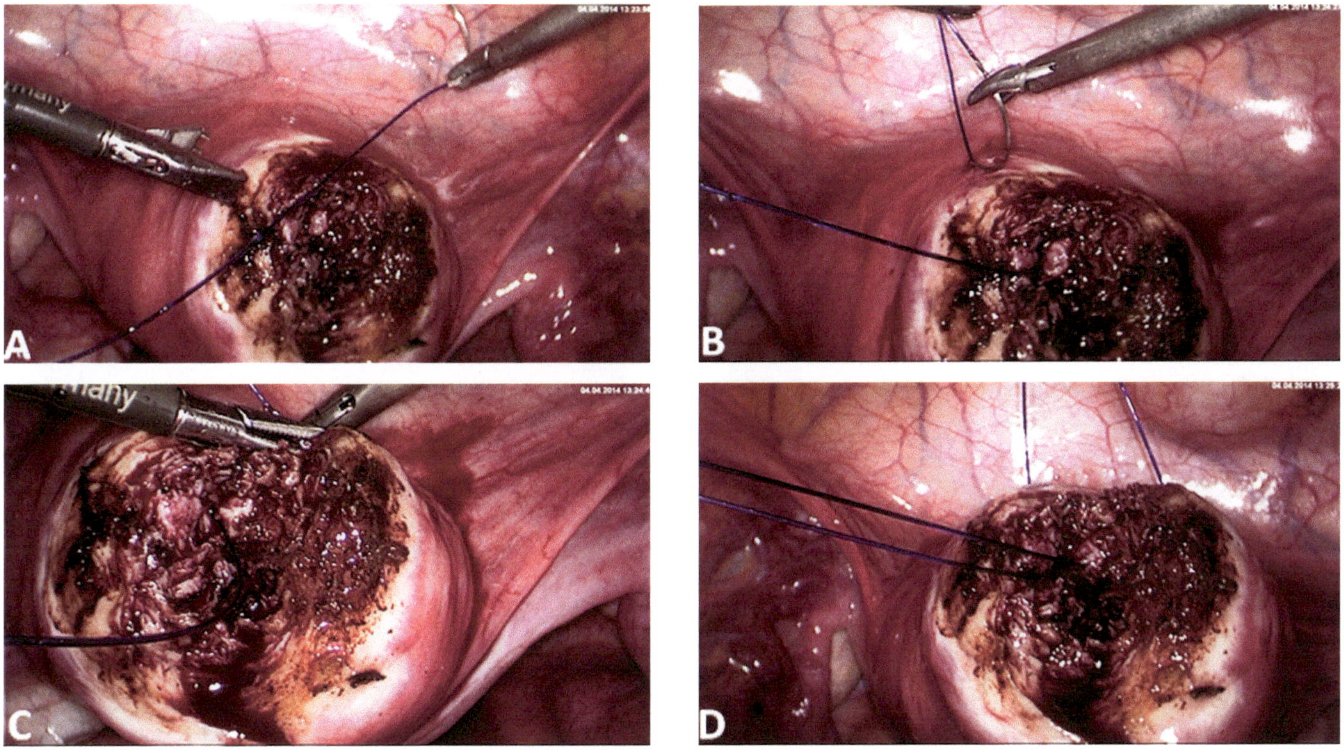

FIGURE 10.4 Laparoscopic myoma enucleation. (A) Final coagulation of the capsule vessels. (B) Double belly fibroid after complete enucleation. (C) Minimal coagulation of bleeding vessels under suction and irrigation. (D) Approximation of wound edges with either straight or round, sharp needle and a monofilar late-absorbable suture.

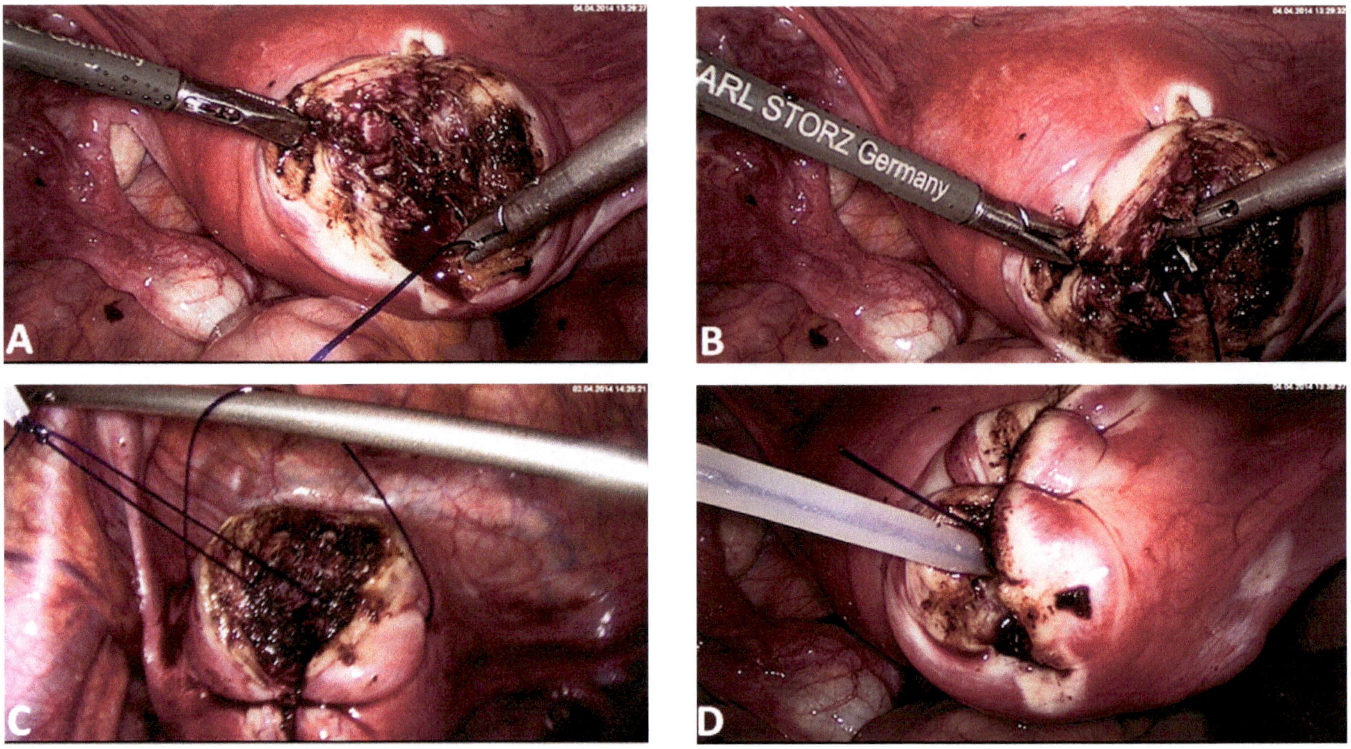


**FIGURE 10.5** Laparoscopic myoma enucleation. (A) Advantage of round needle stitch. The wound angle is elevated safely and completely by elevating it with a Manhes-forceps. Deeper layers of the myometrium can be grasped more easily using a round needle. (B) Needle exit and simplified regrasping with the right needle holder. (C) Final stitch to invert the knot. (D) Extirpation of the needle and completion of the extracorporeal knot and preparation to push down the extracorporeal knot.

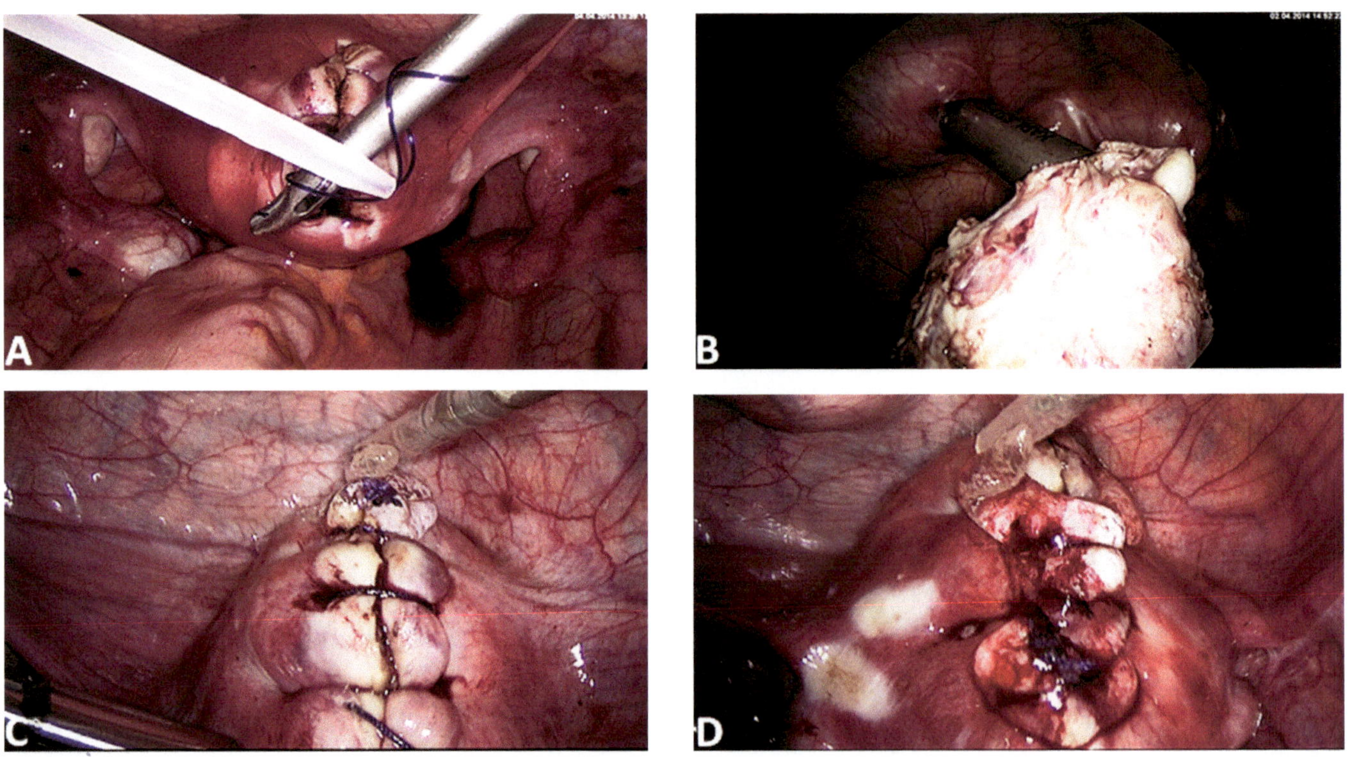


**FIGURE 10.6** Laparoscopic myoma enucleation. (A) Second single stitch starting as deep as possible in the uterine wound. (B) Exiting of the needle on the left wound margin (just next to the Manhes forceps). (C) Completion of the stitch and preparation of the extracorporeal von Leffern knot. The needle holder elevates the thread to avoid tearing of the uterine wall while pulling through the monofilar thread (PDS). (D) The extracorporeal knot is pushed down with a plastic push-rod and deposited deep in the wound minimizing the external suture part.

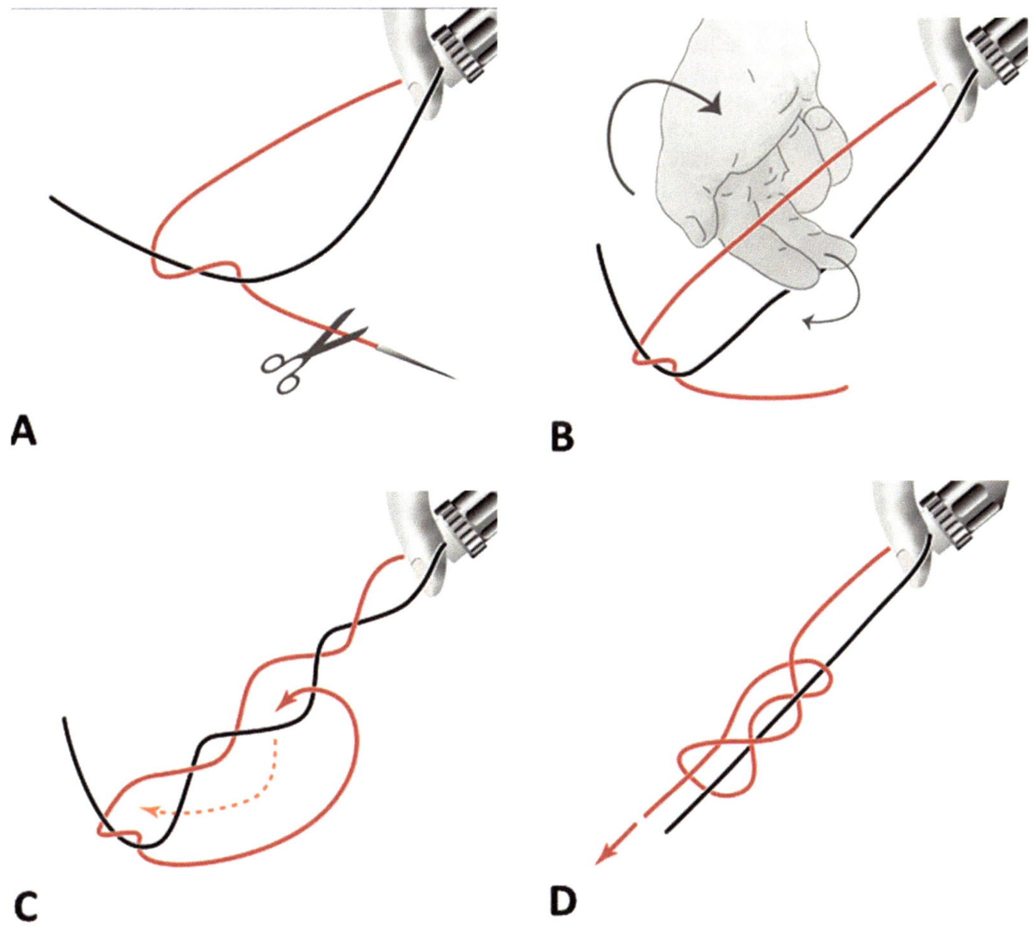


FIGURE 10.7 Laparoscopic myoma enucleation. (A) Intracorporeal safety knot of the knot performed extracorporeally. (B) Morcellation of the fibroid with the Rotocut morcellator (Storz) in an apple-peeling manner. (C) Final situs showing the extracorporeal sutures to adapt the uterine wound edges. (D) Application of Hyalo Barrier (Nordic Pharma) for adhesion prevention.

risk of mechanical failure [47]. To date no advantage compared to conventional laparoscopy could be demonstrated regarding blood loss or operative duration. A more secure myometrial closure has not yet been proven [45]. In obese patients robot-assisted surgery might be beneficial [48].

### *Hysterectomy*

Fibroids are the most common indication for hysterectomy (30% of hysterectomies in white and 50% of hysterectomies in black women). Any of the previously mentioned indications can lead to a hysterectomy. The decision is dependent on the wish of the patient, her health status and whether childbearing has been completed. Only, if the patient suffers from metrorrhagia does the disorder need to be examined further as this may be a sign of endometrial cancer or sarcoma. Nevertheless, evaluation of malignancy alone is not an indication for hysterectomy in most women with fibroids. Magnetic resonance imaging (MRI) or laparoscopy can lead to a more specific diagnosis of rapidly growing uterine masses and the lower abdomen (e.g., adnexa) in the case of a leiomyomatous uterus. In those cases where malignancy is not unlikely, laparotomy can be selected as the surgical approach.

Hysterectomy is recommended for the following indications:

- Acute hemorrhage with non-response to other therapies.
- Completion of family planning and current or increased future risk of other diseases, such as cervical intraepithelial neoplasia, endometrial hyperplasia or an increased risk of uterine or ovarian cancer. Precondition for the indication for hysterectomy is that these risks can be eliminated or decreased by hysterectomy.
- Failure of previous treatment.
- Completion of family planning and significant symptoms (e.g., multiple fibroids or adenomyosis) and the desire for a definitive solution.

The main advantage of hysterectomy over all other therapeutical possibilities is the definitive solution in eliminating all existing symptoms and the risk of recurrence. Nevertheless, the advantage of a definitive solution that allows freedom from future problems can be an obstacle if family planning has not been completed or the patient has a personal inhibition against the removal of the central genital female organ [49]. These issues must be discussed in advance with the patient before the decision for a hysterectomy is taken. Furthermore, for a solitary submucous, subserous, pedunculated or intramural myoma, the complication rate of a hysterectomy has to be compared with the complication rate of a myomectomy. The operational risks have to be compared to the operational risks of hysteroscopy, laparoscopic enucleation or conservative management. With the advances in cervical cancer screening the prevention of future cervical or uterine pathologies is no longer a relevant indication for hysterectomy. The decision must be tailored to meet the needs of each individual patient.

Laparoscopic hysterectomy was first introduced in 1989 with the aim of reducing the morbidity and mortality of abdominal hysterectomy to the level reached with vaginal hysterectomy. Laparoscopic assistance for vaginal hysterectomy can be of advantage if there is a need for adhesiolysis, a need to treat endometriosis simultaneously, a need to treat large leiomyomas and to ensure an easier and safer adnexectomy. If feasible, vaginal hysterectomy allows a more rapid and less painful recovery than open or laparoscopic surgery and is much cheaper [50].

### Removal of ovaries and/or fallopian tubes

Generally, the ovaries are not removed when a hysterectomy is performed for uterine fibroids. Removing the uterus alone will cure the bleeding and the size-related symptoms caused by the fibroids. When treating fibroids it is not necessary to remove the ovaries as is sometimes the case when treating other diseases, such as endometriosis or gynecologic cancers.

According to new research presented at the Annual Clinical Meeting of the American College of Obstetricians and Gynecologists, bilateral salpingectomy at hysterectomy, with preservation of the ovaries, is considered a safe way of potentially reducing the development of ovarian serous carcinoma. Removing the fallopian tubes does not cause the onset of menopause, as does the removal of the ovaries. Furthermore, prophylactic removal of the fallopian tubes during hysterectomy or sterilization would rule out any subsequent tubal pathology, such as hydrosalpinx, which is observed in up to 30% of women after hysterectomy. Women undergoing hysterectomy with retained fallopian tubes or sterilization have at least double the risk of subsequent salpingectomy. Removal of the fallopian tubes at hysterectomy should therefore generally be recommended [51].

As the indication for abdominal hysterectomy in benign diseases has become very rare, it is not discussed in this article. Furthermore, robot-assisted laparoscopy has not yet shown any advantage for the experienced surgeon in the treatment of hysterectomy and therefore is not recommended by the American Association of Gynecologic Laparoscopists (AAGL) to replace conventional laparoscopic or vaginal procedures [52].

### Vaginal hysterectomy

Before starting a vaginal hysterectomy a bimanual pelvic examination is performed to assess uterine mobility and descent, and to exclude unsuspected adnexal pathology. Only then can a final decision be made whether to proceed with a vaginal or abdominal approach. The operation starts with entry into the cul-de-sac. The uterosacral ligaments are identified and clamped including the lower portion of the cardinal ligaments. In the next step, the vesicovaginal space is opened and after identification of the peritoneal fold it is cut and the cardinal ligaments are ligated, including the uterine vessels. Most adnexa can be removed by grasping the ovary and clamping the infundibulopelvic ligament. The uterus can then stepwise be enucleated from the remaining peritoneal fold at a safe distance from the bladder. The peritoneum can either be closed or left open and the vaginal epithelium is reapproximated in either a vertical or a horizontal manner. A myomatous uterus has to be morcellated in a piecemeal manner. Sometimes it is necessary to enucleate solitary large myomas or to perform intramyometrial coring, especially in cases of diffusely enlarged uteri [53, 54].

### Laparoscopic supracervical hysterectomy (LSH)

The supracervical hysterectomy was first described in 1990 by Lyons and in another technique by Semm. The operative technique is similar to the total laparoscopic hysterectomy. Only after occluding the ascending branch of the uterine artery is the uterine corpus resected as a reverse conus down to the endocervical canal [55]. For LSH and LTH (total laparoscopic hysterectomy) the trocar placement is the same as for laparoscopic myomectomy (see above). There is no need to perform ureterolysis at the beginning of the operation as the ureter is at a safe distance if the suturing line is kept strictly at the uterine wall. The infundibulo pelvic ligament and the round ligament are divided from the pelvic side wall and, if the adnexa are to remain in situ, division of the adnexa from the uterus. The broad ligament is then opened, dissected and each leaf separately coagulated. The bladder is separated from the uterus by opening the vesico uterine ligament and pushing the bladder downwards for about 1–2 cm. This is followed by presentation of the ramus ascendens of the uterine artery and division of the uterine pedicles with the same stepwise dissection of the left adnexa. A thorough inspection of the cervix then takes place. The cervix is separated from the uterus with the help of the electric cutting loop or any other cutting instrument. This is followed by coagulation of the cervical canal and closure of the peritoneum over the remaining cervical stump for infection and adhesion prevention. Afterward, morcellation of the uterine body is performed and, if the adnexa are also resected, they should be put into an endo bag for extraction.

### Total laparoscopic hysterectomy (LTH)

Laparoscopic supracervical hysterectomy should be avoided if adenomyosis uteri is suspected because part of the endometrial glands remain in the cervical and paracervical channel. These can cause an early recurrence or persistence of the symptoms although the few existing data offer no direct confirmation of this view [56, 57].

The surgical steps are identical to the LSH, the only difference being that a uterine manipulator is placed in the vagina before the operation. After separation of the bladder from the uterus, the bladder is pushed and dissected down 2–3 cm to clearly visualize the rim of the cervical cap. In cases of post-cesarean section, a gentle, blunt and intermediate sharp dissection has to be carried out. The uterus is lateralized by pushing up the manipulator. The uterine artery and vein with collateral arteries are completely coagulated near the cervix and dissected. The vagina is resected from the cervix with the monopolar hook by firmly stretching the manipulator cranially and carefully performing an intrafacial dissection leaving the sacro-uterine ligaments almost completely in place. This is in accordance with the CISH technique introduced by Kurt Semm [58]. The uterus is then retracted through the vagina while still fixed to the manipulator. If the uterus is too large, it has to be morcellated either intra-abdominally or transvaginally. The vagina is closed with 2 corner sutures and 1 or 2 sutures in between the corner sutures. The sacro-uterine ligaments and the middle portion of the vagina are stitched and elevated to prevent vaginal prolapse or enterocele formation at a later time. Peritonealization and drainage are not required.

With the improvement of endoscopic surgery and above all the improvement in endoscopic suturing laparoscopic-assisted vaginal hysterectomy has become obsolete, especially as this technique does not include a suspension of the cardinal and sacro-uterine ligaments.

## Conclusion

Treatment options for uterine leiomyomas vary. The choice of treatment should be made on an individual basis taking into account the following factors: the patient's level of suffering due to bleeding disorders or displacement-caused pain, the status of family planning and the patient's preferences regarding the different treatment options.

In *asymptomatic women* expectant management is suggested except for hydronephrosis caused by displacement or hysteroscopically resectable submucous fibroids in women who pursue pregnancy.

In *postmenopausal women* without hormonal therapy fibroids usually shrink and become asymptomatic. Therefore, expectant management is the method of choice. However, sarcoma should be excluded if a new or an enlarging pelvic mass occurs in a postmenopausal woman. Surgical treatment is the option of choice if the leiomyomas are symptomatic. If there are contraindications to operative procedures or hysterectomy is declined by the patient for personal reasons, any of the alternative treatment options can be considered (medical, embolization or guided ultrasound).

In *premenopausal women* appropriate submucosal leiomyomas should be resected hysteroscopically if the women wish to preserve their childbearing potential and/or they are symptomatic (e.g. bleeding, miscarriage). Intramural and subserosal leiomyomas in women who wish to preserve their fertility can be removed laparoscopically. Nevertheless, an appropriate surgical technique and advanced laparoscopic skills are necessary. If this cannot be guaranteed, abdominal myomectomy has to be recommended or referral to a laparoscopic center to maximize the possibility and safety of pregnancy after uterine reconstruction. The risk of uterine rupture in pregnancy following myomectomy needs to be discussed with the patient.

Robotic assistance might make laparoscopic suturing easier; however, to date there are too few data to support this contention.

For *women who have completed their family planning,* hysterectomy is the definitive procedure for relief of symptoms and prevention of recurrence of fibroid-related problems. With increasing experience in laparoscopic hysterectomies, the risk of side effects has become manageable. In relation to the compliance and individuality of the patient, the suitable solution can be laparoscopic supracervical or total laparoscopic hysterectomy.

## Acknowledgment

The authors thank Dawn Rüther for editing the manuscript.

## References

1. Buttram VC, Jr., Reiter RC. Uterine leiomyomata: etiology, symptomatology, and management. Fertil Steril. 1981;36(4):433–45.
2. Lefebvre G, Vilos G, Allaire C, Jeffrey J, Arneja J, Birch C, et al. The management of uterine leiomyomas. J Obstet Gynaecol Can. 2003;25(5):396–418; quiz 9-22.
3. Alkatout I, Mundhenke C, Maass N, Schem C. Die Rolle der Angiogenese und seiner Inhibitoren in der Gynäkologie. Der Gynäkologe. 2012;in press.
4. Peddada SD, Laughlin SK, Miner K, Guyon JP, Haneke K, Vahdat HL, et al. Growth of uterine leiomyomata among premenopausal black and white women. Proc Natl Acad Sci USA. 2008;105(50):19887–92. doi:0808188105 [pii] 10.1073/pnas.0808188105.
5. Laughlin SK, Hartmann KE, Baird DD. Postpartum factors and natural fibroid regression. Am J Obstet Gynecol. 2011;204(6):496 e1–6. doi:S0002-9378(11)00181-5 [pii] 10.1016/j.ajog.2011.02.018
6. Zaima A, Ash A. Fibroid in pregnancy: characteristics, complications, and management. Postgrad Med J. 2011;87(1034):819–28. doi:postgradmedj-2011-130319 [pii] 10.1136/postgradmedj-2011-130319
7. Marjoribanks J, Lethaby A, Farquhar C. Surgery versus medical therapy for heavy menstrual bleeding. Cochrane Database Syst Rev. 2006(2):CD003855. doi:10.1002/14651858.CD003855.pub2
8. Al-Hendy A, Lee EJ, Wang HQ, Copland JA. Gene therapy of uterine leiomyomas: adenovirus-mediated expression of dominant negative estrogen receptor inhibits tumor growth in nude mice. Am J Obstet Gynecol. 2004;191(5):1621–31. doi:S000293780400417X [pii] 10.1016/j.ajog.2004.04.022.
9. Edwards RD, Moss JG, Lumsden MA, Wu O, Murray LS, Twaddle S, et al. Uterine-artery embolization versus surgery for symptomatic uterine fibroids. N Engl J Med. 2007;356(4):360–70. doi:356/4/360 [pii] 10.1056/NEJMoa062003.
10. van der Kooij SM, Bipat S, Hehenkamp WJ, Ankum WM, Reekers JA. Uterine artery embolization versus surgery in the treatment of symptomatic fibroids: a systematic review and metaanalysis. Am J Obstet Gynecol. 2011;205(4):317 e1–18. doi:S0002-9378(11)00325-5 [pii] 10.1016/j.ajog.2011.03.016.
11. Kim HS, Baik JH, Pham LD, Jacobs MA. MR-guided high-intensity focused ultrasound treatment for symptomatic uterine leiomyomata: long-term outcomes. Acad Radiol. 2011;18(8):970–6. doi:S1076-6332(11)00196-6 [pii] 10.1016/j.acra.2011.03.008.
12. Funaki K, Fukunishi H, Sawada K. Clinical outcomes of magnetic resonance-guided focused ultrasound surgery for uterine myomas: 24-month follow-up. Ultrasound Obstet Gynecol. 2009;34(5):584–9. doi:10.1002/uog.7455.
13. Gynaecologists RCoOa. Preventing entry-related gynaecological laparoscopic injuries. RCOG Green-top Guideline. 2008; 49:1–10.
14. Wallach EE, Vlahos NF. Uterine myomas: an overview of development, clinical features, and management. Obstet Gynecol. 2004; 104(2):393–406. doi:10.1097/01.aog.0000136079.62513.39.
15. Kim MS, Uhm YK, Kim JY, Jee BC, Kim YB. Obstetric outcomes after uterine myomectomy: Laparoscopic versus laparotomic approach. Obstet Gynecol Sci. 2013;56(6):375–81. doi:10.5468/ogs.2013.56.6.375.
16. Lonnerfors C, Persson J. Pregnancy following robot-assisted laparoscopic myomectomy in women with deep intramural myomas. Acta Obstet Gynecol Scand. 2011;90(9):972–7. doi:10.1111/j.1600-0412.2011.01207.x.
17. Mettler L, Schollmeyer T, Tinelli A, Malvasi A, Alkatout I. Complications of uterine fibroids and their management, surgical management of fibroids, laparoscopy and hysteroscopy versus hysterectomy, haemorrhage, adhesions, and complications. Obstet Gynecol Int. 2012;2012:791248. doi:10.1155/2012/791248.
18. Di Spiezio Sardo A, Mazzon I, Bramante S, Bettocchi S, Bifulco G, Guida M, et al. Hysteroscopic myomectomy: a comprehensive review of surgical techniques. Hum Reprod Update. 2008; 14(2):101–19. doi:dmm041 [pii] 10.1093/humupd/dmm041.
19. Emanuel MH, Hart A, Wamsteker K, Lammes F. An analysis of fluid loss during transcervical resection of submucous myomas. Fertil Steril. 1997;68(5):881–6. doi:S001502829700335X [pii].
20. Wamsteker K, Emanuel MH, de Kruif JH. Transcervical hysteroscopic resection of submucous fibroids for abnormal uterine bleeding: results regarding the degree of intramural extension. Obstet Gynecol. 1993;82(5):736–40.
21. Hart R, Molnar BG, Magos A. Long term follow up of hysteroscopic myomectomy assessed by survival analysis. Br J Obstet Gynaecol. 1999;106(7):700–5.
22. Mettler L, Sammur W, Alkatout I, Schollmeyer T. Imaging in gynecologic surgery. Womens Health (Lond Engl). 2011;7(2):239–48; quiz 49-50. doi:10.2217/whe.11.6.
23. Varma R, Soneja H, Clark TJ, Gupta JK. Hysteroscopic myomectomy for menorrhagia using Versascope bipolar system: efficacy and prognostic factors at a minimum of one year follow up. Eur J Obstet Gynecol Reprod Biol. 2009;142(2):154–9. doi:10.1016/j.ejogrb.2008.10.006.
24. Loffer FD, Bradley LD, Brill AI, Brooks PG, Cooper JM. Hysteroscopic fluid monitoring guidelines. J Am Assoc Gynecol Laparosc. 2000;7(3):438.
25. Jansen FW, Vredevoogd CB, van Ulzen K, Hermans J, Trimbos JB, Trimbos-Kemper TC. Complications of hysteroscopy: a prospective, multicenter study. Obstet Gynecol. 2000;96(2):266–70.
26. Propst AM, Liberman RF, Harlow BL, Ginsburg ES. Complications of hysteroscopic surgery: predicting patients at risk. Obstet Gynecol. 2000;96(4):517–20.

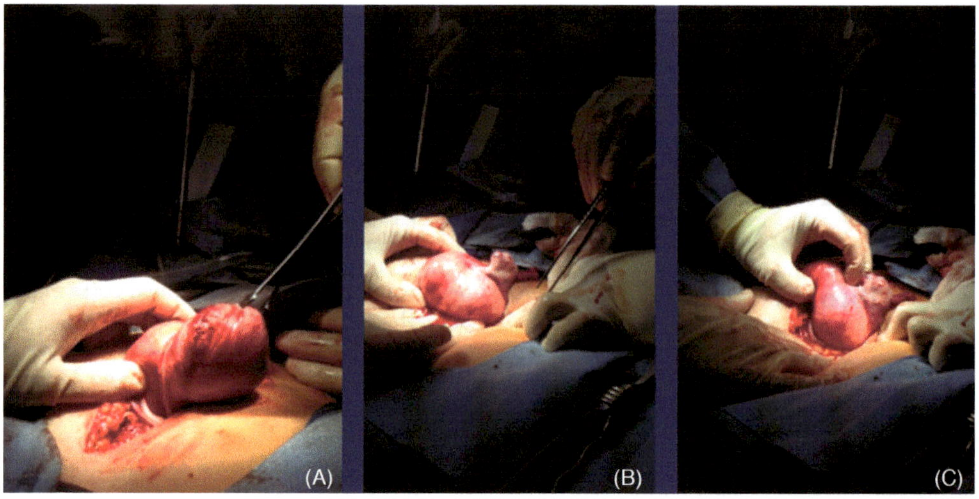


**FIGURE 11.2** (A–C) Abdominal myomectomy, large intramural and subserosal fibroids being removed via laparotomy. (Courtesy of Prof. Botros Rizk.)

Surgery remains the main modality (**Figure 11.2**) for many patients especially in cases of subfertility. However, there are a variety of treatment options including expectant management, hormonal management and non-surgical interventions such as uterine artery embolization (**Figure 11.3**) [6].

## History of robotic myomectomy

Throughout the last three decades, gynecological surgeries have seen a surge in the utilization of minimally invasive surgery (MIS). Several clinical trials and studies have demonstrated the superiority of MIS to open approaches in estimated blood loss, length of hospital stay, complications and surgical outcomes [7]. Robotic surgery is a subset of MIS and it was first approved by the Food and Drug Administration (FDA) to be used in gynecology in 2005. The da Vinci surgical system is currently the only robotic system used in surgery [8]. As mentioned earlier, surgery is one treatment option for symptomatic uterine fibroids. The choice of MIS versus an open approach depends on multiple factors including but not limited to the number, size, location of fibroids (**Figure 11.4**), surgeon's skill and patient preference [9]. There is an increasing use of the da Vinci system as it addresses some of the limitations of traditional laparoscopic myomectomy such as dexterity, EndoWrist technology, elimination of hand tremor, three-dimensional vision, superior suturing and dissection and convenient learning curves [10].

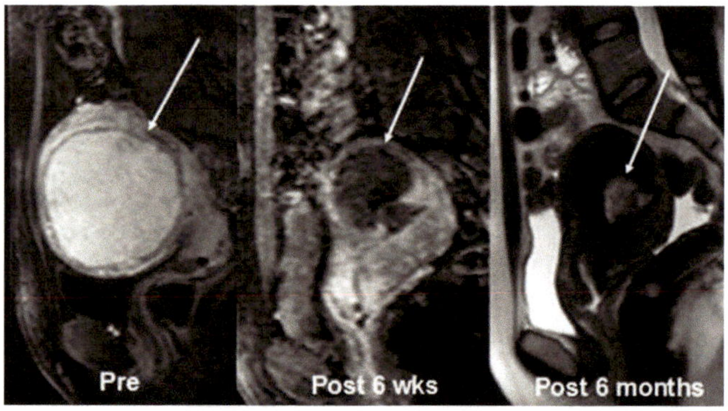


**FIGURE 11.3** Contrast-enhanced sagittal MRI depicts response of leiomyoma to UAE. (Reproduced with permission from Badawy SZA, Henning H, Singer B. Uterine artery embolization for the treatment of uterine fibroids. In Rizk B and Puscheck E, (Eds), *Ultrasonography in Gynecology*, CUP, Cambridge, 2014, Chapter 13, 132–137.)

## Indications and patient selection

There are several indications for myomectomy. The most common are abnormal uterine bleeding, chronic pelvic pain, changes in urinary habits [11] and fibroids causing subfertility or pregnancy loss [12].

There is a consensus on general guidelines that favor MIS in myomectomies over an open approach. In general, it is preferred for intramural and subserosal fibroids when the number of fibroids is usually limited to 5. It is also preferred when the diameter of the largest fibroid is generally <15 cm, and the uterus is <16 weeks in size [13]. MIS demands more surgical skill if the fibroid is in proximity to the cervix, uterine arteries, broad ligament and the uterine cornua [14]. It is also more convenient to resect an anterior fibroid through laparoscopy compared to a posterior one. If there are multiple fibroids in different positions and several incisions have to be made, then an open approach is preferred since uterine reconstruction will be significant [15]. Intracavitary and submucosal fibroids on the other hand can be removed hysteroscopically.

### Preoperative preparation

A thorough and detailed preoperative planning is recommended before the patient is scheduled for a robotic myomectomy. It includes a medical history, physical examination, laboratory tests and diagnostic imaging [11].

The medical history should include details of the menstrual cycle, history of pelvic or abdominal pain, changes in urinary or bowel habits, previous surgeries and any pertinent medical condition especially coagulopathies. The physical examination consists of a bimanual exam to directly palpate the fibroids. A complete blood count and a pregnancy test are also recommended.

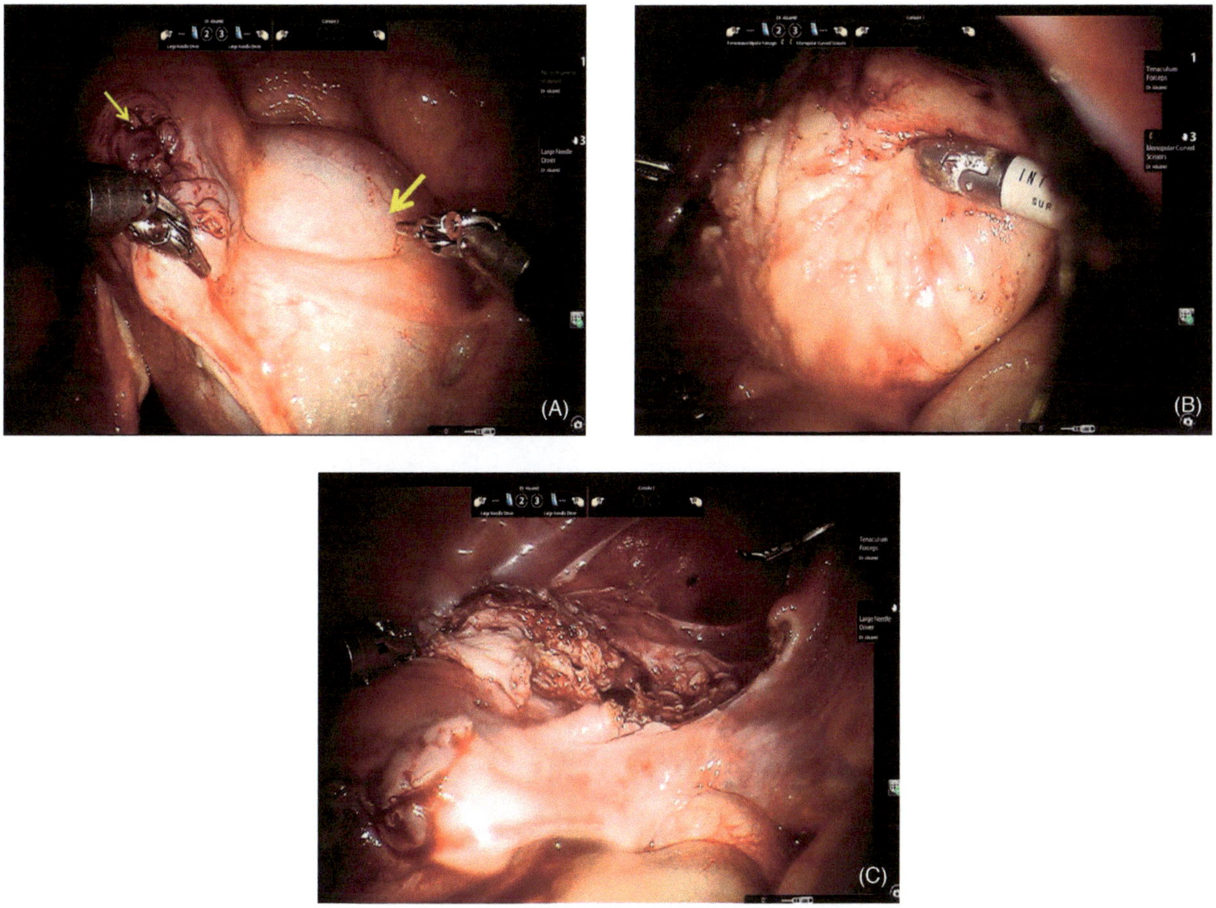


**FIGURE 11.4** Laparoscopic pictures using da Vinci laparoscope and camera showing (A) a large broad ligament fibroid pushing the uterus to the left (large arrow); an area where a 5 cm fibroid was dissected and removed from the fundal region of the uterus is seen (small arrow); (B) the fibroid being dissected from the broad ligament; (C) a gap in the broad ligament after removal of the fibroid. (Reproduced with permission from Abuzeid M, Joseph S. Transvaginal ultrasonography of uterine fibroids. In Rizk B, Puscheck E (Eds), *Ultrasonography in Gynecology*, CUP, Cambridge, 2014, 80–97.)

Preoperative imaging is mainly by transvaginal ultrasound (**Figure 11.5**) and saline infusion sonohysterography is particularly important for MIS to accurately locate fibroids since haptic feedback is absent in robotic myomectomy. Magnetic resonance imaging (MRI) is the most accurate modality used to detect the number and position of fibroids, as well as their relation to adjacent structures [16].

### Tumor size reduction

There are several preoperative interventions to control the severity of symptomatic fibroids. Gonadotropin releasing hormone agonists (GnRHa) are notable agents used to reduce fibroid size and minimize blood loss during surgery [6]. Some patients are also supplemented with estrogen therapy to control for side effects of GnRHa such as hot flashes, vaginal dryness and osteopenia [15]. However, GnRHa may distort the fibroid planes and complicate the surgical procedure. Therefore, some prefer to use these agents only in the case of anemia secondary to fibroids [17].

There are other available options that can achieve similar outcomes, including receptor modulators such as ulipristal acetate (UPA). It causes few side effects, and thus it can be used if GnRHa are not tolerated by the patient [18]. It can be combined with an aromatase inhibitor like letrozole as this combination has been proven to reduce operative time and blood loss during myomectomy [19].

## Surgical technique

The following steps should be followed for a successful robotic myomectomy (**Figure 11.6**) [17, 20].

### Port placement

- Patient is placed in a dorsal lithotomy position. The padded patient's arms and hands are tucked next to her torso to avoid any nerve or muscle injury.
- The vagina and abdomen are sterilized to allow the insertion of a temporary Foley catheter and a uterine manipulator.
- The umbilicus is used an entry point to the abdominal cavity using a 5–10 mm trocar. An alternative entry point is Palmer's point in the left upper quadrant below the subcostal margin along the mid-clavicular line.
- Insufflation with carbon dioxide allows two 8-mm robotic trocars to be placed. They are inserted 8–10 cm lateral from the umbilical port at an angle of 10–15 degrees.
- The umbilical port is switched to a 12-mm port to accommodate for the robotic camera.
- A 12-mm assistant port is placed in the right lower quadrant. It is used to exchange needles and suctioning.
- Needle exchange can also be performed using a trocar through a gelport cover. This method has the advantage of

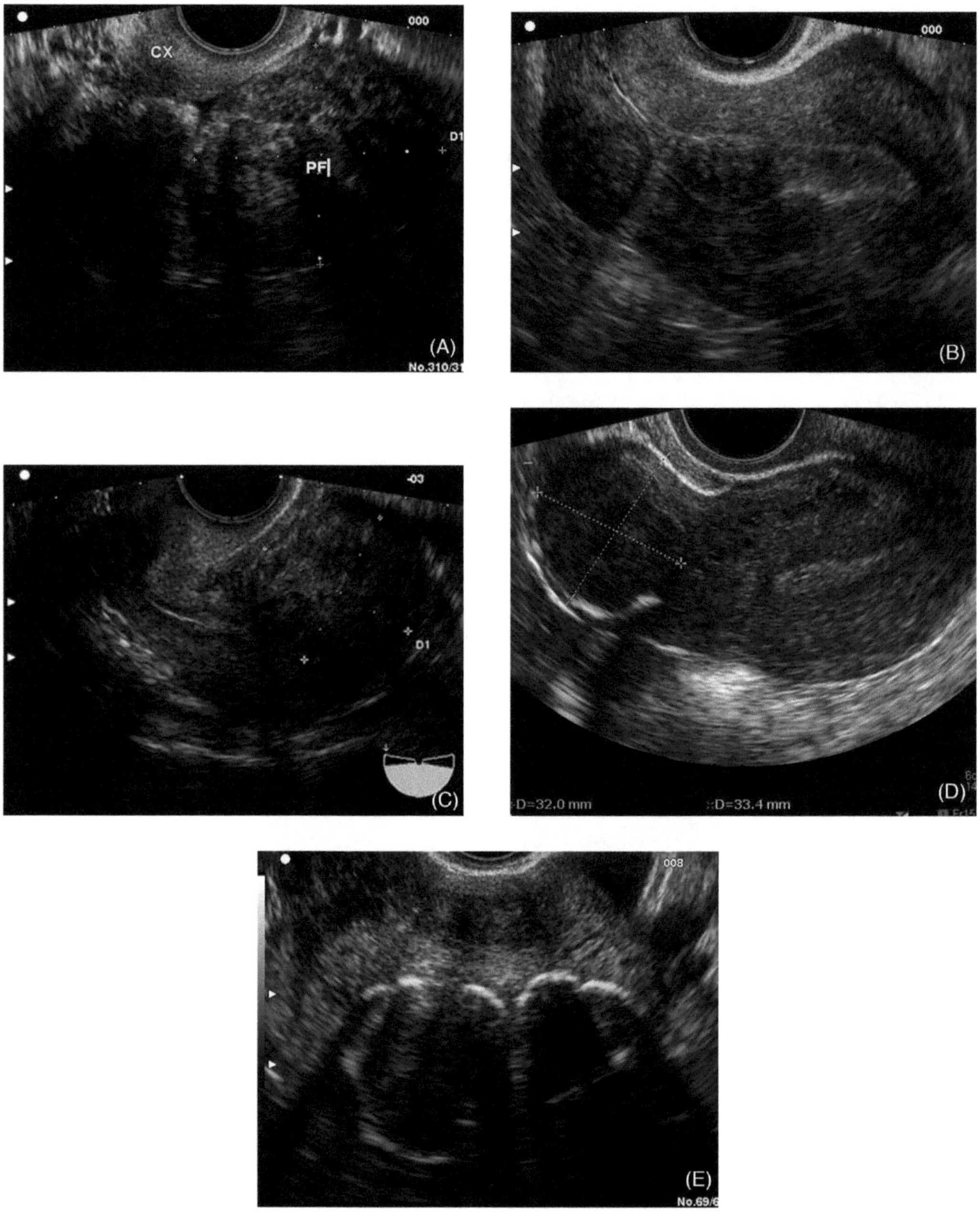


**FIGURE 11.5** Ultrasonography of uterine fibroids. (A) Pedunculated fibroid; (B) submucosal fibroid; (C) intramural fibroid; (D) subserosal fibroid; (E) posterior wall intramural fibroids with calcified outlines. (Reproduced with permission from Clough, Khalaf Y. Ultrasonography of uterine fibroids. In Rizk B (Ed), *Ultrasonography in Reproductive Medicine and Infertility*, CUP, Cambridge, 2010, 87–97.)

observing needle entry and exit from the lower abdomen, which helps in case of an accidental needle drop.

- A 5-mm assistant port can be placed in the right or left upper quadrant lateral to the rectus abdominis muscle. It is used for traction and manipulation of fibroids.

## Uterine incisions

- It is encouraged to minimize the number of uterine incisions to promote better scar healing and reduce the risk of uterine rupture. In case multiple fibroids are in proximity to each other, a single incision is sufficient to extract them.
- The incision is usually transverse to facilitate laparoscopic suturing (**Figure 11.7**). It should not be close to the uterine cornua or adnexa.
- A harmonic scalpel is used to dissect the serosa and myometrium.

## Enucleation

- This requires a robotic tenaculum and a harmonic scalpel.
- The position of the fibroid again plays an important role. If the fibroids are in a posterior position, for example, the surgeon may opt to use the manipulator to push the uterus forward to adequately dissect the fibroid away from

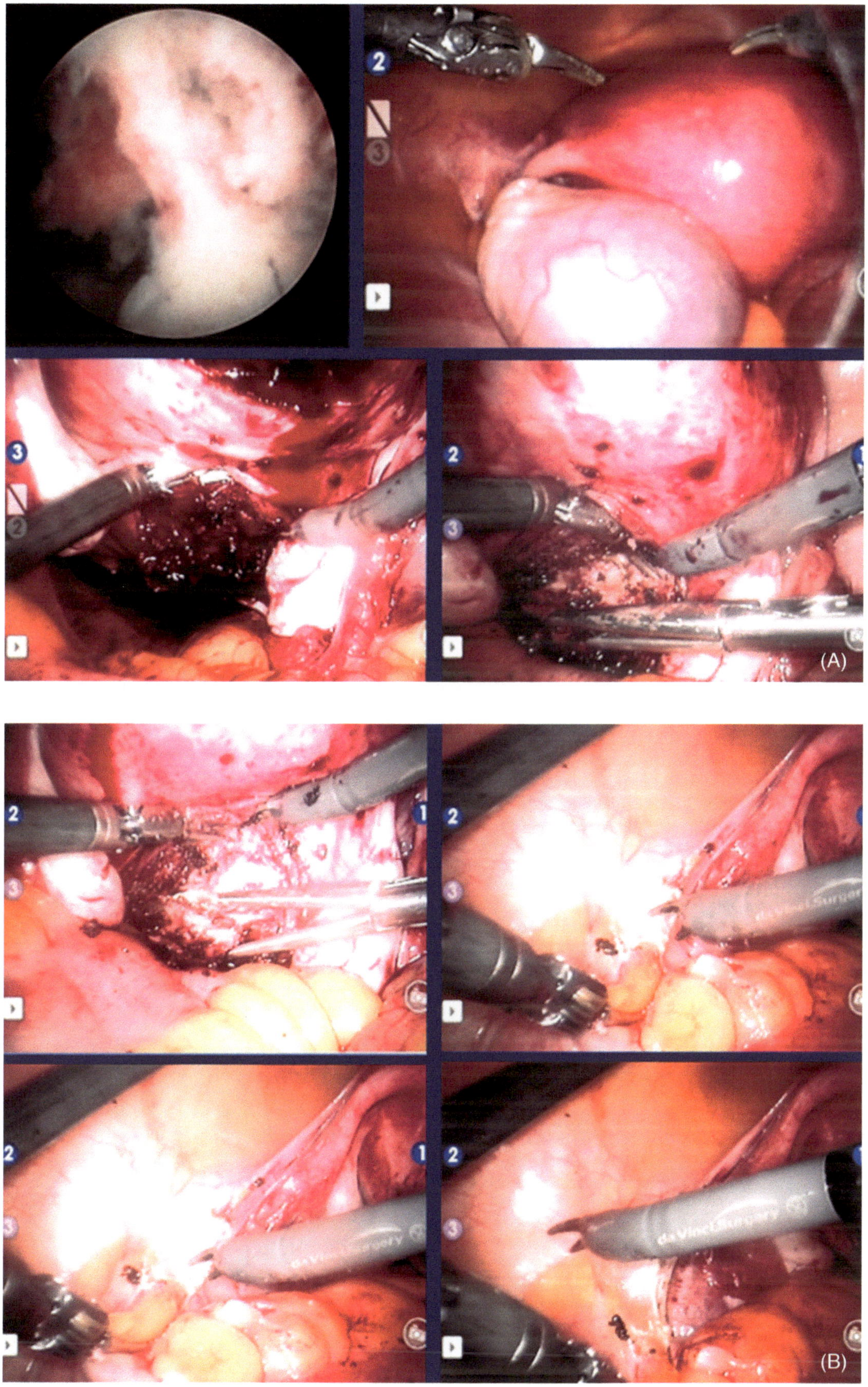


**FIGURE 11.6** (A–B) Robotic myomectomy, step by step. (Courtesy of Prof. Botros Rizk.)

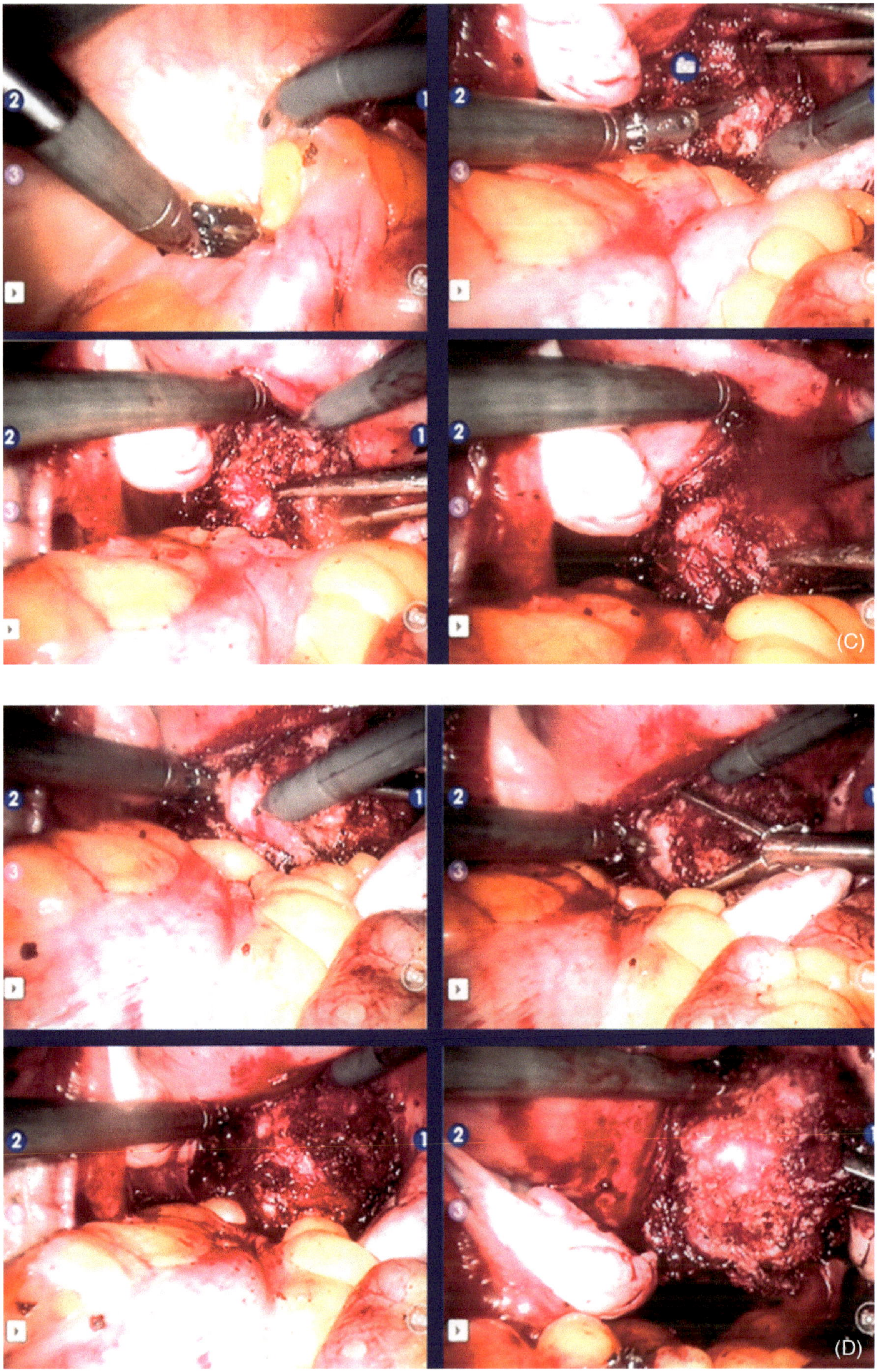


**FIGURE 11.6** (C–D) Robotic myomectomy, step by step. (Courtesy of Prof. Botros Rizk.)

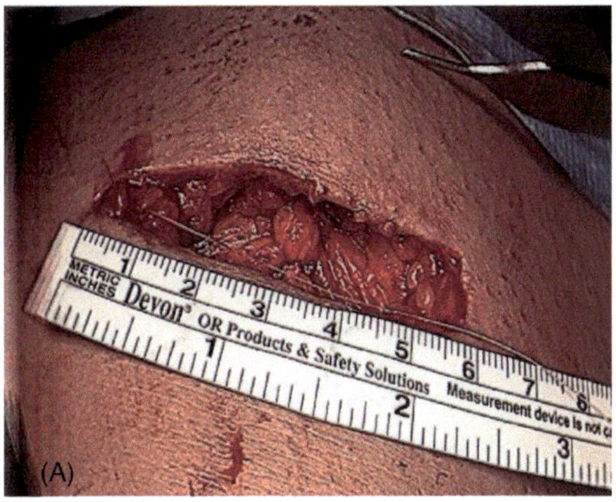


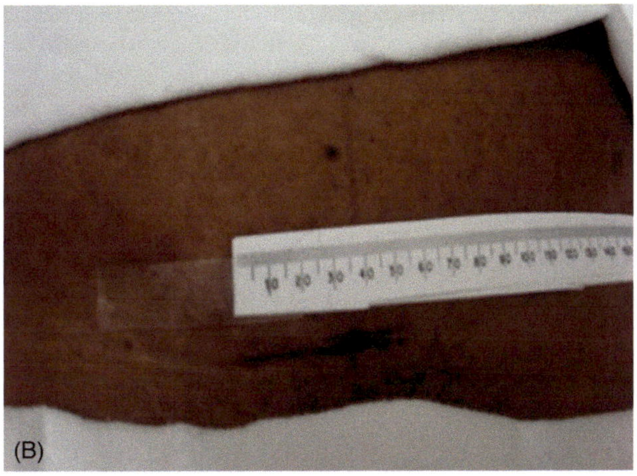


**FIGURE 11.7** (A) 5 cm transverse suprapubic mini-laparotomy incision through which the repair of a large myometrial defect in the posterior wall of the uterus was performed. (B) Postoperative scar. (Reproduced with permission from Abuzeid M, Joseph S, Transvaginal ultrasonography of uterine fibroids. In Rizk B and Puscheck E (Eds), *Ultrasonography in Gynecology*, CUP, Cambridge, UK, 2014, 80–97.)

the rectosigmoid. Intramural fibroids may risk the dissection of the endometrial cavity. Methylene blue can be used intraoperatively to check the integrity of the cavity.

### Morcellation

- Power morcellation was the usual standard to extract fibroid tissue after enucleation. It has the risk, however, of dissemination of occult malignancies such as sarcomas [17].
- Alternative contained morcellation techniques have emerged to counter this problem.
- The first is manual morcellation inside a laparoscopic bag. The bag is pulled through a port incision and the fibroid is dissected into pieces by alternative coring.
- The second is making an incision in the posterior cul-de-sac. This can be achieved either through the uterosacral ligaments to retract the rectosigmoid colon or vaginally.
- There is also a decreased risk of injury to the gastrointestinal system in contained morcellation.

### Suturing of myometrium and serosa

- The myometrium is sutured in multiple layers using barbed sutures to reduce risk of uterine rupture in subsequent pregnancies.
- The serosa is sutured with 3-0 monofilament sutures.
- In case of endometrial cavity breach, it is closed with 3-0 or 4-0 suture.

### Minimizing blood loss during surgery

- There are several intraoperative interventions that can minimize blood loss.
- The two most common agents used are misoprostol applied rectally and intravenous vasopressin.

## Limitations of robotic myomectomy

There are two noteworthy limitations of robotic myomectomy. Its first drawback is the absence of haptic feedback and tactile sensation. In open myomectomies, surgeons can palpate the uterus and appreciate the location and nature of each fibroid including the minor ones. This is not the case in robotic myomectomy, and as a result some fibroids may be missed. Its second drawback is difficulty determining the strength needed for suturing. Improper suturing can lead to poor wound healing and increase risk of uterine rupture in future pregnancies [7].

Increased total operative time is another limitation of robotic myomectomy. This will be discussed later.

## Intraoperative ultrasound guidance

In order to overcome the absence haptic feedback, intraoperative ultrasound guidance can be used to locate fibroids including intramural and submucosal ones [21, 22]. It can be utilized in two ways: (i) by introducing an ultrasound probe into a laparoscopic port [20] or (ii) by inserting a transvaginal ultrasound, which has been documented to be as effective as the ultrasound probe. These techniques have improved surgical outcomes of myomectomies by detecting minor fibroids and reducing the rate of fibroid recurrence to a minimum [22].

## Comparison between robotic myomectomy versus laparoscopic myomectomy and abdominal myomectomy

Myomectomies can be performed through three routes: An Abdominal Myomectomy (AM), Laparoscopic Myomectomy (LM) and Robotically Assisted Laparoscopic Myomectomy (RALM). Wang et al. conducted a meta-analysis of twenty studies comparing RALM to LM and AM. There were 1852 female patients in studies comparing RALM to AM, and 1000 patients in studies comparing RALM to LM [23].

RALM showed a statically significant decrease in estimated blood loss (EBL) and conversion rate to AM in comparison with LM. There was no difference in length of hospital stay (LHS), operative time (OT), size of the largest fibroid removed, fertility rate post-surgery, transfusion rate or reoperation rate. Five studies showed a decrease in complication rate in RALM compared to LM while three studies showed no significant difference.

RALM also showed a statistically significant decrease in EBL, transfusion rate, LHS, complication rate and postoperative pain compared to AM. The OT was significantly longer in RALM, and there was no difference in the size of the largest fibroid [23].

## Total operative time

As mentioned earlier, the total operative time is significantly longer in RALM than AM. This puts a strain on the cost and efficiency of RALM, as well as the number of cases a gynecologist can perform in a single day. The increase in operative time can be partially explained by the difficult technicality of RALM compared to AM [24]. Movilla et al. conducted a cross-sectional retrospective study to determine the factors that increase the total operative time (TOT). They found that younger patients with a personal history of Diabetes Mellitus 2 (DM) and a greater uterine volume are at a higher risk. Other critical factors include the diameter of the fibroid, the total number of fibroids, the number of fibroids >3 cm and limited surgeon experience. The authors also noted that although body mass index (BMI) was not a statistically significant factor, obesity was associated with a prolonged TOT [25].

## Financial impact of robotic surgery

Despite its advantages, critics of robotic-assisted surgery argue that its financial burden outweighs its benefits. There are several attempts to quantify the added cost of robotic surgery. However, this is not a straightforward process as there are multiple direct and indirect factors that come into play [26].

There are the fixed costs, which include the initial purchase of the da Vinci system and its maintenance. The robotic system costs around $1 to $2.3 million, and its maintenance can range between $100,000 and $180,000 [27]. Additional costs also arise from ancillary equipment, such as robotic forceps, robotic ports, camera drape, etc. [28].

Postoperative complications such as infections can also add to the overall costs of care. In fact, they can add up to $11,000 to the original cost [29]. Since robotic surgery is associated with a significant decrease in intraoperative and postoperative complications, there is a reduction in the overall cost. Similarly, since the LHS is reduced in RALM, extra charges associated with length of stay such as laboratory tests, pain medications and the room fee are significantly reduced [26]. The financial burden of any surgery can also be judged based on the recovery time the patient needs [30]. Patients undergoing robotic hysterectomies for example often return to their baseline routine sooner than their counterparts [31], adding to the financial benefits.

The length of surgery is another crucial component of the overall cost. It is hypothesized that the increased expenses of robotic myomectomies are largely due to the long operative time [24]. There are other factors, however, that come into play including surgeon experience and the familiarity of the surgical staff with the da Vinci system [32]. In fact, the staff efficiency in setting up the robotic system can significantly alter the operation time regardless of the surgeon experience [24]. Thus, the TOT and overall cost of robotic myomectomy can be reduced with staff training and experience.

## Future of robotic surgery in gynecology

The da Vinci system is currently the only FDA approved robotic system used. This monopoly will not hold in the future, as new systems will be introduced. The cost of robotic-assisted surgery will therefore decrease due to market competition [33]. One example is the REVO-I robotic system (Meerecompany Inc., Seongnam, South Korea), which was shown to be safe and efficient in tubal reanastomosis [34]. It also has a unique feature of reusable instruments that can further reduce the cost of MIS [35]. Another innovative system is the Senhance surgical robotic system, and it offers an advantage over the da Vinci system by providing haptic feedback and follows the surgeon's eye movements to provide camera control [36]. Such innovations will reshape gynecological surgery and improve patient care.

## References

1. Yoshino O, Hayashi T, Osuga Y, Orisaka M, Asada H, Okuda S, et al. Decreased pregnancy rate is linked to abnormal uterine peristalsis caused by intramural fibroids. Hum Reprod. 2010;25(10):2475–9.
2. Baird DD, Dunson DB, Hill MC, Cousins D, Schectman JM. High cumulative incidence of uterine leiomyoma in black and white women: ultrasound evidence. Am J Obstet Gynecol. 2003; 188(1):100–7.
3. Bulun SE. Uterine fibroids. N Engl J Med. 2013;369(14):1344–55.
4. Cardozo ER, Clark AD, Banks NK, Henne MB, Stegmann BJ, Segars JH. The estimated annual cost of uterine leiomyomata in the United States. Am J Obstet Gynecol. 2012;206(3):211 e1–9.
5. Munro MG, Critchley HO, Broder MS, Fraser IS, Disorders FWGoM. FIGO classification system (PALM-COEIN) for causes of abnormal uterine bleeding in nongravid women of reproductive age. Int J Gynaecol Obstet. 2011;113(1):3–13.
6. Kashani BN, Centini G, Morelli SS, Weiss G, Petraglia F. Role of medical management for uterine leiomyomas. Best Pract Res Clin Obstet Gynaecol. 2016;34:85–103.
7. Barakat EE, Bedaiwy MA, Zimberg S, Nutter B, Nosseir M, Falcone T. Robotic-assisted, laparoscopic, and abdominal myomectomy: a comparison of surgical outcomes. Obstet Gynecol. 2011;117(2 Pt 1): 256–65.
8. Visco AG, Advincula AP. Robotic gynecologic surgery. Obstet Gynecol. 2008;112(6):1369–84.
9. Kim S, Luu TH, Llarena N, Falcone T. Role of robotic surgery in treating fibroids and benign uterine mass. Best Pract Res Clin Obstet Gynaecol. 2017;45:48–59.
10. Cho JE, Nezhat FR. Robotics and gynecologic oncology: review of the literature. J Minim Invasive Gynecol. 2009;16(6):669–81.
11. Moon AS, Garofalo J, Koirala P, Vu MT, Chuang L. Robotic surgery in gynecology. Surg Clin North Am. 2020;100(2):445–60.
12. Pritts EA, Parker WH, Olive DL. Fibroids and infertility: an updated systematic review of the evidence. Fertil Steril. 2009;91(4):1215–23.
13. Chen CC, Falcone T. Robotic gynecologic surgery: past, present, and future. Clin Obstet Gynecol. 2009;52(3):335–43.
14. Prentice A, Taylor A, Sharma MA, Magos A. Laparoscopic versus open myomectomy for uterine fibroids. Cochrane Database of Systematic Reviews. 2004;1:1465–1858.
15. Donnez J, Dolmans MM. Uterine fibroid management: from the present to the future. Hum Reprod Update. 2016;22(6):665–86.
16. Parker WH. The utility of MRI for the surgical treatment of women with uterine fibroid tumors. Am J Obstet Gynecol. 2012;206(1):31–6.
17. Flyckt R, Coyne K, Falcone T. Minimally invasive myomectomy. Clin Obstet Gynecol. 2017;60(2):252–72.
18. Levy BS. Modern management of uterine fibroids. Acta Obstet Gynecol Scand. 2008;87(8):812–23.
19. Leone Roberti Maggiore U, Scala C, Venturini PL, Ferrero S. Preoperative treatment with letrozole in patients undergoing laparoscopic myomectomy of large uterine myomas: a prospective non-randomized study. Eur J Obstet Gynecol Reprod Biol. 2014; 181:157–62.
20. Wu H, Frost, A., and Borahay, AM. Laparoscopic and robotic-assisted myomectomy. Fibroids and Reproduction. [Book Chapter] (in press). 2020.
21. Lin PC, Thyer A, Soules MR. Intraoperative ultrasound during a laparoscopic myomectomy. Fertil Steril. 2004;81(6):1671–4.

22. Shimanuki H, Takeuchi H, Kikuchi I, Kumakiri J, Kinoshita K. Effectiveness of intraoperative ultrasound in reducing recurrent fibroids during laparoscopic myomectomy. J Reprod Med. 2006; 51(9):683–8.
23. Wang T, Tang H, Xie Z, Deng S. Robotic-assisted vs. laparoscopic and abdominal myomectomy for treatment of uterine fibroids: a meta-analysis. Minim Invasive Ther Allied Technol. 2018; 27(5):249–64.
24. Nash K, Feinglass J, Zei C, Lu G, Mengesha B, Lewicky-Gaupp C, et al. Robotic-assisted laparoscopic myomectomy versus abdominal myomectomy: a comparative analysis of surgical outcomes and costs. Arch Gynecol Obstet. 2012;285(2):435–40.
25. Movilla P, Orlando M, Wang J, Opoku-Anane J. Predictors of prolonged operative time for robotic-assisted laparoscopic myomectomy: development of a preoperative calculator for total operative time. J Minim Invasive Gynecol. 2020;27(3):646–54.
26. Wu CZ, Klebanoff JS, Tyan P, Moawad GN. Review of strategies and factors to maximize cost-effectiveness of robotic hysterectomies and myomectomies in benign gynecological disease. J Robot Surg. 2019;13(5):635–42.
27. Pasic RP, Rizzo JA, Fang H, Ross S, Moore M, Gunnarsson C. Comparing robot-assisted with conventional laparoscopic hysterectomy: impact on cost and clinical outcomes. J Minim Invasive Gynecol. 2010;17(6):730–8.
28. Advincula AP, Xu X, Goudeau St, Ransom SB. Robot-assisted laparoscopic myomectomy versus abdominal myomectomy: a comparison of short-term surgical outcomes and immediate costs. J Minim Invasive Gynecol. 2007;14(6):698–705.
29. Donnez O, Jadoul P, Squifflet J, Donnez J. A series of 3190 laparoscopic hysterectomies for benign disease from 1990 to 2006: evaluation of complications compared with vaginal and abdominal procedures. BJOG. 2009;116(4):492–500.
30. Hanstede MM, Wise LA, Stewart EA, Feldman S. The relation of annual surgeon case volume to clinical outcomes and resource utilization in abdominal hysterectomy. J Reprod Med. 2009; 54(4):193–202.
31. Sarlos D, Kots L, Stevanovic N, von Felten S, Schar G. Robotic compared with conventional laparoscopic hysterectomy: a randomized controlled trial. Obstet Gynecol. 2012;120(3):604–11.
32. Barnett JC, Judd JP, Wu JM, Scales CD, Jr., Myers ER, Havrilesky LJ. Cost comparison among robotic, laparoscopic, and open hysterectomy for endometrial cancer. Obstet Gynecol. 2010;116(3):685–93.
33. Lim CS, Griffith KC, Travieso J, As-Sanie S. To robot or not to robot: the use of robotics in benign gynecologic surgery. Clin Obstet Gynecol. 2020;63(2):327–36.
34. Abdel Raheem A, Troya IS, Kim DK, Kim SH, Won PD, Joon PS, et al. Robot-assisted Fallopian tube transection and anastomosis using the new REVO-I robotic surgical system: feasibility in a chronic porcine model. BJU Int. 2016;118(4):604–9.
35. Kim DK, Park DW, Rha KH. Robot-assisted partial nephrectomy with the REVO-I robot platform in porcine models. Eur Urol. 2016;69(3):541–2.
36. Peters BS, Armijo PR, Krause C, Choudhury SA, Oleynikov D. Review of emerging surgical robotic technology. Surg Endosc. 2018; 32(4):1636–55.

# 12

# METHODS FOR MASS TISSUE REMOVAL BY MINIMALLY INVASIVE REPRODUCTIVE SURGERY

**Magdi Hanafi**

## Introduction

Infertility affects millions of women around the world. However, an unknown number of women who experience infertility are not aware of their status, primarily due to a failure to pursue evaluation by a medical professional. In addition, women are often unaware that a failure to conceive after having unprotected sexual intercourse for over one year [1] may be due to etiological medical reasons in one or both partners. Infertility is a very common problem worldwide, with the prevalence highest in South Asia, Sub-Saharan Africa, North Africa/Middle East, and Central/Eastern Europe and Central Asia [2]. According to a study performed in 2010, 1.9% of women aged from 20 to 44 were unable to have their first child and 10.5 percent of women who already had one child were unable to have a second one. Due to population growth, the number of couples affected by infertility increased from 42.0 million (39.6 million, 44.8 million) in 1990 to 48.5 million (45.0 million, 52.6 million) in 2010 [2]. The infertility factors contribute to 35 percent of the measurable causes of infertility [3]. For example, some identifiable female factors include ovulatory disorders, endometriosis, leiomyomas, pelvic adhesions, adenomyosis, ovarian cysts, tubal blockage, hyperprolactinemia, advanced age, and congenital anatomical disorders of the uterus, fallopian tubes and ovaries [84, 85]. The underlying medical problems can often be corrected medically, surgically or through the use of more progressive approaches including advanced reproductive technology (ART), for example, in vitro fertility (IVF).

For patients who require minimally invasive surgery of the reproductive organs, for example, the uterus, ovaries and fallopian tubes, to excise lesions, tumors, cysts, endometriosis and adhesions, a safe effective method of tissue removal out of the peritoneal and or uterine cavity is required. The methods for removal of the tumors, lesions, endometriosis, adhesions and cysts depend on the size, texture, contents of the cyst, and the surrounding organs and tissue.

## Laparoscopic tissue removal from the peritoneal cavity

Main objectives:

- Safe complete removal of the affected tissue without injury to the small or large bowel, bladder, ureters and major blood vessels (iliac, hypogastric, aortic vessels)
- Maintain the aesthetic appearance of the skin, and minimize the size, and number of the skin incisions in the abdominal wall
- Minimize the incidence of postoperative incisional hernias.
- Inhibit the spread of potential malignancies arising as a result of tissue removal.
- Minimize the chances of surgical site infection
- Reduce blood loss from the surrounding organs of the tissues removed

The size, consistency (cystic versus solid component) and the risk of malignancy are essential factors influencing the route of specimen retrieval [53]. The risk of spillage (especially in suspected early malignancy) has to be considered during excision and retrieval. When there is suspected malignancy, it is best to choose the removal method that yields the least chance of inadvertent dispersion, dermoid cysts, for example.

### Uterine lesion tissue extractions (mostly fibroid tumors (leiomyomata) and adenomyosis

Uterine masses or lesions that may require removal include uterine fibroids (**Figure 12.1**), adenomyosis, polyps, or the presence of a septate uterus. **Uterine leiomyoma** (myomas) are among the most common tumors of the female reproductive tract [4].

Approximately 30%–50% of women have fibroid tumors (uterine leiomyoma), which are typically benign, non-cancerous growths of muscle in the uterus. While most fibroid tumors are asymptomatic, and thus go undetected, some can grow during the reproductive years [18]. Depending on their size and location,

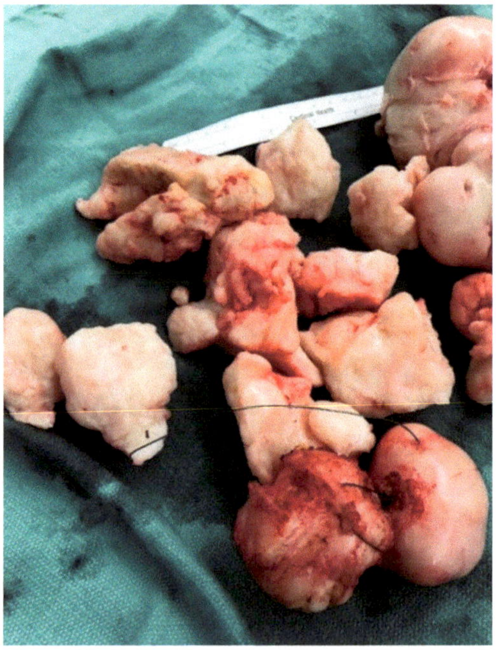

**FIGURE 12.1** Fibroid tumor tissue removed (same patient as **Figure 12.5**).

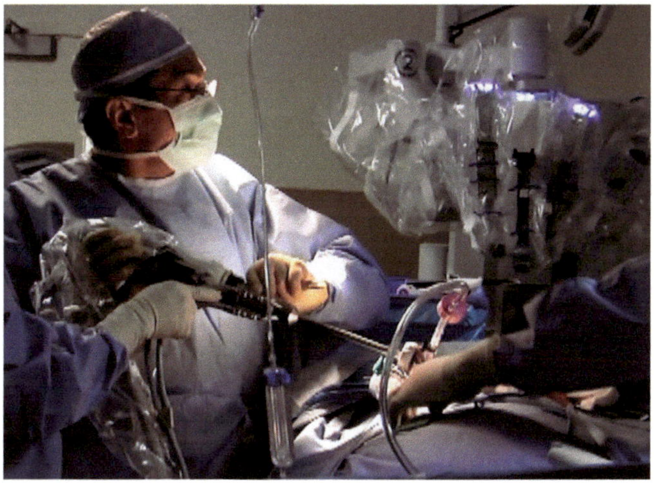

FIGURE 12.2 da Vinci Robotic System before the arms dock in the trocars. (Robotic Laparoscopic Myomectomy, RLM.)

fibroid tumors can cause infertility, recurrent miscarriages, excessive uterine bleeding, pain and pressure, or severe anemia [84]. Fibroids are most common in women between their 30s and their early 50s, and are more common with advancing in age. If fibroids occur during pregnancy, they may cause complications such as miscarriage and preterm birth. A study of 100 hysterectomy specimens found myomas in 77% of uterine specimens. Most women had multiple myomas, with an average of 7.6 fibroids per individual [5].

By utilizing the da Vinci Robotic System (**Figures 12.2** and **12.3**), laparoscopic myomectomy can be accomplished with multiple advantages over conventional laparoscopic myomectomy for the following advantages:

- Precise enucleation of the tumor
- Suturing the uterine wall incisions precisely by the use of robotic needle holders with good dexterity
- Excellent ergonomically for the surgeons
- Less blood loss
- Shorter hospital stays

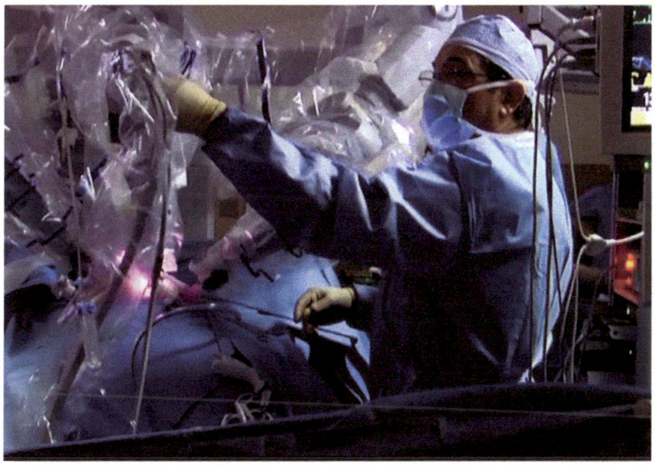

FIGURE 12.3 da Vinci Robotic System after the arms dock in the trocars. (Robotic Laparoscopic Myomectomy, RLM.)

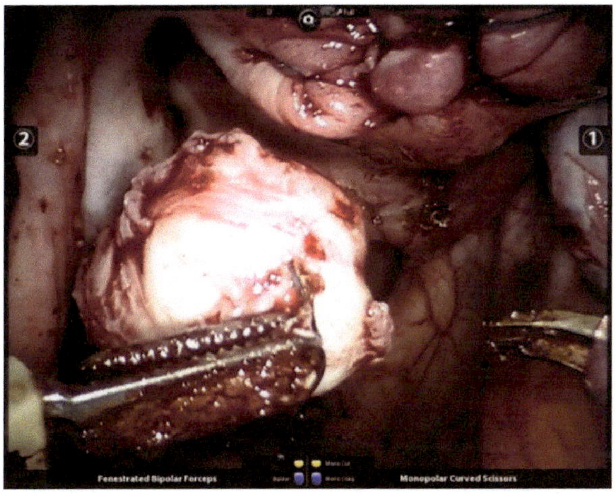


FIGURE 12.4 Removal of small fibroid tumor through accessory port trocar.

Enabling cutting of some of the fibroid tumors and tissue extraction through the 12-mm trocar with or without endoscopic bag (**Figure 12.4**)

For larger fibroid tumors, Hanafi AUI (Video 12.1) was made in the upper fold of the umbilicus which increased the wound size significantly without compromising the appearance of the umbilicus after closure of the incision. An excision of a small portion of the skin (0.5–1.5 inches) was made, which allowed more space for retraction of the upper edge of the incision up to 2.5 inches above the umbilical fascia attachment. This opened a small longitudinal fascia incision (1.5–2.0 inches above the umbilicus) for the laparoscopic camera trocar (Hasson trocar insertion). This incision provides more space between the tip of the laparoscope (camera) and the tumors for easier excision and suturing. It also gives the surgeon more incision space for tissue extraction of larger fibroid tumors. If the tumor is much larger than the skin incision size and is hard in texture, cutting the fibroid tumors into two to four pieces in sequences after bagging the tumors with their attached sutures and protecting the bowels with wet laps (hold their blue tapes clamped with hemostat outside the patient umbilical incision). Pull each tumor tissue with its attached suture with towel clips against the umbilical incision tightly. Then cut as big cones of the tumor tissue using blade size 11, one after the other if needed, until you are able to deliver the larger tumor tissue through the AUI. This method possibly reduces the incidence of additional Pfannenstiel incision for removing the larger tumors.

The opening of the parietal peritoneum was completed closed with zero polyglactin 0 in CT1 needle.

Special attention should be given in closing the annular umbilical incision in order to accomplish the desired cosmetic appearance and to avoid herniation of the umbilicus. The fascial midline incision was closed securely with PDSII size 0 with multiple figure of eight sutures. Subcutaneous tissue was closed in two layers. The deep layer was sutured by interrupted figure eight multiple polyglactin size 0 in CT1 needle, sutures anchored to the fascia after excision of the excess fat, and tailored to approximate the upper and lower edges of the skin incision. The superficial layer was sutured by Monocryl dyed sutures 4-0 in a PS-2 needle, which are used to close the skin in a continuous subcuticular or interrupted superficial skin suture.

Adenomyosis occurs when the cells that produce endometrial tissue move beyond the lining of the uterus and lodge within the muscles of the uterine wall. Due to the displacement of the

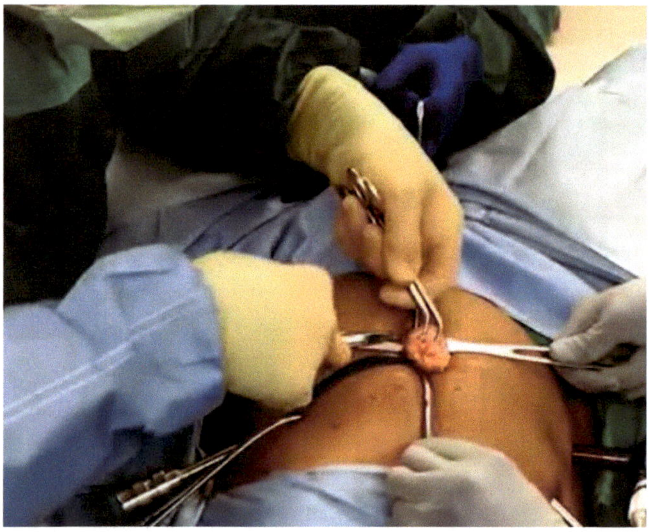

**FIGURE 12.5** Fibroid tumor tissue extraction through Hanafi AUI after RLM.

uterine wall, this condition can cause enlargement of the uterus. Although the etiology remains unknown, it is associated with increased levels of estrogen. Women with this condition may experience severe pain and abnormal uterine bleeding. The condition varies from patient to patient, and the cells may be localized to one area of the uterus, diffuse with involvement of large areas of the uterine muscle, scattered or clustered.

A combination of fibroid tumors and adenomyosis are present in 57% of the diagnosed fibroid cases by histopathological evaluation of the surrounding uterine muscular uterine wall tissue (Hanafi et al.) [85]. It is advisable to remove the adenomyosis suspicious uterine wall tissue surrounding the fibroid tumors as much as possible without compromising the uterine cavity size and shape. The size and the texture of the tumor or the adenomyosis uterine wall tissue. If the tissue is less than 2 cm you can remove it through the 12 mm assistant trocar with no difficulty (**Figure 12.5**). For the calcified tissue and/or less than 4 cm, you can remove it through the umbilical incision (Hanafi AUI) with visualization by placing the laparoscopic camera on the 12-mm assistant trocar access.

For larger tumors, hard texture, you suture the tumors together like a big family by 0 V lock suture in one, two or three groups for easily identified and removal through the annular umbilical incision (Hanafi AUI; Video 12.1).

For calcified tumors, it depends on the size; if they are 1–6 cm, they can be removed through the annular umbilical incision (Hanafi AUI); if the tumor diameter is larger than 6 cm (**Figure 12.6**), it should be extracted through a mini Pfannenstiel incision because the tumor cannot be cut or morcellated or compressed due to the hard nature of the tumor calcified capsule which feels mostly like a piece of a rock. If the tumor looks suspicious of any malignancy (severely discolored or highly vascular, bleeds easily with any touch) multiple sites biopsies from the tumor for frozen section urgent pathological evaluation should be done before myomectomy is performed. If these tumors are benign, the tissue must be contained in an endoscopic bag with exit through Hanafi AUI. Any malignant tumors cannot be excised and surgery should be postponed until complete work up is done to determine the extended of the malignancy and the distant metastases status and to inform the patient with the options of treatment and consult the gynecological oncologist accordingly.

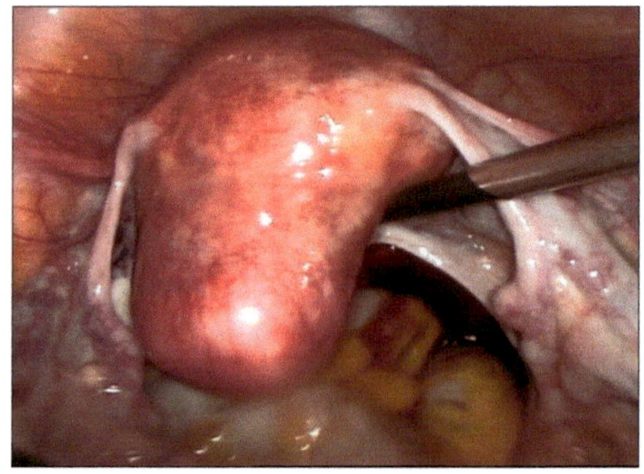

**FIGURE 12.6** Posterior uterine wall with large fibroid tumor (different patient).

Advantages of Hanafi AUI are:

1. Enabling the insertion of the open laparoscopic trocar about 2–3 inches above the umbilical insertion in the rectus fascia and subsequently give more space between the tip of the camera and the pelvic organs especially larger fibroid tumors, ovarian cysts, etc.
2. Allow inspection, dissection and excision of the pelvic lesions, controlling of the bleeders and suturing precisely and efficiently laparoscopically.
3. Facilitate the inspection of the fimbria of fallopian tubes for chromo perturbation procedure with Indigo Carmin diluted saline, which is important in infertility patient.
4. Allow the tissue removal of larger or calcified fibroid tumor, ovarian lesions/tumors by expanding the rectus fascia and peritoneum incision longitudinally and may extend the skin incision slightly laterally without compromising in the esthetic appearance of the umbilical incision or the need of an additional mini laparotomy incision.

Morcellation facilitates tissue extraction of large tissue masses during minimally invasive approaches to surgery [75]. Tissue masses that are too large to be removed can be broken down by two types of morcellation: power morcellation (electromechanical) and manual [38]. A power morcellator is typically a sharp rotating cylindrical blade inside a tube. It cuts the tissue into strips to be extracted through the sheath of the morcellator [83]. There are recent restrictions in power morcellator usage and concerns regarding its association with both benign and malignant tissue dispersal, with the United States FDA releasing a warning statement discouraging the use of power morcellation in women undergoing hysterectomy and myomectomy based on the safety concerns [40]. Morcellation within a containment bag provides an option for removal with decreased chances of specimen dispersion and an updated FDA statement release recommended a tissue containment system when using power Morcellation when the tissue is not suspected [41, 42]. As the usage of a morcellator may include the risk of spreading unrecognized malignancies, discussing such risks with the patient is recommended. Contained manual morcellation can be done via mini-laparotomy or posterior colpotomy.

In the mid-1980s and early 1990s, it was common for tissue to be extracted through posterior colpotomy. This is not surprising, given that we were trained to perform transvaginal tubal ligation and to use colpotomy to drain turbo-ovarian abscesses, which are now uncommonly performed, in order to avoid injury to the rectum, ureters and iliac vessels. Tissues, e.g. large masses, are now

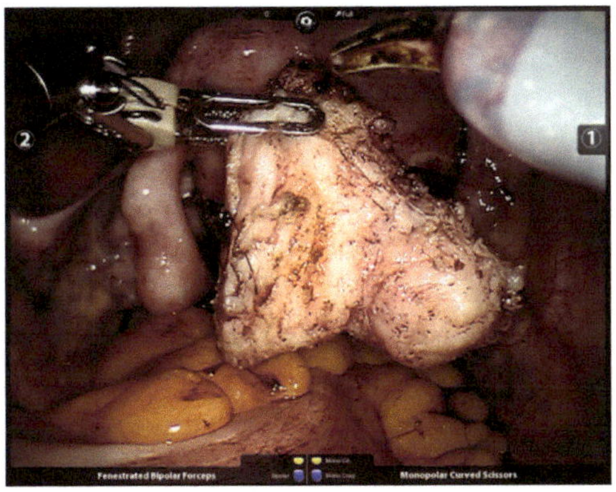

FIGURE 12.7 Cutting fibroid tumor by monopolar robotic scissors for tissue removal.

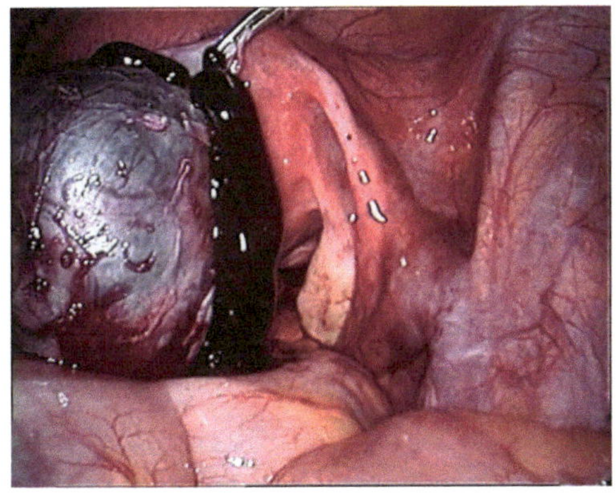

FIGURE 12.8 Endometriomas or chocolate cyst.

removed through the trocar, primarily through the laparoscopic camera port (Hanafi AUI **Figure 12.5**), after removal of Hassan operative trocar (**Figures 12.1** and **12.7**, **Videos 12.2** and **12.3**). First, remove the Hassan trocar and extend the rectus fascia longitudinally and if possible the skin incision slightly, to accommodate the size of the tissue mass to be removed through the Hanafi AUI.

Posterior colpotomy proved to be problematic in situations that required the removal of multiple masses while still attempting to maintain laparoscopic visualization [30]. In 1995, an oophorectomy method was proposed that combined a posterior colpotomy and a nylon drawstring bag. The bag itself became the closing valve to the vaginal opening, decreasing the removal time and preventing loss of $CO_2$ gas and subsequent visibility impairment. The bag also allowed for removal of any suspected ovarian malignancies without puncture or morcellation [34]. Though not as widely used today, a posterior colpotomy incision has been shown as a safe, effective and technically feasible alternative to extending umbilical or accessory abdominal ports for transvaginal specimen retrieval while avoiding concomitant hysterectomy [26, 35]. There have also been novel developments based on obstetric forceps as extraction tools to remove end bag-contained specimens [29]. Most physicians now prefer removal through the umbilical incision laparoscopic port. Before widespread availability of laparoscopic bags and morcellators, removal of tissue trapped in the flap valve of trocars and large masses requiring port removal posed potential problems with this method. Although a morcellator can reduce the risk of hernia formation associated with large mass removal, since there is less tearing and stretching of fascia, the use of power morcelator has its own caveats [37].

## Ovarian cysts and ovarian tumors

Ovarian cysts including endometriomas (**Figure 12.8**, **Video 12.4**), benign ovarian cystic tumors (serous or mucinous cyst adenoma; **Figure 12.9**, **Video 12.5**), should be drained with a large-gauge needle or through a small capsular incision tightly closed by suture over the suction tip. This will reduce the spillage of the cyst fluid content into the peritoneal cavity to reduce the amount of postoperative adhesions and the development of myxedema peritonei in mucinous cysts or chemical peritonitis in dermoid cysts (**Figure 12.10**). The cyst wall must be peeled off the remaining ovarian tissue to reduce the amount of bleeding and technically faster and easier to cut only the severely adherent points. Preservation of the ovarian wall as much as possible because good amount of the wall contains viable active ovarian tissue which maintains the patient's hormonal and ova needs. The ovarian wall can be reconstructed with fine continuous suture like 3-0 V lock. Ample irrigation with warm saline of the peritoneal cavity and meticulous hemostasis are important to reduce adhesion formation between the ovary and adjacent tissues like the fallopian tubes are very important especially for infertility patients. The cysts wall can be removed in an endoscopic bag through Hanafi AUI. Second look by the laparoscope and

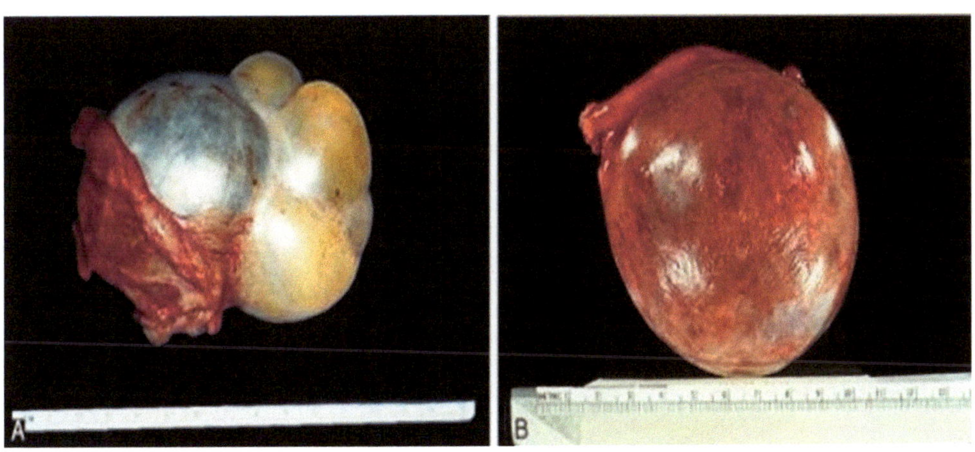


FIGURE 12.9 Gross appearance of a mucinous (A) and serous (B) cystadenoma of the ovary.

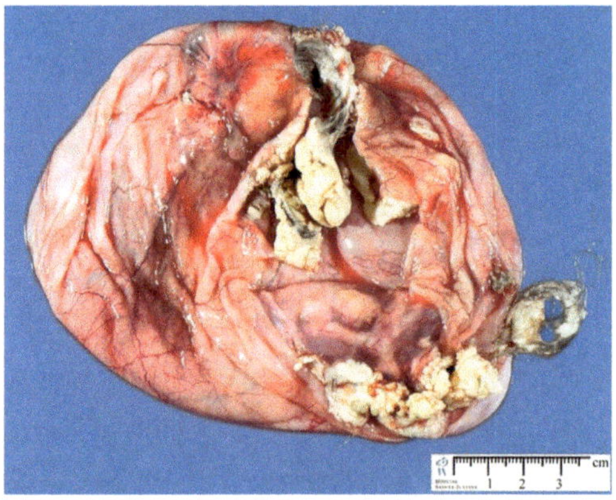

**FIGURE 12.10** Dermoid cysts are also known as mature cystic teratomas are congenital abnormalities that may be removed laparoscopically. Extraction involves aspiration of the cyst using a vacuum aspirator using a verses needle.

irrigation is very important to be sure that the entire cyst wall tissue was removed, complete hemostasis has been accomplished and the bowel is intact. With any suspicious malignancy, the entire cyst is sent for frozen section for immediate pathological diagnosis. The peritoneal wash is taken before the excision of the cyst sent for malignant cells detection for proper staging of the malignant condition if present.

Endometriomas and large simple serous and mucinous cysts must be drained before excision and/or enucleating to reduce the size of the cyst and to prevent spillage of the contents in the peritoneal cavity which can cause postoperative pelvic adhesions including the bowels and severe consequences of pelvic pain and possible bowel obstruction. The most effective treatment of endometriomas is excision [68]. Laparoscopy is the most common and advanced procedure used to diagnose and excise mild to moderate endometriosis [72].

### Tubal conditions include acute (ruptured or unruptured), sub-acute or chronic ectopic pregnancy, tubal lesions, adhesions and cysts

The surgical approach to an ectopic pregnancy (**Figure 12.11**) is guided by the location of the pregnancy in the fallopian tube, tubal integrity and the patient's desire concerning future childbearing. Surgical management of an unruptured ectopic pregnancy is highly dependent on the number of weeks of gestation. When tubal ectopic pregnancy is less than 3 cm in diameter, a linear salpingostomy can be carried out on the anti-mesenteric side of the fallopian tube. Desiccation of the serosal vessels along the anticipated incisional line should be performed using a bipolar fine tip needle electrosurgical device. Between 5 and 10 cc of 10 IU vasopressin diluted in 100 mL of injectable saline can be injected into the antimesenteric border to decrease blood loss. A linear incision should be made over the portion of the tube contains the gestational sac at the area of maximum distension. If the myosalpingeal contraction that expels the gestational products does not occur after three minutes, external compression may be gently performed using forceps. Once the contents are expressed, they should be removed using a secondary site. Lavage should then be used to cleanse the abdomen, and bleeding controlled with electrocautery. The benefit to the patient in utilizing a laparoscopic salpingostomy is the preservation of reproductive function of the tube. Checking the patency of both tubes by indigocarmin diluted solution in injectable saline must be performed and ample saline irrigation of the pelvic and abdominal organs is essential to prevent future pelvic adhesions.

For a ruptured ectopic pregnancy, the presence of intra-abdominal blood can be determined by aspirating the contents of the rectouterine pouch of Douglas which is not needed now after the use of high-resolution pelvic ultrasound technology. A salpingectomy may be required for rapid treatment and the prevention of further morbidity. Laparoscopic partial salpingectomy may be performed by desiccation or through the application of ligatures or harmonic scalpel across the tube that is proximal and

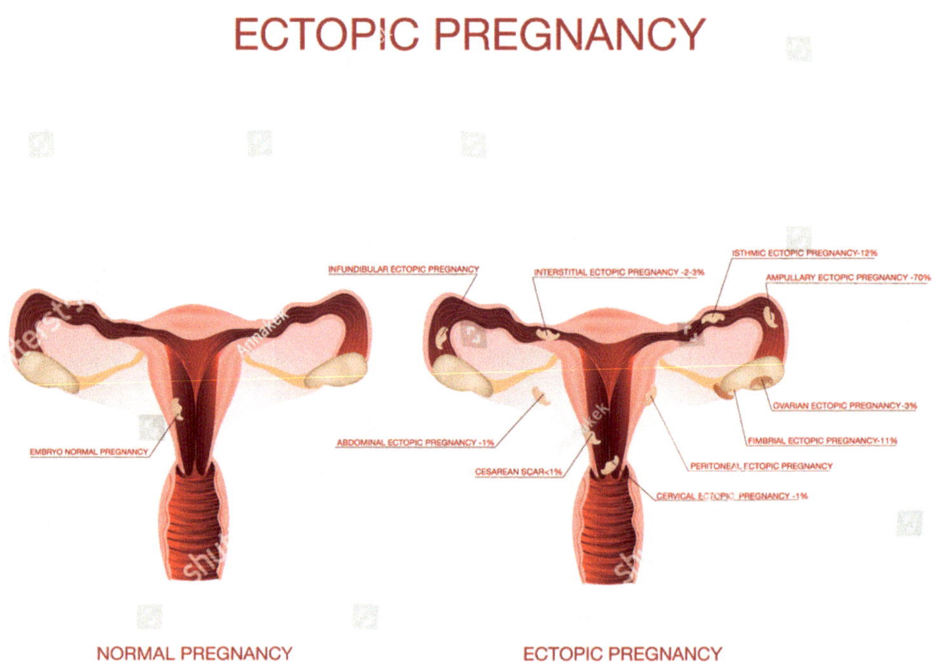


**FIGURE 12.11** Types of ectopic pregnancy.

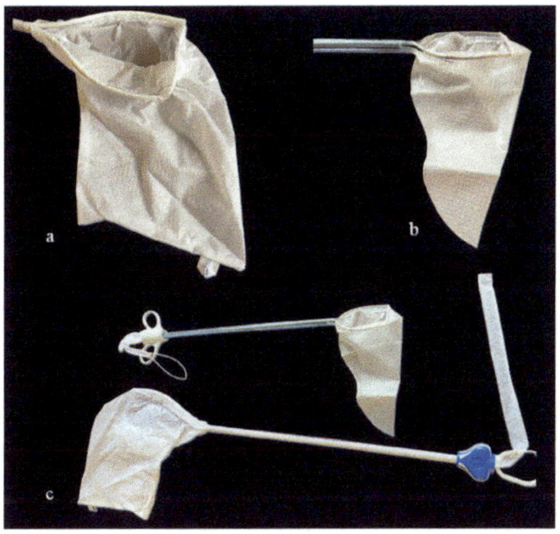


**FIGURE 12.12** Automatic opening specimen bags with (a) larger diameter bag, (b) smaller diameter bag, and (c) medium diameter bag.

distal to the gestational mass. The mesosalpinx is ligated along this portion of the tube or the use of harmonic scalpel. The specimen is excised using Hanafi AUI with the use of endoscopic bag. If the gestational mass is greater than 5 cm, morcellation may be performed inside an endoscopic pouch or bag.

Fallopian adhesions are usually treated using adhesiolysis, a laparoscopic approach in which bipolar electrocautery or harmonic scalpel is used. Well-developed adhesions may be highly vascularized, and care must be taken to ensure adequate hemostasis, whether adhesiolysis is performed using electrocautery, ligation, or harmonic scalpel.

Laparoscopic salpingectomy is usually necessary in hematosalpinx, as the presence of blood, trophoblastic tissue, and disrupted tubal tissue cause an inflammatory response, resulting to intraluminal adhesions and subsequent tubal obstruction or ectopic pregnancy or pyosalpinx.

Specimen retrieval bags (**Figure 12.12**) are used for contained removal of mass tissue [27]. The currently available bags differ in diameter (usually from 10 to 15 cm) and the technique consists of opening and deploying the bag, whereby some open automatically and others require manual opening using two graspers on the bag edges [28]. Industry-made bags also differ in durability, with variable resistance to manipulation and puncture [29]. The availability of bags in a range of sizes allows for selection based on the type of mass being removed. Laparoscopic bags offer greater advantage when the extracted tissue is soft, such as with a dermoid cyst, or ovary, while dense tissue, such as a partially calcified leiomyomata, is more difficult to manage [30]. Examples of industry-made laparoscopic tissue retrieval bags include E-Sac, Pleat man Sac, End bag and ENDO CATCH [29]. Some surgeons construct their own bags using sterile medical baggies or gloves [31–33]. These self-made approaches to retrieval bags have been shown to reduce costs and appear to even be associated with less postoperative pain in some instances, although more research is required on this aspect [32].

## Pelvic peritoneal lesions include endometriosis and adhesions in cul-de-sac and pelvic wall

Endometriosis of the peritoneum should be excised in its entirety rather than fulgurated by cautery in order to obtain a viable tissue to be examined by the pathologist microscopically for accurate diagnosis (**Figure 12.13**). Tissue removal of the endometriotic

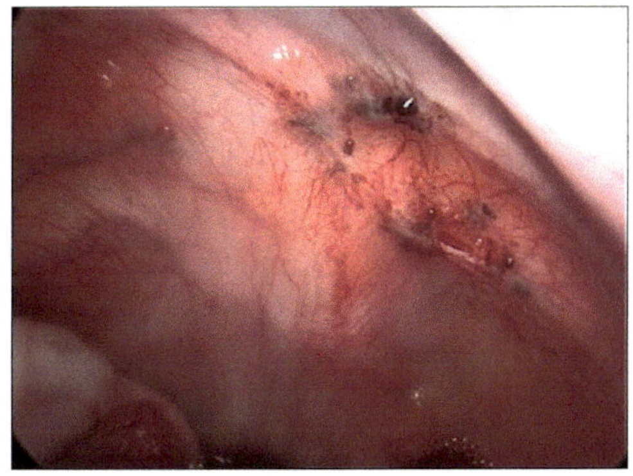

**FIGURE 12.13** Endometriosis associated with the peritoneum. Endometriosis is defined as the growth, adhesion and progression of endometrial tissue outside of the uterine cavity.

lesions of the peritoneum mostly are easily passed through the 12 mm trocar or camera umbilical incision, Larger endometrioma or severely fibrotic harder lesions can be removed through Hanafi AUI or a mini Pfannenstiel incision.

Endometriosis occurs within roughly 5% to 10% of women [7]. Endometriosis is a condition where tissue that normally lines the uterus develops outside the uterine cavity in abnormal locations such as the ovaries, fallopian tubes and abdominal cavity (**Figures 12.13** and **12.14**). Symptoms may depend on the location of the excess tissue development and can cause pelvic pain (often worsening during the menstrual cycle), painful intercourse and infertility [81]. Treatment, such as hormone therapy, surgery or both, may help relieve the pain associated with endometriosis and restore the patient's fertility. Factors associated with an increased risk of endometriosis include nulliparity [5], prolonged exposure to endogenous estrogen (e.g., early menarche before age 11–13 years [7] or late menopause) [13], shorter menstrual cycles (defined as ≤27 days) [5], heavy menstrual bleeding [5], obstruction of menstrual outflow, for example, Müllerian anomalies [13], exposure to diethylstilbestrol in utero [14], height greater than 68 inches, lower body mass index [5], exposure to severe physical and/or sexual abuse in childhood or adolescence [54], and a high consumption of trans unsaturated fat [55].

The most effective treatment of endometriomas is excision [68]. Laparoscopy is the most common and advanced procedure used to diagnose and excise mild to moderate endometriosis [72]. Small bowel endometriosis affected portion resection tissue can

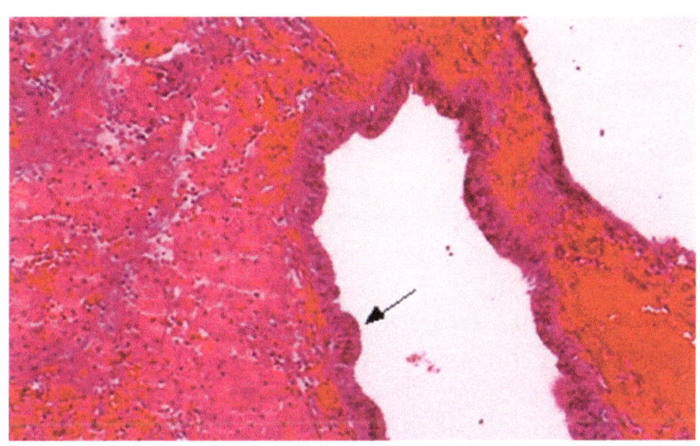

**FIGURE 12.14** Light microscopy of implanted peritoneal endometriosis implant shows endometrial glandular epithelium (arrow) and surrounding stroma.

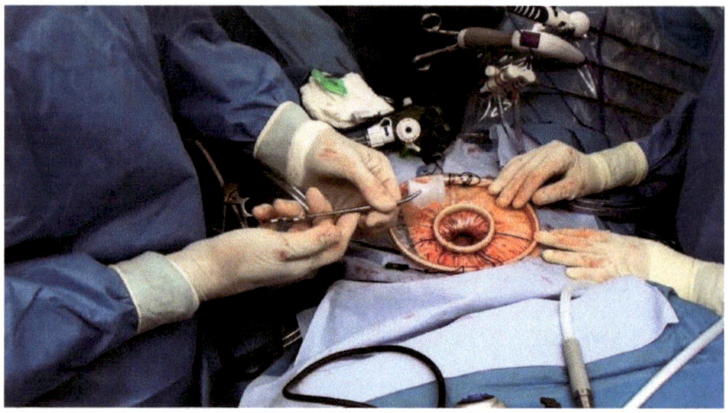

**FIGURE 12.15** Minilaporatomy Pfannestiel incision for extraction of large and/or calcified fibroid tumor tissues.

be easily removed through umbilical incision and placing the specimen in an endoscopic bag. Large bowel specimen tissue removal is done through the rectum or mini Pfannenstiel incision (**Figure 12.15**). Any part of the bowel should be removed in an endoscopic bag to reduce the amount of bowel contents and subsequent infection [85].

## Hysteroscopic tissue removal from the uterine cavity

Main objectives:

- Safe complete removal of the lesion tissue without uterine perforation by proper selection of cases, only type zero and one submucous fibroid tumors, no suspicion of malignancy, no additional pelvic or abdominal issues like intramural fibroid tumor, severe adenomyosis, ovarian lesions or endometriosis, pelvic adhesions, which can leads to uterine wall perforation and the loss of intrauterine fluid pressure, loss of the view, possible injury to bowel, urinary bladder, ureter, major blood vessels.
- Reduce the blood loss by the use of selective fine point diathermy applicator, injecting diluted vasopressin (Pitressin-ADH) solution, preoperative Leuprolide (Lupron) by injection or possibly Elagolix (Orilissa) orally.
- Reduce the chances of damaging the interstitial portion of the fallopian tubes mostly by diathermy, which leads to blockage of the fallopian tubes.

Polyps of the female reproductive tract have a prevalence ranging from 8% to 50% of women, and are usually benign. Cervical polyps are most commonly found in women over the age of 20 who have already given birth. While the cause is not yet known, they are associated with cervical inflammation. Ectocervical polyps develop from the outer surface layer cells of the cervix, whereas endocervical polyps develop from the cervical glands inside the cervical canal. Uterine polyps develop from the endometrium, and may flatten to fit the cavity of the uterus supply [14]. Hysteroscopic instruments that may be used to remove a polyp include: grasping forceps, microscissors, electrosurgical loop (i.e., resectoscope), morcellator, or a bipolar electrosurgical probe [58].

Submucous fibroid tumors type 0 & 1 can be removed by several methods. The most common method is hysteroscopic resectoscope, MyoSure and others.

Types 2 and 3 must be removed through the laparoscopic approach which enables suturing the uterine wall after myomectomy procedure.

## VIDEOS FOR CHAPTER

The following videos may be accessed by readers of this text at:

http://resourcecentre.routledge.com/books/9780367188320

- **Video 12.1:** Robotic Laparoscopic Myomectomy: The Hanafi Annular Umbilical Incision
- **Video 12.2:** Robotic Laparoscopic Myomectomy: Chromopertubation Tissue Extraction through the Annular Umbilical Incision (Hanafi AUI)
- **Video 12.3:** Robotic Laparoscopic Myomectomy: Extraction of a Smaller Fibroid Tumor through a 12-mm Lateral Trocar
- **Video 12.4:** Drainage of Large Endometriomas of the Left Ovary through the Annular Umbilical Incision before Robotic Laparoscopic Excision of the Cyst Wall
- **Video 12.5:** Robotic Laparoscopic Excision of Large Ovarian Cyst Wall after Drainage of the Fluid Content

## References


1. Practice Committee of the American Society for Reproductive Medicine. Definitions of infertility and recurrent pregnancy loss. Fertil Steril. 2008;90(S5):S60.
2. Mascarenhas MN, Flaxman SR, Boerma T, Vanderpoel S, Stevens GA. National, regional, and global trends in infertility prevalence since 1990: a systematic analysis of 277 health surveys. PLoS Med. 2012;9(12):100–356.
3. Recent advances in medically assisted conception. Report of a WHO Scientific Group. World Health Organ Tech Rep Ser. Geneva, Switzerland. 1992;820:1–111.
4. Baird DD, Dunson DB, Hill MC, Cousins D, Schectman JM. High cumulative incidence of uterine leiomyoma in black and white women: ultrasound evidence. Am J Obstet Gynecol. 2003; 188(1):100–107.
5. Cramer SF, Patel A. The frequency of uterine leiomyomas. Am J Clin Pathol. 1990;94(4):435–438.
6. Purohit P, Vigneswaran K. Fibroids and Infertility. Curr Obstet Gynecol Rep. 2016;5:81–88.
7. Advincula AP, Xu X, Goudeau S, Ransom SB. Robot-assisted laparoscopic myomectomy versus abdominal myomectomy: a comparison of short-term surgical outcomes and immediate costs. J Minim Invasive Gynecol. 2007;14(6):698–705.
8. Fader AN, Escobar PF. Laparoendoscopic single-site surgery (LESS) in gynecologic oncology: technique and initial report. Gynecol Oncol. 2009;114(2):157–161.
9. Koo Y-J. Recent advances in minimally invasive surgery for gynecologic indications. Yeungnam Univ J Med. 2018;35(2):150–155.
10. Yang YS. Robotic natural orifice transluminal endoscopic surgery (NOTES) hysterectomy as a scarless and gasless surgery. Surg Endosc. 2020;34(1):492–500
11. Yoshiki N. Review of transvaginal natural orifice transluminal endoscopic surgery in gynecology. Gynecol Minim Invasive Ther. 2017;6(1):1–5.
12. Jallad K, Walters MD. Natural Orifice Transluminal Endoscopic Surgery (NOTES) in Gynecology. Clin Obstet Gynecol. 2017; 60(2):324–329.

13. Hald K, Langebrekke A, Kløw NE, Noreng HJ, Berge AB, Istre O. Laparoscopic occlusion of uterine vessels for the treatment of symptomatic fibroids: Initial experience and comparison to uterine artery embolization. Am J Obstet Gynecol. 2004;190(1):37–43.
14. Goldfarb HA. Laparoscopic coagulation of myoma (myolysis). Obstet Gynecol Clin North Am. 1995;22(4):807–819.
15. Carranza-Mamane B, Havelock J, Hemmings R, Cheung A, Sierra S, Carranza-Mamane B, Case A, Cathie D, Graham J, Havelock J, Hemmings R, Liu K, Murdock W, Vause T, Wong B, Burnett M. The management of uterine fibroids in women with otherwise unexplained infertility. J Obstet Gynaecol Can. 2015;37(3):277–285.
16. Tanos V, Berry KE, Frist M, Campo R, DeWilde RL. Prevention and management of complications in laparoscopic myomectomy. BioMed Res Int. 2018;2018.
17. Nathani F, Clark TJ. Uterine polypectomy in the management of abnormal uterine bleeding: A systematic review. J Minim Invasive Gynecol. 2006;13(4):260–268.
18. Cruz De La MSD, Buchanan EM. Uterine fibroids: diagnosis and treatment. Am Fam Physician. 2017;95(2):100–107.
19. Orozco LJ, Tristan M, Vreugdenhil MM, Salazar A. Hysterectomy versus hysterectomy plus oophorectomy for premenopausal women. Cochrane Database Syst Rev. 2014;(7).
20. van Wessel S, Coryn N, van Vliet H, Schoot B, Weyers S, Hamerlynck T. Reproductive and obstetric outcomes after hysteroscopic removal of retained products of conception. J Minim Invasive Gynecol. July 2019.
21. Ahmad G, Baker J, Finnerty J, Phillips K, Watson A. Laparoscopic entry techniques. Cochrane Database Syst Rev. 2019;2019(1). doi: 10.1002/14651858.CD006583.pub5
22. Thepsuwan J, Huang K-G, Wilamarta M, Adlan A-S, Manvelyan V, Lee C-L. Principles of safe abdominal entry in laparoscopic gynecologic surgery. Gynecol Minim Invasive Ther. 2013;2(4):105–109.
23. Carter JE. Surgical treatment for chronic pelvic pain. JSLS. 1998; 2(2):129–139.
24. Park K-H, Kim J-Y, Shin J-S, et al. Treatment outcomes of uterine artery embolization and laparoscopic uterine artery ligation for uterine myoma. Yonsei Med J. 2003;44(4):694–702.
25. Księżakowska-Łakoma K, Żyła M, Wilczyński J. Removal of uterine fibroids by mini-laparotomy technique in women who wish to preserve their uterus and fertility. Videosurgery Miniinv. 2015; 10(4):561.
26. Clark LE, Menderes G, Tower AM, Silasi D-A, Azodi M. A simple approach to specimen retrieval via posterior colpotomy incision. JSLS. 2015;19(2):e2015.00222.
27. Amer N, Amer M, Mishra R. Different techniques of tissue retrieval from abdominal cavity during minimal access surgery. World J Laparosc Surg. 2013;6(2):63–68.
28. Smorgick N. Laparoscopic specimen retrieval bags. J Obstet Gynaecol India. 2014;64(5):370–372.
29. Schellpfeffer MA. A novel laparoscopic tissue retrieval device. JSLS. 2011;15(4):527–532
30. Bieber E. Laparoscopic tissue extraction: pros and cons of 4 techniques. OBG Manag. 2004;16(3):17–27.
31. Akdemir A, Ergenoğlu AM, Akman L, Yeniel AÖ, Şendağ F, Öztekin MK. A novel technique for laparoscopic removal of the fallopian tube after ectopic pregnancy via transabdominal or transumbilical port using homemade bag: a randomized trial. J Res Med Sci. 2013;18(9):777–781.
32. Güngördük K, Aşıcıoğlu O, Gülseren V, et al. Evaluation of the optimal laparoscopic method for benign ovarian mass extraction: a transumbilical route using a bag made from a surgical glove versus a lateral transabdominal route employing a standard endobag. J Obstet Gynaecol. 2020;40(3):378–381
33. Zhang N-N, Chen S-L, Zuo N, Sun T-S, Yang Q. Laparoscopic myomectomy using self-made retrieval bag to contain tissue extraction. Fertil Steril. 2020;113(3):679–680.
34. Bratschi HU, Heiz B. Total pelviscopic removal of ovarian tumors in a bag bag posterior colpotomy. Geburtshilfe Frauenheilkd. 1995; 55(7):383–386.
35. Uccella S, Cromi A, Bogani G, Casarin J, Serati M, Ghezzi F. Transvaginal specimen extraction at laparoscopy without concomitant hysterectomy: our experience and systematic review of the literature. J Minim Invasive Gynecol. 2013;20(5):583–590.
36. Clark NV, Cohen SL. Tissue extraction techniques during laparoscopic uterine surgery. J Minim Invasive Gynecol. 2018; 25(2):251–256.
37. Miller CE. Methods of tissue extraction in advanced laparoscopy. Curr Opin Obstet Gynecol. 2001;13(4):399–405.
38. Taylan E, Sahin C, Zeybek B, Akdemir A. Contained morcellation: review of current methods and future directions. Front Surg. 2017;4:15.
39. Smorgick N, Barel O, Fuchs N, Ben-Ami I, Pansky M, Vaknin Z. Hysteroscopic management of retained products of conception: meta-analysis and literature review. Eur J Obstet Gynecol Reprod Biol. 2014;173:19–22.
40. Winner B, Biest S. Uterine morcellation: fact and fiction surrounding the recent controversy. Mo Med. 2017;114(3):176–180.
41. Gilmeno-Gil A, Laberge PY, Lemyre M, Gorak E, Maheux-Lacroix, S. Morcellation during total laparoscopic hysterectomies: implications of the use of a contained bag system. J Obstet Gynaecol Can. 2020; S1701-2163(19)30985–5.
42. The Tissue Extraction Task Force Members. Morcellation during uterine tissue extraction: an update. J Minim Invasive Gynecol. 2018;25(4):543–550.
43. Lambat ES, Pluchino N, Petignat P, Tille JC, Pache JC, Pinto J, Botsikas D, Dubuisson J. Cell spillage after contained electromechanical morcellation using a specially designed in-bag system for laparoscopic myomectomy: Prospective Cohort Pilot Study. J Minim Invasive Gynecol. 2019; 26(7):1351–1356.
44. Cohen SL, Einarsson JI, Wang KC, Brown D, Boruta D, Scheib SA, Fader AN, Shibley T. Contained power morcellation within an insufflated isolation bag. Obstet Gynecol. 2014;124(3):491–497.
45. Goggins ER, Greenberg JA, Cohen SL, Morris SN, Brown DN, Einarsson JI. Efficacy of contained tissue extraction for minimizing tissue dissemination during laparoscopic hysterectomy and myomectomy [66]. Obstet Gynecol. 2015;125:29S.
46. Herman A, Duraiswamy N, Nandy P, Myers MR, Price V, Gibeily G, Hariharan P. In vitro leakage testing of tissue containment bags when subjected to power morcellation forces. J Minim Invasive Gynecol. 2020;27(3):655–664
47. Detorakis S, Vlachos D, Athanasiou S, Grigoriadis T, Domali A, Chatzipapas I, Stamatakis E, Mousiolis A, Patrikios A, Antsaklis A, Loutradis D, Protopapas A. Laparoscopic cystectomy in-a-bag of an intact cyst: Is it feasible and spillage-free after all? Minim Invasive Surg. 2016;2016: 8640871.
48. Hizkiyahu R, Yahav L, Yakovi S, Davidesko S, Abecassis A, Weintraub AY. Short- and long-term outcomes of intraoperative spillage during laparoscopic removal of benign ovarian cysts. Surg Endosc. October 2019.
49. Stavroulis A, Memtsa M, Yoong W. Methods for specimen removal from the peritoneal cavity after laparoscopic excision. Obstet Gynaecol. 2013;15(1):26–30.
50. Montz F, Holschneider C, Munro M. Incisional hernia following laparoscopy: a survey of the American Association of Gynecologic Laparoscopists. Obstet Gynecol. 1994;84:881–884.
51. Liu FW, Galvan-Turner VB, Pfaendler KS, Longoria TC, Bristow RE. A critical assessment of morcellation and its impact on gynecologic surgery and the limitations of the existing literature. Am J Obstet Gynecol. 2015;212(6):717–724.
52. Laparoscopic Hysterectomy - In-Bag Morcellation. https://www.youtube.com/watch?v=prv939GgBWc. Accessed March 27, 2020.
53. Policy Statement: Guidelines for the laparoscopic management of the adnexal mass. J SOGC. 1998;20(10):983–989.
54. Allaf M, Patriciu A, Mazilu D, Kavoussi L, Stoianovici D. Overview and fundamentals of urologic robot-integrated systems. Urol Clin North Am. 2004;31(4):671–682.
55. Dharia SP, Falcone T. Robotics in reproductive medicine. Fertil Steril. 2005;84(1):1–11.

56. Chan YY, Jayaprakasan K, Zamora J, Thornton JG, Raine-Fenning N, Coomarasamy A. The prevalence of congenital uterine anomalies in unselected and high-risk populations: a systematic review. Hum Reprod Update. 2011;17(6):761–771.
57. Health C for D and R. UPDATE: The FDA recommends performing contained morcellation in women when laparoscopic power morcellation is appropriate. FDA. February 2020. http://www.fda.gov/medical-devices/safety-communications/update-fda-recommends-performing-contained-morcellation-women-when-laparoscopic-power-morcellation. Accessed March 20, 2020.
58. Preutthipan S, Herabutya Y. Hysteroscopic polypectomy in 240 premenopausal and postmenopausal women. Fertil Steril. 2005; 83(3):705–709.
59. Yassaee F. Tuboplasty as a reversal macrosurgery for tubal ligation, is pregnancy possible? A case series. Iran J Reprod Med. 2014; 12(5):361–364.
60. Transvaginal NOTES Tubal Reanastomosis: A Novel Route for Tubal Surgery. https://www.youtube.com/watch?v=BCeU_lN-Rz0. Accessed March 27, 2020.
61. Liu J, Lin Q, Blazek K, Liang B, Guan X. Transvaginal natural orifice transluminal endoscopic surgery myomectomy: a novel route for uterine myoma removal. J Minim Invasive Gynecol. 2018; 25(6):959–960.
62. Wiley Publication. Diagnostic accuracy and potential limitations of transvaginal sonography for bladder endometriosis. Ultrasound Obstet Gynecol. 2009;34(5):595–600.
63. Hachim EG, Ashour GS, Amer AA, Shaikhoon MM, Khojah MI. Review of 244 cases of ovarian cysts. Saudi Med J. 2015;36(7):834–838. doi:10.15537/smj.2015.7.11690
64. Rhodes, RA. Laparascopic trocar complications. Prevention and Management of Laparoendoscopic Surgical Complications. 3rd Ed.
65. Stoica RA, Bistriceanu I, Sima R, Iordache N. Laparascopic myomectomy. J Med Life. 2014;7(4):522–524.
66. Sinha R, Sundaram M. Laparascopic management of large myomas. J Gynecol Endosc Surg. 2009;1(2):73–82. doi:104103/0974-1216.71611.
67. Flyct R, Soto E, Nutter B, Falcone T. Comparison of long-term fertility and bleeding outcomes after laparoscopic and abdominal myomectomy. Obstet Gynec Int. 2016;2016:2789201.
68. Rimbach S, Ulrich U, Schweppe KW. Surgical therapy of endometriosis: challenges and controversies. Geburtshilfe und Frauenheilkunde. 2013;73(9):918–923.
69. Van Lieshout L, Steenbeek MP, De Hullu JA, Vos MC, Houterman S, Wilkinson J, Piek JMJ. Hysterectomy with salpingectomy versus hysterectomy alone. Cochrane Database Syst Rev. 2019:8.
70. Finco A, Centini G, Lazzeri L, Zupi E. Surgical management of abnormal uterine bleeding in women. Womens Health (Lond). 2015;11(4):513–525.
71. Duffy JMN, Arambage K, Correa FJS, Olive D, Farquhar C, Garry R, Barlow DH, Jacobson TZ. Laparoscopic surgery for endometriosis. Cochrane Database Syst Rev. 2014; 4.
72. Ezzati, M, Norian JM. Management of uterine fibroids in the patient pursuing assisted reproductive technologies. Womens Health (Lond Engl). 2009;5(4):413–421.
73. Wilczyński M, Cieślak J, Malinowski A. Supracervical hysterectomy—the vaginal route. Videosurgery Miniinv. 2014;(2):207–212. doi:10.5114wiitm.2014.41633.
74. American College of Obstetricians and Gynecologists. Uterine morcellation for presumed leiomyomas. ACOG Committee Opinion No. 770. Obstet Gynecol. 2019;133e238–48.
75. Arian SE, Munoz JL, Kim S, Falcone T. Robot-assisted laparoscopic myomectomy: current status. Robot Surg. 2017; 4:7–18.
76. Tanos, Vasilios, Berry KE, Seikkula J, Raad EA, Stavroulis A, Sleiman Z, Campo R, Gordts S. The management of polyps in female reproductive organs. Int J Surg.2017; 43: 7–16.
77. Chao X, Wang X, Xiao Y, Ji M, Wang S, Shi H, Fan Q, Zhu L, Leng J, Sun D, Lang J. Effects of hysterectomy with simultaneous bilateral salpingectomy on the subsequent pelvic mass. J Ovarian Res. 2019; 12:27.
78. Patil E, Jensen JT. Update on permanent contraception options for women. Curr Opin Obstet Gynecol. 2015; 27(6): 465–470.
79. Kim Y-W, Park B-J, Kim T-E, Ro D-Y. Single-port laparoscopic salpingectomy for surgical treatment of tubal pregnancy: comparison with multi-port laparoscopic salpingectomy. Intern J Med Sci. 2013;10(8)-1073–1078.
80. Boyd CA, Riall TS. Unexpected gynecological findings during abdominal surgery. Curr Probl Surg. 2012;49(4):195–251.
81. Moniz, MH, Chang T, Heisler M, Admon L, Gebremariam A, Dalton VK, Davis, MM. Inpatient postpartum long-acting reversible contraception and sterilization in the United States, 2008–2013. Obstet Gynecol. 2017;129(6):1078–1085.
82. Boe EI, Woie K, Hordnes K. Transcervical endometrial resection: long-term results of 390 procedures. Acta Obstetricia et Gynecologica Scandinavica. 2006; 85: 82–87.
83. Fakhrolmoulouk Y. Tuboplasty as a reversal macrosurgery for tubal ligation, is pregnancy possible? A case series. Iran J Reprod Med. 2014;12(5):361–364.
84. Abrao MS, Muzii L, Marana R. Anatomical causes of female infertility and their management. Int J Gynecol Obstet. 2013; 123(S2):1–7.
85. Unane D, Tournaye H, Velkeniers B, Poppe K. Endocrine disorders and female infertility. Best Pract Res Clin Endocrin Metab. 2011;25:861–873.
86. Jones S, O'Donovan P, Toub D. Radiofrequency ablation for treatment of symptomatic uterine fibroids. Obstet Gynecol Int. 2012:194839.
84. Farghaly SA. Current diagnosis and management of ovarian cysts. Clin Exp Obstet Gynecol. 2014;41(6):609–612.
85. Hanafi M. Ultrasound diagnosis of adenomyosis, leiomyoma, or combined with histopathological correlation. J Human Reprod Sci. 2013; 6(3):189–193.

# 13

## SURGICAL MANAGEMENT OF CERVICAL FIBROID

**Huda Afaneh, Salem K. Joseph, and Mostafa I. Abuzeid**

### Introduction

The exact incidence of uterine leiomyomas is thought to be underestimated due to the presence of asymptomatic leiomyomas in women of all ages. Generally, incidence is reported to be at least between 20% and 25%, and has been cited to comprise about 27% of gynecologic complaints in the office [1]. Uterine fibroids account for a substantial number of indications for hysterectomy and myomectomy in the United States [2]. Cervical leiomyomas account for less than 5% of uterine leiomyomas [3, 4]. Reported incidence appears to be 0.6%–2% in some case reports and there continues to be a limited number of case reports in the literature [5].

### Classification of cervical leiomyomas

Cervical leiomyomas can be classified based on their location within the cervical canal, its relation to the vagina (supravaginal vs. vaginal), as well as the extent of involvement into the pelvic structures. Classifications based on the size of a cervical leiomyoma are not clearly defined. In the literature, some authors refer to cervical leiomyomas 20 cm in diameter or more as "very large" [6]. The size and location play a definite role in the clinical presentation in patients affected by cervical leiomyoma. We can further categorize cervical leiomyoma into supravaginal and vaginal types (**Table 13.1**) [7].

A supravaginal cervical leiomyoma may be anterior, posterior, lateral, deep-rooted and/or central in nature, based on the location of the cervix that is encompassed by much of the leiomyoma [8, 9]. The central type, which occupies the entire cervical canal and displaces the uterus superiorly, is very rare, and the most difficult type of cervical myoma to manage. Cervical leiomyomas can be submucosal, intramural or subserous, much like the uterine leiomyoma. In addition, they can be pedunculated or sessile in nature [10]. Further specifications have been described when considering lateral extension of supravaginal cervical leiomyomas involving the broad ligament. In such cases it can be referred to as a broad ligament cervical fibroid [9]. Intracervical vaginal cervical leiomyomas refer to a submucosal leiomyoma (pedunculated or sessile) arising from the cavity of the cervical canal and it can extend into the vaginal canal [11] (**Table 13.1**). On the other hand, extra cervical vaginal myoma (intramural or subserous) arises from wall of the cervical canal and protrudes into the vaginal canal.

TABLE 13.1: **Classification of Cervical Fibroids**

| Supravaginal Portion of the Cervix | Vaginal Portion of the Cervix |
|---|---|
| Anterior | Intracervical (Submucosal)<br>Arising from the cavity of the cervical canal (Pedunculated or Sessile) |
| Posterior | Extracervical (Intramural or subserous) |
| Lateral | |
| Deep-Rooted | Arising from the cervical canal wall (Pedunculated or Sessile) |
| Central* | |

* Surrounding the entire cervical canal and lying centrally in the pelvis displacing the uterus superiorly.

### Anatomical considerations

Cervical leiomyomas are a truly remarkable phenomena when considering the composition of the cervix, which is primarily made up of connective tissue and much less smooth muscle [1]. The exact location of a fibroid involving the cervical stroma may have different symptoms and impact on the patient's livelihood both in the acute and chronic setting. Certain locations are associated with specific symptoms defined by involved organs, such as urinary retention and constipation with anteriorly and posteriorly located fibroids, respectively. Cervical fibroids involving the broad ligament have profound surgical implications, as they obstruct access to the uterine arteries and are near the ureters. The specific location of the fibroid alters the pelvic anatomy thus impacting surgical approaches and increasing the risk of surgical complications. When considering factors that facilitate removal in the case of myomectomy, the base or stalk of the leiomyoma plays a major role. A base along the cervical canal that is more visible and accessible through the vaginal route may suggest a less complicated surgery and increased ease of myomectomy. Chang et al. (2010) [9] also had the additional classification of deep-rooted cervical myoma in their study, representing a cervical myoma which extends deeply in the vagina [9]. The myomectomy techniques discussed in their study were specific depending on the location and will be discussed in more detail later in the text [9].

### Clinical presentation

The characteristics of cervical leiomyomas create a variety of clinical presentations. Based on our review of the available literature, cervical leiomyomas tend to be solitary entities rather than a conglomerate of masses that can sometimes be seen in the uterine corpus. Much like the uterine corpus fibroids, cervical fibroids can be associated with prolonged or intermenstrual bleeding, as well as bulk symptoms. Several case reports publish cases of cervical fibroids both in pregnant and non-pregnant populations. Symptoms vary from vague abdominal and pelvic discomfort symptoms to significant bleeding requiring blood transfusion. Vaginal leiomyomas can present with symptoms of a vaginal bulge and prolapse [12]. In some cases, with larger leiomyomas protruding into the vagina, the patient can present with massive hemorrhage and abdominal pain [13]. In the study by Matsuoka et al. (2010) [14], out of 16 patients, eight experienced increased menstrual bleeding, three experienced pressure-like symptoms, two were primarily concerned with their infertility, and one had chronic back pain [14]. In addition, 7 of the 16 were nulliparous [14]. The average cervical myoma diameter was 6.9 ± 1.6 cm measured by MRI imaging [14]. Similarly, Chang et al. (2010) [9] discussed 28 cases with various symptoms including dysmenorrhea, tenesmus and urinary symptoms [9]. A proportion of the presented patients also had a history of pregnancy loss and infertility [9].

The presence of a cervical leiomyoma in pregnancy is a rare entity, but the implications that this can have on a pregnancy are important to consider [15]. Keriakos and Maher (2013) [15] reported a case of a cervical fibroid more than doubling in size from a diameter of 5–12 cm between preconception and about 36 weeks gestation illustrating the hormonal influences that may play a role in the reproductive population, although this pattern of growth is not typical [15]. Gandhi et al. (2014) [16] reported a patient who had an 8 cm × 8 cm cervical leiomyoma in pregnancy that was an incidental finding, illustrating the possibility of a cervical fibroid producing no symptoms at all [16]. Antepartum considerations include risks of severe hemorrhage, preterm prelabor rupture of membranes and preterm delivery [15–19]. Cervical leiomyoma (sessile or pedunculated) protruding into the cervical canal are more associated with symptoms of prolapse and abnormal bleeding [20, 21]. The size and location of the leiomyoma can influence the mode of delivery and MRI may be necessary to map the specific myoma location [6].

Tian and Wensheng (2012) [6] studied cervical leiomyoma management in pregnancy and post-partum [6]. In some instances, with cervical leiomyomas greater than 20 cm in size, hysterectomy was unavoidable, due to massive hemorrhage [6]. Cervical fibroids greater than 10 cm required a transfusion during myomectomy, which raises the question of leaving cervical fibroids in situ following a cesarean section (CS) delivery rather than performing the myomectomy at the same time of a CS delivery [6]. However, during involution, the cervical fibroid may undergo degeneration, thus increasing the possibility of infection from a necrosed cervical leiomyoma. The management decisions are individualized and based on the specific clinical presentation of the patient and will be discussed later in this chapter [6]. Degenerating fibroids can create concerns for malignancy in both premenopausal and postmenopausal patients [22]. Necrotic degenerating fibroids have also been documented in some rare cases to present as a severe infection necessitating removal, or even in some cases, hysterectomy [15, 23].

## Diagnostic modalities

After a thorough patient history is obtained and a complete physical examination is performed, traditionally transvaginal and/or trans-abdominal ultrasound scan, saline sonohysterography, hysteroscopy and magnetic resonance imaging (MRI) are used to diagnose uterine leiomyomas. The same principles can be applied during the work up of cervical leiomyoma. Transvaginal and trans-abdominal ultrasound scan offer an inexpensive way to evaluate the presence and location of cervical leiomyoma. Transvaginal ultrasound is effective in locating even very small uterine leiomyomas, but an extremely displaced uterus or retroverted uterus may be more difficult to evaluate [24]. Transvaginal ultrasound scan with saline sonohysterography can be more helpful in visualizing any lesions within the uterine cavity. The specificity of the mass in the uterus is limited, as it may be difficult to differentiate leiomyomas from hematometra or polyps. These studies can vary depending on the experience of the operator performing the study and patient's tolerance [24]. In the setting of vaginal cervical leiomyoma, it is perhaps not helpful or even possible to distend the uterine cavity with saline in the majority of cases.

In cases of cervical leiomyomas, MRI is arguably the most appropriate diagnostic tool, despite its increased cost, knowing the exact location and categorizing the leiomyoma based on anatomy would be invaluable to the gynecologic surgeon [22]. Furthermore, the classification of supravaginal, vaginal cervical leiomyoma and broad ligament cervical fibroid extension can be attained much easily using MRI. Matsuoka et al. (2010) [14] heavily relied on MRI in classifying cervical leiomyomas based on their location for surgical planning prior to laparoscopic myomectomy [14, 25]. We conclude that MRI would be the more appropriate tool to differentiate between supravaginal and vaginal types of leiomyomas as well as for surgical mapping and planning. The MRI imaging modality is also crucial in determining possible embolization techniques when vascularity of the leiomyoma is evaluated.

## Surgical treatment

The management of the cervical myoma will depend mainly on the patient's desire of future fertility, size of the myoma and presence or absence of symptoms. If the patient has completed her family, and the size of the myoma is large and/or the patient has significant symptoms, hysterectomy is the surgical treatment of choice. In addition, hysterectomy may be the only surgical option that can be offered, irrespective of fertility desire, if the cervical myoma is very large, or in cases of a large central supravaginal cervical myoma occupying the entire cervical canal. On the other hand, if fertility preservation is desired, myomectomy can be considered if surgically feasible. Myomectomy is the only conservative approach for such pathology, as some studies show a decreased efficacy in uterine artery embolization of cervical fibroids [26]. Kim et al. (2012) [26] reported that uterine artery embolization (UAE) has been used unsuccessfully to treat cervical fibroids with only 20% showing complete necrosis after embolization [26]. However, more recently, DeMeritt et al. (2018) [27] reported the first successful treatment of a patient with a small (4 cm in diameter) supravaginal posterior cervical myoma using bilateral superselective cervicovaginal artery embolization using 100–300-μm Embospheres, along with cone beam CT to confirm nontarget tissue exclusion to avoid the hypothetical risk of vaginal and/or labial ischemia and necrosis [27]. Smaller beads size was used instead of the standard 500–700-μm beads, usually used during UAE, in view of the smaller size of the terminal cervical arterial arcades and perifibroid plexus [27].

Due to the anatomy of the cervix, a cervical myoma would be located in close proximity of important organs and structures such as the ureters, uterine vessels, bladder and rectum. This fact makes surgical treatment with either hysterectomy or myomectomy a risky procedure compared to the same surgery when done for uterine fibroids in other locations. In addition, the risk for hysterectomy at the time of planned myomectomy is much higher due to the possibility of excessive bleeding.

Adequate preoperative preparation is essential when considering management of a cervical fibroid. Appropriate imaging with ultrasound or MRI, as discussed previously, is helpful in mapping out the cervical fibroid origin and involvement with surrounding structures. Although cervical fibroids may interfere with conception, many reports suggest that pregnancy can occur, even in the presence of a large cervical fibroid [6, 19]. However, the possible impact of cervical fibroids on fertility potential and the complications that can occur prior to and during delivery and the post-partum period are considerable enough to proceed with treatment before attempting conception [6]. Myomectomy is the procedure of choice with the hope to address uterine factor infertility and to reduce the risks and complications associated with such pathology during pregnancy, delivery and the post-partum. It may also be helpful to consider GnRH agonist therapy with leuprolide acetate for 3–6 months prior to surgery to decrease the volume of the cervical fibroid, which can make both myomectomy and even hysterectomy technically more feasible and safer.

## Hysterectomy

The specific hysterectomy approach, whether that be abdominal, laparoscopic or vaginal does depend on the surgeon's level of skill when approaching a very technically difficult surgery and type, location and size of the cervical leiomyoma. However, vaginal approaches in the literature usually included small cervical leiomyomas or large leiomyomas with a base that was completely visualized and could be effectively ligated. One could expect large distortions in the anatomy when approaching the surgery abdominally, whether proceeding via laparoscopy or laparotomy. Specifically, one must be cognizant of the ureters as they may be displaced from the usual location in the medial leaf of the broad ligament, and instead be proximal to the base of the fibroid. During a hysterectomy, a uterine manipulator or a colpotomy cup cannot be placed due to the presence of the leiomyoma. The cervical fibroid also makes access to the uterine arteries much more difficult.

Depending on the type, location and size of the myoma, certain modification should be adopted before hysterectomy [14]. Such modification should include both preoperative and intra-operative measures. Preoperative measures should include attempts at reducing the myoma size by treatment with GnRH analog agonist or aromatase inhibitor, and ensure adequate level of hemoglobin (HB) and hematocrit (HCT) [14, 28–30]. Other preoperative measures should include the use of iron infusion, if needed, to improve HB/HCT and consider autologous blood transfusion planning. Uterine artery embolization can be used prior to the myomectomy in an attempt to reduce blood loss during surgery [31]. The safety of such procedure in patients who desire to preserve their fertility potential is not fully evaluated and there is concern of possible increased morbidity during pregnancy. In addition, the efficacy of uterine artery embolization of cervical fibroids has been shown to be decreased [26]. Although, temporarily embolization of the uterine artery using an endovascular balloon occlusion catheter has been described in the literature, it has not yet become acceptable for general use [14, 32, 33]. Intra-operative measures to reduce bleeding should include the use of vasopressin injection (20 IU in 60 cc of normal saline), and ligation of the uterine artery at its origin [34–36]. Cell–salvage systems can be used in selected cases, especially in the presence of a large myoma [37, 38]. In addition, some authors suggested that temporarily clipping of the uterine artery is an effective reversible method to control blood loss during myomectomy for cervical fibroid [14]. Depending on the size and location of the cervical myoma, a myomectomy may be needed first, even when total hysterectomy is to be performed. If myomectomy is to be done first via laparotomy, a temporary placement of vascular bulldog clamps on the infundibulopelvic ligaments during myomectomy can be performed to reduce the total blood loss.

There are several video presentations on the safe use of laparoscopic hysterectomy for the large cervical fibroid with some valuable insight on how to avoid injuries to near-by structures and reduce bleeding during the procedure [11, 39–50]. For example, in a video presentation by Ecker et al. (2013) [39], they described strategies and techniques of a laparoscopic hysterectomy for a patient with large cervical fibroid. They presented a 43-year-old gravida 2, para 2 woman with menometrorrhagia and pelvic pressure. On exam, she had an enlarged fibroid uterus with a 7 cm fibroid replacing most of the cervix, causing it to be dilated to 2 cm with 90% effacement [39]. She desired definitive management with hysterectomy. These strategies included placement of ureteral stents, ligation of the superior vaginal artery and of the uterine artery at its origin, ureterolysis and placement of a vaginal retractor to aid in successfully completing the hysterectomy [39].

## Myomectomy

A myomectomy might be the procedure of choice in order to preserve fertility, or to make carrying out the steps of a hysterectomy easier. The principles of surgery applied to myomectomy for cervical fibroid are the same as those applied as discussed in the hysterectomy section. It is appropriate to place ureteral stents prior to initiating the surgery. Filling the bladder with sterile milk or saline to locate the bladder location during anterior dissection is helpful for delineating planes at the anterior surface of the cervical fibroid. Diluted vasopressin is an important consideration when approaching the cervical fibroid, as profound bleeding will make visualization difficult. Ligating the uterine artery at the origin at the hypogastric artery, either by ligation or surgical clipping will decrease chances of excessive bleeding. Locating the hypogastric artery can be difficult in this scenario, and the literature discusses using the medial umbilical ligament to orient oneself followed by dissecting towards the uterine artery origin [39]. During a myomectomy, it has also been described in some case reports that the cervical fibroid is morcellated while attached to the uterus after using a myoma screw to elevate the myoma away from the vulnerable structures around the myoma. Following enucleation and removal of the leiomyoma, the closure of the myoma bed may also be technically challenging. The cervix may also need reconstruction and the patient should be seen by a high-risk specialist to screen for cervical shortening and possible prophylactic cervical cerclage in future pregnancies.

### Supravaginal cervical fibroid

In the presence of a supravaginal posterior cervical fibroid, a laparoscopic myomectomy is feasible if the fibroid is small and sessile subserous in nature (**Figure 13.1**) or if the fibroid is pedunculated in nature (**Figure 13.2**). However, in general, performing myomectomy for supravaginal cervical myoma can be associated with increased surgical morbidity due to the increased risk of injuries to the uterine vessels, ureters, urinary bladder and rectum as a result of a distorted anatomy. This is especially the case during an attempt at laparoscopic myomectomy, although minimally invasive surgeries have their known benefits [4, 25]. Injury to the uterine vessels leads to excessive blood loss and increases the risk of injury to the ureters or the bladder during attempts to control the bleeding [51, 52]. In the presence of a large cervical myoma, the laparoscopic approach in such cases may be challenged by the deep position of the operative field and the associated difficulty during suturing of the myoma bed [9]. Therefore, the surgical approach for myomectomy of a supravaginal cervical myoma should depend on the location, size and experience of the surgeon. The role of da Vinci robotic-assisted laparoscopic myomectomy for supravaginal cervical myoma has not been defined. However, at least in theory, the use of the robotic approach by an

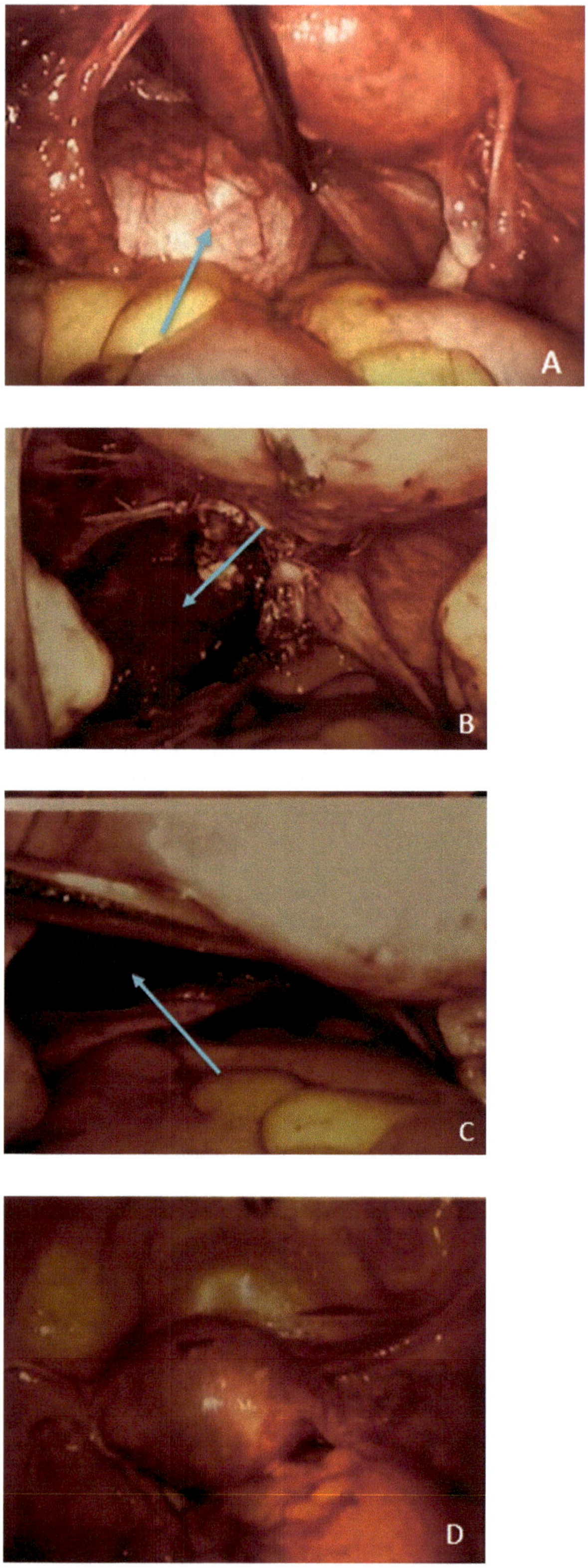


FIGURE 13.1 (A) Supravaginal sessile subserousposterior cervical fibroid with broad base (blue arrow). (B) The gap at the base of the left broad ligament and the left side of the pouch of Douglas, after excision of the cervical fibroid (blue arrow). (C) The gap at the base of the left broad ligament and the left side of the pouch of Douglas, after securing hemostasis (blue arrow). (D) Laparoscopic picture at the end of the procedure. (Courtesy of Dr. M Abuzeid.)

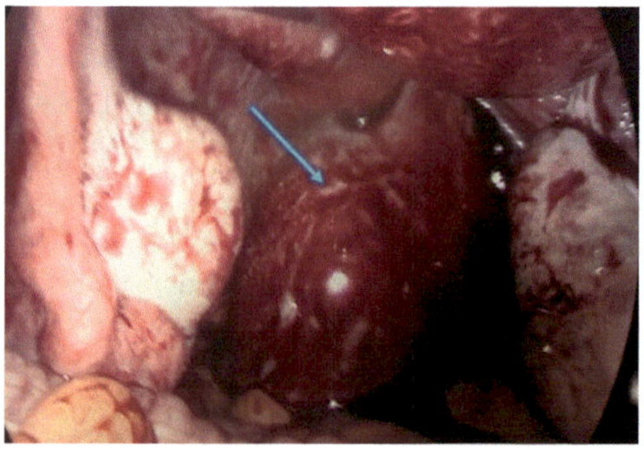

FIGURE 13.2 Laparoscopic picture showing a supravaginal pedunculated subserous posterior cervical fibroid (blue arrow) seen at the time of laparoscopy for leaking ectopic pregnancy. (Courtesy of Dr. M Abuzeid.)

experienced robotic surgeon during laparoscopic myomectomy for cervical myoma may facilitate both dissection and suture repair of the myoma bed.

Laparotomy via a vertical midline incision is probably the best surgical approach for patients with a very large supravaginal cervical myoma who desire myomectomy. Booher et al. (2018) [10] reported their management of a very large (20 cm in diameter) solitary cervical fibroid [10]. The cervical myoma was sessile, subserous and located in the posterior wall of the cervix [10]. The authors performed a myomectomy via laparotomy [10]. A midline vertical skin incision was planned to optimize visualization [10]. This was done in an attempt to reduce the risks of bleeding from uterine vessels, injury to the ureters and the need for a hysterectomy [10]. The patient was counseled about the high chance of hysterectomy and received a consult with a gynecologic oncologist and had blood products available in the operating room [10]. Diluted vasopressin was used to reduce blood loss and a vertical incision was made along the serosa of the cervical myoma to avoid injury to the ureters [10]. The procedure was successful and they reported an uneventful postoperative period [10]. They recommended cesarean delivery for any future pregnancies [10].

On the other hand, other documented cases illustrate a successful laparoscopic myomectomy of a similar cervical myoma without any complications [53]. In one case, the surgeon morcellated the large myoma at the end of the procedure using myoma morcellator device [53]. This technique has been banned in the United States, due to risks of possible occult malignancy. However, if one adopts a similar technique, the myoma can be removed through a posterior colpotomy or by extending the umbilical incision and then one can morcellate the myoma within a specimen bag and remove the tissue from the incision. Nuri et al. (2017) [54] in a video manuscript, illustrated a successful laparoscopic myomectomy for what appeared to be a posterior wall cervical fibroid [54].

In a case series of 28 patients of supravaginal cervical myoma, Chang et al. (2010) [9] described their experience of laparoscopic myomectomy of supravaginal cervical myoma [9]. Most of the lesions were anterior supravaginal cervical myoma (43%) and posterior supravaginal cervical myoma (32%) [9]. The remaining were supravaginal central cervical myoma (4%), supravaginal lateral cervical myoma (14%) and deep rooted cervical myoma (7%) [9]. The investigators outlined their strategies to achieve a successful outcome for each of the above [9]. The authors and others alluded to the fact that hemorrhage is a major concern during myomectomy for cervical myoma, especially in the presence of an aberrant blood

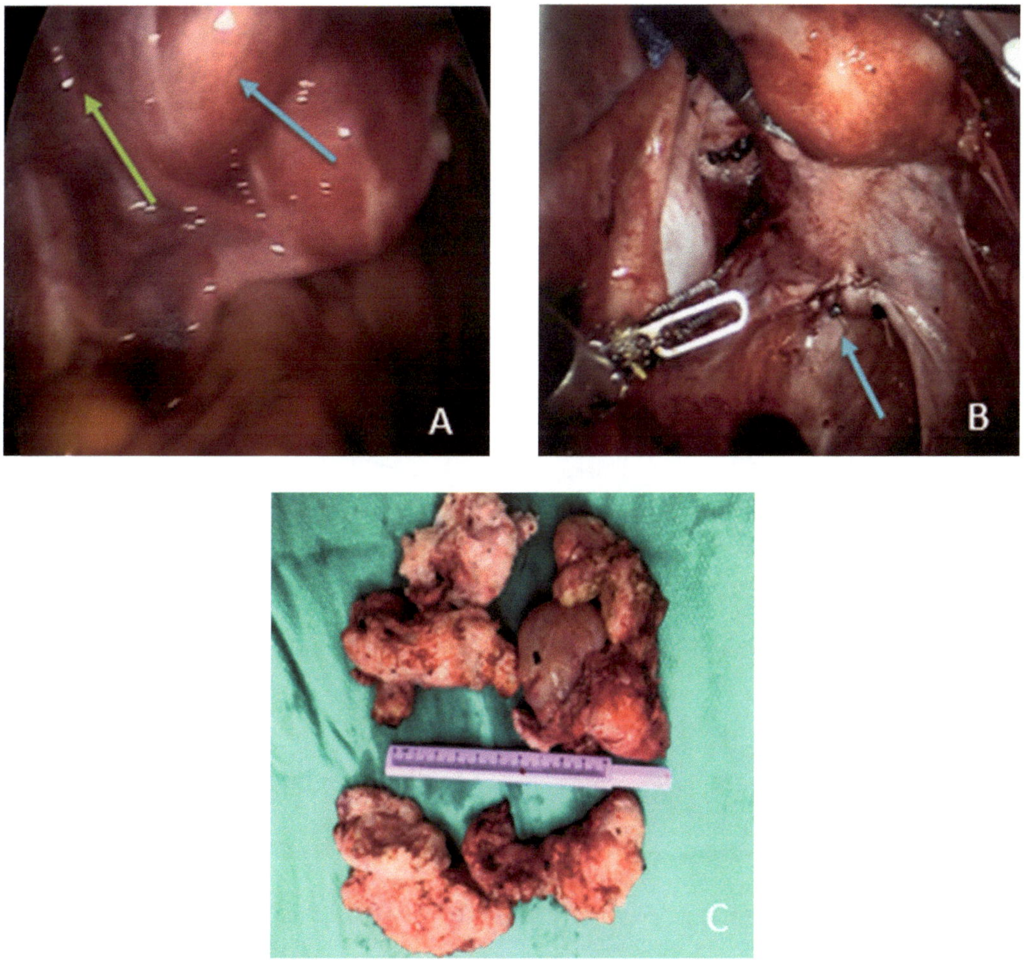


**FIGURE 13.3** (A) Laparoscopic picture showing a large anterior supravaginal cervical myoma. The large myoma (blue arrow) is in close proximity with the urinary bladder (green arrow). (B) Laparoscopic pictures using da Vinci laparoscope and camera showing the end result after myomectomy and repair of the myoma bed (not seen) and the repair of the posterior colpotomy (blue arrow) after the myoma was marcelated and removed. (C) Marcerated myoma. (Courtesy of Dr. M Abuzeid.)

supply [9, 55]. Chang et al. (2010) [9] used ligation of the uterine artery and diluted vasopressin injection in all cases and reported minimal blood loss [9]. For both anterior and posterior lesions, they advised to do a transverse incision at the junction between the myoma and the uterine corpus [9]. This was done to prevent injury to the bladder and rectum respectively and to facilitate the repair of the myoma bed during suturing [9]. One of our patients were found to have a large sessile anterior supravaginal cervical fibroid and it was determined that she would benefit from a da Vinci-assisted laparoscopic myomectomy (unpublished data), (**Figure 13.3**). She subsequently underwent a successful da Vinci robotic-assisted laparoscopic myomectomy by a gynecologic oncologist (**Figure 13.3**). In another case series, Matsuoka et al. (2010) [14] described their laparoscopic techniques to successfully perform laparoscopic myomectomy for supravaginal cervical fibroid [14].

In rare cases, the cervical myoma may be deeply rooted with the myoma present within the cervical wall above the vagina but also greatly protruding into the vaginal canal (**Figure 13.4**). In such cases it is difficult to enucleate the entire myoma via laparoscopy. Such deeply rooted supravaginal cervical myoma accounted for 7% of the case series of Chang et al. (2010) [9]. Such myomas were managed by making a 4–5 cm incision to expose the cervical myoma and the incision was extended if needed to visualize the entire myoma (**Figure 13.4**). The large myoma was pushed upwards manually in the direction of the abdominal cavity by the fingers of an assistant inserted into the vagina (**Figure 13.4**). This was followed by morcellation of the myoma before separating it from the cervix (**Figure 13.4**). This usually facilitates the dissection of the entire myoma laparoscopically. In patients with deep-rooted cervical myoma, any attempt at vaginal myomectomy can be very hazardous [25, 56]. In a case series of 22 patients, Pelosi and Pelosi (1997) [56] described a combined approach of laparoscopic myomectomy and posterior colpotomy which allowed them to do digital repair and visual inspection via laparoscopy [56]. In addition, Chang et al. (2010) [9] reported one patient with supravaginal central cervical fibroid that was removed laparoscopically [9]. However, this type of leiomyoma can be very difficult to be removed without damaging the entire cervical canal [9]. Chang et al. (2010) [9] concluded that laparoscopic myomectomy performed for supravaginal cervical fibroid by an experienced surgeon at the appropriate facility is safe, providing some modifications are made as described under myomectomy section [9]. Supravaginal lateral cervical fibroid accounted for 14% of cases in Chang et al. (2010) report [9]. The authors described the surgical technique utilized and reported a successful outcome with laparoscopic myomectomy [9]. This type of cervical fibroid will be

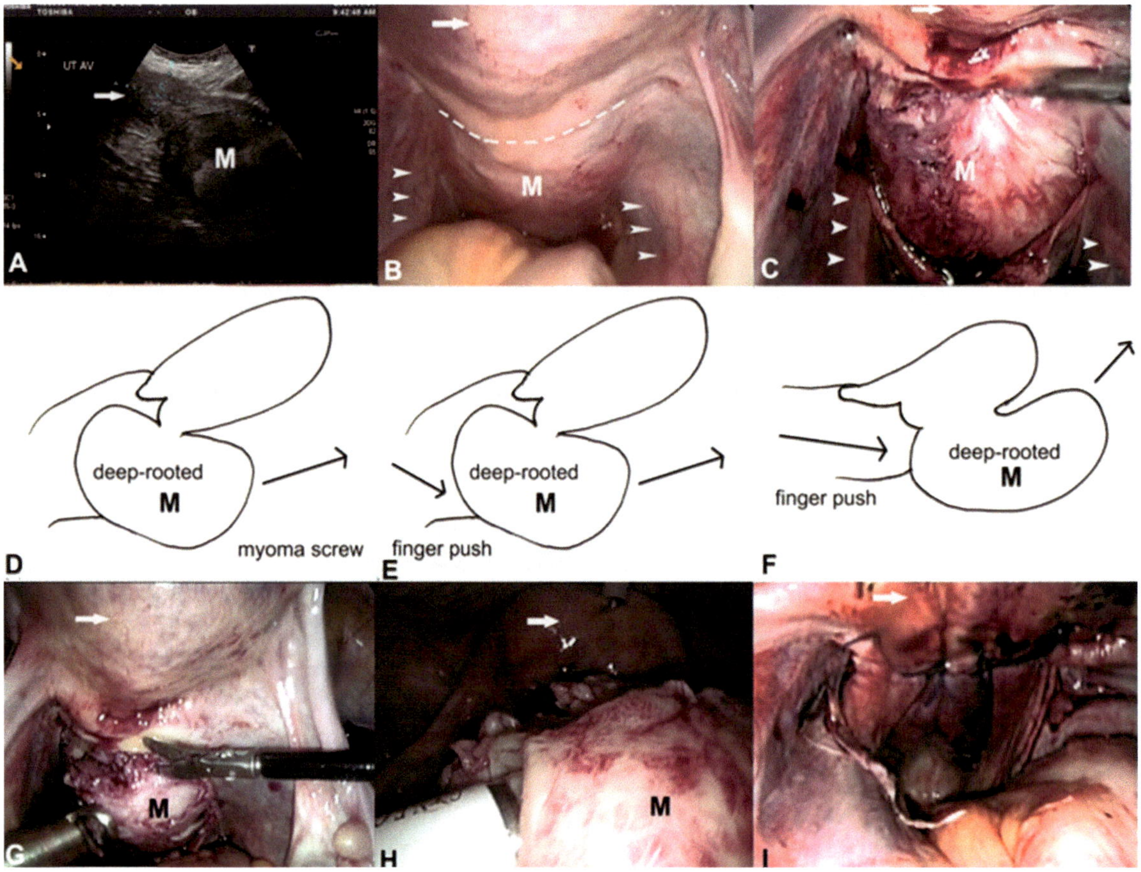


**FIGURE 13.4** Laparoscopic myomectomy in a deep-rooted cervical myoma. (A) Preoperative ultrasonographic image shows the myoma projecting into the vagina (arrow ¼ uterine body; M ¼ myoma). (B) The main part of myoma is deep rooted in the vagina. The dotted line indicates the incision and the arrowheads indicate the bilateral ureters. (C) A transverse incision is made just below the uterine body. (D, G) Attempts to expose the myoma with the aid of a myoma screw have failed. (E, F) The cervical myoma is pushed upward manually in the direction of abdominal cavity. (H) Morcellation is performed. (I) The wound is sutured with two-layer interrupted sutures. (By permission from Chang et al. 2010.)

discussed under the heading of broad ligament fibroid and cervical myoma.

## Broad ligament fibroid and cervical myoma

Fibroids that are located in the broad ligament are called broad ligament fibroids. The presence of leiomyomas in such locations may present both diagnostic and management dilemmas to the gynecologist. Although, trans-abdominal and transvaginal ultra sound scans can help in making the diagnosis, MRI is considered the gold standard for the diagnosis of such leiomyomas. Considering the location of the fibroid in relation to the uterine vessels and the ureter, the surgical management of patients with broad ligament fibroids is fraught with risks and complications, irrespective whether the patient is undergoing myomectomy or hysterectomy. Some of these fibroids arise from the cervical canal wall. Therefore, the lesions are referred to as supravaginal lateral cervical fibroids [9]. The fibroid can be attached to the cervical wall by a pedunculated or sessile pedicle. Bhardwaj (2015) [11] used the name "false broad ligament fibroid" to describe broad ligament fibroids that originated from the lateral walls of the uterus or the cervix [11]. In a video presentation by Bhardwaj (2015) [11], 16 cases of false broad ligament fibroids were described. All were removed through laparoscopic route with very minimal blood loss and no complications [11]. The reconstruction of the ectocervical canal was gratifying and resulted in anatomical and functional results although laparoscopic suturing was challenging [11]. In Bhardwaj's series, two patients underwent successful elective cesarean deliveries at term [11]. Chang et al. (2010) [9] reported four cases with lateral cervical fibroids which were pedunculated subserosal myoma extending into the broad ligament [9]. Although they described successful laparoscopic myomectomy in all four cases, they indicated that ligation of uterine vessels prior to enucleation of a very large lateral cervical myoma could prove to be difficult [9]. They suggested decompression of the lateral cervical myoma by partial enucleation and morcellation using an electric morcellator while still attached to the uterus, a technique that was also described by other investigators [9, 57, 58]. Thereafter, they proceeded with ligation of the uterine artery [9, 32, 59]. The cervical myoma was then completely enucleated, and complete morcellation was performed [9]. In our practice, we managed two cases of large broad ligament fibroids. Both were arising from the lower uterine segment and cervical canal. In both patients, the large myomas were successfully removed laparoscopically. In one case, a da Vinci robotic-assisted laparoscopic myomectomy was performed (**Figure 13.5**) [60]. In the second case, a laparoscopic myomectomy was successfully performed (unpublished data), (**Figure 13.6**). A third case encountered by our

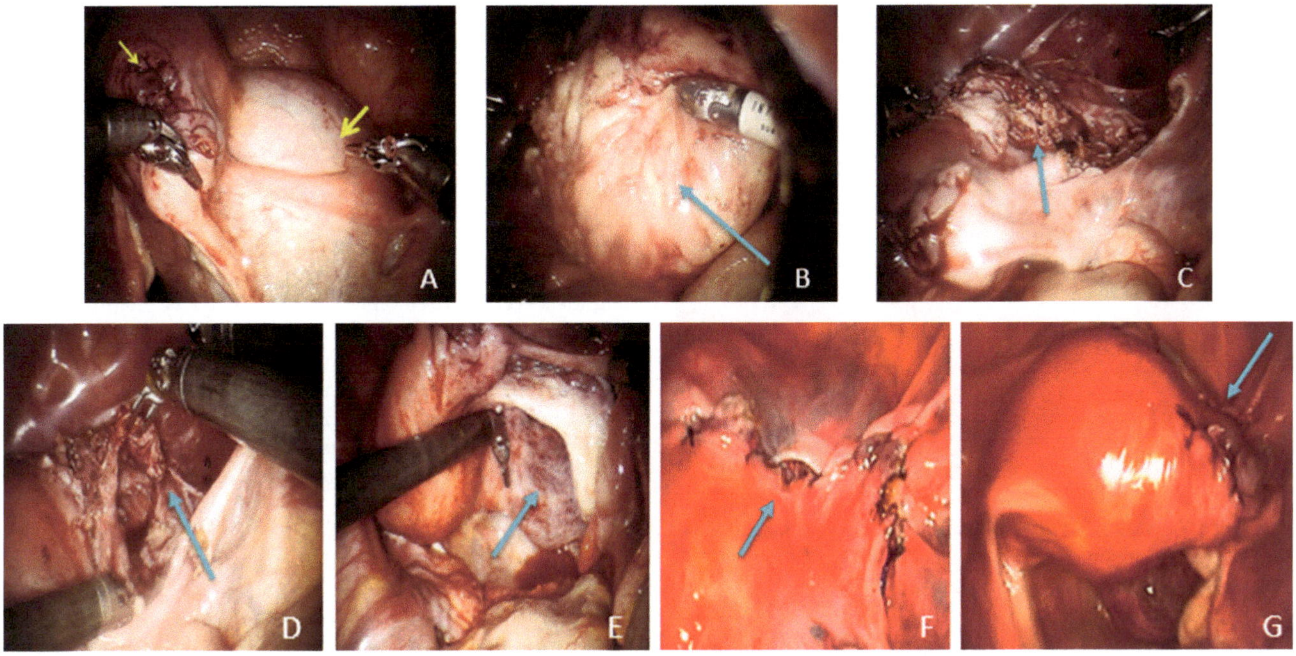


**FIGURE 13.5** Laparoscopic pictures using the da Vinci laparoscope and camera showing (A) a large broad ligament supravaginal cervical fibroid pushing the uterus to the left after diluted Vasopressin injection (large yellow arrow). An area where a 5-cm fibroid was dissected and removed from the fundal region of the uterus in seen (small yellow arrow); (B) the fibroid being dissected from the broad ligament (blue arrow); (C) a gap in the broad ligament after removal of the fibroid (blue arrow); (D) careful inspection of the gap in the broad ligament to insure homeostasis (blue arrow); (E) the posterior leaf of the broad ligament is seen intact (blue arrow); (F) the anterior leaf of the broad ligament is repaired (blue arrow); and (G) an apparently normal uterus and pelvic anatomy at the conclusion of the procedure (blue arrow). (Reproduced with permission from Abuzeid M, Joseph S. In: Rizk B, Puscheck EE (Eds.) *Ultrasonography in Gynecology*, Cambridge University Press, 2014, Chapters 9, 90–91.)

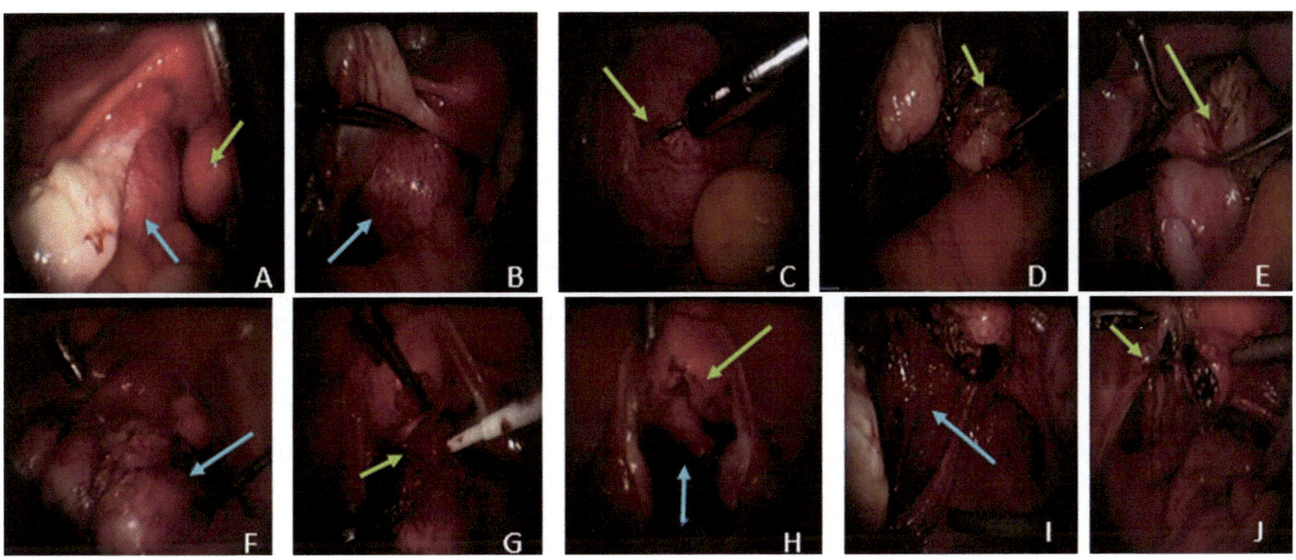


**FIGURE 13.6** Laparoscopic pictures showing: (A) A large left broad ligament supravaginal cervical fibroid pushing the uterus to the right (blue arrow) and a small subserous pedunculated fibroid attached to posterior wall of the upper uterine segment (green arrow). (B) The large left broad ligament supravaginal cervical fibroid is clearly seen (blue arrow) after the left ovary was lifted up with a metal probe. (C) Diluted vasopressin injection in the fibroid (green arrow). (D) and (E) The fibroid being dissected from the broad ligament (green arrow). (F) The broad ligament supravaginal cervical fibroid after it was dissected from the broad ligament (blue arrow), but it remained attached to the posterior wall of the supravaginal portion of the cervical canal. (G) The wide pedicle that attach the fibroid to the wall of the cervical canal (green arrow) is being divided using a spatula with monopolar cautery (70 watts cutting current and 50 watts coagulation current). (H) Hemostasis was secured from the pedicle (blue arrow) and a figure of 8 suture using 0 vicryl was placed after removal of the small myoma (green arrow). (I) and (J) Depicts the gape in the posterior wall of the left broad ligament before (blue arrow) and after repair (green arrow).

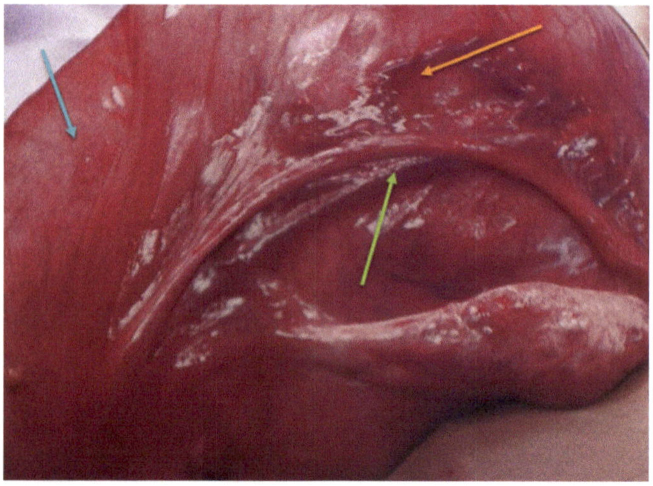

**FIGURE 13.7** Laparoscopic picture depicting a large broad ligament fibroid (orange arrow) originated from both the uterine body and cervical canal pushing the uterus (blue arrow) to the left side. Notice that the right fallopian tube is stretched over the large fibroid (green arrow). (Reproduced with permission from Abuzeid M, Joseph S. In: Rizk B, Puscheck EE (Eds.) *Ultrasonography in Gynecology*, Cambridge University Press, 2014, Chapters 9, 89.)

practice included a large broad ligament myoma originated from both the uterine body and cervical canal was removed via laparotomy without any complications (**Figure 13.7**) [61].

## Vaginal cervical myoma

The specific surgical procedure for removal of vaginal cervical myoma will depend on its type and location (**Table 13.1**).

### Intracervical (submucosal): Myoma arising from the cavity of the cervical canal

Vaginal cervical myoma arising from the cavity of the cervical canal is usually pedunculated, with the myoma protruding into the vagina. Such pathology was reported to be rare compared to a pedunculated myoma originating from the ectocervix [62]. The pedicle can be seen below the external cervical os or may be present inside the cervical canal. If the pedicle is seen in the vagina, and the size of the myoma is not very large and the procedure can be done in a procedure room in the office. If the pedicle is not thick, the protruded myoma can simply be removed by twisting the myoma using a ringed-forceps. After a vaginal speculum is placed and adequate exposure of the myoma is obtained, a 0-Vicryl Endoloop (Ethicon US, LLC part of Johnson & Johnson, New Jersey) passed around the myoma, the pedicle is tied and the suture is cut. The myoma is then removed and homeostasis should be secured from the pedicle. If the need arises, another Endoloop can be placed higher at the base of the pedicle in the cervical canal. However, such procedure should be performed in the operating room under anesthesia if the myoma is very large or there is significant difficulty visualizing the pedicle, or difficulty in passing the Endoloop around the myoma. Furthermore, one needs to perform the procedure in the operating room if the pedicle is thick or vascular. In such cases, a LigaSure (Medtronic, Minneapolis, MN) device could be used to coagulate and cut the pedicle and secure homeostasis. There are few case reports in the literature discussing the clinical presentation and management of huge myomas originating from the cervical canal and protruding through the vagina with or without uterine prolapse or incarcerated procidentia [7, 23, 63].

Patients with vaginal cervical myomas that arise in the cervical canal with a sessile attachment, usually present both a diagnostic and surgical dilemma to the gynecologist. This is especially challenging with patients with underlying anemia secondary to hemorrhage. The challenge of a critically anemic patient is compounded with an already present surgical challenge. Once the diagnosis is confirmed on MRI, tamponade as a hemostatic technique can be attempted by inserting a Foley's catheter into the uterine cavity and inflating its balloon until permanent surgical management can be performed. Alternatively, if deemed necessary, uterine artery embolization or balloon insertion can be performed by an interventional radiologist. Once the leiomyoma bleeding is controlled and the patient is hemodynamically stable, definitive treatment can be performed. Hysterectomy may be performed if the patient does not desire fertility preservation. If fertility preservation is needed, hysteroscopic myomectomy by an experienced gynecologist is an option. We recently managed a patient with a myoma that was partially protruding through the cervical os. The patient presented to the emergency department with severe lower abdominal pain, excessive vaginal bleeding and a low HB (6 g/dl). MRI suggested a sessile cervical myoma (3 cm in diameter) arising from the posterior wall of the cervical canal near the internal os (**Figure 13.8**). The patient was stabilized with intravenous hydration and 4 units of packed red blood cells. She underwent a successful hysteroscopic myomectomy. An 8 French Pediatric Foley catheter was inserted into the uterine cavity and its balloon was inflated with 4 cc of normal saline to reduce postoperative bleeding (**Figure 13.8**). The procedure was uneventful, and the patient did well postoperatively and was discharged home after 24 hours with the Foley catheter still in place. The catheter was removed after 4 days. The pathology report confirmed the diagnosis of a benign leiomyoma. The patient did well and had no evidence of any recurrence of the cervical myoma 3 months after surgery. Abha and Kavneet (2012) [64] reported a similar case in a 17-year-old patient who was managed in a similar manner after 3 days of misdiagnosing her with abnormal uterine bleeding secondary to anovulatory cycles [64]. Eventually they discovered a cervical polyp measuring 2.5 × 2.5 × 1.5 cm, with a sessile broad base distending the external os but not protruding into the vagina. The leiomyoma was electrocauterized at its base and histopathology confirmed a Myomatous polyp [64].

### Extracervical (intramural or subserous): Myoma arising from the wall of the vaginal portion of the cervical canal

Pedunculated vaginal cervical myomas arising from the wall of the cervical canal should be managed the same way as described for the pedunculated myoma arising from the cavity of the cervical canal. The choice of the technique will again depend on the size, location, thickness and vascularity of the pedicle as described previously. On the other hand, if the vaginal cervical myoma is sessile in nature, it needs to be excised from the cervical canal followed by meticulous reconstruction of the cervical canal wall. It is crucial to completely remove the myoma and avoid occluding the cervical canal during suturing and repairing of the cervical wall. We recently operated on a patient that had a recurrent large sessile myoma arising from the entire anterior wall of the vaginal portion of the cervical canal. The patient had

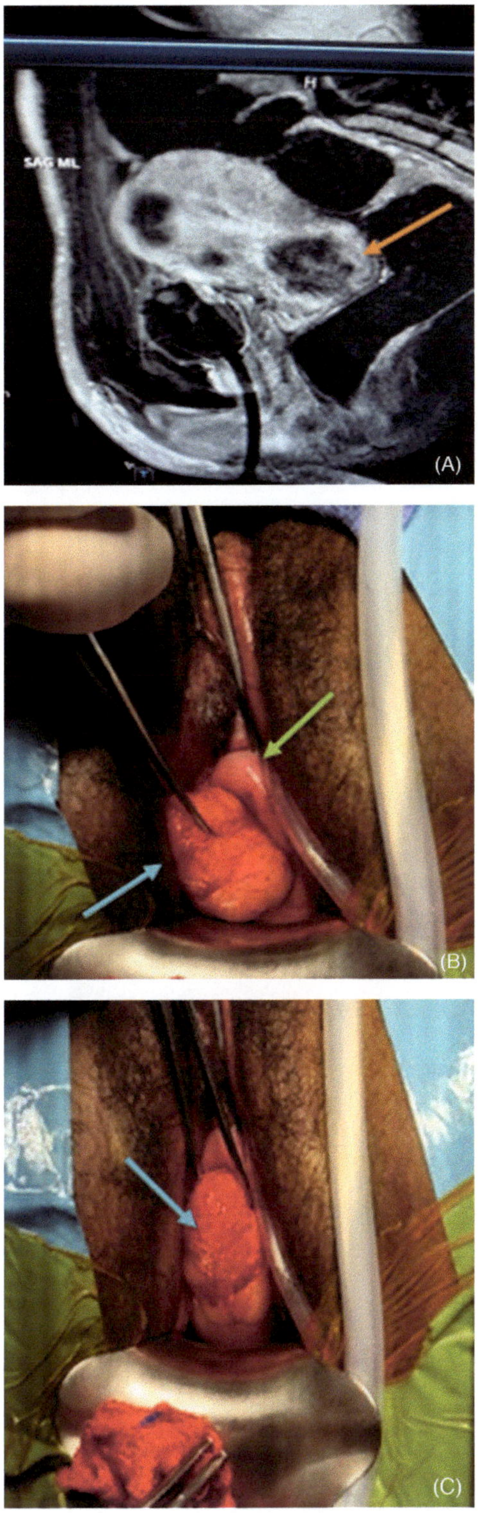


**FIGURE 13.8** (A) An MRI showing a large low T2 signal intensity mass in the endocervical canal which measured 4.0 × 3.5 × 3.2 cm compatible with pedunculated uterine fibroid attached to the posterior wall of the cervical canal (orange arrow). Pictures (B) and (C) depict a sessile cervical myoma arising from the posterior wall of the cervical canal near the internal os. (B) The myoma (blue arrow) was partially protruding through the external os (green arrow). (C) The myoma was lifted up with single toothed tenaculum to try visualize the pedicle, but it was not seen (blue arrow). (Courtesy of Dr. M Abuzeid.)

a previous excision at another clinic, but it recurred within a few months possibly as a result of incomplete removal. **Figure 13.9** illustrates the steps of the myomectomy. The myoma bed was repaired with 2-0 Vicryl using interrupted figure-of-8 sutures for the first layer and in a continuous running manner for the superficial layer (**Figure 13.9**). A Pediatric Foley catheter (size 8 French) was introduced into the endometrial cavity, and its balloon was inflated with 3 cc of normal saline and catheter was secured to the inner side of the patient's thigh to avoid scarring of the external os (**Figure 13.9**). The catheter was removed after 3 days. The pathology report was consistent with a benign myoma. Following her surgery, the patient had uneventful recovery with no evidence of any recurrence of the vaginal cervical myoma 3 months after surgery. There was no evidence of scarring of the external os. However, there was a slight distortion in the overall position of the external os as it was directed more towards the right lateral fornix.

However, the management of moderate and large sessile myoma of the vaginal portion of the cervix can be a surgical challenge to many gynecologists, who would counsel for hysterectomy as opposed to myomectomy due to the risks associated with uncontrollable bleeding. In addition, the hysterectomy may have many surgical challenges and risks as well. Such cases should be referred to a specialized center with experience in management of such rare pathology.

Uterine artery embolization (UAE) is discussed as a treatment option for cervical leiomyoma in some studies. However, UAE has displayed less effectiveness, with only 20% showing complete necrosis after embolization [26]. More recently, DeMeritt et al. (2018) [27] reported the first successful treatment of a symptomatic patient with a 4 cm cervical myoma occupying the entire posterior wall of the cervix, which was not amenable to surgical excision by myomectomy [27]. The patient presented with history of menorrhagia and episodes of persistent vaginal bleeding requiring blood transfusion [27]. Her gynecologist initially recommended a hysterectomy, but the patient wanted to preserve her fertility potential [27]. The authors performed bilateral superselective cervicovaginal artery embolization using 100–300-µm Embospheres, along with cone beam CT to confirm nontarget tissue exclusion to avoid the hypothetical risk of vaginal and/or labial ischemia and necrosis [27]. Smaller beads size was used instead of the standard 500–700-µm beads, usually used during UAE, in view of the smaller size of the terminal cervical arterial arcades and perifibroid plexus [27]. The patient became pregnant 3 months after her treatment. The pregnancy was uncomplicated and she delivered a healthy male at 38-weeks gestation. MRI at 3 months and 14 months following selective cervicovaginal artery embolization showed a 91% and a 96% reduction in fibroid volume respectively [27].

In some rare situations, the vaginal cervical myoma can be large enough to entirely replace the cervical canal. In our practice, a 31-year-old female nulligravida who wanted to preserve her fertility potential presented to our clinic. She has a 10-cm vaginal cervical myoma arising from the anterior and lateral walls of the cervical canal (unpublished data). The external cervical os was palpable with difficulty behind the vaginal cervical myoma which protruded in the vagina and encompassed the entire vagina. The patient presented with symptoms of pelvic pressure, urinary frequency and dyspareunia. She was referred by her primary care physician to our clinic for evaluation and management after she was told by her gynecologist that hysterectomy is the only possible management for her pathology. Transvaginal ultrasound revealed a large anterior fibroid (8.7 × 7.9 × 9.1 cm) replacing the

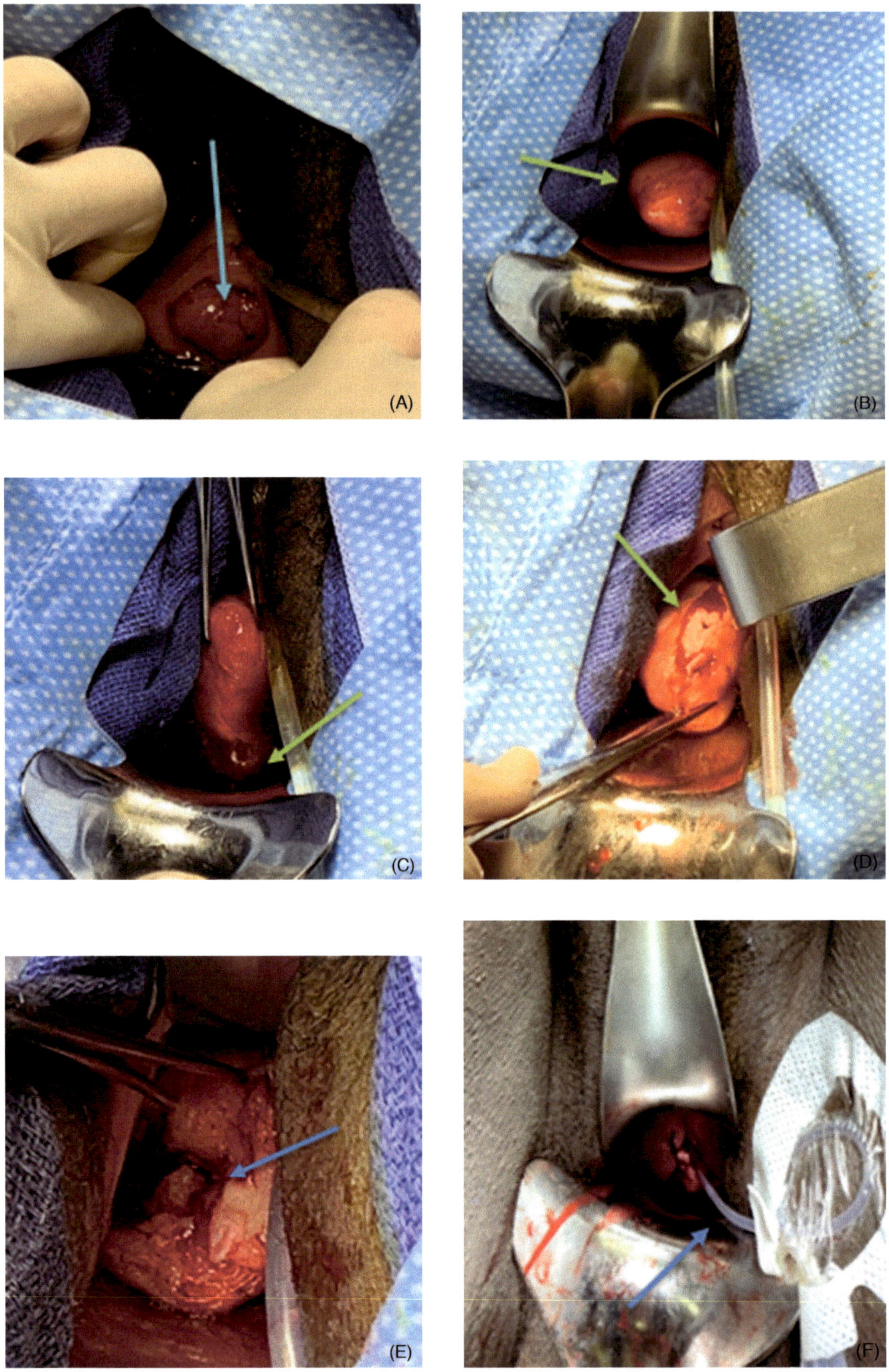


**FIGURE 13.9** A large sessile myoma arising from the entire anterior wall of the vaginal portion of the cervical canal. (A) The myoma is seen protruding through the introitus (blue arrow). (B) and (C) The myoma position in relation to the external os (green arrow). (D) A vertical incision is made along the mucosa covering the myona (green arrow). (E) The myoma bed after excision of the myoma (blue arrow). (F) Pediatric Foley's catheter size 8 French was introduced into the endometrial cavity, balloon was inflated with 3 cc of normal saline and catheter was taped to the inner side of the thigh to avoid scarring of the external os (blue arrow). The catheter was removed after 3 days. (Courtesy of Dr. M Abuzeid.)

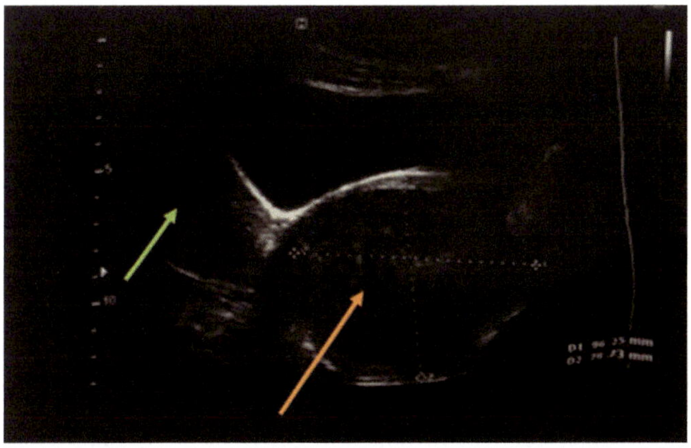

**FIGURE 13.10** Transvaginal ultrasound picture depicting a large anterior fibroid (8.7 × 7.9 × 9.1 cm) replacing the entire cervix (orange arrow) which was not visualized. The uterus is seen on the left side of the picture (green arrow). (Courtesy of Dr. M Abuzeid.)

entire cervix which was not visualized (**Figure 13.10**), and MRI confirmed the diagnosis. No other leiomyomas were identified. This was also confirmed during examination under anesthesia and a diagnostic laparoscopy. Following her initial diagnostic surgery, a gynecologic oncologist was consulted and the plan was to attempt a robotic-assisted laparoscopic myomectomy. However, the patient was counseled for possible vaginal myomectomy and hysterectomy in light of the challenges anticipated. Robotic-assisted bilateral ureterolysis and bladder dissection off the anterior surface of the uterus and cervix were performed. There was only partial exposure of the myoma after the anterior colpotomy was performed. At that stage, it was determined that a vaginal approach is the only option to complete the myomectomy. After injection of diluted vasopressin (20 units in 60 cc normal saline) into the myoma, vaginal myomectomy was performed by morcellating the myoma while it was still attached to the cervical canal. This was followed by excision of the remaining pedicle of the myoma from the cervical canal. The cervical canal was then repaired using 2-0 Vicryl in an interrupted figure-of-8 suture. Care was taken to avoid obliterating the cervical canal. Hemostasis was secured. Cystoscopy was normal with no evidence of ureteral or bladder injuries. Estimated blood loss was 700 mL and no complications were encountered postoperatively. Pathology confirmed a benign leiomyoma. Postoperatively, the patient experienced normal periods and relief of previous symptoms, indicating patency of the cervical canal. Transvaginal 2D and 3D US with and without saline sonohysterography revealed a normal cervical canal and uterine cavity demonstrating excellent postoperative results. The patient conceived naturally 6 months after surgery, and she is currently at 20-week gestation.

## Management of cervical fibroids in pregnancy

Cervical fibroid is very rare during pregnancy. This is partly due to the possibility that patients with cervical fibroids have difficulty conceiving. However, the discovery of cervical fibroid during pregnancy poses a significant management dilemma in consideration of maternal and fetal risks. Most of the literature is in the form of case reports describing the treatment strategy for the specific case. The proposed strategy in each case depended on the clinical presentation, its severity, type, location and size of the cervical fibroid, gestational age and patient's desire for fertility preservation. Management strategies in the literature include conservative or surgical treatment. Myomectomy was performed during pregnancy, at time of delivery or after delivery. Hysterectomy was usually performed at time of cesarean delivery, or in the postpartum period following complications such as severe hemorrhage or infection. In addition, there are two case reports of superselective embolization of the cervicovaginal arteries, as conservative method of management of supravaginal cervical fibroid. One of those cases was performed prior to pregnancy and the other during pregnancy at 20-week gestation [19, 27].

## Sessile vaginal cervical fibroid during pregnancy

The presence of sessile vaginal cervical fibroid during pregnancy is very rare. These leiomyomas can increase in size during pregnancy, or present with excessive vaginal bleeding requiring blood transfusion. Antenatal complications can include, preterm prelabor rupture of membranes and postpartum vaginal prolapse [15–18]. Cervical fibroids do tend to undergo degeneration in the postpartum period as a result of thrombosis of the feeding vessels which usually leads to reduction in the size of the fibroid. This may allow for continued observation or vaginal myomectomy becomes a viable option without increased risk of hysterectomy [15, 16]. However, degeneration of fibroids in the postpartum period could be associated with increased risk of infection, which may require an emergent hysterectomy [17]. Gandhi et al. (2014) [16] reported a successful conservative management of a sessile vaginal posterior wall cervical fibroid during pregnancy [16]. Although the fibroid increased in size during pregnancy, the patient remained asymptomatic until she delivered by cesarean delivery. Four days following her delivery, the patient presented with vaginal prolapse of the fibroid. The authors decided to continue with conservative management by using a simple rubber ring pessary to support the prolapsed fibroid. After 6 weeks, the fibroid decreased in size to 3 cm in diameter which allowed the authors to continue with observation and avoid surgical treatment altogether [16].

In another case report, Keriakos and Maher (2013) [15] proceeded with conservative management in a patient with a vaginal sessile posterior cervical fibroid measuring 5 cm in diameter [15]. The patient attempted to conceive and avoided myomectomy, due to the fear of the associated risk of hysterectomy. In addition, uterine artery embolization was not pursued [15]. The fibroid continued to increase in size and patient had several episodes of vaginal bleeding, with one episode requiring blood transfusion. However, the authors continued conservative management safely [15]. The patient delivered via cesarean section at 37-week gestation. As expected, the cervical myoma underwent degeneration and decreased in size after 6 weeks, which allowed the authors to perform a vaginal myomectomy without difficulty [15].

Sengupta et al. (2006) [65] reported a patient with a large (12 × 14 cm) sessile vagina cervical fibroid arising from the anterior, left lateral and posterior part of the cervix that prolapsed outside the vagina at 36-week gestation. The patient was delivered by emergency cesarean section and a vaginal myomectomy was successfully performed concomitantly following her delivery [65].

Tripathi et al. (2013) [66] removed a 7 × 8 cm right vaginal cervical fibroid with a 2 cm attachment to the cervix at 37-week gestation without any complications [66]. This allowed the patient to have a vaginal delivery 10 days later; therefore, avoiding cesarean delivery and possible complications that may occur in cervical fibroid after delivery [66].

## Pedunculated prolapsed vaginal cervical myoma during pregnancy

There are six cases in the literatures reporting the procedure of vaginal myomectomy for pedunculated prolapsed myomas during pregnancy. Tigdi and Chan (2019) [20] described a vaginal myomectomy for 5–6 cm fibroid protruding through the cervix into the vagina arising from the level of the internal os of the cervix [20]. The patient was a 28-year-old G1 P0 at 18-week gestation who had confirmed diagnosis of trisomy 18 [20]. Dilatation and evacuation was planned, however, the pedunculated vaginal cervical leiomyoma complicated a safe cervical dilatation [20]. She received cervical ripening agents with laminaria dilators and a Foley catheter. Afterwards, the pedicle was felt to be attached to the cervical canal [20]. The stalk was transected and cauterized to achieve homeostasis. Dilation and evacuation were performed without difficulty [20]. Four other pregnant patients underwent vaginal myomectomy for pedunculated prolapsed cervical fibroids by twisting or clamping of the base of a pedunculated myoma. In two of these patients, the pregnancy continued, and the patients delivered at full term [67]. Another patient had preterm prelabor rupture of membranes and subsequent miscarriage at 15-week gestation 2 weeks after surgery [68]. A patient with a pregnancy at 22-week gestation also had preterm prelabor rupture of membranes, 4 weeks after the surgery [67]. MRI prior to such procedures is crucial to ensure that the stalk of the myoma arises from the cervical canal and not from the endometrial cavity. In addition, prophylactic antibiotics should be used to reduce the incidence chorioamnionitis and preterm prelabor rupture of membranes [21].

Obara et al. (2013) [21] reported a pregnant patient with a semi-pedunculated myoma (6 × 4 cm) who required vaginal myomectomy at 13-weeks gestation for severe vaginal bleeding secondary to the myoma [21]. The authors indicated that the stalk was too wide, making twisting and clamping of the base impossible [21]. MRI confirmed that the vaginal myoma was submucosal in nature originating from the posterior wall of the uterine cervix with a closed internal os [21]. An incision was made in the surface of the vaginal portion of the leiomyoma, and the myoma was removed [21]. Systemic and local antibiotics were used postoperatively [21]. The myoma bed was sutured and homeostasis was ensured. Postoperative course was uneventful and the patient had a vaginal delivery at term [21].

### Supravaginal cervical fibroid in pregnancy

The discovery of cervical fibroid during pregnancy should raise concerns such as regarding possible complications such as antepartum hemorrhage obstruction of labor, and degeneration and possible infection in the postnatal period. Once the diagnosis of cervical fibroid in pregnancy is made, MRI should be performed to confirm the diagnosis, and determine the exact location and type of the cervical fibroid. Cesarean delivery is the usual mode of delivery in the majority of patients with a cervical fibroid. Tian and Wensheng (2012) [6] published a paper addressing the management of 17 patients with a solitary supravaginal cervical fibroid during pregnancy and delivery [6]. They reported a frequency of 0.03% in the population studied [6]. One patient with an intramural supravaginal cervical fibroid delivered vaginally without complications. The remaining 16 patients delivered by C-section [6]. In their report myomectomy was performed in 9 patients at the time of cesarean delivery. Hysterectomy was performed in 3 patients with a very large cervical myoma (>20 cm in diameter) [6]. In one of these patients, cesarean hysterectomy was performed because of severe hemorrhage [6]. In 2 patients, (with leiomyoma > 20 cm in diameter) the myoma was left in place [6]. Both patients had a hysterectomy after delivery, one for severe postpartum hemorrhage and one for severe and persistent post-partum infection despite medical treatment [6]. The authors reported a positive correlation between the total blood loss and the size of the cervical myoma [6]. Cervical fibroids greater than 10 cm required a transfusion during myomectomy, which raises the question of leaving cervical fibroids in situ following cesarean delivery rather than combining the two procedures in the same surgery. However, during involution the cervical fibroid may undergo degeneration thus increasing the possibility of infection from a necrosed cervical leiomyoma. Based on the data of the Tian and Wensheng (2012) [6], proceeding with surgical management of supravaginal cervical myoma at the time of delivery will depend on the size of the myoma. Cesarean hysterectomy by an experienced surgeon, preferably in the presence of a gynecologic oncologist is necessary if the myoma is very large [6]. In addition, the data in this report suggest that myomectomy for small supravaginal cervical myoma can safely be performed at the time of cesarean section by experienced gynecologists [6]. The need for blood products is always an important consideration. Furthermore, in 7 patients in this case series the diagnosis of supravaginal cervical myoma was diagnosed prior to conceiving [6]. These patients should be advised to have myomectomy, if feasible, before pregnancy in order to reduce the risks that can occur during pregnancy and delivery.

### Superselective embolization of the cervicovaginal arteries for a bleeding cervical fibroid in pregnancy

Lohle et al. (2015) [19] reported a successful treatment and pregnancy outcome after performing superselective cervicovaginal artery embolization in a 20-week pregnant woman. She had life-threatening vaginal bleeding as a result of a supravaginal large (9 cm) intramural anterior cervical fibroid [19]. It was calculated that the estimated absorbed radiation dose by the fetus during the embolization was 40 mGy, much lower than the dose threshold of 100 mGy, which can lead to severe mental disability [19]. The authors reported immediate cessation of bleeding and the remainder of her antenatal care was uncomplicated. The patient delivered a healthy male at 38-week gestation [19]. MRI performed 2 months after delivery, revealed an almost complete infarction of the cervical fibroid [19]. Three years post-delivery, the child's physical and mental development was normal [19]. These preliminary reports on the use of superselective cervicovaginal artery embolization for treatment of supravaginal cervical fibroids that are not amenable to surgery and/or in patients in whom surgery is contraindicated or associated with more risk are promising [19, 27]. However, more data is needed before the safety and efficacy of this procedure is determined.

## Conclusion

The various clinical presentations of cervical leiomyoma depend on the size, location, characteristics and have various impacts on fertility potential and antepartum care, as well as symptoms of abnormal uterine bleeding and pelvic prolapse. The importance of utilizing the diagnostic modalities to accurately map the cervical fibroid location and preoperative planning is paramount. The gynecologic surgeon must be prepared to anticipate potential surgical complications such as managing an acutely anemic patient should hemorrhage arise, avoiding injury of surrounding organs and structures, and whether the surgery will be best carried out through a vaginal or abdominal approach. The patient presentations in the literature allow us to derive diagnostic clues and specific surgical techniques when the decision is made to approach a cervical leiomyoma medically, through superselective embolization or surgically via myomectomy, hysterectomy or both.

The population of pregnant individuals who present with cervical leiomyoma teach us the importance of an accurate and thorough diagnostic workup prior to conception if possible, or during the pregnancy in order to plan out the appropriate management in a timelier fashion. The number of cases presented and reviewed in the literature limits the evidence with regards to the best approach to treatment, but there is evidence that supports conservative management, embolization and surgical approaches in pregnancy.

## References


1. Pelvic Mass. In: Hoffman BL, Schorge JO, Bradshaw KD, Halvorson LM, Schaffer JI, Corton MM. eds. *Williams Gynecology, 3rd ed.* McGrawHill, New York, NY, 2016.
2. Berek JS, Novak E. Eds. In: *Berek and Novak's Gynecology.* Wolters Kluwer, Philadelphia, 2015.
3. Stovall T. Myomectomy. In: Mann WJ ST, ed. *Gynecologic Surgery.* New York, NY: Churchill Livingstone, 1996:445–461.
4. Stencheerv M, Droegemueller W, Herbst A, Mishell D. In: *Comprehensive Gynecology.* 4th ed. St. Louis, MO: Mosby Inc., 2001.
5. Tiltman, AJ. Leiomyomas of the uterine cervix: A study of frequency. *Int J Gynecol Pathol.* 1998;17(3):231–234.
6. Tian J, Wensheng H. Cervical leiomyomas in pregnancy: report of 17 cases. *Aust Nz J Obstet Gyn.* 2012;52(3):258–261.
7. Kanash S, Priscilla S, Manju P. A Huge pedunculated cervical fibroid polyp with sepsis - a case report. *J. Evol. Med. Dent. Sci.* 2016; 5(99):7305–7306.
8. Mendiratta S, Dash S, Mittal R, Dath S, Sharma M, N. Sahai R. Cervical fibroid: an uncommon presentation. *Int J Reprod Contracept Obstet Gynecol.* 2017;6(9):4161.
9. Chang WC, Chen SY, Huang SC, Chang DY, Chou LY, Sheu BC. Strategy of cervical myomectomy under laparoscopy. Fertil Steril 2010;94(7):2710–2715.
10. Booher M, Edelson M, Jaspan D, Goldberg J. Myomectomy of a large cervical fibroid in a patient desiring future fertility. *OBG Management* 2018;30(10):20–24.
11. Bhardwaj P. Laparoscopic management of broad ligament and cervical fibroids with reconstruction of ectocervical canal. *JMIG* 2015;22(6):S1-S253:425.
12. Sangwan N, Duhan N, Sirohiwal D, Rajotia N. Cervical fibroid mimicking prolapse. *JK Sci.* 2010;12(1):51.
13. Ramya R, Narayanaswamy M. Prolapsed giant posterior cervical leiomyoma. *Global J Med Public Health,* 2013;2(4): ISSN 2277-9604 (Online). https://doaj.org/toc/2277-9604 (external link) http://www.gjmedph.org/uploads... (external link) https://doaj.org/article/5b750.
14. Matsuoka S, Kikuchi I, Kitade M, et al. Strategy for laparoscopic cervical myomectomy. *JMIG* 2010;17(3):301–305. https://doi:10.1016/j.jmig.2009.12.020
15. Keriakos R, Maher M. Management of cervical fibroid during the reproductive period. *Case Rep Obstet Gynecol.* 2013;984030. https://doi.org/10.1155/2013/984030
16. Gandhi AC, Hemant I., Dugad HI, Shah Y. A rare presentation of cervical fibroid in pregnancy. *Ann. Afr. Med.* 2014;13(2):88.
17. Abitbol MM, Madison RL. Cervical fibroids complicating pregnancy. *Obstet Gynecol* 1958;12(4):397–398.
18. Erian J, El-Toukhy T, Chandakas S, Kazal O, Hill N. Rapidly enlarging cervical fibroids during pregnancy: a case report. *J Obstet Gynaecol* 2004;24(5):578–579.
19. Lohle PNM, Boekkooi PF, Fiedeldeij CA, et al. Selective embolisation of a heavily bleeding cervical fibroid in a pregnant woman. *Cadiovasc Intervent Radiol* 2015;38:1649–1653.
20. Tigdi J, Chan C. A case report of overcoming an obstructive, pedunculated cervical fibroid at the time of uterine evacuation. *Case Rep Obstet Gynecol* 2019;2651680. https://doi.org/10.1155/2019/2651680
21. Obara M, Hatakeyama Y, Shimizu Y. Vaginal myomectomy for semipedunculated cervical myoma during pregnancy. *AJP Rep* 2014;4(1):37–40.
22. Goel N, Shikha S. An unusual case of cervical fibroid masquerading as ovarian tumor. *J Mid-Life Health.* 2016;7(3):144–146.
23. Khade SA, Jadhav B, Raut R. Huge cervical pedunculated leiomyoma with uterine prolapse: a case report. *Int J Reprod Contracept Obstet Gynecol.* 2019;8(2):772–775.
24. Khan AT, Shehmar M, Gupta JK. Uterine fibroids: current perspectives. *Int J Women's Health* 2014;6:95–114.
25. Takeuchi H, Kitade M, Kikuchi I, et al. A new enucleation method for cervical myoma via laparoscopy. *JMIG.* 2006;13(4):334–336.
26. Kim MD, Lee M, Jung DC, et al. Limited efficacy of uterine artery embolization for cervical leiomyomas. *J Vasc Interv Radiol.* 2012; 23:236–240.
27. DeMeritt JS, Waiswol E, Wattamwar A. Pregnancy after superselective embolization of the cervicovaginal arteries for a bleeding cervical fibroid. *Lett Editor* 2019;30(10):1639. https://doi.org/10.1016/j.jvir.2018.09.036
28. Parsanezhad ME, Azmoon M, Alborzi S, et. al. A randomized, controlled clinical trial comparing the effects of aromatase inhibitor (letrozole) and gonadotropin-releasing hormone agonist (triptorelin) on uterine leiomyoma volume and hormonal status. *Fertil Steril* 2010;93(1):192–198.
29. Lethaby A, Vollenhoven B, Sowter M. Efficacy of preoperative gonadotrophin hormone releasing analogues for women with uterine fibroids undergoing hysterectomy or myomectomy: a systematic review. *BJOG* 2002;109(10):1097–1108.
30. Vercellini P, Trespidi L, Zaina B, Vicentini S, Stellato G, Crosignani PG. Gonadotropin-releasing hormone agonist treatment before abdominal myomectomy: a controlled trial. *Fertil Steril* 2003;79(6):1390–1395.
31. The Practice Committee of the American Society for Reproductive Medicine in collaboration with the Society of Reproductive Surgeons: myomas and reproductive function. *Fertil Steril.* 2008;90(5 Suppl):S125–S130. https://doi:10.1016/j.ferilstert.2008.09.012
32. Takeda A, Koyama K, Imoto S, Mori M, Sakai K, Nakamura H. Temporary endovascular balloon occlusion of the bilateral internal iliac arteries for control of hemorrhage during laparoscopic-assisted myomectomy in a nulligravida with a large cervical myoma. *Fertil Steril* 2009;91(3):935.e5–e9.
33. Campian CE, Weinreb SJ, Tatalovich JM, Jan AG. Uterine artery embolization prior to total laparoscopic hysterectomy for large fibroid uterus. *J Minim Invasive Gynecol* 2012;19, S71–S122, 367 Video Session 11 Advanced Endoscopy.
34. Shimanuki H, Takeuchi H, Kitade M, Kikuchi I, Kumakiri J, Kinoshita K. The effect of vasopressin on local and general circulation during laparoscopic surgery. *J Minim Invasive Gynecol* 2006;13(3):190–194.
35. Alborzi S, Ghannadan E, Alborzi S, Alborzi M. A comparison of combined laparoscopic uterine artery ligation and myomectomy versus laparoscopic myomectomy in treatment of symptomatic myoma. *Fertil Steril.* 2009;92(2):742–747.
36. Warty NR, Sawant RM, Parikh KP, Warty TR, Puntambekar SP. Changing anatomical relationships in lateral cervical fibroids. *J Minim Invasive Gynecol* 2016;23(7), S1–S252, 307 Video Session 4 - Reproductive Issues.
37. Wu HY, Yen TT, Singh B, et. al. Cell salvage system use in minimally invasive myomectomy. *J Minim Invasive Gynecol.* 2019; 26(7):S1–S97, S33 Open Communications 4: Laparoscopy.
38. Son M, Evanko JC, Mongero LB, et. al. Utility of cell salvage in women undergoing abdominal myomectomy. *Am J Obstet Gynecol* 2014;211(1):28.e1–e8.
39. Ecker AM, Lum D, Lee TTM. Laparoscopic hysterectomy for cervical fibroids - strategies and techniques. *J Minim Invasive Gynecol.* 2013;20(6), S1–S49, 93 Video Session 3 - Hysterectomy.
40. Ramirez CI, Lee TTM. Laparoscopic hysterectomy for cervical fibroid: surgical tips. *J Minim Invasive Gynecol.* 2017;24(7), S1–S201, 28 Plenary 4 - Laparoscopy.

41. Riley K, Harkins G, Davies M. Laparoscopic hysterectomy complicated by large cervical fibroid. *J Minim Invasive Gynecol.* 2011; 18(6):S114–S115, 387 Video Session 12 Laparoscopy.
42. Istre O, Springborg H. Laparoscopic hysterectomy in cervical fibroids. *J Minim Invasive Gynecol.* 2012;19(6), S71–S122, 366 Video Session 11 Advanced Endoscopy.
43. Leroy L, Topete VM, Lara Viesca T, Castellon RM, Casso VA. Laparoscopic total hysterectomy with cervical fibroid. *J Minim Invasive Gynecol.* 2012;19(6):S179–S188, 613.
44. Deimling T, Harkins G, Davies M. Laparoscopic trachelectomy with cervical fibroid and endometriosis. *J Minim Invasive Gynecol.* 2011;18(6):S71–S90, 294 Video Session 9 Laparoscopy.
45. Nahas S and Magrina JF. Robotic excision of right cervical fibroid. *J Minim Invasive Gynecol.* 2012;19(6):S179–S188, 645.
46. Azari A. Single port TLH+BS for 16 weeks enlarged uterus with cervical fibroid and abdomen-pelvic adhesion. *J Minim Invasive Gynecol* 2014;21(6):S191–S227, 688 Poster Video: Laparoscopic Surgeries.
47. Kliethermes C, Guan X. Single-incision robotic hysterectomy with anterior cervical fibroid. *J Minim Invasive Gynecol* 2016;23(7): S1–S252, 343 Video Session 8 - Robotics.
48. Lee EM, Delgado S, Hendessi P. Surgical approach to a large cervical fibroid. *J Minim Invasive Gynecol* 2019;26(7):S1–S97.
49. Atkin RP, Nimaroff ML, Prabakar C, Egbuniwe M. Total laparoscopic hysterectomy to remove a large cervical fibroid. *J Minim Invasive Gynecol* 2010;17(6), S152–S177, 547.
50. Holloran-Schwartz MB. Total laparoscopic hysterectomy with a large cervical fibroid. *J Minim Invasive Gynecol* 2018;18(6), S71–S90, 254 Video Session 8 Robotics.
51. Kongnyuy EJ, Wiysonge CS. Interventions to reduce haemorrhage during myomectomy for fibroids. Cochrane Database Syst Rev 2009; 3: CD005355. https://doi:10.1002/14651858.CD005355.pub3.
52. Neilson JP. Interventions to reduce haemorrhage during myomectomy for fibroids. *Obstet Gynecol* 2007;109(5):1197–1198.
53. Mishra RK. Laparoscopic removal of posterior cervical fibroid. https://youtu.be/3S82KqfpTFw.
54. Nuri P, Gundogan S, Sendag F. Laparoscopic management of huge cervical myoma. *J Minim Invasive Gynecol.* 2017;24(3):345–346.
55. Sinha R, Sundaram M, Lakhotia S, Hegde A. Cervical myomectomy with uterine artery ligation at its origin. *J Minim Invasive Gynecol.* 2009;16(5):604–608.
56. Pelosi MA and Pelosi MA. Laparoscopic-assisted trans vaginal myomectomy. *J Am Assoc Gynecol Laparosc.* 1997;4:241–246.
57. Torng PL, Hwang JS, Huang SC, Chang WC, Chen SY, Chang DY, Hsu WC. Effect of simultaneous morcellation in situ on operative time during laparoscopic myomectomy. *Hum Reprod* 2008;23(10):2220–2226.
58. Sinha R, Hegde A, Warty N, Mahajan C. Laparoscopic myomectomy: enucleation of the myoma by morcellation while it is attached to the uterus. *J Minim Invasive Gynecol.* 2005;12(3):284–289.
59. Sinha RY, Hegde A, Mahajan C, Dubey N, Warty N, Jain R. Laparoscopic devascularization of uterine myomata followed by enucleation of the myomas by direct morcellation. *J Am Assoc Gynecol Laparosc* 2004;11:99–102.
60. Ahmed Abdelaziz A, Joseph S, Abuzeid M. Broad ligament uterine fibroid: management with da Vinci robotic myomectomy. *MEFSJ* 2016;21(1):65–68.
61. Abuzeid M, Joseph S. Transvaginal ultrasonography of uterine fibroids. In: Ultrasound in Gynecology. Editors: Botros Rizk and Elizabeth Puscheck Cambridge University Press 2014, Chapter 9, 80–93.
62. Breech LL, Rock JA. Leiomyomata uteri and myomectomy. In: *Te Linde's Operative Gynecology.* Rock and Jones III Editors10th ed. Chapter 31, 2014:687–726.
63. Suneja A, Taneja A, Guleria K, Yadav P, Agarwal N. Incarcerated procidentia due to cervical fibroid: an unusual presentation. *Aust N Z J Obstet Gynecol* 2003;43:252–253.
64. Abha M, Kavneet G. Severe adolescent menorrhagia due to cervical fibroid. *J Obstet Gynecol India* 2012;62(5):575–576.
65. Sengupta S, Reddy K, Pillai M. Prolapsed cervical fibroid in pregnancy: a challenging obstetric dilemma. *J Obstet Gynaecol* 2006; 26(8):823–824. https://doi:10.1080/01443610600994684
66. Tripathi U, Agrawal V, Pradhan S. Vaginal myomectomy of a cervical fibroid in term pregnancy. *J Evolution Med Dent Sci* 2013; 2(22):4009–4012.
67. Straub HL, Chohan L, Kilpatrick CC. Cervical and prolapsed submucosal leiomyomas complicating pregnancy. *Obstet Gynecol Surv* 2010;65(9):583–590.
68. Kilpatrick CC, Adler MT, Chohan L. Vaginal myomectomy in pregnancy: a report of two cases. *Southern Med J* 2010; 103(10):1058–1060.

# 14

## SURGICAL MANAGEMENT OF RARE LOCATIONS OF UTERINE FIBROIDS

**Brian F.G. Tesler, Renee Sundstrom, and Mostafa I. Abuzeid**

### Introduction

Leiomyomas of the uterus, or fibroids, are a regular finding in today's gynecological and obstetric setting. They are cited as the most common form of tumor growth in women, and subsequently a leading cause of hysterectomy in the United States. Although morbidity is variant and dependent upon size, location and the number of leiomyomas bring many women to seek care from their gynecologist. It is estimated that a third of all women with fibroids will become symptomatic by the end of their reproductive years [1, 2]. The transformation to a malignant process is rare, however, they still impact lifestyle, sexual interactions, fertility, pregnancy and productivity in a woman's life.

Approximately 75% of uterine leiomyomas are found within or adjacent to the uterine corpus. The locations most noted are [1, 3, 4]:

- Submucosal: Found to protrude in the endometrial cavity
- Intramural: Found embedded within the myometrium
- Subserosal: Under the serosa of the uterus

Occurrences in other locations are known. However, cervical and broad ligament leiomyomas are the most common sites [2–4]. Following the International Federation of Obstetrics and Gynecology (FIGO) system of leiomyoma sub-classification these would fall in the "O – Other" category at number 8 [5]. The occurrences of these rare location leiomyomas are cervical ranging from approximately 2%–3%, and broad ligament representing less than 1% [1, 3, 4]. Other sites can include parasitic, defined as leiomyomas that are not connected to or part of the uterine corpus or immediate adjacent structures. Parasitic type leiomyoma's blood flow is separate, from that which supplies the uterus. These are rare and are often cited as iatrogenically seeded from a myomectomy or other surgery involving non-parasitic processes [6–8]. Other rare locations include vaginal leiomyomas, leiomyoma in a uterine septum and leiomyomatosis peritonealis disseminata.

This chapter will explore the various forms of rare locations of leiomyoma. They will be discussed in accordance to the pathogenesis, diagnosis and management of each type.

### Cervical leiomyomas

As the more common of the rare locations, cervical leiomyomas are found in 2%–3% of leiomyoma cases [1, 4]. These tumors are further classified related to their location (anterior, posterior, lateral and central) (**Figures 14.1** and **14.2**). Some growth of the cervical form can also be found to have an interstitial or a subperitoneal component. Extension and growth in the vaginal canal have also been noted (**Figure 14.3**) [1, 4, 9, 10].

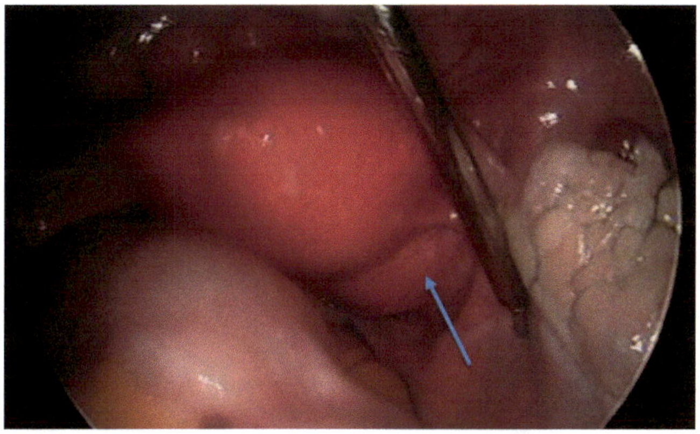

FIGURE 14.1 Large supravaginal sessile subserous posterior cervical fibroid with broad base on the right side (blue arrow).

#### Symptoms and presentation

Patients with cervical leiomyoma can present with various gynecological complaints of a benign or usual nature. Complaints vary from pelvic pain, abnormal bleeding, menstrual irregularities, dyspareunia [1, 3, 11]. The location of the cervical tumor may also produce specific findings. Those with anterior placement often produce urinary symptoms such as retention or frequency; which varies with involvement of the urethra. A posterior placement can elicit rectal pressure and constipation [1, 3, 11]. An obstetric complication of dystocia is uniquely related to the cervical form of these leiomyoma as they can obstruct the vaginal outlet [1, 11]. Lateral growth or displacement from mass effect can lead to nerve or lymphatic complications of the pelvic and lower extremity regions adjacent to the growth [11].

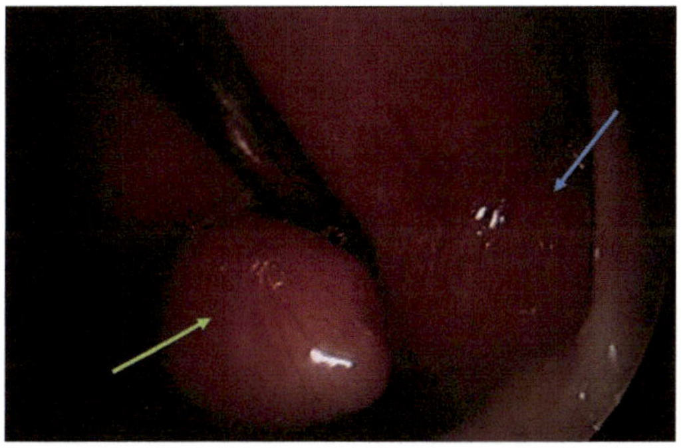

FIGURE 14.2 A close up of the posterior cervical fibroid (blue arrow) in **Figure 14.1** and a small pedunculated cervical subserous fibroid is also seen medial and superior to the sessile cervical fibroid (green arrow).

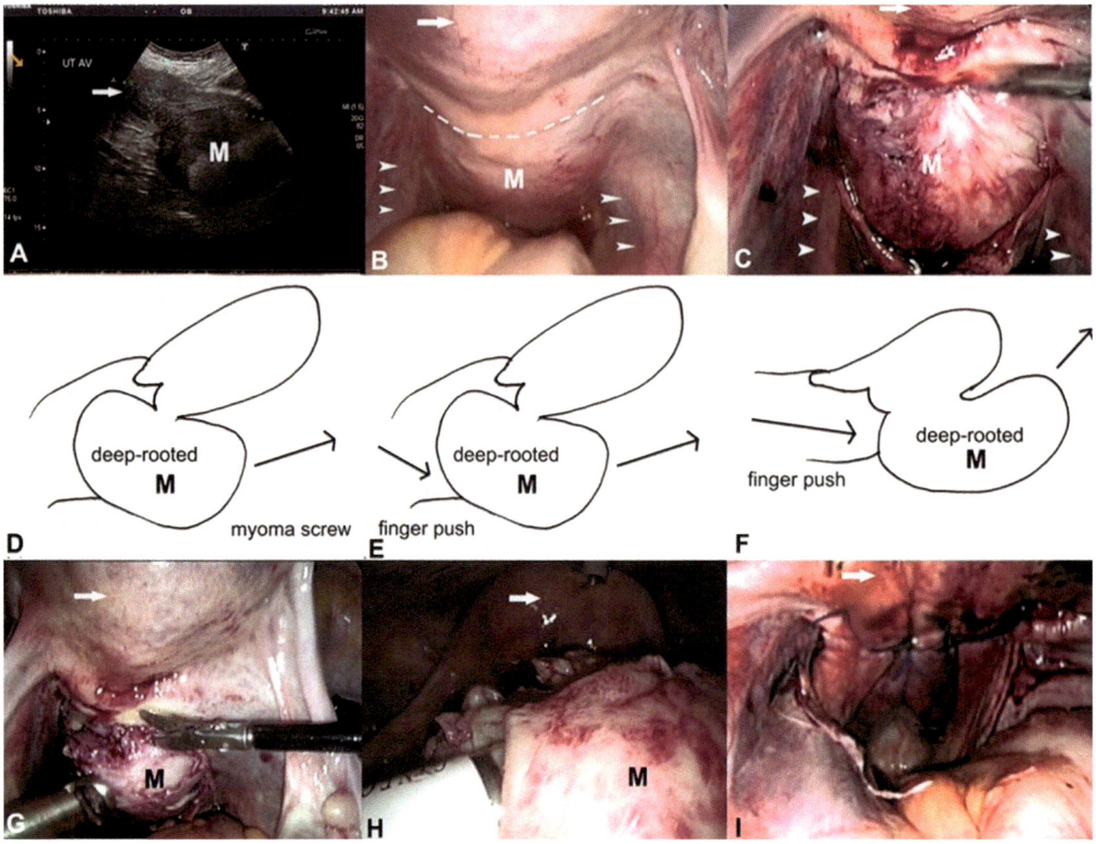


FIGURE 14.3 Laparoscopic myomectomy in a deep-rooted cervical myoma. (A) Preoperative ultrasonographic image shows the myoma projecting into the vagina (arrow, ¼ uterine body; M, ¼ myoma). (B) The main part of myoma is deep-rooted in the vagina. The dotted line indicates the incision and the arrowheads indicate the bilateral ureters. (C) A transverse incision is made just below the uterine body. (D, G) Attempts to expose the myoma with the aid of a myoma screw have failed. (E, F) The cervical myoma is pushed upward manually in the direction of abdominal cavity. (H) Morcellation is performed. (I) The wound is sutured with two-layer interrupted sutures. (By permission from Chang WC et al. Fertil Steril. 2010:94(7)2710–5.)

### Diagnosis and differential

The cervical location lends itself to a differential diagnosis of:

- Cervical polyp
- Pedunculated submucosal fibroid
- Cervical malignancy
- Malignancy of adjacent organs
- Melanoma of the vaginal origin with cervical involvement (Rare)

The diagnosis would be achieved through clinical evaluation followed by imaging if not evident in the examination. Procedural biopsy or surgical removal would give sampling for histopathological examination and confirmation.

### Imaging

The location of these masses does not change the most accepted imaging modality for leiomyoma examination using ultrasonography (US) and magnetic resonance imaging (MRI) [11]. The use and low cost of ultrasound allows for location inspection and proximity and involvement in adjacent structures. An MRI is known for providing detailed evaluation regarding the origin of cervical submucosal fibroids and its location relative to the rest of the uterus and surrounding structures. Another added benefit of the MRI is a more precise evaluation of involvement of rectum, bladder and endometrium [4, 11].

### Management

Before proceeding with surgical intervention, a shared decision-making model should be used regarding the patient's desire for future fertility. After this decision is made, next considerations would be the size, location and involvement with adjacent structures. The sessile and well circumscribed, accessible tumor can be managed with vaginal approach myomectomy. The more accessible tumor originates from the vaginal effacing portion of the cervix. If pedunculated, a polypectomy approach may be taken for its removal [1, 11]. Lateral masses can also have myomectomy attempted if they lend themselves to access and involvement in the tissues beyond the cervix is known. The latter can usually be done through imaging evaluation preoperatively.

If fertility is no longer desired or access is limited by anatomy, then hysterectomy is used as the most common approach. The central cervical tumor is usually approached in the aforementioned manner. The blood supply to the actual leiomyoma by anatomical development is low. However, the cervix and adjacent tissues are rich in vascularity [1, 11, 12].

## Broad ligament leiomyomas

Broad ligament leiomyomas, also known as intra-ligamentary, are a rare form of leiomyoma. Found within or adjacent to the broad ligament they represent approximately less than 1% of

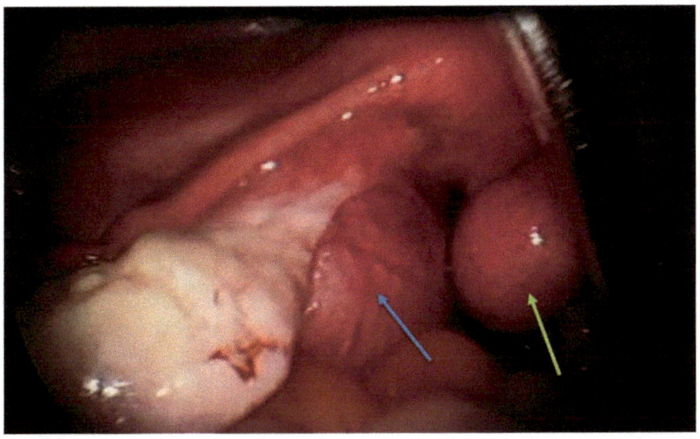

**FIGURE 14.4** A large left broad ligament supravaginal cervical fibroid pushing the uterus to the right (blue arrow) and a small subserous pedunculated fibroid attached to posterior wall of the upper uterine segment (green arrow).

leiomyoma. Based on the origin of the broad ligament leiomyoma, such tumors are divided into two main categories: true broad ligaments and false broad ligaments leiomyomas. True broad ligaments leiomyomas are derived from the muscular fibers of the mesometrium and are commonly located in the round ligament, utero-ovarian ligament, within supporting connective tissue of the ovary and the uterine vessels. The false broad ligament tumors originate from the lateral wall of the uterus and cervix (**Figure 14.4**) [1, 4, 12, 13].

## Symptoms and presentation

Broad ligament tumors are found to often be symptomatic with abdominal distension, menstrual irregularities, dysmenorrhea, dyspareunia. These presentations are due to mass related effects. However, unique to broad ligament tumor is the lateral extension towards the ureters (**Figure 14.4**). The compression effect on the ureters may lead to ipsilateral hydroureter, hydronephrosis, increased frequency of urinary tract infection and other urological symptoms [1, 13].

The broad ligament tumors present special complications related to their size and location. The following can be uniquely related to these tumors [13]:

- Ovarian torsion
- Cystic degeneration that appears as ovarian malignancy
- Pseudo-Meig's syndrome
- Acute abdomen presentation from large growing tumors
- Hydroureter and hydronephrosis

## Diagnosis and differential

The location of the broad ligament lends itself to a differential diagnosis of [1, 4, 13]:

- Tubo-ovarian mass
- Ovarian neoplasm (with solid components)
- Ovarian malignancy
- Brenner tumor
- Ligamentous mesenchymal tumors
- Neurofibromatosis pelvic tumor
- Pedunculated subserosal with lateral or projection towards the broad ligament
- Parasitic leiomyoma that has involvement with the broad ligament
- Hydrosalpinx
- Ectopic pregnancy

The diagnosis would be achieved through clinical evaluation followed by imaging if not evident in the examination. Procedural biopsy or surgical removal would give sampling for histopathological examination and confirmation.

## Imaging

Transvaginal 2D ultrasound (TV 2D US) is usually the first imaging study to be done once a pelvic mass is found on pelvic examination. Once a broad ligament leiomyoma is suspected on TV 2D US, more imaging studies are needed to confirm the diagnosis and to help in the management. With broad ligament leiomyoma the imaging modality frequently utilized is MRI [4, 13]. The ability to examine multiplanar views increases the ability to find the origin location and involved structures. An important distinction derived from MRI is whether the mass is involved with the cervix, ureters, bladder, ovaries, tubes or a combination of these structures.

Often intravenous pyelography accompanies other imaging modalities to further evaluate the urinary tract, as often uterine anomalies accompany anomalies of the urinary tract. Concurrent urinary tract anomalies have been cited with incidence as high as 30% [1, 4, 13].

## Management

Often the management of the true broad ligament fibroids, with narrowing or delineation from the cervix and uterus is myomectomy. This is especially true in larger fibroids causing compression syndromes, no other fibroids of uterine origin, signs of degeneration, and those that wish to preserve fertility [1, 12, 13].

If hysterectomy is being considered this is often due to requests of definitive management from the patient, with or without simultaneous uterine originated tumors. If there is any suspicion of malignancy, a hysterectomy is usually performed and often with a gynecological oncologist's co-management. Other findings that suggest hysterectomy as treatment is involvement of endometrial or cervical lesions.

## Leiomyoma in a uterine septum

One of the rarest forms of leiomyoma locations is in the uterine septum. Uterine septum is the most common of all Müllerian anomalies, as it accounts for 55% of such anomalies [14]. The incidence of uterine septum is estimated to be 3.9% in infertile patients [15]. Published data indicate an improvement in reproductive outcome after hysteroscopic division of uterine septum [16, 17]. Previous reports suggested that it may be difficult to diagnose uterine septum on TV 3D US in the presence of leimyoma [18, 19]. The presence of a leiomyoma in a uterine septum is very rare in the literature. In fact, there are only five case reports of such association in the English literature (three manuscripts and two published abstracts) [20–24].

## Clinical presentation

Patients who have a complete uterine septum, an incomplete uterine septum or a significant arcuate uterine anomaly may present with history of infertility, recurrent pregnancy loss or history of bad obstetric history [22]. However, some of these patients may have had no difficulty conceiving and a normal obstetric history. If the patient is not trying to conceive, she may be asymptomatic and such anomalies may only be diagnosed during TV 2D or 3D US. However, patients with both uterine septum and leiomyoma in the septum may also present with symptoms and signs related to the fibroid. Such clinical presentation may include menorrhagia, dysmenorrheal and pelvic pain depending on size, location and type of fibroid.

## Diagnosis

TV 2D and 3D US with and without saline infusion sonohysterography (SIH) are the first line for diagnosis of uterine fibroid and uterine septum. However, previous investigators suggested that TV 3D US may not be accurate in the diagnosis of uterine septum in the presence of uterine fibroid [18]. In addition, other investigators reported on the difficulty encountered during the diagnosis of uterine septum in the presence of uterine fibroids [19]. MRI may help in detecting such anomalies (when suspected) in patients who were found to have leiomyoma on TV 2D and 3D US. In addition, MRI will help in determining the location of the fibroid and its type. MRI may clearly show if a submucosal fibroid is Type II (with more than 50% of the fibroid is in the myometrium), according to the European Society for Gynecological Endoscopy (ESGE) classification and FIGO classification [5, 25]. Such information is needed to determine whether it can be removed hysteroscopically, or whether it is safer to remove it laparoscopically. Diagnostic hysteroscopy is needed to confirm the diagnosis of uterine septum or significant uterine anomaly [26, 27]. In fact, the presence of a leiomyoma in the uterine septum or at the base of the septum can only be confirmed during operative hysteroscopy and hysteroscopic division of the uterine septum/arcuate uterine anomaly [23, 24].

## Treatment

The management of concurrent uterine fibroids and uterine septum or significant arcuate uterus will depend on a patient's clinical presentation, her desire for future fertility and size and type of the fibroid. If the patient has no desire for further fertility, and has no symptoms one may continue observation. Observation may also be adopted if the patient has no symptoms and such concomitant pathology is not affecting her reproductive performance. On the other hand, surgical treatment should be considered if a patient with this concurrent pathology is symptomatic, having difficulty conceiving or maintaining a pregnancy or had an unexplained bad obstetric history [22–24]. Diagnostic hysteroscopy should be done first to confirm the diagnosis, which should be followed by hysteroscopic division of the uterine septum or the significant arcuate uterine anomaly as previously described [16]. In brief, a straight resectoscope loop electrode is used to divide the uterine septum in its mid portion, utilizing a monopolar system. A zero degree or 12-degree hysteroscope should be used. Glycine 1.5% or any other non-electrolyte solution should be used as a distension medium if monopolar current is used. Normal saline can be used if bipolar current is utilized. The authors of this chapter suggest a cutting current of 70 watts and a coagulation current of 50 watts with a blend of 1. The procedure of septum division is considered complete when the operator is able to move the tip of the straight resectoscope loop electrode from the area of one tubal ostium to the other without any resistance. The authors of this chapter prefer to use an ACMI hysteroscope (Division of Olympus; Maple Grove, MN, USA). Once the uterine fibroid that is embedded at the base of the uterine anomaly is visualized a hysteroscopic myomectomy should be performed in a routine fashion as described previously [23, 24]. In brief, the straight resectoscope loop can be used to slice the fibroid into 2 pieces (**Figure 14.5**). Thereafter, a straight or a right angled resectoscope loop can then be utilized to re-sect the fibroid free from the base of the uterine septum (**Figure 14.6**). If the fibroid that is present at the base of the septum is large or is near the serosal layer, it is imperative to do the hysteroscopic myomectomy under laparoscopic observation of the uterine fundus to avoid uterine perforation and other complications. A Pediatric Foley catheter (size 8 French) should be placed inside the endometrial cavity and its balloon should be filled with 3 cc of normal saline at the conclusion of the procedure in an attempt to reduce intra uterine scar tissue formation [28]. The catheter should be removed after 7 days. Oral Estrogen should be started 2 days after surgery and continued for 6 weeks. Oral Progestogen should be added during the last 10 days of Estrogen course. The patient should undergo a TV 2D and 3D US with SIH 8 weeks after surgery for evaluation of the endometrial cavity.

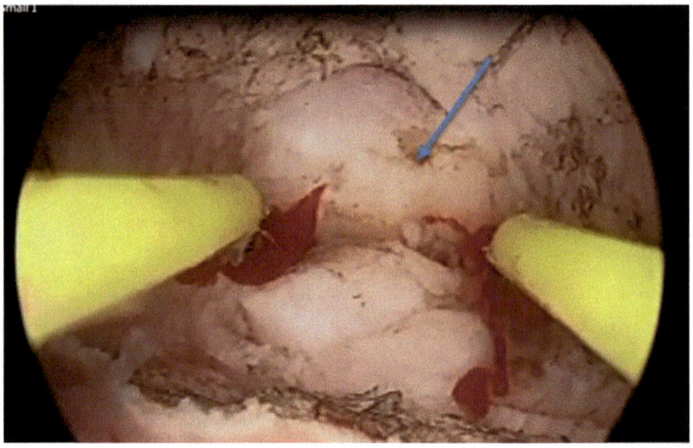

**FIGURE 14.5** Use of a straight resectoscope loop to slice the fibroid embedded at the base of the divided uterine septum into two pieces (blue arrow).

Reproductive surgeons should also be aware, that operative hysteroscopy is the most accurate method to make the diagnosis of this concurrent pathology. Therefore, the authors of this chapter believe that reproductive surgeons and gynecologists should be familiar with this scenario prior to performing hysteroscopic division of a uterine septum. This is especially the case, if there is evidence of uterine fibroids somewhere else in the uterus and division of the septum is being performed using a hysteroscopic scissor. The operator should be prepared to change the operative hysteroscope to a hysteroscopic resectoscope to be able to complete the procedure and remove the fibroid as described above.

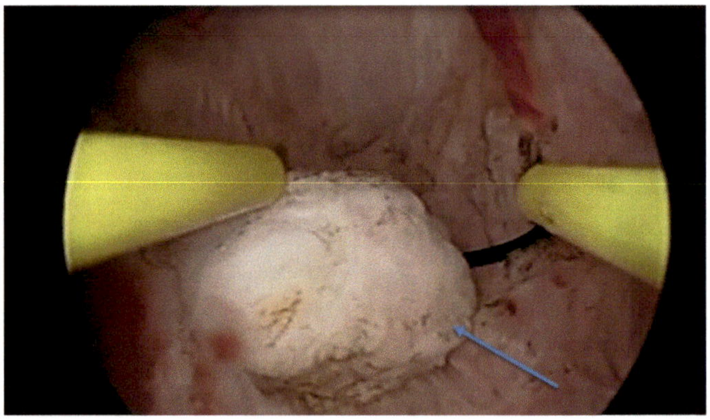

**FIGURE 14.6** Use of a straight resectoscope loop to resect one portion of the fibroid sliced into two pieces in **Figure 14.5** (blue arrow).

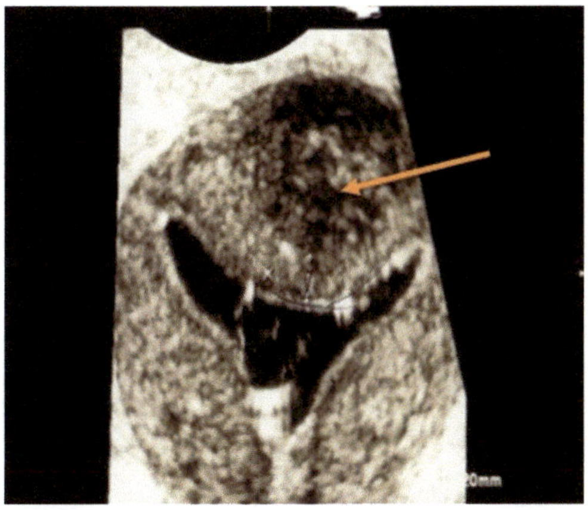

**FIGURE 14.7** Transvaginal 3D ultrasound with saline infusion hysterosonography showing a 3 × 2 cm submucosal intramural subserosal fundal fibroid (Type II submucosal fibroid by ESGE classification and Type 2-5 by FIGO classification) (orange arrow). (From Abuzeid, M., and Joseph, S. (2014). Transvaginal ultrasonography of uterine fibroids. In B. Rizk and E. Puscheck (Eds.), *Ultrasonography in Gynecology* (pp. 80–93). Cambridge: Cambridge University Press. doi:10.1017/9781139342544.010. With permission.)

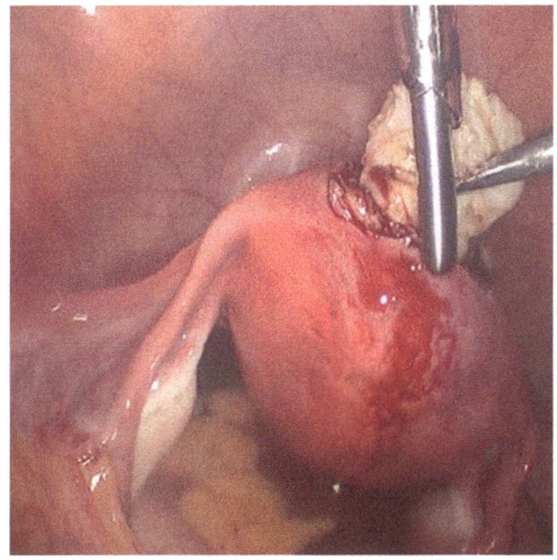

**FIGURE 14.9** Laparoscopy of dissection of the fundal uterine fibroid, seen in **Figure 14.8**. (From Abuzeid, M., Joseph, S. (2014). Transvaginal ultrasonography of uterine fibroids. In B. Rizk and E. Puscheck (Eds.), *Ultrasonography in Gynecology* (pp. 80–93). Cambridge: Cambridge University Press. doi:10.1017/9781139342544.010. With permission.)

Another scenario of this concurrent pathology can occur with a fundal fibroid that is large and Type II submucosal fibroid in nature according to the ESGE classification or type 2-5 according to FIGO classification (**Figure 14.7**) [22]. A submucosal fibroid type 2-5 by FIGO classification is a hybrid leiomyoma that impact both endometrium and serosa. In such patient surgical correction should be attempted if the patient desires future fertility or has a history of infertility or an unexplained recurrent pregnancy loss. In such cases surgical correction requires a two-step procedure. The first procedure should be a laparoscopic or robotic-assisted laparoscopic myomectomy (**Figures 14.8–14.12**) [22]. Three to four months later one may proceed with hysteroscopic division of uterine septum or significant arcuate uterus (**Figure 14.13 a,b**). A previous report detailed the surgical management of a patient with recurrent pregnancy loss secondary with an incomplete uterine septum and a large Type II submucosal fibroid by ESGE classification (Type 2-5 by FIGO classification) [22]. The patient had a two-step procedure as described above [22]. She subsequently was able to deliver two babies.

## Vaginal leiomyomas

The vagina is indeed a rare location for leiomyomas. Since first recognized by Denys de Leyden in 1733, approximately 300 cases have been reported in the literature. Vaginal leiomyomas

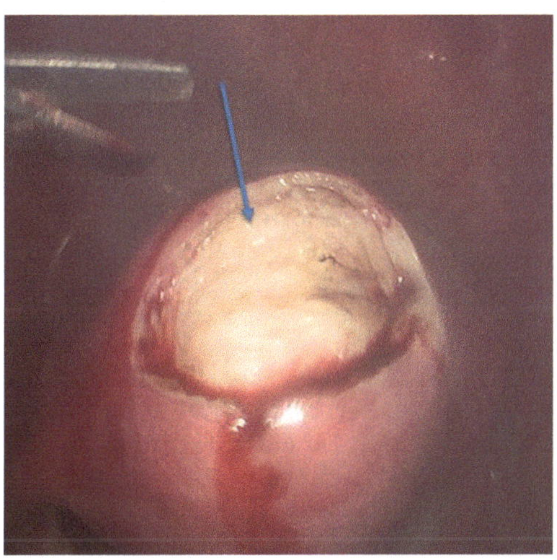

**FIGURE 14.8** Laparoscopy of the upper portion of the fibroid seen in **Figure 14.7** (blue arrow) after a transverse incision is made in the fundal region.

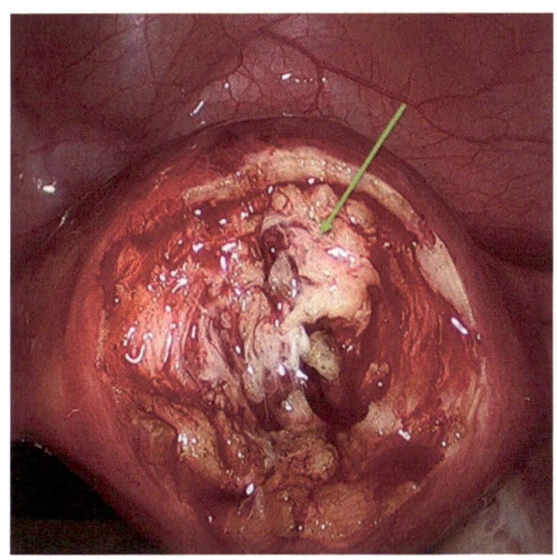

**FIGURE 14.10** Laparoscopy of the myometrial defect after removal of the fundal uterine fibroid seen in **Figure 14.9** (green arrow). (From Abuzeid, M., Joseph, S. (2014). Transvaginal ultrasonography of uterine fibroids. In B. Rizk and E. Puscheck (Eds.), *Ultrasonography in Gynecology* (pp. 80–93). Cambridge: Cambridge University Press. doi:10.1017/9781139342544.010. With permission.)

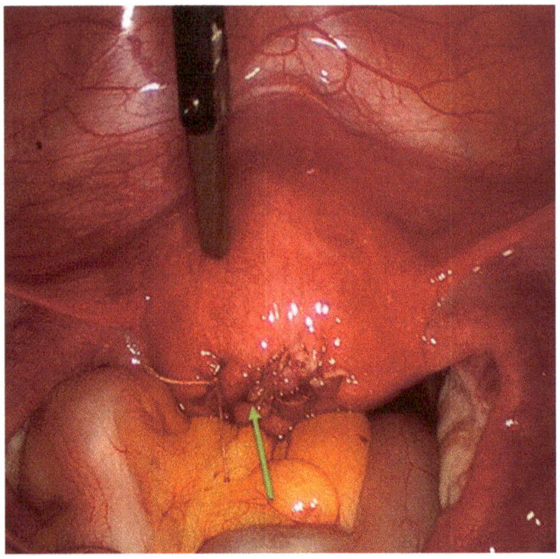

**FIGURE 14.11** Laparoscopy of the end result after the myometrial defect seen in **Figure 14.10** was sutured in two layers (green arrow). (From Abuzeid, M., Joseph, S. (2014). Transvaginal ultrasonography of uterine fibroids. In B. Rizk and E. Puscheck (Eds.), *Ultrasonography in Gynecology* (pp. 80–93). Cambridge: Cambridge University Press. doi:10.1017/9781139342544.010. With permission.)

generally present in women between the ages of 30 and 50, with greater incidence in Caucasian women. This is in contrast to uterine leiomyoma, which are more common in non-Caucasian females [9, 29].

## Symptoms and presentation

Vaginal leiomyomas arise most commonly from the midline anterior vaginal wall, and less often from the posterior or lateral walls. They typically present as a single, well-circumscribed mass and may be near the bladder or urethra. Because of the anterior wall location, these masses may be misdiagnosed as a urethral diverticulum or paraurethral cyst [30]. Although most leiomyomas of the vagina are within the wall and expand into the vagina, in some instances they may be pedunculated and protrude into the vagina, attached to the wall by a stalk. The appearance may vary from the classic solid tumor to a mass with solid and cystic components. They are generally benign and slow-growing; rapid growth may indicate a sarcomatous tumor [9]. Similar to their uterine counterparts, vaginal myomas are thought to be estrogen-dependent because they demonstrate growth in pregnancy and the reproductive years, but regress after menopause [31, 32].

The size and location of vaginal leiomyomas determine the symptomatology. With an intravaginal location of a myoma many patients are asymptomatic until the myoma reaches a fairly large size. At this point the patient may complain of low abdominal, pelvic, low back pain, or a combination of these. Symptoms of vaginal pressure, vaginal bleeding or dyspareunia may signal a vaginal mass [9]. Leiomyomas within the vaginal wall can protrude from the vagina, mimicking a uterine prolapse [32]. Tumors arising in the lower anterior vaginal wall may present with urinary symptoms such as dysuria, frequency, urgency and urinary obstruction [33].

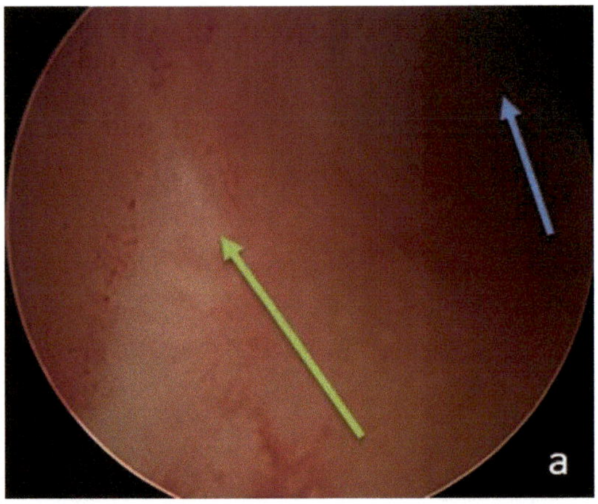

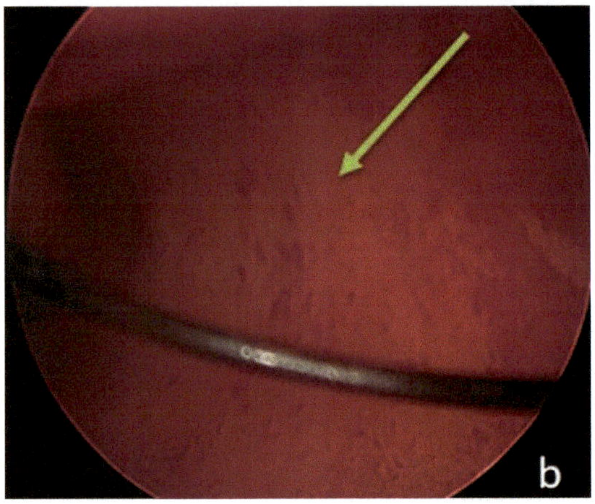

**FIGURE 14.13** (a) Hysteroscopy 18 months after laparoscopic myomectomy showing the left cornual region with tubal ostium (blue arrow) and left portion of an incomplete short uterine septum (green arrow). (b) Hysteroscopy 18 months after laparoscopic myomectomy showing a straight resectoscope loop just before starting dividing the incomplete short uterine septum (green arrow).

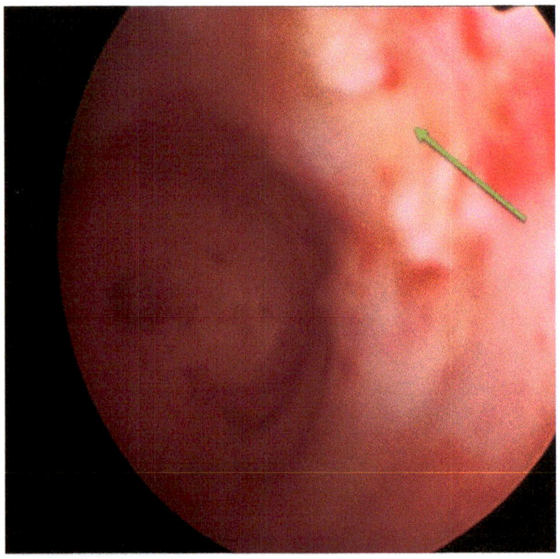

**FIGURE 14.12** Hysteroscopy of the conclusion of the laparoscopic myomectomy showing the right cornual region with tubal ostium and right portion of a possible incomplete short uterine septum (green arrow). (From Abuzeid, M., Joseph, S. (2014). Transvaginal ultrasonography of uterine fibroids. In B. Rizk and E. Puscheck (Eds.), *Ultrasonography in Gynecology* (pp. 80–93). Cambridge: Cambridge University Press. doi:10.1017/9781139342544.010. With permission.)

### Diagnosis and differential

The diagnosis of a vaginal leiomyoma is made by physical examination in conjunction with imaging [34]. On visual inspection and palpation, the mass is typically smooth, firm, non-tender and non-fluctuant. In some instances, vaginal bleeding may be present because of an exposed, pedunculated or prolapsed myoma.

The rare nature of leiomyomas in this area may make the diagnosis more challenging. The differential diagnosis varies with the location of the myoma and includes urethral diverticulum, polyp, cystocele, Skene duct abscess, or even vaginal malignancy. Cystic masses such as Gartner duct cysts, vaginal cysts and Bartholin gland cysts should also be included in the differential [33, 34].

Tissue biopsy may be indicated when the diagnosis is unclear or there is concern for malignancy [33]. Ultimately, histopathologic diagnosis of the excised mass is necessary to confirm benign leiomyoma and is considered the gold standard [9, 29].

### Imaging

Ultrasonography is one modality used for diagnosis, and a transvaginal 2-D or 3D approach may provide a better image due to the location. MRI is considered the best imaging technique and shows a classic whorled appearance within a well-circumscribed mass. The myoma demonstrates a hypointense or isointense signal compared with muscle on T1-weighted images. T2-weighted images demonstrate a hyperintense to isointense signal. Administration of gadolinium contrast results in homogeneous uptake. Degenerating myomas may take on a more heterogeneous appearance due to edema, cystic change and myxoid degeneration. Leiomyosarcomas and other vaginal malignancies also appear irregular and heterogeneous, due to necrosis and hemorrhage [10].

### Management

In the majority of clinical situations involving vaginal leiomyomas, surgical excision is the recommended treatment. This is usually accomplished with a vaginal approach. With the anterior vaginal wall location being most common, the surgeon must take care to protect the urethra and bladder. Placement of a Foley catheter during surgery helps delineate these structures [9, 33, 35].

Larger fibroids located in the upper portion of the vagina may require a combined abdomino-perineal approach or a laparoscopic-perineal approach. A case report of a vaginal leiomyosarcoma in the upper portion of the vagina was successfully treated with a robotic-assisted radical hysterectomy and upper vaginal tumor resection [36]. These more difficult cases may benefit from preoperative procedures to decrease the size of the myoma and potentially decrease surgical blood loss. These preoperative adjuncts include embolization of the mass [30], or the use of a pharmacologic agent such as a gonadotropin-releasing agonist/antagonist or selective progesterone-receptor modulator [34].

Recurrence of vaginal leiomyoma is uncommon, but the practitioner should be aware of this possibility and consider this in the evaluation of a new mass in the same region. If the leiomyoma is recurrent, it has been suggested that bilateral oophorectomy may be indicated in a premenopausal woman to reduce estrogen levels and prevent further issues [32].

## Parasitic leiomyomas

Another rare entity, parasitic leiomyomas may arise spontaneously or may be the result of an iatrogenic process. The classic definition of a parasitic leiomyoma is a subserosal fibroid, usually pedunculated, which twists on its stalk and becomes detached from the uterus. It then attaches to intra-abdominal structures and acquires new blood supply from those structures [6]. Common sites for the development of these tumors are the broad ligament and omentum [6, 7, 37]. However, case reports in the literature describe parasitic myomas with blood supply from vascular structures such as the iliac artery, the inferior epigastric artery, bowel and mesentery [7, 37–39].

The advent of minimally invasive surgical techniques for myomectomy and hysterectomy has introduced the potential for iatrogenic parasitic fibroids [40]. Non-confined morcellation of fibroids, whether via powered instrumentation or traditional morcellation techniques, creates small fibroid fragments which may adhere to abdominal structures, become vascularized, and grow [40].

### Symptoms and presentation

The location and size of parasitic leiomyomas drives symptomatology. When the fibroids are small, they are asymptomatic and may be an incidental finding on imaging or during surgery for another indication [39]. Larger myomas may cause abdominal or pelvic pain, pelvic/abdominal pressure, abdominal distention, urinary symptoms, constipation, dyspareunia and sometimes vaginal bleeding [8, 39]. Myomas located within or near the anterior abdominal wall may present with a palpable abdominal mass [38, 41]. Unusual presentations include small bowel obstruction and laparoscopic port-site masses [39, 40].

Parasitic myomas may be found throughout the abdomen with common sites being the abdominal wall, pelvic cavity/wall, small intestines, cecum, rectum, vaginal cuff or cervical stump [8]. The widespread nature of these sites of implantation is explained by the seeding that can occur with morcellation at the time of hysterectomy or myomectomy. The cited incidence of parasitic fibroids following laparoscopic myomectomy is approximately 0.2%–1.25% with a median time to diagnosis being around 48 months [8]. It is noted that a laparoscopic procedure carries a greater risk of postoperative parasitic myomas compared to a laparotomy [38].

### Diagnosis and differential

The diagnosis of a parasitic leiomyoma begins with a thorough history and physical exam with focus on surgical history because of the relation to leiomyoma morcellation [41]. The differential diagnosis includes both benign and malignant tumors of the uterus, ovary, intestine, musculature and other intra-abdominal or retroperitoneal organs depending on the location of the mass or masses [37, 41].

Imaging is an important diagnostic tool used to pinpoint the location of the myoma and assess characteristics that may raise suspicion of malignancy. In some instances, tumor markers such as CA-125, alpha-fetoprotein, and CA 19-9 may be helpful in ruling out a malignant process [8]. Biopsy of the mass is an option and may be beneficial in planning treatment, but the final diagnosis is made by histologic evaluation and confirmation of benign leiomyoma [8, 37].

### Imaging

Imaging modalities for parasitic leiomyomas are similar to those used to evaluate the pelvic organs. Abdominal and pelvic ultrasound may be the initial choice, as well as computed tomography scanning of the abdomen and pelvis [8, 37]. However, MRI is the best choice for delineation of the mass from soft tissues in the abdomen and pelvis [37]. As with vaginal leiomyomas, parasitic myomas are typically well-circumscribed and demonstrate a whorled appearance. The T1-weighted images demonstrate low to intermediate signal intensity with T2-weighted images also showing a low intensity signal. Variations in signal intensity are seen with degeneration of the myoma and cystic or myxomatous changes [37].

### Management

Parasitic myomas are best treated with surgical exploration and excision. If the mass or masses are small and asymptomatic, close follow-up with symptom surveillance, examination, and imaging may be appropriate [8]. However, larger symptomatic masses will require surgical intervention. The size, multiplicity and location of the mass or masses will dictate an open laparotomy or minimally invasive laparoscopic approach [40]. The availability of a multidisciplinary surgical team may be advisable depending on the location of the myoma and which adjacent structures may be involved [8]. The excised mass should be sent for histopathologic evaluation to confirm the diagnosis of benign parasitic leiomyoma.

Given the association of iatrogenic parasitic leiomyomas with morcellation (especially power morcellation) of fibroids at laparoscopic myomectomy or hysterectomy, the use of a specimen bag for contained morcellation is a reasonable option. Inspection and irrigation of the pelvis and abdomen may aid in identification and removal of any remaining fragments of fibroid tissue that could potentially seed the abdominal cavity [8]. The American College of Obstetricians and Gynecologists recommend that preoperative discussions should include the potential for spread and implantation of tissue when planning the surgical approach for myomectomy or hysterectomy in a patient with uterine fibroids [7].

### Leiomyomatosis peritonealis disseminata

Leiomyomatosis Peritonealis Disseminata (LPD) is one of the rarest forms of extrauterine pathology. Very few cases to date have been reported. This is the presence of multiple sub peritoneal and peritoneal surface myomatous nodules. Common findings in this location include peritoneal surfaces and the omentum [42]. The process is usually reported in premenopausal women and found to be benign. Although there are variances in reporting, these tumors are found to be of smooth muscle in origin and co-existing with and without uterine fibroids concurrently [42].

### Symptoms and presentation

Most documented case presentations note the lesions are found incidentally by examination, or more commonly, in imaging initiated for other pathological work-up [42]. If symptoms were reported, they were often described as abdominal girth increase, abdominal mass or distension [42]. Due to the rare presentation of the disease, and being mostly found incidentally, it is most likely underdiagnosed.

### Diagnosis and differential

The differential for this process is often isolated to ruling out malignancy and metastatic processes when noted. Included in this work-up would include pathology such as carcinomatosis peritonealis and abdominal disseminated malignancy possibly related to a gastrointestinal or ovarian source [42]. However, the disease is not part of the differential in most cases. Because of this, it does not usually appear with signs and symptoms, and if it does, they are broad in nature.

The diagnosis relies on identification of lesions during the examination or imaging. Once noted, then an invasive means of collecting tissue, such as a biopsy, would be completed followed by histopathological examination which would reveal findings consistent with smooth muscle tumors [42].

### Management

As stated, few cases present with complications or complaints and are often incidentally noted. The ascertainment of definitive diagnosis would be warranted if found to rule out a malignant process. Some authors favor open surgical forms of sampling as opposed to interventional radiology methods because vascular lesions tend to be quite dynamic when bleeding occurs [42, 43].

## Conclusion

This chapter has explored some of the leiomyoma encountered in rare locations. In general, these tumors are handled through medical, and surgical intervention much like their more traditionally located uterine corporal lesions. However, the unique complications, considerations for patient fertility and surgical management are well noted in the literature. This lends to the demand for increased knowledge, and practice that we have reviewed here.

## References


1. Berek JS. In: Berek & Novak's Gynecology, Lippincott Williams & Wilkins, Philadelphia, 2007.
2. Kumar P, and Malhotra N. Jeffcoate's Principles of Gynecology. 7th ed. Jaypee Brothers Medical Publishers (P) Ltd., New Delhi, 2008.
3. Buttram VC Jr and Reiter RC. Uterine leiomyomata: etiology, symptomatology, and management. *Fertil Steril.* 1981;36:433–45.
4. Arleo EK, Schwartz PE, Hui P, McCarthy S. Review of leiomyoma variants. *AJR.* 2015;205(4):912–21.
5. Munro MG, Critchley HOD, Broder MS, Fraser IS. FIGO classification system (PALM-COEIN) for causes of abnormal uterine bleeding in nongravid women of reproductive age. *Int J Gynecol Obstet.* 2011;113(1):3–13. https://doi-org.proxy2.cl.msu.edu/10.1016/j.ijgo.2010.11.011
6. Dashraath P, Lim LM, Huang Z, Llancheran A. Parasitic leiomyoma. *AJOG.* 2016;215(5):665.e1–665.e2.
7. Khan A, Shawl, A, Leung PS. Parasitic leiomyoma of the greater omentum presenting as small bowel obstruction. *J Surg Case Rep.* 2018; 2018(7):rjy164. https://doi.org/10.1093/jscr/rjy164
8. Putran J, Khaled K. Parasitic leiomyomas: two case reports and review of literature. *Gynecol Surg.* 2010;7:383–4.
9. Chakrabarti I, De A, Pati S. Vaginal leiomyoma. *J Midlife Health.* 2011;2(1):42–3. https://doi:10.4103/0976-7800.83274
10. Hubert KC, Remer EM, Rackley RR, Goldman HB. Clinical and magnetic resonance imaging characteristics of vaginal and paraurethral leiomyomas: can they be diagnosed before surgery? *BJU Int.* 2010;105(12):1686–88.
11. Tiltman, AJ. Leiomyomas of the uterine cervix: a study of frequency. *Int J Gynecol Pathol.* 1998;17:231–4.
12. American College of Obstetricians and Gynecologists (ACOG) Committee on Practice Bulletins—Gynecology with the assistance of Elizabeth A. Stewart, MD., Clinical Management Guidelines for Obstetricians Gynecologists, Practice Bulletin 96, 2008.
13. Monaghan JM, Lopes T, Naik R. Total hysterectomy for cervical and broad ligament fibroids. In: Bonney's Gynecological Surgery, 10th ed. Wiley-Blackwell Publishing, 2004.
14. Acien P. Reproductive performance of women with uterine malformations. *Hum Reprod.* 1993;8:122–6.
15. Saravelos SH, Cocksedge KA, Li TC. Prevalence and diagnosis of congenital uterine anomalies in women with reproductive failure: a critical appraisal. *Hum Reprod Update.* 2008;14(5):415–29.
16. Abuzeid M, Ghourab G, Abuzeid O, Mitwally M, Ashraf M, Diamond M. Reproductive outcome after IVF following hysteroscopic division of incomplete uterine septum/arcuate uterine anomaly in women with primary infertility. *Facts Views Vis Obgyn.* 2014;6(4):194–202.
17. Daly DC, Maier D, Soto-Albors C. Hysteroscopic metroplasty: six years experience. *Obstet Gynecol.* 1989;73:201–529.

18. Kupesic S. Clinical implications of sonographic detection of uterine anomalies for reproductive outcome. *Ultrasound Obstet Gynecol.* 2001;18:387–400.
19. Abdulaziz A, Zaghmout O, Ashraf M, Abuzeid M. The preoperative dilemma in establishing the diagnosis of uterine anomalies when simultaneously present with fibroids. *J Minim Invasive Gynecol.* 2014, 21, S91-S135:446.
20. Caliskan E, Cakiroglu Y, Turkoz E, Corakci A. Leiomyoma on the septum of a septate uterus with double cervix and vaginal septum: a challenge to manage. *Fertil Steril.* 2008;89:456.e3–7.
21. Iwase A, Goto M, Manabe S, Kobayashi H, Kondo M, Kikkawa F. Surgical management of a septate uterus constricted with leiomyomas: hysteroscopic metroplasty using a Foley catheter. *Arch Gynecol Obstet.* 2013;287:835–6.
22. Javaid H, Ashraf M, Abuzeid M. Management dilemma of concurrent fundal submucous fibroid and incomplete uterine septum in a patient with recurrent pregnancy loss. *Gynecol Surg.* 2013; 29(3):165–8.
23. Abuzeid O, Hebert J, Abuzeid M. Surgical management of small uterine fibroids that were found embedded in a significant arcuate uterine anomaly and in incomplete uterine septum. *J Minim Invasive Gynecol.* 2017;24(7), Supplement, Page S142. https://doi.org/10.1016/j.jmig.2017.08.409
24. Abuzeid O, Hebert J, Abuzeid M. Surgical management of a large leiomyoma embedded in a complete uterine septum. *J Minim Invasive Gynecol.* 2017;24(7), Supplement, Page S180. https://doi.org/10.1016/j.jmig.2017.08.580
25. Wamsteker K, Emanuel MH, deKruif JH. Transcervical hysteroscopic resection of submucous fibroids for abnormal uterine bleeding: results regarding the degree of intramural extension. *Obstet Gynecol.* 1993;82:736.
26. Abuzeid O, LaChance J, Zaghmout O, Corrado J, Hebert J, Ashraf M, Abuzeid MI. The role of diagnostic hysteroscopy in diagnosis of incomplete uterine septum/significant arcuate uterine anomaly in infertile patients in the era of transvaginal 3D ultrasound scan. *Middle East Fertil Soc J.* 2020;25:1.
27. Abuzeid O, LaChance J, Hebert J, Abuzeid MI, Welch R. The role of diagnostic hysteroscopy in diagnosis of incomplete uterine septum in patients with recurrent pregnancy loss in the era of transvaginal 3D ultrasound scan. *Gynecol Surg.* 2019;16:14.
28. Abuzeid OM, Hebert J, Ashraf M, Mitwally M, Diamond MP, Abuzeid MI. Pediatric Foley Catheter after Operative Hysteroscopy Does Not Cause Ascending Infection. *J Minim Invasive Gynecol.* 2018;25(1):133–8.
29. Patil RR, Vijay NR, Joshi S. An unusual presentation of vaginal leiomyoma. *J Midlife Health.* 2019;10(4):204–5.
30. Boskovic V, Vrzic-Petronijevic S, Petronijevic M, Atanackovic J, Bratic D. Removal of a vaginal leiomyoma presenting as tumor previa allowing a vaginal birth. *Eur J Gynaec Oncol.* 2012;33(3):326–7.
31. Wu Y, Wang W, Sheng X, Kong L, Qi J. A misdiagnosed vaginal leiomyoma: case report. *Urol Case Rep.* 2015;3(3):82–3.
32. Goyal LD, Kaur H, Kaur S. An unusual case of vaginal myoma presenting with postmenopausal bleeding. *J Family Reprod Health.* 2013;7(2):103–4.
33. Sim CH, Lee JH, Kwak JS, Song SH. Necrotizing ruptured vaginal leiomyoma mimicking a malignant neoplasm. *Obstet Gynecol Sci.* 2014; 57(6):560–3.
34. Egbd TO, Kobenge FM, Metogo JAM, Wankie EM, Tolefac PN, Belley-Priso E. Vaginal leiomyoma: medical imaging and diagnosis in a resource low tertiary hospital: case report. BMC Women's Health. 2020;20(12). https://doi.org/10.1186/s12905-020-0883-2
35. Akkamahadevi CH, Neekita P, Pooja S, Bhavana N, Prashanth R, Shivakumar S. Benign primary vaginal leiomyoma-A diagnostic challenge: Rare case report. *Eur J Obstet Gynecol Reprod Biol.* 2020;247:261–2.
36. Hagen J, Wilhite A, Tarbunova M, Erickson B. Successful robotic surgery for primary resection of a vaginal leiomyosarcoma: a case report. *Gynecol Oncol Rep.* 2019;30:100503.
37. Fasih N, Shanbhogue AKP, Macdonald DB, et al. Leiomyomas beyond the Uterus: Unusual Locations, Rare Manifestations. *Radiographics* 2008;28(7):1931–48.
38. Temizkhan O, Erenel H, Arici B, Asicioglu O. A case of parasitic myoma 4 years after laparoscopic myomectomy. *J Min Access Surg.* 2014;10(4):202–3.
39. Oindi FM, Mutiso SK, Obura T. Port site parasitic leiomyoma after laparoscopic myomectomy: a case report and review of the literature. *J Med Case Rep.* 2018;12(1):339. https://doi:10.1186/s13256-018-1873-y
40. American College of Obstetricians and Gynecologists (ACOG) Committee Opinion No. 770 Summary: Uterine Morcellation for Presumed Leiomyomas. *Obstet Gynecol.* 2019;133(3):604–5. https://doi:10.1097/AOG.0000000000003127
41. Elagwany AS, Rady HA, Abdeldayem TM. A case of parasitic leiomyoma with serpentine omental blood vessels: an unusual variant of uterine leiomyoma. *J Taibah Univ Med Sci.* 2014;9(4):338–40. https://doi.org/10.1016/j.jtumed.2014.05.002
42. Halama N, Grauling-Halama SA, Daboul I. Familial clustering of leiomyomatosis peritonealis disseminata: an unknown genetic syndrome? *BMC Gastroenterol.* 2005;5:33. https://DOI:10.1186/1471-230X-5-33
43. Papadatos D, Taourel P, Bret PM. CT of leiomyomatosis peritonealis disseminata mimicking peritoneal carcinomatosis. *Am J Roentgenol.* 1996;167(2):475–6. https://doi:10.2214/ajr.167.2.8686629

# 15

## HYSTEROSCOPIC MYOMECTOMY

**Priyanka Sinha, Yehia Shawki, Shima Al Bashi, Osama Shawki, and Botros Rizk**

### Introduction

Uterine myomas are benign encapsulated tumors that originate from the muscle tissue of the uterus. They are the most frequent benign tumors in the female genital tract and occur in 20%–30% of women of the reproductive age, frequently increasing toward the end of the reproductive period [1, 2]. Depending upon their location, they can be classified as subserosal, intramural submucosal, cervical, and broad ligament myoma. Submucosal myomas comprise 5%–10% of uterine fibroids [3].

Submucosal myomas are associated with symptoms of abnormal uterine bleeding, dysmenorrhea, and reproductive problems. The FIGO classification (2011) described eight types of myoma. FIGO (0-2) types are incavitary: Type 0 is a submucosal fibroid pedunculated within the uterine cavity, Type 1 is submucosal with more than 50% of the leiomyoma within the uterine cavity, and Type 2 is submucosal with less than 50% of the leiomyoma within the uterine cavity.

Submucosal myoma is one of the most common indications of hysteroscopic resection. Hysteroscopic resection is currently the gold standard for symptomatic submucosal myoma treatment. The goal of hysteroscopic myomectomy is removal of the entire fibroid without compromising the surrounding myometrium or endometrium. This will result in alleviation of the patient's symptoms without weakening the myometrium or creating intracavitary synechia. Removal of the entire myoma will also decrease the risk of regrowth of the lesion.

Presurgical evaluation includes transvaginal ultrasound scanning (TVS), sonohysterography (SHG), and office hysteroscopy [4–6].

Hysteroscopic resection of leiomyoma can be carried out by electrosurgical as well as mechanical instruments. Available instruments include Mazzon cold loops, Versapoint, MyoSure, Symphion, and Truclear.

Hysteroscopic resection of submucosal myoma greatly improves the prognosis in women with recurrent pregnancy loss and infertility [7].

#### Evolution of hysteroscopic myomectomy

Evolution of endoscopy made these myomas approachable and respectable through the inside of the uterus leading to avoidance of laparotomy and conventional or robotic myomectomy [8, 9].

Initially, the lesions were removed by somewhat harsh methods: ovum forceps were used to twist the pedunculated myoma off their pedicle and scissors were introduced outside the hysteroscopy sheath to cut the myoma pedicle.

Hysteroscopic myomectomy was first performed by Neuwirth and Amin in 1976. They used a urologic resectoscope, monopolar current, and 32% dextran as distension media to resect the leiomyoma.

A gynecological resectoscope was developed in 1987, which was a continuous flow device with 0° optic, cutting current, and 1.5% glycine used as distension media [10].

Due to advances in instruments and refining of techniques, hysteroscopic myomectomy has become a standard minimally invasive procedure for resection of submucosal fibroid [11, 12].

Development of this method leads to avoidance of laparotomy and conventional or robotic myomectomy, which reduces complications, shortens the recovery period, and allows the procedure to be carried out in ambulatory settings.

#### *Significance of submucosal fibroid*

Abnormal uterine bleeding is an important symptom, most commonly described as heavy or prolonged menstrual bleeding. The prevalence of submucosal myoma in women with abnormal uterine bleeding was found to be 23.4%, the majority of these cases being premenopausal women [13]. Abnormal uterine bleeding is presumably caused in these cases by a submucosal fibroid distorting the cavity and increasing the bleeding surface of the endometrium [14].

Infertility can be associated with myoma, with submucosal fibroids having the most deleterious effects on the pregnancy rates [15, 16]. Myoma causes alteration of the uterine cavity contour and abnormal uterine contractility which might impede sperm migration, ovum transport, or embryo implantation [17–19].

The implantation failure and pregnancy loss can be due to endometrial inflammation, endometrial vascular disturbances, secretion of vasoactive substances, or an enhanced endometrial androgen environment [17, 20, 21].

Other symptoms are pelvic pain and dysmenorrhea. Obstetric complications can be miscarriage, preterm labor, and malpresentation.

#### *Patient evaluation or diagnosis*

Multiple modalities exist, with the most widely used being transvaginal ultrasound. The 3D ultrasound provided a further jump in the prediction of submucosal myoma assessment (**Figure 15.1**).

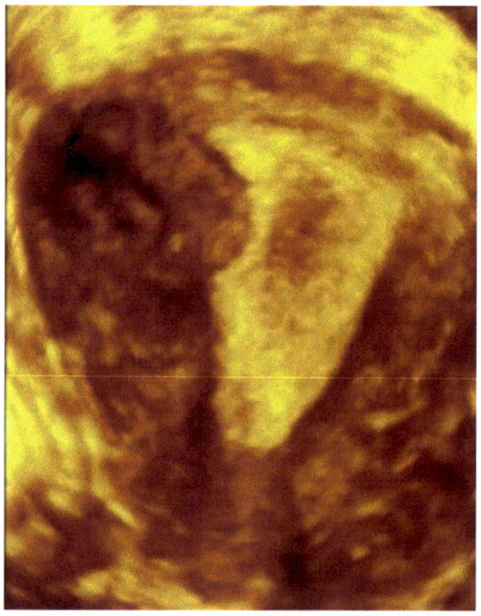

FIGURE 15.1 3D Ultrasound showing submucosal fibroid at right cornual region. (Courtesy of Prof. Botros Rizk.)

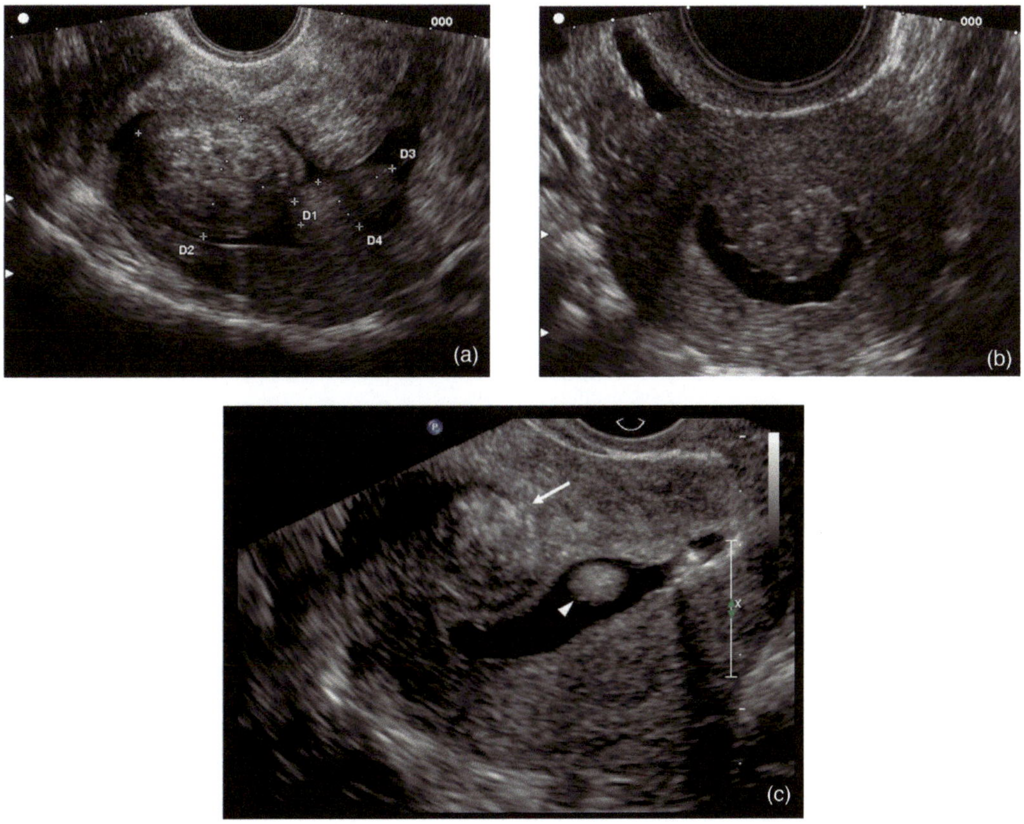


**FIGURE 15.2** Saline infusion sonohysterogram (SIS): (a) Type 0 submucosal fibroid; (b) Type I submucosal fibroid; (c) Type II submucosal fibroid (big arrow). (a, b: From Clough A, Khalaf Y, Ultrasonography of uterine fibroids, in Rizk BRMB, ed., *Ultrasonography in Reproductive Medicine and Infertility*, Cambridge University Press, 2010. With permission. c: From Brown WW, Sonohysterography, in Rizk BRMB, ed., *Ultrasonography in Reproductive Medicine and Infertility*, Cambridge University Press, 2010. With permission.)

It provides the "myometrial-free margin" (thickness of the outer myometrial layer of the myoma) and the presence of any other pathology. Myometrial free margins should be at least 1 cm for submucosal myoma to be reached hysteroscopically [6, 22].

Saline instillation sonography, which includes filling the endometrial cavity with fluid and then performing the ultrasound examination, also aids in distinguishing whether a myoma protrudes into the uterine cavity or not. In **Figure 15.2a–c**, saline instillation sonography demonstrates types 0, 1, and 2 of submucosal fibroid. MRI, in particular, is used to identify the presence and exact number of very small myomas [23].

Hysteroscopy can also be used in a diagnostic capacity to identify the submucosal involvement of any myomas. In fact, hysteroscopy shows a much higher sensitivity in diagnosing submucous myomas when compared to ultrasonography, with the main limitations being availability, cost, and operator dependency [23].

## *Classification*

The old classification of uterine myomas as subserosal, interstitial, or submucosal was progressed in 2011 by the FIGO classification to Type 0-8. This gave a more detailed view on the location of the myoma and the surgical approach best suited to tackle the pathology [24]. The FIGO classification of leiomyomas is [25]:

- Type 0 – submucosal and pedunculated within the uterine cavity
- Type 1 – submucosal with more than 50% of the leiomyoma within the uterine cavity
- Type 2 – submucosal with less than 50% of the leiomyoma within the uterine cavity
- Type 3 – intramural, contacting the endometrium
- Type 4 – intramural, not contacting the endometrium or serosa
- Type 5 – subserosal with more than 50% of the leiomyoma intramural
- Type 6 – subserosal with less than 50% of the leiomyoma intramural
- Type 7 – subserosal and pedunculated
- Type 8 – other location, such as cervix or broad ligament

A more specific classification for submucosal myomas was proposed by Lasmar, dubbed the Lasmar scoring system for submucous myomas (**Table 15.1**). This classification gave more attention to the surgical aspect of the pathology, categorizing myomas into low complexity cases, high complexity cases, and cases where hysteroscopic management is not recommended [6].

## *Preoperative considerations*

Preoperative considerations include cervical ripening and optimizing the endometrium. Because almost one-half of all complications are due to attempting initial hysteroscope entry through the cervix, cervical ripening can assist the provider [26]. Unfortunately, there is no universal consensus regarding agent or timing, but some authors advocate 200–400 µg of vaginal misoprostol approximately 8–12 hours before the procedure [26]. For optimizing the endometrium, timing the procedure for

TABLE 15.1: Lasmar's Presurgical Classification of Submucous Myomas

| Points | Penetration into Myometrium | Fibroid Size (m) | Extension of the Base of Fibroid | Topography | Lateral Wall |
|---|---|---|---|---|---|
| 0 | 0 | ≤2 | ≤1\3 | Lower | |
| 1 | ≤50% | > 2–5 | > 1\3–2\3 | Middle | + 1 |
| 2 | > 50% | > 5 | > 2\3 | Upper | |
| Score | + | + | + | + | + |
| Score | Group | Complexity and therapeutic option. | | | |
| 0–4 | I | Low complexity hysteroscopic myomectomy. | | | |
| 5–6 | II | High complexity hysteroscopic myomectomy: consider the use of GnRH analogue and/or two-stage hysteroscopic myomectomy. | | | |
| 7–9 | III | Hysteroscopic myomectomy not indicated: consider an alternative non-hysteroscopic technique. | | | |

*Source:* From Di Spiezio Sardo A, et al. Hum Reprod Update. 2008;14(2):101–19 [23]. With permission.

the proliferative stage can be an advantage, but requires careful scheduling. The use of GnRH agonists, selective progesterone receptor modulators, and anti-progestins to otherwise achieve optimal intrauterine conditions has been studied, but no consensus exists as to the balance of risks versus benefits [23, 26].

Preoperative GnRH agonist use has some benefits; a reduction of endometrial thickness, of size, and of vascularisation of the myoma results in improved visibility for the operator by limiting blood loss [27]. The most useful effects of GnRH agonists are reduced operating time and decreased hysteroscopic fluid resorption (through a reduction of uterine blood flow) [28]. Their main proven benefit is that they can reduce menstrual blood loss and correct anemia prior to surgery [27, 29].

The procedure can be scheduled as patients do not necessarily need to be operated in the early proliferative phase [28].

### *Intraoperative medical management*

Intraoperative use of vasopressin causes vasoconstriction within the myoma and the surrounding myometrium [30, 31]. Studies have demonstrated that intracervical injection of dilute vasopressin reduces fluid intravasation and operative blood loss [32, 33]. Injection of dilute vasopressin into the cervical stroma improved visual clarity [34]. The recommended maximum concentration of vasopressin for intraoperative use is 0.4 U/mL [35].

### *Instruments and devices*

An operative hysteroscope is the instrument used to resect submucosal myoma under direct visualization. Its working element can be electrosurgical loops, mechanical cold loops, or morcellator technology. Two main approaches exist to tackle submucous myomas: cold energy and electrocautery. The commonly used form of cold energy is 5 Fr hysteroscopic scissors which can be used to cut the base of a small submucous myoma and intrauterine morcellators. Which of the various hysteroscopic myomectomy techniques is used depends on the specific patient, and there are no universally accepted guidelines [26]. Electrocautery allows for attempting more challenging cases such as myomas with intramural components and larger sizes. The most suitable insert for myomas is the loop insert, which allows a good grasp on the myoma and slicing the fibroid into strips.

Electrosurgical systems can be monopolar or bipolar. Monopolar instruments are those in which current flows from the extremity of resectoscope to plate [23]; nonconducting distension media (sorbitol 5% or glycine 1.5%) is used for monopolar electrodes [23]. Due to development of superior bipolar resectoscope and growing concern over nonconductive media, the bipolar resectoscope has become the treatment of choice for submucosal myoma types 0-2. The hysteroscopic mechanical morcellator was subsequently developed to overcome some of the restraints of the resectoscope [23]. There are no universally accepted guidelines for preference of use between the various hysteroscopic morcellation techniques [23]. Some proponents believe that Type 0 leiomyomas are more amenable to morcellation while Type 2 leiomyomas are better treated with bipolar resectoscopy [23]. Electrosurgical techniques are better than morcellators for complete resection of myoma > 4 cm with a significant intramural component [36–37].

### Bipolar resectoscope

Bipolar instruments are those in which both electrodes are introduced into the thermal loop (**Figure 15.3**). Bipolar instruments are safe as current only passes through the tissue with which the loop comes into contact. Bipolar diathermy allows the use of isotonic conductive fluid (normal saline) [23]. It has an external sheath with two different sizes—7 mm and 9 mm—with 9 mm being commonly used for submucosal myoma resection. The inner sheath contains a U-shaped wired electrode, which uses 130–170 W cutting current [26]. Each pass of the current removes 3–5 mm of tissue under direct visualization [26]. The standard gynecological resectoscope is a passive model, which consists of the working element in a resting state. Activating the working element will push the loop insert outside the sheath and toward the desired pathology.

Bipolar current is activated by a foot pedal just prior to contact with the tissue. Resection starts at the highest point on the myoma, moving toward the surgeon. Tissue fragments should be

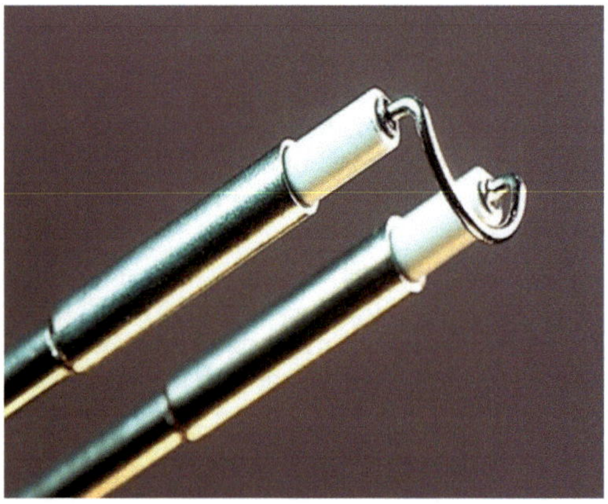

FIGURE 15.3 Bipolar resectoscope showing the cutting loop. (From Hologic with permission.)

periodically removed to provide a clear field of view. Resectoscope wire or polyp forceps can be used for pulling out tissue fragments [26]. Removal and reinsertion of the resectoscope might lead to air embolism [26]. Intermittent or coagulation current of 70–100 W can be used for hemostasis [26]. The most commonly used bipolar resectoscope is Versapoint by Ethicon.

## Intrauterine morcellators

Hysteroscopic morcellators progressively cut the myoma with immediate removal of the tissue. Normal saline is used as distension media for mechanical morcellators. Three hysteroscopic intrauterine morcellators currently exist on the market: MyoSure (Hologic, Bedford, MA), Symphion (Boston Scientific, Marlborough, MA), and TRUCLEAR (Smith & Nephew, Andover, MA) [38]. Mechanical energy is used by MyoSure and TRUCLEAR. Symphion utilizes electrical energy [38]. The inner sheath has a side-facing resection window with a hollow cylindrical blade which is inserted into the external sheath. It is incorporated with vacuum suction that aspirates tissue fragments [26]. The tissue cutting and removal is done in a single step as the blade resects the myoma while the vacuum suction removes tissue and clears a bloody field, improving visibility and reducing the risk of perforation [26].

### *MyoSure system*

The MyoSure hysteroscopic tissue removal system (**Figure 15.4**) is a fast, convenient way to remove intrauterine pathology like submucosal myoma, polyp, uterine septum, and uterine adhesions hysteroscopically. A fluid control function means it can quickly remove submucosal myoma while maintaining uterine form and functions [37, 39]; as the MyoSure tissue removal device simultaneously cuts and removes intrauterine tissue, the Aquilex fluid control system balances steady fluid inflow with active suction to optimize uterine distention and provide a clear field of view free from tissue debris.

The MyoSure device has a sideshaver window with a hollow cylindrical cutting blade, presenting with an outer bevel. The system includes a tissue trap that is connected to the tissue removal device through a regulated vacuum. Constant regulated isotonic electrolyte solution irrigation maintains target intrauterine distension pressure, with continuous aspiration of resected tissues [38].

Under hysteroscopic guidance, the standard unit's cutting blade contacts target tissue through a 14 mm long and 2.4 mm deep side channel on the morcellator distal shaft. Foot pedal-controlled activation retracts the blade guard covering the window and engages the stainless steel blade's dual cutting motion, rotating at up to 8,075 rpm while oscillating at 3 cycles/second [38]. There are various types of MyoSure, such as MyoSure Lite, XL, and Reach; the Reach and XL are intended specifically for myoma resection.

MyoSure Classic and MyoSure XL differ in the size of their external sheath, with 7.25 mm for XL and 6.25 mm for Classic. The working channel outer diameter for MyoSure Reach and MyoSure XL is 3 mm and 4 mm, respectively [26]. MyoSure Reach was designed to access hard-to-reach areas, including the upper third of the uterine cavity, removing fibroid of ≤3 cm; XL removes ≤ 5 cm [26]. **Figure 15.5a** shows the cutting window of the MyoSure device.

### *The truclear system*

Truclear uses mechanical energy. There are three types of truclear device: Truclear INCISOR, Truclear INCISOR Plus 4.0, Truclear ULTRA Plus with the Truclear INCISOR Plus 4.0, and Truclear ULTRA Plus mainly used for submucosal myomectomy. The external sheath size for Truclear is 9 mm and the working channel outer diameter is 4 mm [26]. Truclear INCISOR Plus is designed to remove fibroid ≤3 cm and ULTRA plus ≤5 cm. The tissue removal rate for Truclear ULTRA Plus is 2.96 g/min for fibroid tissue [26]. **Figure 15.5c** shows the cutting window of Truclear incisor plus and Truclear Ultra plus.

## Advantages of mechanical morcellators

1. Preserves uterine function: As mechanical resection is carried out, radiofrequency energy is not used and the uterine form, histology, and functions are preserved so the specimens can be collected intact [26, 37, 39].

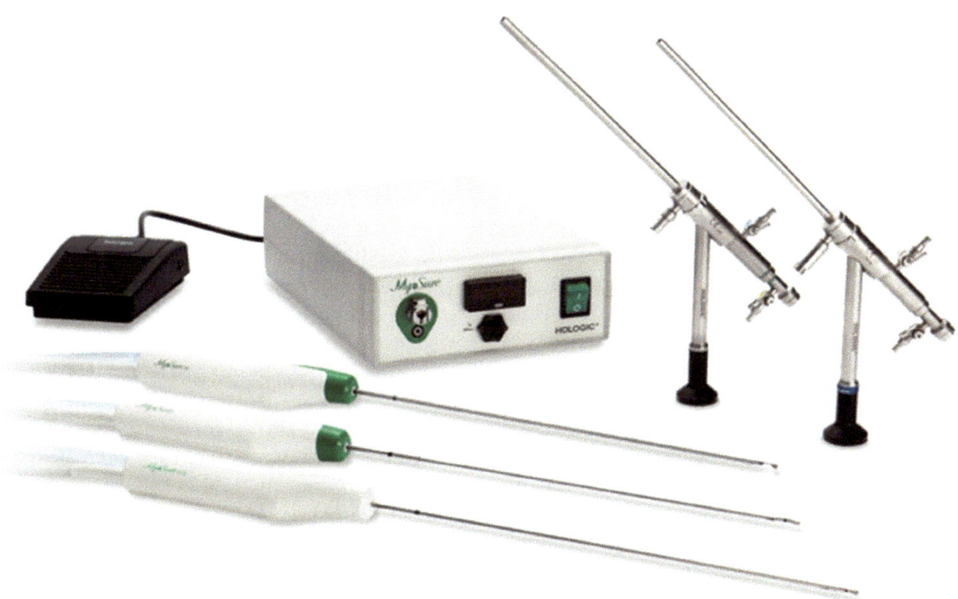


**FIGURE 15.4** MyoSure hysteroscopic tissue removal system. (From Hologic with permission.)

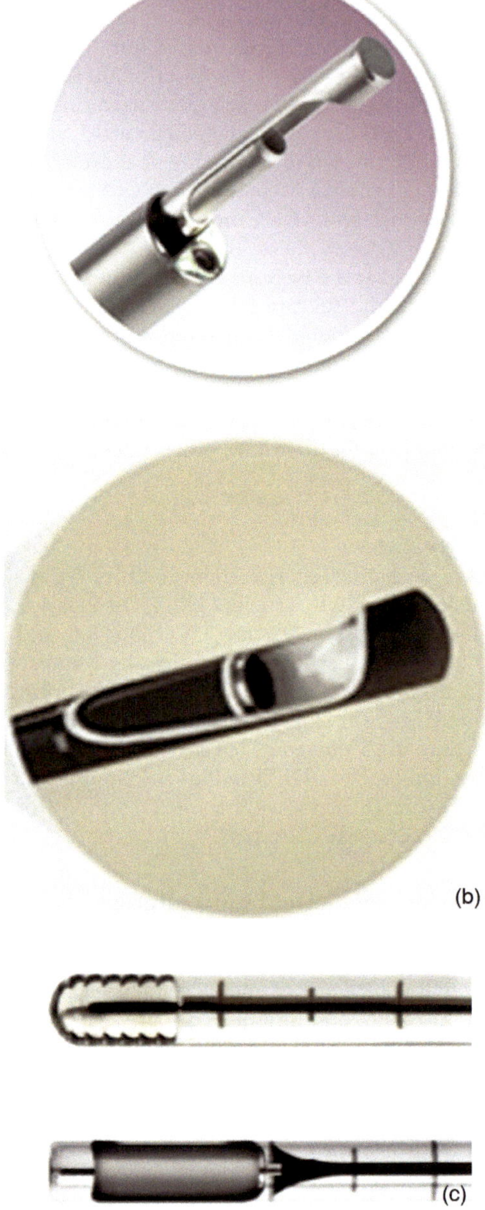


**FIGURE 15.5** Intrauterine morcellators showing the cutting window: (a) MyoSure device, (b) Symphion device, and (c) Truclear device. (From Hologic with permission.)

2. Performs tissue cutting and removal in a single step: While the stainless steel blade resects the myoma tissue, the fluid management system simultaneously removes tissue as well as clears a bloody field using suction, thereby improving visibility and reducing the risk of perforations. The device combined with suction continuously aspirates resected tissue through the device [39]. The tissue removal rate for MyoSure Reach, MyoSure XL, and Truclear Ultra plus is 1.5 g/min and 4.3 g/min, and 2.96 g/min for fibroid tissue, respectively [26].
3. Includes a side-facing cutting window: The side-facing cutting window provides better tissue contact for efficient removal and minimizes the risk of perforation [26, 39].
4. Minimizes procedure time: Rapidly achieving and holding constant distention independent of hysteroscope diameter provides optimal visualization for the surgeon, leading to reduced length of anesthesia and a lower risk of intravasation [26, 39, 40].

## Symphion tissue removal device

The Symphion Tissue Removal Device is a disposable, hand held, bipolar radiofrequency device designed for the resection and aspiration of uterine pathology. It has a 3 mm OD hysteroscope, a closed loop molecular filtration system, and a 3.6 mm radiofrequency bipolar tissue resection device. This closed loop filtration system uses only one three-liter bag of saline which is recirculated through a 15 kilodalton (5.0 nanometer) molecular filtration system that removes viruses, bacteria, proteins, cytokines, endotoxins, and cells.

This design volumetrically limits fluid overload. Additionally, the combination of the direct intrauterine pressure monitoring allows the system to monitor pressure from within the cavity and adjust the fluid flow to help prevent cavity collapse [41]. **Figure 15.5b** shows the cutting window of the Symphion device.

The Mazzon technique uses a cold loop for removal of submucosal myoma, with 88% success in the one-step removal of Type 1 and 2 fibroids. It minimizes thermal damage to healthy myometrium, thereby reducing synechiae formation [42].

Zayed et al. described another technique for fibroids with intramural component removal in one stage: a U-shaped cutting device slices down the fibroid to the endometrium and a loop is then inserted into the cleavage plane between the myoma and the myometrium to remove myoma. This has a 95% success rate for removal of Type II fibroids less than 6 cm [43].

## *Surgical steps*

Symptomatic uterine myomas are usually tackled hysteroscopically through a transcervical approach. The procedure can be performed under office conditions with minimal or no anesthesia, under regional anesthesia or general anesthesia in the operating room. This will depend on the preference of the patient and the feasibility and availability of equipment. The timing of the procedure should be postmenstrual in premenopausal women. Myomas of type 0 and 1 (up to 5 cm in diameter) and type 2 (up to 4 cm) can be removed hysteroscopically [44, 45].

The hysteroscopy tower consists of three main systems, namely:

1. A visual system composed of the monitor, endoscopy camera, and an optic lens. This lens usually exists in two sizes: a 2.9 mm for office sheaths and procedures and a larger 4 mm lens for operative sheaths and resectoscopes. The lens can be 0°, 12°, or 30° (which is the most commonly used for hysteroscopy) [23].
2. An illumination system which is composed of a light source and light cable connecting to the optic lens.
3. A distension system which consists of a fluid medium with or without a fluid pump connected to the hysteroscopy sheath intended to distend the uterine cavity.

Identification of the myoma's pseudocapsule is imperative to be able to cut the myoma from its base. This also leaves the nerve component intact and allows for optimal healing following expulsion of the myoma [46].

The patient is placed in the dorsal lithotomy position with the surgeon operating through the vagina as a natural orifice. The hysteroscopy tower can be placed on either side of the patient or ideally, the monitor could be mounted to the ceiling and descend centrally above the patient.

Electrolyte (isotonic) media is used for cold surgeries or bipolar electrocautery, with saline being the most widely used. Nonelectrolyte (hypotonic) media is saved for monopolar electrocautery, with glycine being the proposed medium. Both forms of fluid media are liable to produce fluid overload; however, more electrolyte imbalance and glycinemia occur with the nonelectrolyte media, and thus the suggested cut off limit of fluid deficit is lower with nonelectrolyte media [23].

The procedure usually starts with a diagnostic hysteroscopy with the minimal diameter hysteroscope. This allows for dilation of the cervical canal under vision and understanding of the direction of the cervix and uterine cavity, followed by examination of the uterine cavity and assessment of the exact site, number, and submucous extension of any myomas. The submucous extension can be confirmed by lowering the pressure inside the uterine cavity and seeing the myoma bulge into the cavity.

Depending on the diameter of the resectoscope used, dilation of the cervix is then performed, with care taken not to impact the myomas or injure the endometrium, which could cause shredding of the endometrium and impair visualization during the hysteroscopic procedure.

This is followed by introduction of the hysteroscope and the procedure begins. In order to maximize the success rates of the surgery, proper distension of the cavity is necessary to separate the uterine walls and create the necessary space to operate on the myoma. In cases when fluid pressure is suboptimal, the surgeon will operate in a cramped space with the uterine walls in contact with the myoma and will possibly be hampered by bleeding from the myoma once cutting into the myoma begins. There is no distinct number to set the pressure to, as the uterus is a dynamic organ with continuous sources of leakage (namely the fallopian tubes and the cervix). The ideal pressure is that which provides optimal visualization for the surgeon and allows for competent access to the myoma.

### *Type 0 myoma*

Pedunculated Type 0 myomas can be cut from the base stalk and left to be expelled spontaneously [23]. Alternatively, they can also be decompressed and cut into long strips by the resectoscope or morcellator. The key to success in this particular case is identifying the base and origin of the myoma, which should be done during the diagnostic portion of the procedure [23]. With this information the surgeon can access the base by the resectoscope. A hysteroscopic view from a patient with a type 0 fibroid is shown on **Figure 15.6**, with a stepwise approach with the MyoSure device for hysteroscopic myomectomy of Type 0 myoma in **Figure 15.7**.

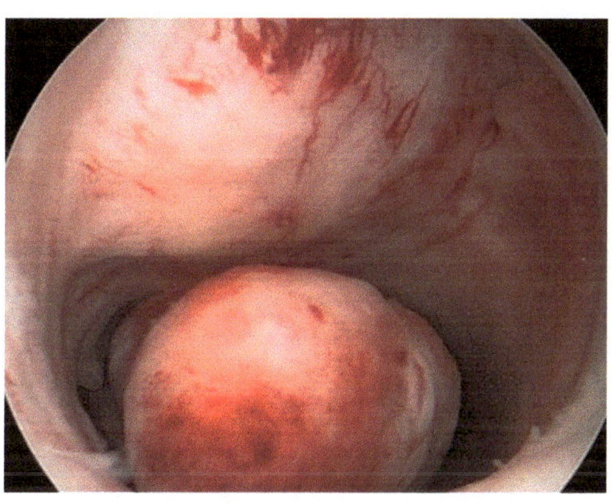

**FIGURE 15.6** Hysteroscopic view of patient showing type I submucosal myoma (top half of the image) and type 0 submucosal myoma (lower half of image). (Courtesy of Prof. Botros Rizk.)

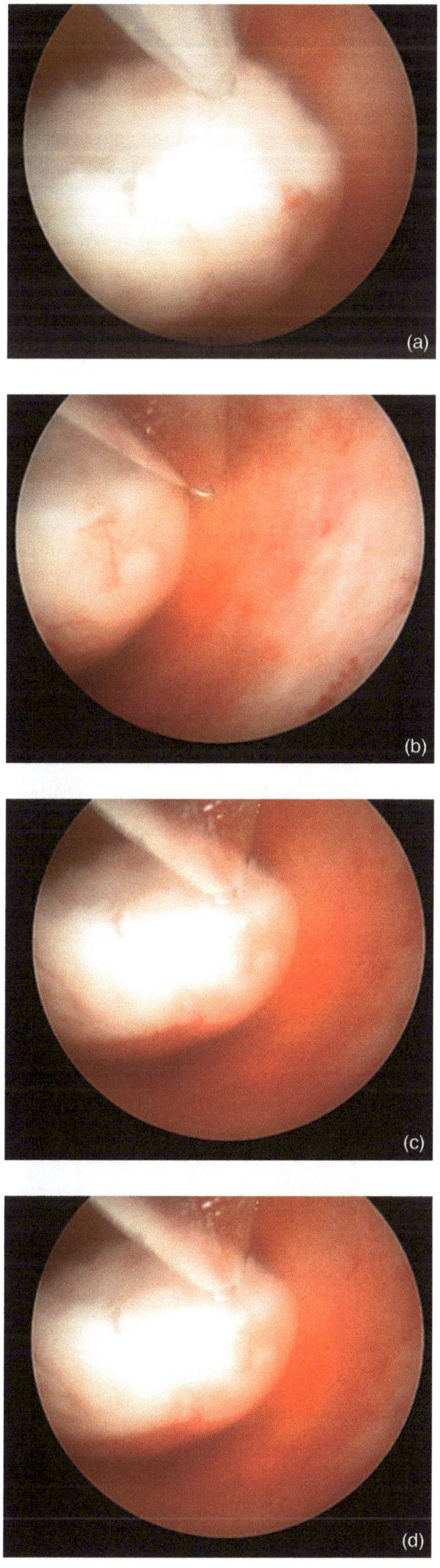


**FIGURE 15.7** Stepwise approach with MyoSure device during hysteroscopic myomectomy. (Courtesy of Prof. Botros Rizk.)

Hysteroscopic myomectomy using the MyoSure device for type 0 submucosal myoma is shown in **Figure 15.8**, with a stepwise demonstration in **Figure 15.9**.

### *Type 1 myoma*

A myoma with less than a 50% intramural component will usually have an acute angle with the uterine wall from which it arises. Two approaches can be utilized:

1. Beginning to cut the myoma into strips from its lateral end, going from one side to the other [23].
2. Cutting the myoma into strips in the center, effectively bisecting the fibroid [23].

Some surgeons prefer to continuously remove the strips from the uterine cavity, which is useful in avoiding crowding of the uterine cavity by myoma strips; however, this is time-consuming and runs the risk of introducing air into the uterine cavity. It may also take time to regain a proper distension and adequate visualization of the uterine cavity before cutting the myoma can resume. These problems can be avoided by using intrauterine morcellators that simultaneously cut and remove intrauterine tissue, with the fluid control system balancing a steady fluid inflow with active suction to optimize uterine distention and provide a clear

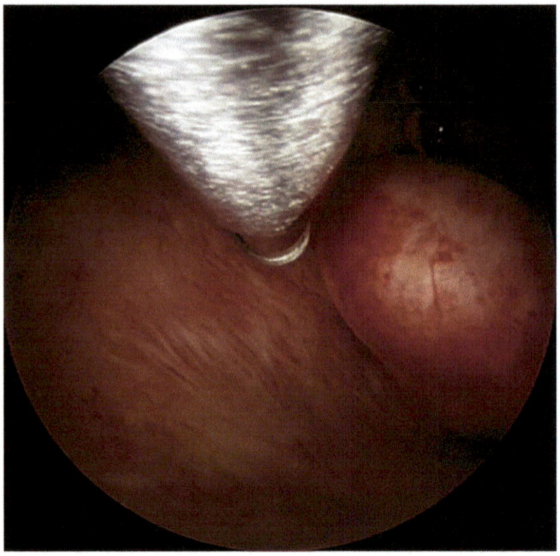

**FIGURE 15.8** Hysteroscopic myomectomy using MyoSure device for type 0 submucosal myoma. (Courtesy of Prof. Botros Rizk.)

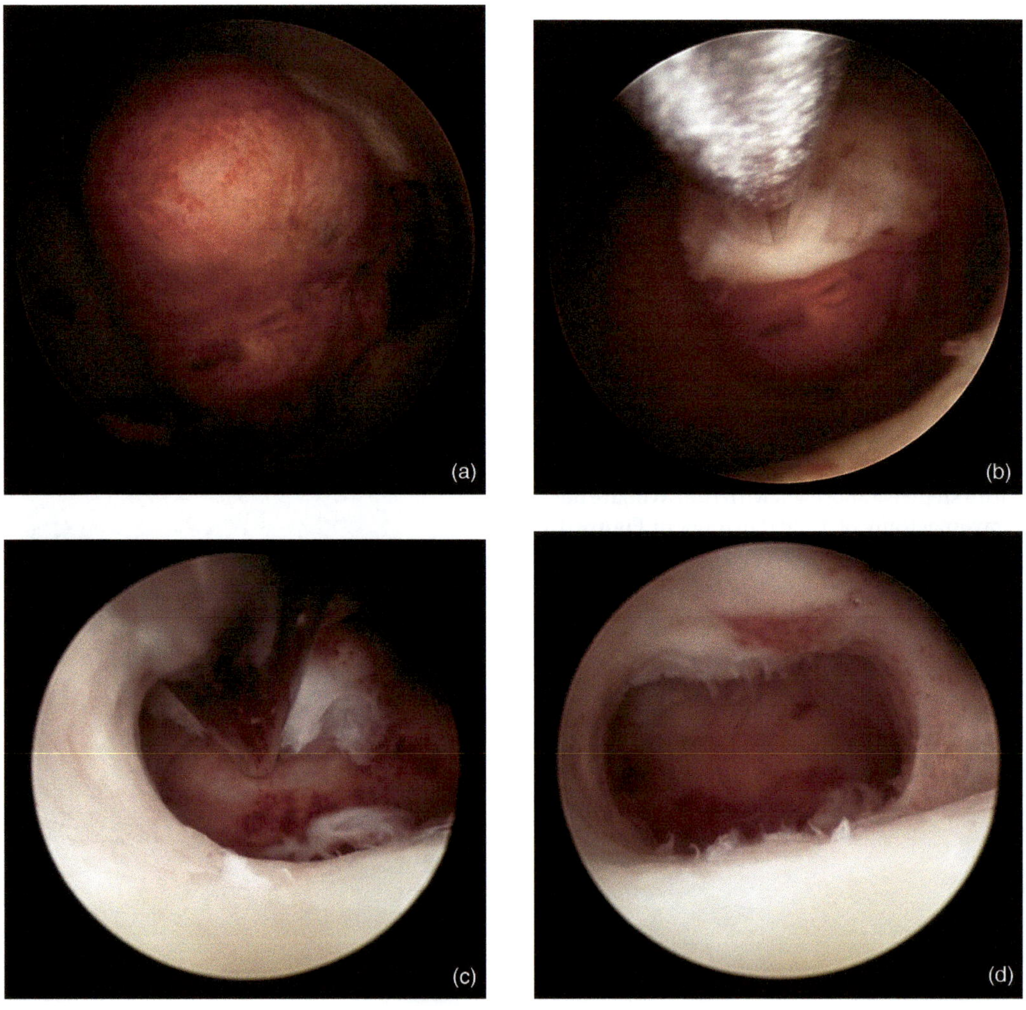


**FIGURE 15.9** Stepwise demonstration of hysteroscopic myomectomy using MyoSure device for type 0 submucosal fibroid. (Courtesy of Prof. Botros Rizk.)

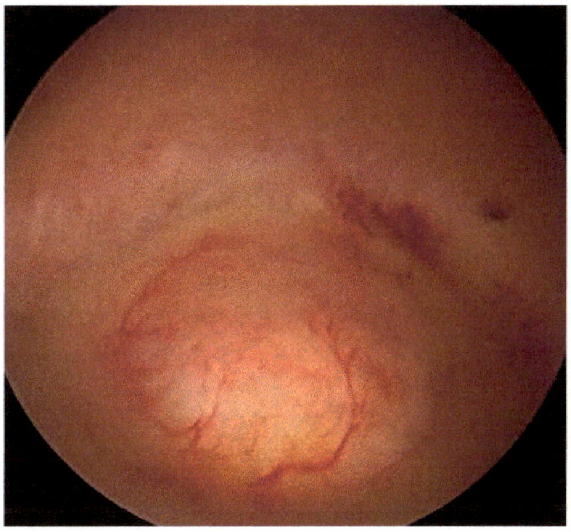

FIGURE 15.10 Type 2 myoma in regular fluid pressure settings. (Courtesy of Dr. Osama Shawki.)

field of view. A hysteroscopic view of a type 1 fibroid is shown on **Figure 15.6**.

### *Type 2 myoma*

Myomas with more than a 50% intramural component provide more challenging cases as resection must continue deep into the myometrium to fully excise the myoma. The key to success here is identifying the cut off limit for resection, which is when the surgeon reaches the pseudocapsule. The myoma fibers are white, whorled fibro-muscle, while the pseudocapsule and the myometrium are pink, compressed interlacing muscle fibers. The resectoscope loop is used to dig deep into the intramural component of the myoma, excising it in chips [23].

Alternatively, the procedure can be divided into multiple steps, with the first step including resection of the submucous component and waiting for expulsion of the intramural component into the uterine cavity (to be resected in a second procedure).

This stepwise approach may also be necessary for large myomas where the surgery is limited by fluid deficit for patient safety. A hysteroscopic view of a type 2 fibroid in regular pressure setting is shown in **Figure 15.10**; the Type 2 myoma is more clearly visualized when intrauterine pressure is lowered, as shown in **Figure 15.11**. **Figure 15.12** describes the identification of the pseudocapsule.

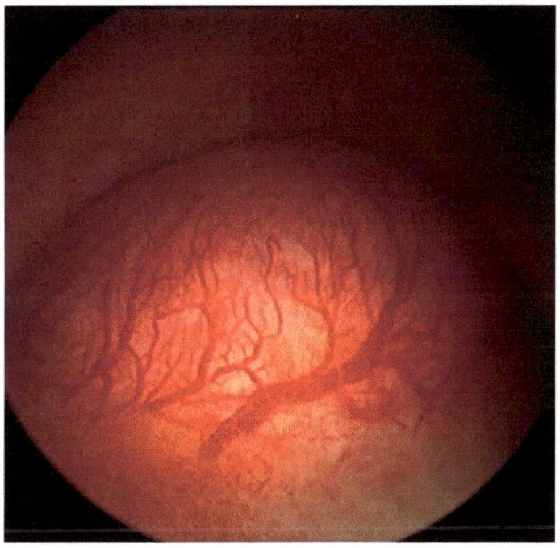

FIGURE 15.11 Type 2 myoma seen in **Figure 15.10** visualized more clearly when the intrauterine pressure is lowered. (Courtesy of Dr. Osama Shawki.)

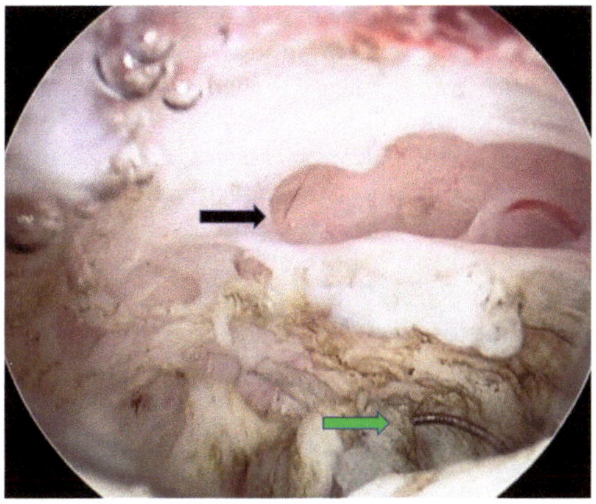

FIGURE 15.12 Identification of the pseudocapsule demarcated by the black arrow. The myoma tissue is demarcated by the green arrow, with the resectoscope loop seen cutting the myoma into strips. (Courtesy of Dr. Osama Shawki.)

### *Office myomectomy*

Office hysteroscopy is suitable and safe for both diagnosis and sometimes treatment of small intrauterine pathologies. Office hysteroscopy can be performed with a hysteroscope < 5 mm in diameter with working channels and continuous flow system which reduces the risk of cervical dilatation, the need for anesthesia, and the cost [26]. Patients can resume normal activities immediately after the procedure. Office myomectomy can be performed for type 0-1 fibroids < 1.5 cm under direct vision. The most common complications associated with office hysteroscopy include vasovagal reaction, local anesthesia toxicity, uterine perforation, bleeding, and false passages [47].

## Complications

The complications of hysteroscopic myomectomy are minimal, but can be very dangerous when encountered. The rate of complications from operative hysteroscopy is approximately 1%, with 50% of those complications related to the initial entry of the hysteroscope through the cervix [26, 48]. These complications are generally associated with operative hysteroscopy, ranging from perforation, infection, to bleeding, but the specific complications with myomectomy are fluid overload and adhesions formation [26].

The main preventive measure against fluid overload is measuring fluid deficit. This also includes using isotonic media when feasible, completing the procedure in the minimum time necessary, and avoiding opening large vascular channels. However, because nonconductive distension media is hypotonic, complications can include hyponatremia, pulmonary edema, and cerebral edema [26]. Conductive distension media, like normal saline, however, are used for bipolar resectoscopy and tend to have less risk of metabolic complications [26]. The consensus is that the maximum fluid deficits for nonconductive media and conductive media are 1000 mL and 2500 mL, respectively, in otherwise healthy patients [26]. In women with significant medical comorbidities, the consensus is 750 mL fluid deficit for both types of distension media [26].

The post-procedure incidence of intrauterine adhesions for the monopolar and bipolar resectoscope are 35%–40% and 7.5%. The adhesion rate after cold loops is 4%, a value closer to what we may expect with morcellation [49].

To avoid adhesion formation, it is necessary to avoid any injury to the surrounding endometrium, specifically by electrocautery. It is also prudent not to resect two fibroids on opposing surfaces (which are dubbed kissing fibroids). Hormonal therapy postoperative has been suggested; anti-adhesion barriers, while promising, are still unproven and therefore require more studies to assess their efficacy [50, 51].

Gas embolism is most likely to occur with resectoscopy as the electric current interacts with tissue and forms a variety of gases which may enter the venous system and cause cardiovascular collapse [26]. Gas embolism manifests as a decrease in end tidal $CO_2$, tachycardia, hypoxia, hypotension, and eventually cardiac arrhythmias. The procedure should be discontinued if gas embolism is suspected and the patient resuscitated as medically mandatory [26]. Steps used to reduce the possibility of gas embolism are: reduce operative time, avoid the Trendelenburg position, use preoperative GnRHa in select patients for volume reduction, and retain intrauterine pressure at or below mean arterial pressure [26].

Obstetric uterine rupture after septum removal has been reported in the literature and appears to be related to excessive excision, myometrium invasion, excessive laser or cautery use, and uterine perforation during the procedure [52].

### Outcome

Bipolar resectoscopy appears to have similar success rates of complete resection as mechanical morcellators [26]. In terms of operative time, the evidence is conflicting and not robust enough to determine superiority of any one brand or type [26]. Finally, patient satisfaction is similar [26].

Patients undergoing hysteroscopic myomectomy using MyoSure had the following outcomes: 71% of women had complete resection, 67% had complete resolution of symptoms, and 27% required subsequent additional surgery [44]. Eighty-four percent of women were still satisfied with the procedure [44]. Patients undergoing hysteroscopic myomectomy using a resectoscope had the following long-term outcomes: 71% of patients were satisfied with the procedure and 20% required surgery in the subsequent 4 years [53].

Hysteroscopic myomectomy, either by resectoscopy or morcellation, is associated with high patient satisfaction and a low risk of needing a subsequent surgery for women with abnormal uterine bleeding [26].

After assessing and handling all other causes of infertility, fertility outcomes after hysteroscopic myomectomy are improved, with an increase in pregnancy rate, higher live birth rates, and fewer miscarriages [54]. Post-hysteroscopic myomectomy, patients should wait for 2–3 weeks to recommence fertility attempts in order to secure uterine cavity healing.

## Conclusion

Hysteroscopic myomectomy is quick and cost-effective, and excellent results have been found with regard to irregular bleeding and fertility improvement. It is a remarkable advance in the field of hysteroscopic surgery and continues to progress with the development of new devices and techniques. Currently, bipolar resectoscope and mechanical morcellators are the most commonly used hysteroscopic myomectomy techniques in women with abnormal uterine bleeding. Large-scale studies have been done to determine which techniques are better in terms of complete myoma resection, shortest operative time, greatest ease of use, and most successful long-term patient outcomes; however, the data remain unclear on which technology is superior. Resectoscopes are preferred for type 2 submucosal myoma. The success of the procedure must always be individualized to the patient's risk factors (the number, type, size, and location of fibroids) and the goal of the procedure. Morcellators are preferred for large type 0 intracavitary myomas at risk of incomplete resection because of the potential decreased operative time and thus decreased fluid intravasation and its associated risks.

## References


1. Fernandez H, Sefrioui O, Virelizier C, Gervaise A, Gomel V, Frydman R. Hysteroscopic resection of submucosal fibroids in patients with infertility. Hum Reprod 2001;16:1489–1492.
2. Valle RF, Baggish MS. Hysteroscopic myomectomy. In: Baggish MS, Valle RF, Guedj H (eds). Hysteroscopy. Visual Perspectives of Uterine Anatomy, Physiology and Pathology Diagnostic and Operative Hysteroscopy, 3rd ed. Philadelphia: Lippincott Williams & Wilkins, a Wolters Kluwer business, 2007, 385–404.
3. Ubaldi F, Tournaye H, Camus M, Van der Pas H, Gepts E, Devroey P. Fertility after hysteroscopic myomectomy. Hum Reprod Update 1995;1:81–190.
4. Fedele L, Bianchi S, Dorta M, Brioschi D, Zanotti F, Vercellini P. Transvaginal ultrasonography versus hysteroscopy in the diagnosis of uterine submucous fibroids. Obstet Gynecol 1991;77:745–748.
5. Fukuda M, Shimizu T, Fukuda K, Yomura W, Shimizu S. Transvaginal hysterosonography for differential diagnosis between submucous and intramural fibroid. Gynecol Obstet Invest 1993;35:236–239.
6. Lasmar RB, Barrozo PR, Dias R, Oliveira MA. Submucous fibroids: a new presurgical classification to evaluate the viability of hysteroscopic surgical treatment–preliminary report. J Minim Invasive Gynecol 2005;12:308–311.
7. Pritts E. Fibroids and infertility: a systematic review of the evidence. Obstet Gynecol Survey. 2001;56:483–491.
8. Walker CL, Stewart EA. Uterine fibroids: the elephant in the room. Science 2005;308:1589–1592.
9. Bradley LD. Abnormal uterine bleeding. Nurse Pract 2005; 30:38–42.
10. Hallez JP. Single-stage total hysteroscopic myomectomies: indications, techniques, and results. Fertil Steril 1995;63:703–708.
11. Vercellini P, Zaina B, Yaylayan L, Pisacreta A, De Giorgi O, Crosignani PG. Hysteroscopic myomectomy: long-term effects on menstrual pattern and fertility. Obstet Gynecol 1999;94:341–347.
12. Takeda A, Manabe S, Hosono S, Nakamura H. Preoperative evaluation of submucosal fibroid by virtual hysteroscopy. J Am Assoc Gynecol Laparosc 2004;11:404–409.
13. van Dongen H, de Kroon CD, Jacobi CE, Trimbos JB, Jansen FW. Diagnostic hysteroscopy in abnormal uterine bleeding: a systematic review and meta-analysis. BJOG. 2007;114:664–675.
14. Maher PJ. Endoscopic management of fibrofibroidta. Rev Gynecol Pract 2003;3:41–45.
15. Pritts EA. Fibroids and infertility: a systematic review of the evidence. Obstet Gynecol Surv 2001;56:483–491.
16. Donnez J, Jadoul P. What are the implications of fibroids on fertility? A need for a debate? Hum Reprod 2002;17:1424–1430.
17. Buttram VC, Jr, Reiter RC. Uterine leiofibroidta: etiology, symptomatology, and management. Fertil Steril 1981;36:433–445.
18. Bettocchi S, Ceci O, Di Venere R, Pansini MV, Pellegrino A, Marello F, Nappi L. Advanced operative office hysteroscopy without anaesthesia: analysis of 501 cases treated with a 5 Fr. bipolar electrode. Hum Reprod 2002;17:2435–2438.
19. Oliveira FG, Abdelmassih VG, Diamond MP, Dozortsev D, Melo NR, Abdelmassih R. Impact of subserosal and intramural uterine fibroids that do not distort the endometrial cavity on the outcome of in vitro fertilization-intracytoplasmic sperm injection. Fertil Steril 2004;81:582–587.

20. Cicinelli E, Romano F, Anastasio PS, Blasi N, Parisi C, Galantino P. Transabdominal sonohysterography, transvaginal sonography, and hysteroscopy in the evaluation of submucous fibroids. Obstet Gynecol 1995;85:42–47.
21. Ng EH, Ho PC. Doppler ultrasound examination of uterine arteries on the day of oocyte retrieval in patients with uterine fibroids undergoing IVF. Hum Reprod 2002;17:765–770.
22. Murakami T, Tamura M, Ozawa Y, Suzuki H, Terada Y, Okamura K. Safe techniques in surgery for hysteroscopic myomectomy. J Obstet Gynaecol Res 2005;31:216–223.
23. Di Spiezio Sardo A, Mazzon I, Bramante S, et al. Hysteroscopic myomectomy: a comprehensive review of surgical techniques. Hum Reprod Update 2008 Mar-Apr;14(2):101–119.
24. Munro MG, Critchley HO, Broder MS, Fraser IS, FIGO Working Group on Menstrual Disorders. FIGO classification system (PALM-COEIN) for causes of abnormal uterine bleeding in non-gravid women of reproductive age. Int J Gynecol Obstet 2011 Apr 1; 113(1):3–13.
25. Laughlin-Tommaso SK, Hesley GK, Hopkins MR, et al. Clinical limitations of the International Federation of Gynecology and Obstetrics (FIGO) classification of uterine fibroids. Int J Gynaecol Obstet. 2017 Nov;139(2):143–148.
26. Friedman JA, Wong JMK, Chaudhari A, et al. Hysteroscopic myomectomy: a comparison of techniques and review of current evidence in the management of abnormal uterine bleeding. Curr Opin Obstet Gynecol 2018 Aug;30(4):243–251.
27. Donnez J, Nisolle M, Grandjean P, Gillerot S, Clerckx F. The role of GnRH agonists in the endoscopic treatment of endometriosis and fibrofibroids. Contracept Fertil Sex 1993;21:59–62.
28. Parazzini F, Vercellini P, De Giorgi O, Pesole A, Ricci E, Crosignani PG. Efficacy of preoperative medical treatment in facilitating hysteroscopic endometrial resection, myomectomy and metroplasty: literature review. Hum Reprod 1998;13:2592–2597.
29. Isaacson K. Hysteroscopic myomectomy: fertility-preserving yet underutilized. OBG Manag 2003;15:69–83.
30. American Association of Gynecologic Laparoscopists (AAGL): Advancing Minimally Invasive Gynecology Worldwide. AAGL practice report: practice guidelines for the diagnosis and management of submucous leiomyomas. J Minim Invasive Gynecol 2012; 19:152–171.
31. Overdijk LE, Rademaker BMP, van Kesteren PJM, et al. The HYSTER study: the effect of intracervically administered terlipressin versus placebo on the number of gaseous emboli and fluid intravasation during hysteroscopic surgery: study protocol for a randomized controlled clinical trial. Trials 2018;19:107.
32. Corson SL, Brooks PG, Serden SP, et al. Effects of vasopressin administration during hysteroscopic surgery. J Reprod Med 1994; 39:419–423.
33. Phillips DR, Nathanson HG, Milim SJ, et al. The effect of dilute vasopressin solution on blood loss during operative hysteroscopy: a randomized controlled trial. Obstet Gynecol 1996;88:761–766.
34. Wong AS, Cheung CW, Yeung SW, et al. Transcervical intralesional vasopressin injection compared with placebo in hysteroscopic myomectomy: a randomized controlled trial. Obstet Gynecol 2014;124:897–903.
35. Munro MG, Storz K, Abbott JA, et al. AAGL practice report: practice guidelines for the management of hysteroscopic distending media. J Minim Invasive Gynecol 2013;20:137–148.
36. Haber K, Hawkins E, Levie M, Chudnoff S. Hysteroscopic morcellation: review of the manufacturer and user facility device experience (MAUDE) database. J Minim Invasive Gynecol 2015; 22(01):110–114.
37. Hamerlynck TW, Dietz V, Schoot BC. Clinical implementation of the hysteroscopic morcellator for removal of intrauterine myomas and polyps. A retrospective descriptive study. Gynecol Surg 2011; 8(02):193–196.
38. Cohen S, Greenberg JA. Hysteroscopic morcellation for treating intrauterine pathology. Rev Obstet Gynecol 2011;4:73.
39. Michael D Scheiber MD, MPH 1 and Serena H. Chen, MD2 A prospective multicenter registry of patients undergoing hysteroscopic morcellation of uterine polyps and myomas. J Gynecol Surg 2016 Dec 1;32(6):318–323.
40. Emanuel MH. New developments in hysteroscopy. Best Pract Res Clin Obstet Gynaecol 2013;27:421.
41. Symphion tissue removal system. Accessed 31/08/2020 at: https://www.bostonscientific.com/content/gwc/en-US/products/uterine-tissue-removal-systems/symphion-system.html
42. Mazzon I, Favilli A, Grasso M, Horvath S, Di Renzo GC, Gerli S. Is cold loop hysteroscopic myomectomy a safe and effective technique for the treatment of submucous myomas with intramural development? A series of 1434 surgical procedures. J Minim Invasive Gynecol 2015;22(05):792–798.
43. Zayed M, Fouda UM, Zayed SM, Elsetohy KA, Hashem AT. Hysteroscopic myomectomy of large submucous myomas in a 1-step procedure using multiple slicing sessions technique. J Minim Invasive Gynecol 2015;22(07):1196–1202.
44. Maheux-Lacroix S, Mennen J, Arnold A, et al. The need for further surgical intervention following primary hysteroscopic morcellation of submucosal leiomyomas in women with abnormal uterine bleeding. Aust N Z J Obstet Gynaecol 2018. [Epub ahead of print]
45. Casadio P, Guasina F, Morra C, et al. Hysteroscopic myomectomy: techniques and preoperative assessment. Minerva Ginecol 2016; 68:154–166. Reinforces strength and limitations of different hysteroscopic myomectomy techniques and that as a whole, hysteroscopic myomectomy is a safe technique.
46. Tinelli A, Favilli A, Lasmar B, Mazzon I, et al. The importance of pseudocapsule preservation during hysteroscopic myomectomy. Eur J Obstet Gynecol Reprod Biol. 2019 Dec;243:179–184.
47. Salazar CA, Isaacson KB. Office operating hysteroscopy: an update. J Minimal Invasive Gynecol 2018; 25(2):199–208.
48. Bosteels J, van Wessel S, Weyers S, et al. Hysteroscopy for treating subfertility associated with suspected major uterine cavity abnormalities. Cochrane Database Syst Rev. 2018 Dec 5;12:CD009461.
49. Bhalani V, Chang, A, Adkins, C, Chen S, Scheiber M. Fertility outcomes after hysteroscopic morcellation of intrauterine leiomyomas and polyps. J Reprod Med 2016;61(4):327–335.
50. Mais V, Cirronis MG, Peiretti M, Ferrucci G, Cossu E, Melis GB. Efficacy of auto-crosslinked hyaluronan gel for adhesion prevention in laparoscopy and hysteroscopy: a systematic review and meta-analysis of randomized controlled trials. Eur J Obstet Gynecol Reprod Biol 2012;160(01):1–5.
51. Bosteels J,Weyers S, Mol BW, D'Hooghe T. Anti-adhesion barrier gels following operative hysteroscopy for treating female infertility: a systematic review and meta-analysis. Gynecol Surg 2014;11:113–127.
52. Practice Committee of the American Society for Reproductive Medicine. Uterine septum: a guideline. Fertil Steril 2016 Sep 1; 106(3):530–540.
53. Hart R, Molnar BG, Magos A. Long term follow up of hysteroscopic myomectomy assessed by survival analysis. Br J Obstet Gynaecol 1999;106:700–705.
54. Pritts EA, Parker WH, Olive DL. Fibroids and infertility: an updated systematic review of the evidence. Fertil Steril 2009;91:1215–1223.

# 16

## HYSTEROSCOPIC REMOVAL OF INTRAUTERINE ADHESIONS AND INTRAUTERINE SEPTUM

**Priyanka Sinha, Shima Al Basha, Isabella Gottlieb, Candice P. Holliday, Ertug Kovanci, and Botros Rizk**

### Introduction

Hysteroscopy evaluates and treats intrauterine pathologies. Appropriate indications for hysteroscopy include infertility, retained intrauterine contraceptives, abnormal uterine bleeding, and Müllerian tract anomalies. Diagnostic hysteroscopy is the gold standard for evaluating the uterine cavity because it allows the provider to have direct visualization [1]. Should the intent of hysteroscopy be both diagnostic and therapeutic, the term operative hysteroscopy is used instead. With recent advances in technology, operative hysteroscopes have a diameter of 4.0–5.5 mm and have up to two instrument channels for grasping forceps, biopsy forceps, scissors, morcellators, myoma fixation instruments, and more [1].

Two common indications for operative hysteroscopy are removal of intrauterine adhesions and uterine septum. A uterine septum occurs when the longitudinal band of muscular tissue between the left and right Müllerian ducts fails to resorb completely prior to the 20th embryonic week.

A uterine septum is an upside down, triangular shaped piece of tissue which divides all or part of the uterine cavity in two. Restoration of the anatomy of the uterus by hysteroscopic septum incision improves pregnancy outcomes [2]. Pregnancy and delivery rates following hysteroscopic septal incision using cold scissors are significantly greater [3].

Intrauterine adhesions are bands of fibrous tissue that form in the endometrial cavity due to uterine procedures. They can manifest as thin strings of tissue or form thick fibrous bands, completely obliterating the cavity. The most common cause of uterine adhesions is trauma following an intrauterine surgical procedure, primarily dilatation and curettage. Hysteroscopic adhesion removal is generally recommended for intrauterine adhesions.

#### Uterine septum

Uterine septum accounts for approximately 80%–90% of congenital uterine malformation and is the most common type of congenital uterine malformation [4]. The septum is composed primarily of muscle fibers and less so connective tissue, as shown by biopsy specimens and magnetic resonance imaging (MRI) [5, 6].

Studies show that poor vascularity, reduced sensitivity of the septal endometrium to preovulatory changes, uncoordinated contractility, and local defect of vascular endothelial growth factor (VEGF) receptors in the septal endometrium make the uterine septum a poor site for embryo implantation [7]. Patients may be asymptomatic or have poor reproductive outcomes [7]. Reproductive failure, obstetrical complications, and an increased incidence of recurrent miscarriage are found in nearly 40% of patients with uterine septum [7].

There are two septum subtypes: partial and complete. A partial septum (subseptate uterus) involves the endometrial canal but not the cervix. In a complete septum, the septum extends from the top of the endometrial cavity and continues through the cervix or extends into a duplicated cervix [8]. The latter may be seen in combination with a longitudinal vaginal septum.

The size and shape of the septum can vary by width, length, and vascularity. The European Society of Human Reproduction and Embryology and the European Society for Gynecological Endoscopy define uterine septum as an internal indentation extending >50% of myometrial wall thickness [9]. A septate uterus should be differentiated from an arcuate or bicornuate uterus for the purposes of prognosis and surgical management.

The American Society of Reproductive Medicine (ASRM) uses the following criteria to differentiate these uterine anomalies:

The arcuate uterus has an angle of tissue indentation of >90 degrees and a depth from the interstitial line to the apex of indentation of <1 cm [10].

The septate uterus has an angle of indentation <90 degrees and a depth from the interstitial line to the apex of indentation of >1.5 cm [10].

The bicornuate uterus has an external fundal indentation of >1 cm. The internal endometrial cavity is similar to the partial uterine septum [10].

#### Intrauterine adhesions

Intrauterine adhesions, also known as intrauterine synechiae and Asherman's syndrome, were first described by Joseph Asherman in 1948 [11]. They are bands of fibrous tissue that form in the endometrial cavity due to intrauterine procedures. They can manifest as thin strings of tissue or form thick fibrous bands, completely obliterating the cavity [12–14]. The endometrium consists of basal and superficial (or functional) layers. The functional layer responds to the cyclical changes of ovarian hormones. Endometrial growth is stimulated in the proliferative phase due to an increase in hormone production, while there is shedding and menstruation in the secretory phase due to a decrease in hormone production. The functional layer is shed during the menstrual cycle while the basal layer is not shed at any time during the menstrual cycle. The basal layer provides the basis for regeneration of the functional layer and regeneration is completed without formation of adhesions. Loss of stroma due to endometrial injury leads to adhesion formation. Fibrous tissue replaces the lost stroma, causing endometrial surfaces to bond to each other and leading to adhesion formation. The basal and functional layers are replaced by an avascular and epithelial monolayer, so the differentiation of these layers is lost, making them unresponsive to hormonal stimulations [15].

## Etiology

### Uterine septum

A uterine septum occurs when the longitudinal band of muscular tissue between the left and right Müllerian ducts fails to resorb completely prior to the 20th embryonic week.

### Intrauterine adhesions

The most common cause of uterine adhesion is trauma following an intrauterine surgical procedure; the most common surgical procedure causing adhesion is dilatation and curettage. Others are myomectomy, cesarean section, endometrial ablation, and septum removal. Adhesions may also form following pregnancy complications such as uterine bleeding after childbirth or miscarriage. Endometritis can also cause adhesions [11].

Adhesions may also form following postpartum or postabortion sharp curettage of the endometrial cavity [16]. In these cases, sharp curettage removes the decidua, which is extremely vulnerable to trauma and infection, and injures the myometrium, ultimately leading to adhesion formation between the anterior and posterior walls of the uterus. The extent of injury determines the amount of adhesion formation. The fundus of the uterus is the most common site for adhesion formation. Other sites are the lower segment, junction of the cervix and uterus, and the cervical canal.

## Patient presentation

### Uterine septum

Patients may be asymptomatic or have poor reproductive outcomes [7]. Reproductive failure, obstetrical complications, and an increased incidence of recurrent miscarriage are found in nearly 40% of patients with uterine septum [7]. A 2018 Cochrane study showed that 1%–4% of women with unexplained infertility had a septate uterus [17].

For women undergoing surgical evaluation for abnormal uterine bleeding, infertility, or pelvic pain, one study found that approximately 33% of these patients had uterine septum [18].

### Intrauterine adhesions

The effect on menstrual history depends on the severity of adhesions [12, 14].

In some cases, adhesion causes no symptoms at all, but the most common symptoms are hypomenorrhea, amenorrhea, dysmenorrhea, infertility, and recurrent pregnancy loss [11]. In patients with amenorrhea, outflow obstruction can cause cyclical pain and retrograde menstruation leading to endometriosis [19].

## Patient evaluation

The methods to diagnose uterine septum and intrauterine adhesions mainly include ultrasonography, hysterosalpingography (HSG), MRI, hysteroscopy, and laparoscopy.

## Hysterosalpingography

### Uterine septum

HSG is often the initial test for diagnosing uterine septum in patients with infertility or recurrent pregnancy loss, but the diagnostic accuracy of the HSG is low for differentiating septate and bicornuate uterus [20].

HSG reveals the size and length of the septum in a "Y" shape. Measuring the angle of fusion at the lower ends of the two horns can differentiate between a septate and bicornuate uterus. An acute angle of less than 90 degree between the uterine horns is suggestive of a septate uterus, while an obtuse angle is more consistent with bicornuate uteri [20].

Unfortunately, the majority of angles of divergence between the horns fall between these ranges, and considerable overlap between the two anomalies is noted. Angle measurements were used prior to the introduction of MRI visualization techniques.

Hysterosalpingogram has a 5.6%–88% accuracy rate for differentiating the septate uterus from the bicornuate uterus [21–24].

### Intrauterine adhesions

The procedure will fail if complete adhesion is present in the cervical canal and lower segment as dye will not be able to pass through the uterine cavity. HSG will show adhesions as multiple linear defects, giving the uterine cavity an irregular appearance when adhesions involve the body and fundus of the uterus. If extensive adhesions occupy the cavity, HSG will show a small uterine cavity [20] (**Figure 16.5**).

## Ultrasound and saline infusion sonohysterography (SIS)

### Uterine septum

Three-dimensional ultrasound with sonohysterography is very accurate in diagnosing septum [10]. The normal uterine cavity has a cone-like appearance on a sagittal view. The external uterine contour of the septate uterus demonstrates a convex, flat, or mildly concave (<1 cm) configuration, while the cavity is separated either partially (subseptate) (**Figure 16.1**) or completely (septate) (**Figure 16.2**) by a midline longitudinal band of tissue of different length and width with intermediate echogenicity (echotexture similar to myometrium) [25]. When planning hysteroscopic metroplasty, the thickness of the septum and the relationship of the septum to fundal myometrium is taken into consideration. Sonohysterography is better at differentiating a septate uterus from a bicornuate uterus [26, 27]. It is very important to differentiate a septate uterus from a bicornuate uterus as the respective

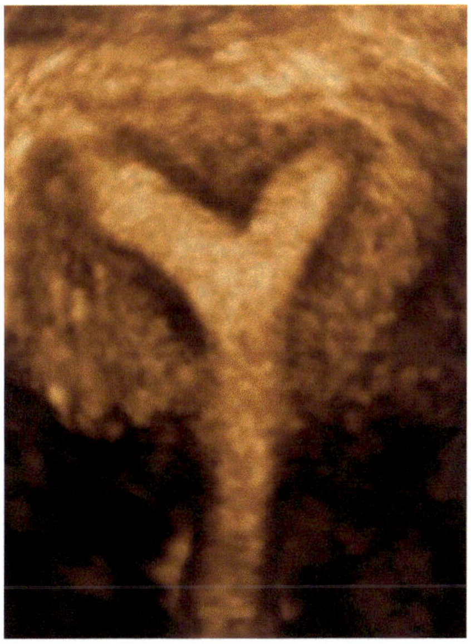

**FIGURE 16.1** Three-dimensional ultrasound showing small uterine septum. (Courtesy of Prof. Botros Rizk.)

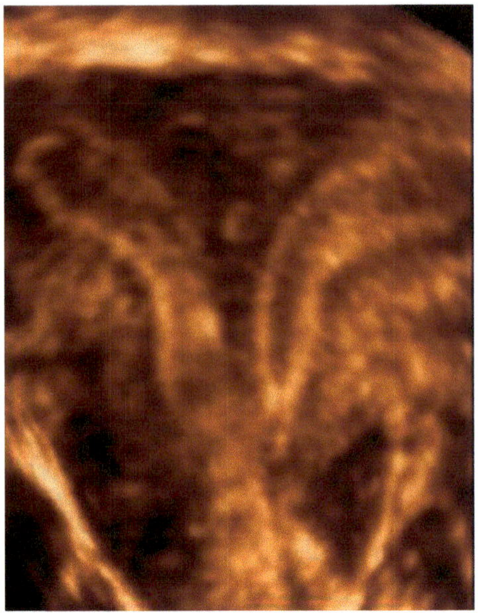

**FIGURE 16.2** Three-dimensional ultrasound showing long uterine septum. (Courtesy of Prof. Botros Rizk.)

corrective surgery for both conditions differs [25]. **Figure 16.3** shows a sonohysterography demonstrating two uterine cavities in the transverse section. The precise measurement of dimensions and volume can be done by three-dimensional ultrasound.

Color doppler may show vascularity in the septum in 70% of cases, which, if present, may be associated with obstetric complication [7]. Some studies suggest that sonohysterography or saline infusion sonography (SIS) is superior to HSG, since it is possible to assess the external as well as internal contour of the uterus.

Studies show that three-dimensional ultrasound combined with saline infusion has a 100% accuracy rate when compared with hysterolaparoscopy [25], and three-dimensional ultrasound without saline infusion has an 88% accuracy rate in diagnosing uterine septum when compared to hysterolaparoscopy [25, 28].

### Intrauterine adhesions

Transvaginal ultrasound may show adhesions as irregular endometrial stripes [24], but alone, it has very restricted diagnostic capability [29].

Sonohysterography demonstrates adhesions as thin, thick, firm, or undulating echogenic connecting bands extending from the anterior to posterior uterine walls on SIS [25]. The lateral walls

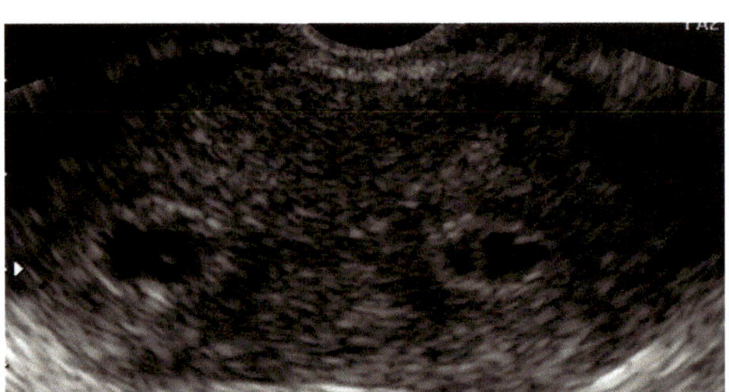

**FIGURE 16.3** Sonohysterography showing two uterine cavity in transverse section. (Courtesy of Prof. Botros Rizk.)

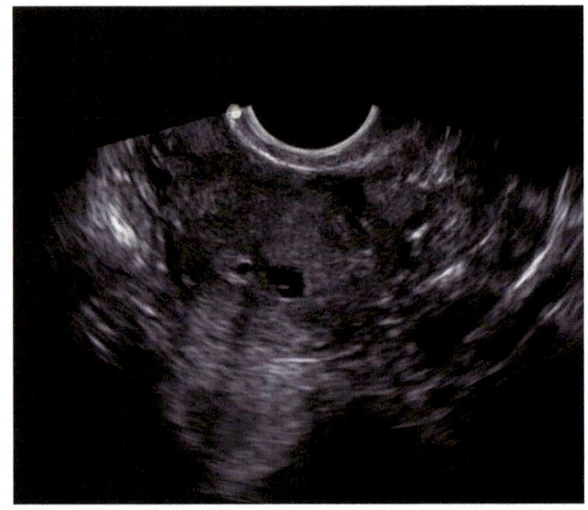

**FIGURE 16.4** Sonohysterography showing intrauterine adhesions in the transverse section. (Courtesy of Dr. Ertug Kovanci.)

and fundus of the uterus also may be involved, and true coronal plane views can help interpret the extent of the disease [25]. Not surprisingly, distension of the cavity may be difficult and require increased injection pressure. The procedure may fail in more severe cases where the endometrial wall is adhered and does not separate during the procedure [25] (**Figures 16.4** and **16.5**).

## MRI

### Uterine septum

MRI is often used for the diagnosis of Müllerian anomalies and is reported to have a high accuracy rate in diagnosing congenital uterine anomalies [10].

MRI allows a simultaneous evaluation of the cavity and fundus of the uterus. MRI of the septate uterus demonstrates a normal uterus with each endometrial cavity appearing smaller than a normal uterine cavity. The septum may be composed of fibrous tissue (low T2 signal intensity), muscular tissue (intermediate signal), or both [8].

The external fundal contour is convex, or flat, or has a slight indentation less than 1 cm deep. The intercornual distance is within the normal range and the intercornual angle is acute. These findings are best seen in oblique long-axis images [8]. A muscular septum has intermediate signal intensity with all pulse sequences, isointense to myometrium. A fibrous septum usually has a lower intensity with all sequences. The muscular or fibrotic nature of an intracavitary septum is assessed more on the basis

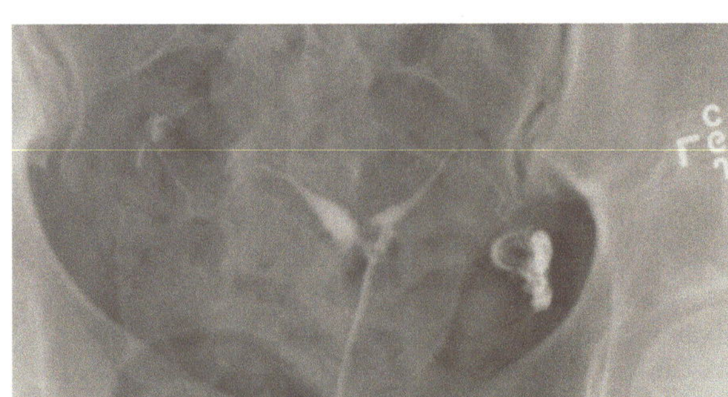

**FIGURE 16.5** Hysterosalpingography (HSG) of the patient in **Figure 16.4**, showing intrauterine adhesions. (Courtesy of Dr. Ertug Kovanci.)

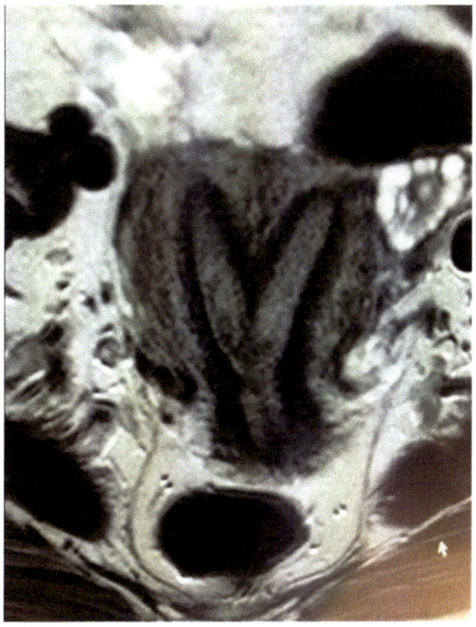

FIGURE 16.6 MRI image of intrauterine septum. (Courtesy of Prof. Botros Rizk.)

of septal thickness than on signal intensity; the fibrous septum is thin and linear [24]. If the septum reaches the internal os, it is complete. If it terminates above the internal os, it is a partial septum [30]. There are few studies comparing the diagnostic accuracy of hysterolaparoscopy with MRI. One study shows that MRI alone has a 70% accuracy rate in diagnosing uterine septum [31]. **Figure 16.6** shows an MRI image of a uterine septum.

### Intrauterine adhesions

Intrauterine adhesions can be diagnosed by MRI, mostly when cervical obstruction is suspected, but there is restricted experience with this technique [15].

## Hysteroscopy/laparoscopy

### Uterine septum

The septate uterine cavity manifests as a typical "cat's eye" shape on hysteroscopy. Hysteroscopy has high diagnostic accuracy, but it is relatively difficult to distinguish a septate uterus from a bicornuate or arcuate uterus on hysteroscopy alone [28, 29]. Conventionally, hysterolaparoscopy was the gold standard method for diagnosing uterine septum, involving direct visualization of the exterior and interior of the uterus. Hysterolaparoscopy can distinguish septate from bicornuate uterus, as it assesses both the outer and inner contour of the uterus. For patients with a uterine septum, a midline, fundal indentation of tissue into the uterine cavity is seen. Due to recent advancement of radiologic methods, the diagnosis of a septate uterus is typically made using radiographic methods rather than surgical techniques [17]. ASRM recommends that less invasive approaches such as hysteroscopy with imaging should be used for diagnosing uterine septum rather than hysterolaparoscopy [17]. **Figure 16.7** shows a hysteroscopic view of a uterine septum.

### Intrauterine adhesions

Conventionally, hysteroscopy was considered the gold standard for the diagnosis of intrauterine adhesions. Hysteroscopy can be performed in the office without anesthesia and allows direct visualization of the uterine cavity. Adhesions appear as thin, flimsy avascular strands, or thick stripes between the anterior

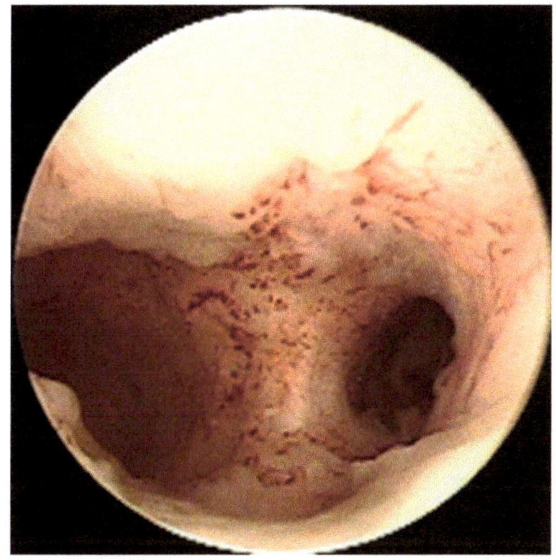

FIGURE 16.7 Hysteroscopic view of intrauterine septum. (Courtesy of Prof. Botros Rizk.)

and posterior walls, or may also appear as adherence of the walls resulting in partial or complete obstruction of the uterine cavity [32-35]. Because hysteroscopy is an invasive test, it should be used in a select group of patients with high likelihood of adhesions. It may be difficult to differentiate adhesions from a unicornuate uterus where only one side of the cavity can only be seen on hysteroscopy.

Hysteroscopy will be difficult in cases where adhesions obliterate the lower part of the uterine cavity. Adhesions in the lower part of the uterine cavity can cause obstruction and make identification of the surgical plane difficult, leading to procedure failure [32–35]. **Figures 16.8**, **16.9**, and **16.10a,b** show a hysteroscopic view of intrauterine adhesions. **Figure 16.11a** shows a hysteroscopic view of severe Asherman's syndrome.

## Preoperative considerations

Preoperative considerations include cervical ripening and optimization of the endometrium. Because almost one-half of all complications occur while inserting the hysteroscope through the cervix, cervical ripening can assist the provider [36]. Unfortunately, there is no universal consensus regarding agent

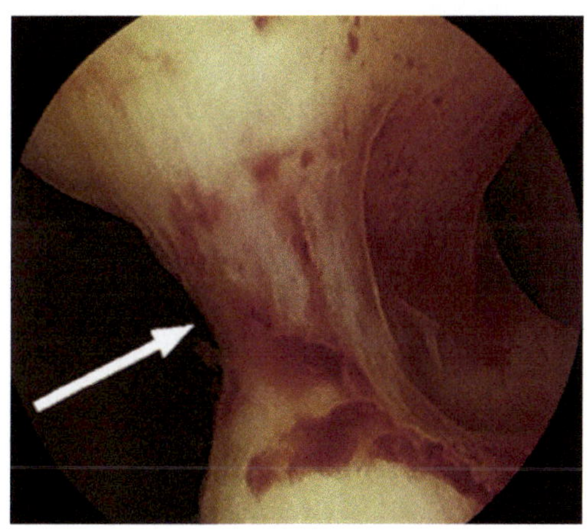

FIGURE 16.8 Hysteroscopic view of intrauterine adhesions. (Courtesy of Prof. Botros Rizk.)

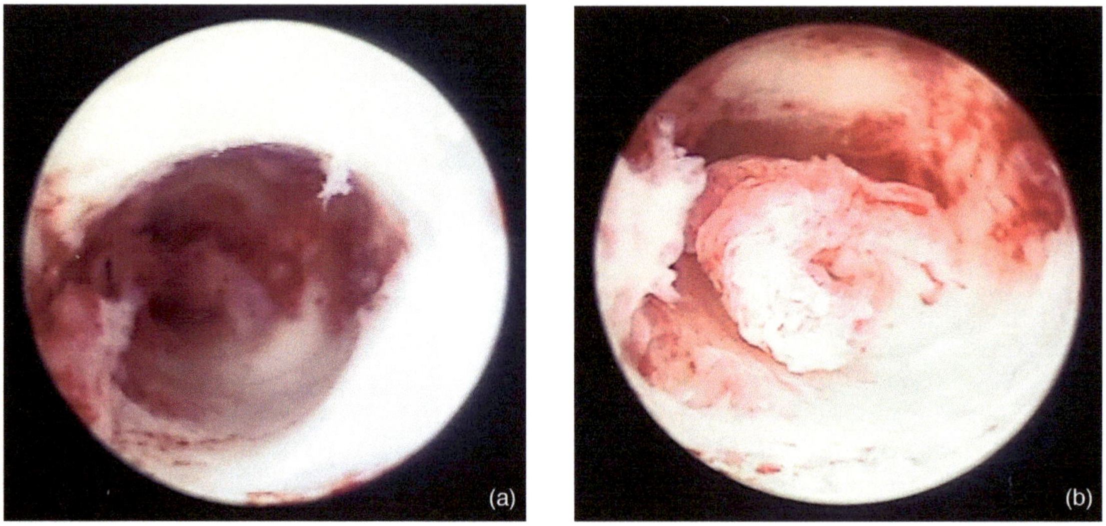

**FIGURE 16.9** Hysteroscopic view of intrauterine cavity of the patient in **Figures 16.4** and **16.5**, showing intrauterine adhesions. (Courtesy of Dr. Ertug Kovanci.)

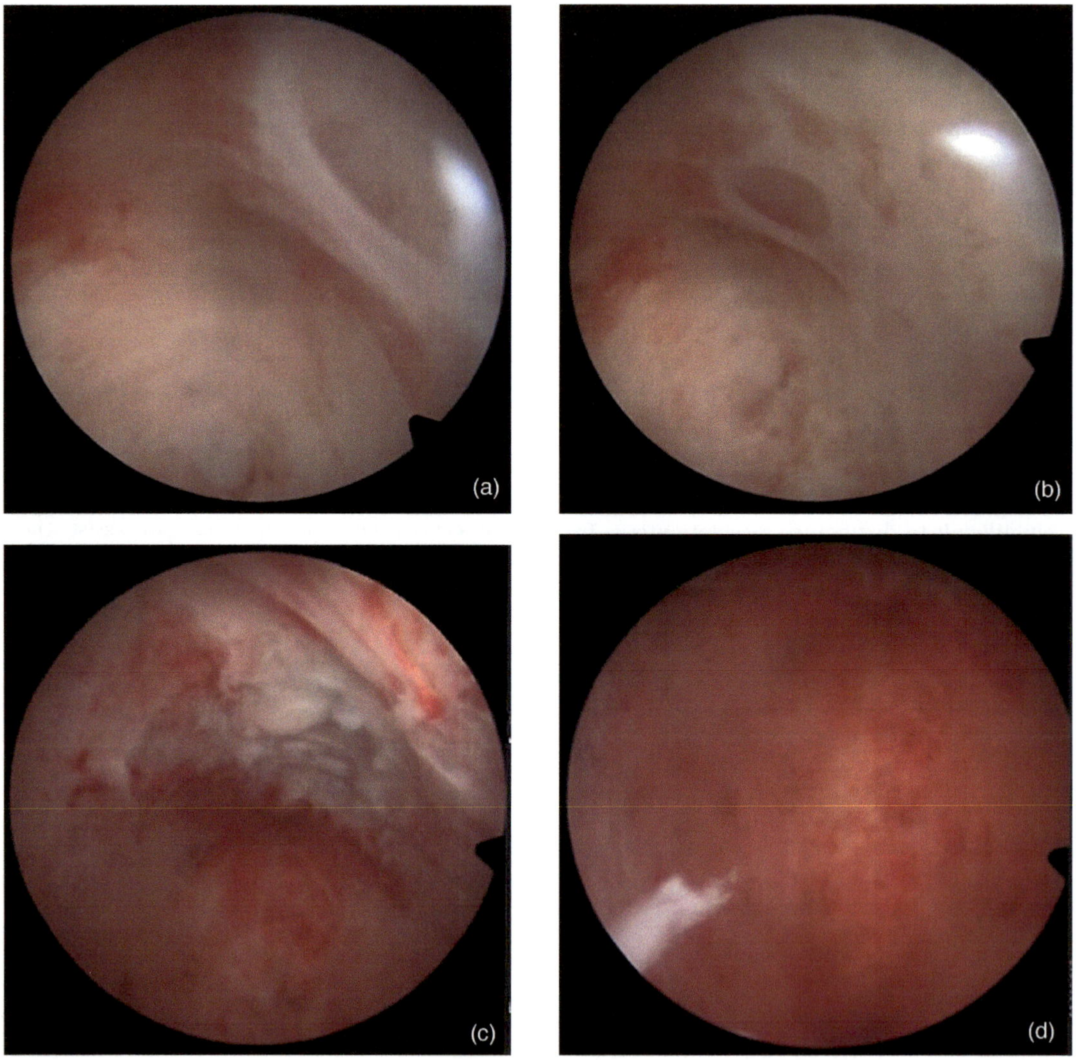

**FIGURE 16.10** (a,b) Hysteroscopic view of intrauterine cavity adhesions; (c,d) hysteroscopic view of intrauterine cavity after hysteroscopic adhesiolysis. (Courtesy of Dr. Carolyn Alexander.)

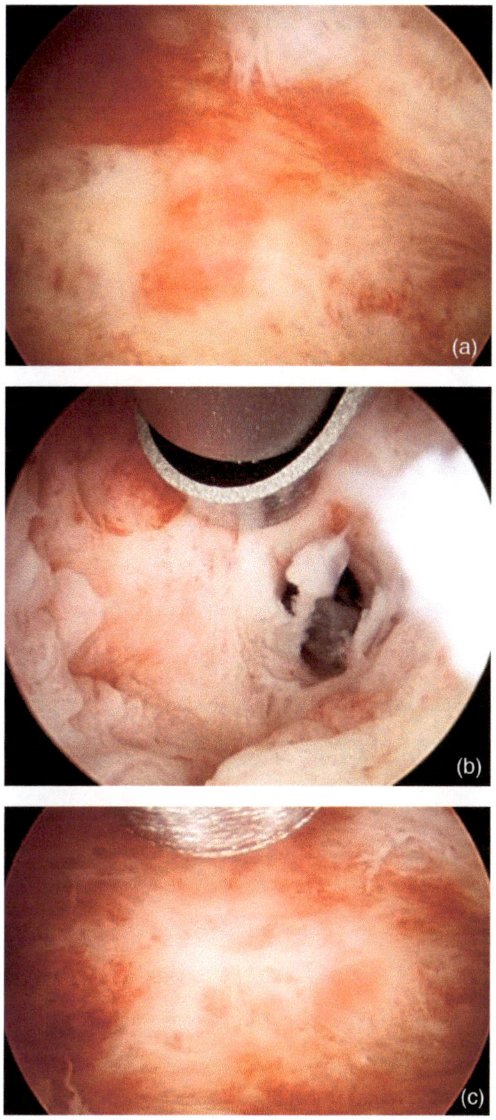


**FIGURE 16.11** (a) Severe Asherman's syndrome demonstrating severe adhesions. (b) MyoSure device introduced in the lower part of the uterine cavity. (c) Normal uterine cavity after removal of adhesions by MyoSure. (Courtesy of Prof. Botros Rizk.)

or timing, but some authors advocate 200–400 μg of vaginal misoprostol approximately 8–12 hours before the procedure [36]. As far as optimizing the endometrium, timing the procedure for the proliferative stage can be advantageous, but requires careful scheduling. Use of GnRH agonists, selective progesterone receptor modulators, and anti-progestins to otherwise achieve optimal intrauterine conditions has been studied, but no consensus exists as to the balance of risks versus benefits [36, 37].

## Operative hysteroscopy

### Uterine septum

Conventionally, the uterine septum was repaired with a laparotomy (Jones or modified Tompkins procedure), but due to advancement of less invasive hysteroscopic techniques, these procedures have been abandoned [10]. Uterine septum can be removed hysteroscopically in the operative room under anesthesia or in an office setting. Commonly used techniques include incision of the septum with cold scissors, unipolar or bipolar cautery, laser, or morcellators. Choice of distension media for hysteroscopy is also important. Nonconductive distension media, like 3% sorbitol or 1.5% glycine, are necessary for monopolar resectoscopes (36). Conductive distension media, like normal saline however are used for bipolar resectoscopy and morcellation [36]. To decrease the risk of uterine perforation and evaluate the complete removal of septum or any other associated anomaly, laparoscopy, or more recently, transabdominal ultrasound can be added [38]. There is no consensus regarding the best method to accomplish removal [11]. Studies comparing unipolar and bipolar techniques have shown no difference in pregnancy delivery rate, preterm delivery, or spontaneous abortion incidence, but operative time, fluid absorption rate, and cervical trauma were significantly greater in unipolar techniques [39]. Studies show that pregnancy and delivery rates are significantly greater in women undergoing septal incision using cold scissors when compared to unipolar techniques [3]. One prospective study demonstrated that ultrasound guidance during hysteroscopic septal incision has similar efficacy and safety compared to laparoscopic observation [40]. **Figure 16.12a–c** show a stepwise approach with a resectoscope during hysteroscopic septum removal for complete uterine septum reaching to the internal os.

The MyoSure Hysteroscopic Tissue Removal System is efficacious in both ambulatory surgical centers and office settings [41]. The MyoSure system is of small enough diameter to allow for use with minimal cervical dilation, which can typically be performed using local anesthesia in the form of a paracervical block. In addition, the MyoSure system uses no electrical energy and is associated with minimal discomfort to patients under local anesthesia [42–44]. MyoSure does not cause thermal damage to surrounding tissues and organs and can reduce the electrosurgical risks and occurrence of water intoxication.

### Septum resection range

Because of the traction effect of the anterior and posterior uterine walls, a slight retraction may occur after uterine septum incision, and normally there is no need for excessive septum resection [45]. If the separation is too deep, damage may be caused to the uterine muscle wall, resulting in heavy bleeding or even uterine perforation; if the separation is too shallow, residual septum may occur, affecting the surgical outcomes [45]. The depth of septum resection is determined by either ultrasound or laparoscopic monitoring, or by the relative position of the incised portion and the uterine horns [45].

Complete septums should be cut from the internal cervical os upward to the fundus; the intracervical septum or uterus didelphys septum should not be resected to avoid cervical incompetence and the artificially increased probability of miscarriage and premature birth caused from it [45]. **Figures 16.13** and **16.14** demonstrate the stepwise progression of hysteroscopic septum removal with the MyoSure device.

### Intrauterine adhesions

Hysteroscopic removal is generally recommended for the treatment of intrauterine adhesions.

Commonly used surgical techniques include adhesiolysis with cold scissors, unipolar or bipolar cautery, laser, or morcellators. Markers of successful treatment are restoration of normal menses, conception, and live birth rate, but many use second-look surgery to estimate the success of treatment [46–49]. Recurrence of intrauterine adhesions is very common despite the use of supplementary treatments, such as postoperative insertion of an intrauterine contraceptive

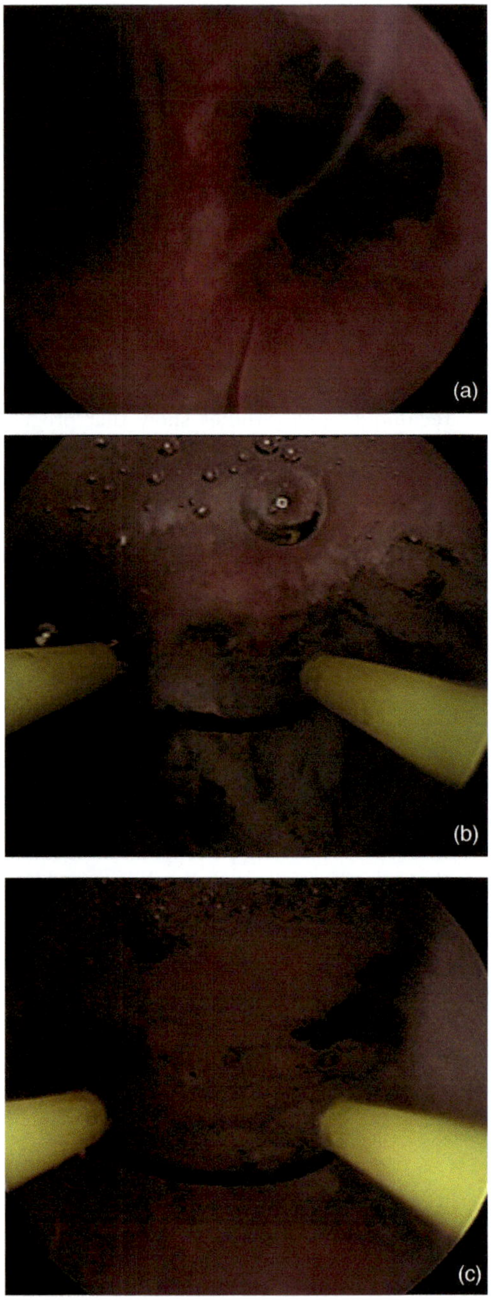


FIGURE 16.12 Stepwise approach with resectoscope during hysteroscopic septum removal for complete uterine septum reaching to the internal os: (a) complete uterine septum reaching to the internal os; (b) septal incision with the resectoscope; (c) uterine cavity at the end of procedure. (Courtesy of Dr. M Abuzeid.)

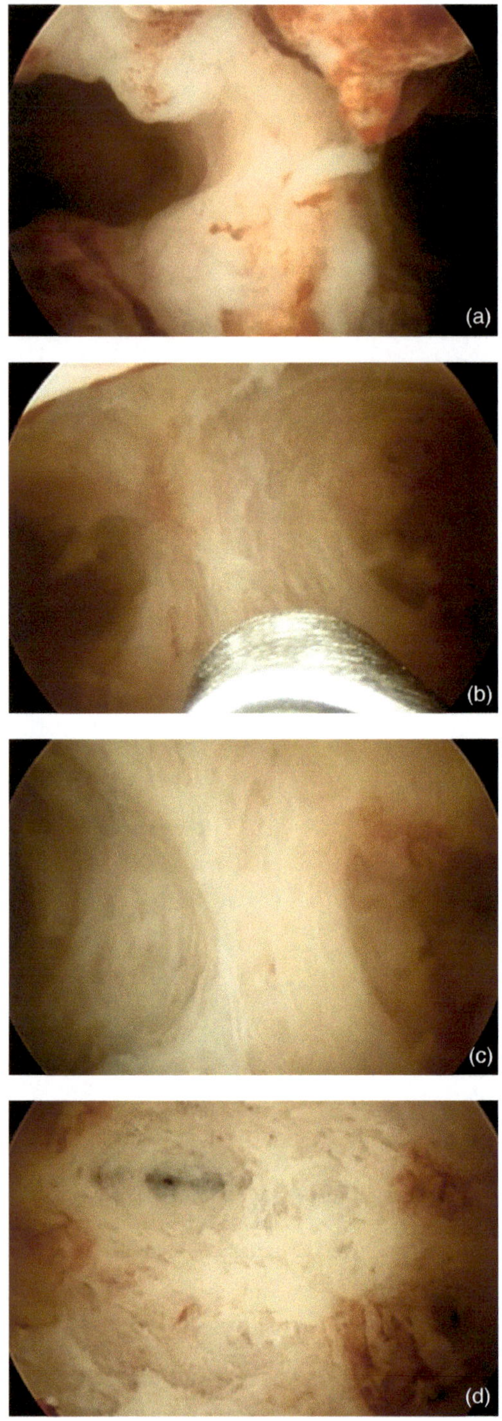


FIGURE 16.13 (a–c) Stepwise approach with the MyoSure device during hysteroscopic septum removal; (d) normal uterine cavity at the completion of procedure. (Courtesy of Prof. Botros Rizk.)

device, anti-adhesive barrier agents, and high dose estrogen. Recurrence rate for intrauterine adhesions varies from 3.1% to 23.5% [50, 51]. Severe forms can have recurrence rates from 20% to 62.5% [51–52]. Multiple surgeries are often required in these patients. Ultrasound can be used to assist difficult hysteroscopic procedures for adhesions. Studies comparing hysteroscopic adhesiolysis using laparoscopic, ultrasound, or no guidance have found that ultrasound is reliable, safe, and cost effective [53]. Postoperative ultrasound can be done to check for recurrent intrauterine adhesions, avoiding the need for routine posttreatment hysteroscopy and eventually reducing the overall cost of treatment and social inconvenience to women. Ultrasound can detect residual adhesions and assist in planning of future treatment. **Figure 16.15** shows a hysteroscopic adhesiolysis with cold scissors. **Figures 16.11a–c** demonstrate the stepwise progression of hysteroscopic adhesiolysis with MyoSure. **Figures 16.10a** and **16.15b** show intrauterine cavity before hysteroscopic adhesiolysis. **Figure 16.10c,d** show intrauterine cavity after hysteroscopic adhesiolysis.

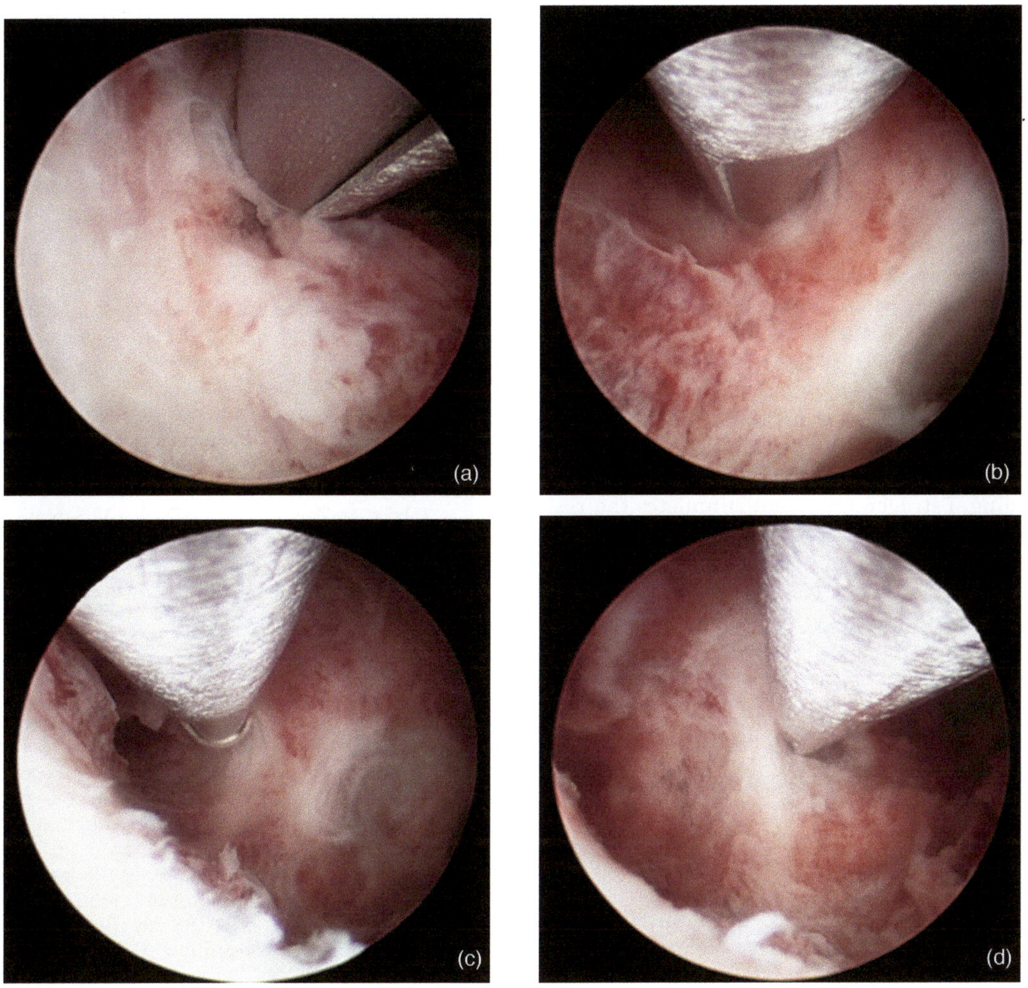


FIGURE 16.14 (a–d) Stepwise approach with the MyoSure device during hysteroscopic septum removal. (Courtesy of Prof. Botros Rizk.)

## Outcomes

### Uterine septum

Various observational studies show improved pregnancy rates after hysteroscopic septum incision in women with infertility [10].

Some limited studies indicate that hysteroscopic removal of septum improves live birth rates and reduces miscarriage rate in patients with a history of recurrent pregnancy loss [10].

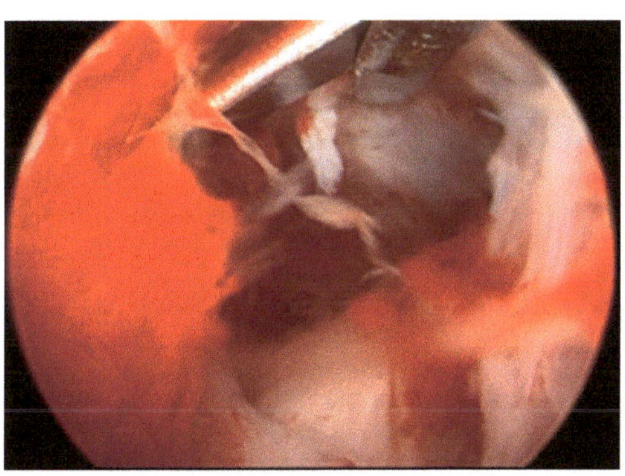

FIGURE 16.15 Hysteroscopic adhesiolysis using cold scissors. (Courtesy of Prof. Botros Rizk.)

Limited studies also indicate that hysteroscopic septum incision improves live birth rates in women with infertility or prior miscarriage [10].

### Intrauterine adhesions

The type and extent of adhesions determines the reproductive outcome after hysteroscopic adhesiolysis. Full-term pregnancy rate after treatment for mild to moderate and severe to extensive adhesions are 70%–80% and 20%–40%, respectively. Menstrual symptoms are frequently reduced after treatment of mild to moderate adhesions. Gestational surrogacy can be suggested to women with extensive adhesions unresponsive to treatment.

## Postoperative considerations

### Uterine septum

The uterine cavity and the covering endometrium become morphologically normal within 8 weeks after a uterine septum surgical resection. However, there is inadequate evidence to recommend a specific time span to attempt conception after the repair [10].

The risk of intrauterine adhesion formation following hysteroscopic septal incision is low, but once formed can have significant consequences. Suggested treatment options to separate the endometrial walls and reduce the risk of postoperative adhesion formation include antibiotics, postoperative estrogen therapy, placement of an intrauterine balloon or device, and use of intrauterine auto-crosslinked hyaluronic acid gel [10]. There is inadequate evidence to propose any specific method or whether to use any postoperative treatment for adhesion prevention following hysteroscopic septum incision [10].

### Intrauterine adhesions

Following adhesion removal, many surgeons recommend using supplementary treatments such as a plastic catheter, intrauterine contraceptive device, anti-adhesive barrier agents, and horonal treatment with estrogen and progesterone to lessen the chance of adhesion formation. Despite the above supplemental treatments, recurrence of intrauterine adhesions is very common. Postoperative patients can be put on estrogen treatment for 6–8 weeks followed by progesterone for 10 days to produce withdrawal bleeding. Estrogen treatment stimulates the residual islands of the endometrium to grow and assist in healing the injury site. Postoperatively, many surgeons use second-look surgery to estimate the success of treatment [46–49]. To avoid the need for operative hysteroscopy, ultrasound can be done to check for recurrent intrauterine adhesions, eventually reducing the overall cost of treatment and social inconvenience to women.

## Common complications

The complications associated with operative hysteroscopy are perforation, infection, bleeding, fluid overload, gas embolism, and adhesions [36].

Nonconductive distension media are hypotonic; complications can include hyponatremia, pulmonary edema, and cerebral edema [10]. Conductive distension media, like normal saline, however, are used for bipolar resectoscopy and morcellation and tend to have less risk of metabolic complications [10]. There is risk of uterine rupture during pregnancy or delivery following septal incision [7]; this risk is correlated with excessive septal incision, penetration of the myometrium, uterine wall perforation, and excessive use of cautery or laser energy during the initial septum incision procedure [7].

## Conclusion

Hysteroscopic removal of uterine septum and adhesions offers an important minimally invasive technique to treat common uterine pathologies. Although there are several different techniques available for each pathology, there are no universally accepted guidelines for which technique to use when; and they are for the most part similar in success and complications.

Diagnosis of uterine septum should be done by imaging or imaging with hysteroscopy rather than hysterolaparoscopy. Hysteroscopic septal incision should be considered in patients with infertility, prior pregnancy loss, or poor obstetrical outcome. Counseling regarding potential risks and benefits of the procedure should be done in patients without infertility or prior pregnancy loss before considering hysteroscopic septal incision. The best method for treating intrauterine adhesions is hysteroscopic adhesiolysis. Hysteroscopic adhesiolysis under ultrasound guidance improves both safety and efficacy of this procedure by providing intraoperative suggestions in difficult cases and fast and objective feedback on the success of surgery, avoiding the need for additional invasive surgery. This has the ability to reduce further the risks linked with repeated surgery, eventually reducing the overall cost of treatment and social inconvenience to women.

## References


1. Bosteels J, van Wessel S, Weyers S, et al. Hysteroscopy for treating subfertility associated with suspected major uterine cavity abnormalities. Cochrane Database Syst Rev. 2018 Dec 5;12:CD009461.
2. Grimbizis GF, Camus M, Tarlatzis BC, Bontis JN, Devroey P. Clinical implications of uterine malformations and hysteroscopic treatment results. *Hum Reprod Update.* 2001;7(2):161–74.
3. Cararach M1, Penella J, Ubeda A, Labastida R. Hysteroscopic incision of the septate uterus: scissors versus resectoscope. Hum Reprod. 1994 Jan;9(1):87–9
4. Troiano RN1, McCarthy SM. Müllerian duct anomalies: imaging and clinical issues. Radiology. 2004 Oct;233(1):19–34. Epub 2004 Aug 18.
5. Dabirashrafi H1, Bahadori M, Mohammad K, Alavi M, Moghadami-Tabrizi N, Zandinejad K, Ghafari V. Septate uterus: new idea on histologic features of the septum in this abnormal uterus. *Am J Obstet Gynecol.* 1995 Jan;172(1 pt 1):105–7
6. Pellerito JS1, McCarthy SM, Doyle MB, Glickman MG, De Cherney AH. Diagnosis of uterine anomalies: relative accuracy of MR imaging, endovaginal sonography, and hysterosalpingography. Radiology. 1992 Jun;183(3):795–800.
7. Valle RF, Ekpo GE. Hysteroscopic metroplasty for the septate uterus: review and meta-analysis. *J Min Invas Gynecol.* 2013;20:22–42
8. Grimbizis GF, Gordts S, Sardo AD, Brucker S, DeAngelis C, Gergolet M, et al. The ESHRE/ESGE consensus on the classification of female genital tract congenital anomalies. *Hum Reprod.* 2013;28:2032–44.
8. Buttram VC Jr, Gibbons WE. Müllerian anomalies: a proposed classification. An analysis of 144 cases. Fertil Steril 1979;32:40–6.
10. Practice Committee of the American Society for Reproductive Medicine. Uterine septum: a guideline. *Fertil Steril.* 2016 Sep 1; 106(3):530–40.
11. Jay M Berman, Intrauterine adhesions. Semin Reprod Med. 2008 Jul;26(4):349–55.
12. Buttram V, Turati G. Uterine synechiae: variation in severity and some conditions which may be conducive to severe adhesions. *Int J Fertil.* 1977;22: 98.
13. Jensen P, Stromme W. Amenorrhea after puerperal curettage. *Am J Obstet Gynecol.* 1971;113:150.
14. Jewelewicz R, Khalaf S, Neuwirth R, et al: Obstetric complications after treatment of intrauterine synechiae (Asherman's Syndrome). *Obstet Gynecol.* 1976;47: 701.
15. Yu D, Wong Y-M, Cheong Y, Xia E, Li T-C. Asherman syndrome – one century later. *Fertil Steril.* 2008;89:759–79.
16. Wamsteker K, De Block S. Diagnostic hysteroscopy: technique and documentation. In *Endoscopic Surgery for Gynecologists.* Sutton C, Diamond M (eds). W. B. Saunders: London, 1998; 511–24.
17. Y.Y. Chan, Jayaprakasan K, Zamora J, Thornton JG, Raine-Fenning N, Coomarasamy A. The prevalence of congenital uterine anomalies in unselected and high-risk populations: a systematic review. Hum Reprod Update. 2011 Nov;17(6):761–71.
18. LaMonica R, Pinto J, Luciano D, et al. Incidence of septate uterus in reproductive-aged women with and without endometriosis. J Minim Invasive Gynecol. 2016 May-Jun;23(4):610–3.
19. March CM. Asherman's syndrome. Semin Reprod Med. 2011; 29:83.
20. Shawky Z, Badawy A, Stuart J, Singer A and Etman A. Hysterosalpingography. *Ultrasonography in Reproductive Medicine and Infertility.* Cambridge University Press, 2010 March; 25(22-33).
21. Mucowski SJ1, Herndon CN, Rosen MP. The arcuate uterine anomaly: a critical appraisal of its diagnostic and clinical relevance. Obstet Gynecol Surv. 2010 Jul;65(7):449–54.
22. Assaf A1, Serour G, Elkady A, el Agizy H. Endoscopic management of the intrauterine septum. *Int J Gynaecol Obstet.* 1990 May;32(1):43–51.

23. Braun P1, Grau FV, Pons RM, Enguix DP. Is hysterosalpingography able to diagnose all uterine malformations correctly? A retrospective study. *Eur J Radiol.* 2005 Feb;53(2):274–9.
24. Saravelos SH, Cocksedge KA, Li TC. The pattern of pregnancy loss in women with congenital uterine anomalies and recurrent miscarriage. Reproductive Biomedicine Online [11 Dec 2009, 20(3):416–22]
25. William WB. Sonohysterography. Ultrasonography in Reproductive Medicine and Infertility, Cambridge University Press, 2010; 42–53.
26. Moini A1, Mohammadi S, Hosseini R, Eslami B, Ahmadi F. Accuracy of 3-dimensional sonography for diagnosis and classification of congenital uterine anomalies. *J Ultrasound Med.* 2013 Jun;32(6):923–7.
27. Ludwin A, Ludwin I, Kudla M, Pitynski K, Banas T, Jach R, et al. Diagnostic accuracy of three-dimensional sonohysterography compared with office hysteroscopy and its interrater/intrarater agreement in uterine cavity assessment after hysteroscopic metroplasty. *Fertil Steril.* 2014;101:1392–9.
28. Alborzi S, Dehbashi S, Parsanezhad ME. Differential diagnosis of septate and bicornuate uterus by sonohysterography eliminates the need for laparoscopy. *Fertil Steril.* 2002;78:176–8.
29. Salle B, Gaucherand P, de Saint Hilaire P, Rudigoz RC. Transvaginal sonohysterographic evaluation of intrauterine adhesions. *J Clin Ultrasound.* 1999;27(3):131–4.
30. Sheth SS, Sonkawde R. Uterine septum misdiagnosed on hysterosalpingogram. Int J Gynaecol Obstet. 2000;69:261–3.
31. El Saman AM1, Shahin AY, Nasr A, Tawfik RM, Saadeldeen HS, Othman ER, Habib DM, Abdel-Aleem MA., Hybrid septate uterus, coexistence of bicornuate and septate varieties: a genuine report. *J Obstet Gynaecol Res.* 2012 Nov;38(11):1308–14.
32. March CM, Israel R, March AD. Hysteroscopic management of intrauterine adhesions. *Am J Obstet Gynecol.* 1978;130:653–7.
33. Nasr AL, Al-Inany HG, Thabet SM, Aboulghar M. A clinicohysteroscopic scoring system of intrauterine adhesions. *Gynecol Obstet Invest.* 2000;50:178–81.
34. The American Fertility Society classifications of adnexal adhesions, distal tubal occlusion, tubal occlusion secondary to tubal ligation, tubal pregnancies, müllerian anomalies and intrauterine adhesions. *Fertil Steril.* 1988;49:944–55.
35. Donnez J, Nisolle M. Hysteroscopic lysis of intrauterine adhesions (Asherman's syndrome). In *Atlas of Laser Operative Laparoscopy and Hysteroscopy.* Donnez J (ed). Parthenon Publishing: New York, 1994; 305–22.
36. Friedman JA, Wong JMK, Chaudhari A, et al. Hysteroscopic myomectomy: a comparison of techniques and review of current evidence in the management of abnormal uterine bleeding. Curr Opin Obstet Gynecol. 2018 Aug;30(4):243–51.
37. Di Spiezio Sardo A, Mazzon I, Bramante S, et al. Hysteroscopic myomectomy: a comprehensive review of surgical techniques. Hum Reprod Update. 2008 Mar-Apr;14(2):101–19.
38. Karande VC, Gleicher N. Resection of uterine septum using gynaeco radiological techniques. Hum Reprod. 1999;14:1226–9.
39. Colacurci N1, De Franciscis P, Mollo A, Litta P, Perino A, Cobellis L, De Placido G. Small-diameter hysteroscopy with Versapoint versus resectoscopy with a unipolar knife for the treatment of septate uterus: a prospective randomized study. J Minim Invasive Gynecol. 2007 Sep-Oct;14(5):622–7.
40. Coccia ME, Becattini C, Bracco GL, Bargelli G, Scarselli G. Intraoperative ultrasound guidance for operative hysteroscopy. A prospective study. J Reprod Med. 2000;45:413–8.
41. Rubino RJ, Lukes AS. Twelve-month outcomes for patients undergoing hysteroscopic morcellation of uterine polyps and myomas in an office or ambulatory surgical center. J Minim Invasive Gynecol. 2015;22:285–90.
42. Shazly SAM, Laughlin-Tommaso SK, Breitkopf DM, et al. Hysteroscopic morcellation versus resection for the treatment of Uterine cavitary lesions: a systematic review and meta-analysis. J Minim Invasive Gynecol. 2016;23(6):867–77.
43. Michael D Scheiber MD, MPH 1 and Serena H. Chen, MD2 A prospective multicenter registry of patients undergoing hysteroscopic morcellation of uterine polyps and myomas. J Gynecol Surg. 2016 Dec 1;32(6):318–23.
44. Arnold A, Ketheeswaran A, Bhatti M, Nesbitt-Hawes E, Abbott J. A prospective analysis of hysteroscopic morcellation in the management of intrauterine pathologies. J Minimal Invasive Gynecol. 2016;23(3):435–41.
45. Wang S, Shi X, Hua X, Gu X, Yang D. Hysteroscopic transcervical resection of uterine septum. JSLS. 2013 Oct-Dec;17(4):517–20.
46. Yang J-H, Chen M-J, Wu M-Y, Chao K-H, Ho H-N, Yang Y-S. Office hysteroscopic early lysis of intrauterine adhesion after transcervical resection of multiple apposing submucous myomas. Fertil Steril. 2008;89(5):1254–9.
47. Yu D, Li T-C, Xia E, Huang X, Liu Y, Peng X. Factors affecting reproductive outcome of hysteroscopic adhesiolysis for Asherman's syndrome. *Fertil Steril.* 2008;89:715–22.
48. Fernandez H, Al-Najjar F, Chauveaud-Lambling A, Frydman R, Gervaise A. Fertility after treatment of Asherman's syndrome stage 3 and 4. *J Minim Invasive Gynecol.* 2006;13:398–402.
49. Zikopoulos KA, Kolibianakis EM, Platteau P, de Munck L, Tournaye H, Devroey P, Camus M. Live delivery rates in subfertile women with Asherman's syndrome after hysteroscopic adhesiolysis using the resectoscope or the Versapoint system. *Reprod Biomed Online.* 2004;8:720–25.
50. Pabuçcu R, Atay V, Orhon E, Urman B, Ergün A. Hysteroscopic treatment of intrauterine adhesions is safe and effective in the restoration of normal menstruation and fertility. *Fertil Steril.* 1997;68: 1141–3.
51. Preutthipan S, Linasmita V. Reproductive outcome following hysteroscopic lysis of intrauterine adhesions: a result of 65 cases at Ramathibodi Hospital. *J Med Assoc Thai.* 2000;83:42–6.
52. Capella-Allouc S, Morsad F, Rongières-Bertrand C, Taylor S, Fernandez H. Hysteroscopic treatment of severe Asherman's syndrome and subsequent fertility. *Hum Reprod.* 1999;14:1230–33.
53. Kresowik JD, Syrop CH, Van Voorhis BJ, Ryan GL. Ultrasound is the optimal choice for guidance in difficult hysteroscopy. *Ultrasound Obstet Gynecol.* 2012;39:715–8.

# 17

# ENDOMETRIAL "SCRATCHING"

## *An Update and Overview of Current Research*

**Veronika Günther and Ibrahim Alkatout**

## Introduction

Approximately one of every six couples is affected by sterility. Procedures of assisted reproduction are currently the method of choice for a number of patients desiring children [1]. Many causes of sterility can be overcome by the aid of in vitro fertilization (IVF), but successful implantation of the embryo still is the major limiting factor. Implantation, also known as nidation, starts on day 5 and ends on day 10 post conception (p.c.). The zona pellucida surrounding the blastocyst ruptures (on day 4 p.c.) due to growth of the blastocyst and enzymatic lysis; the phenomenon is also known as hatching. This is followed by apposition and adhesion of the blastocyst to the endometrium. In this process, the microvilli on the surface of the external trophoblast cells interact with the epithelial cells of the uterus and form junctional complexes with the aid of surface glycoproteins [2]. An essential element of implantation is the estrogen- and progesterone-induced reconstruction of the endometrium during the luteal phase, which is responsible for the receptivity of the endometrium. This episode, which is limited to a period of few days, is referred to as the implantation window [3].

## Recurrent implantation failure

Implantation failure may occur repeatedly. Recurrent implantation failure has been variously defined. One assumes a failure of pregnancy after two to six IVF cycles, following the transfer of at least 10 embryos of good quality [4]. Other authors refer to repeated implantation failure when no clinical pregnancy has occurred after the transfer of at least four embryos in at least three fresh ETs or cryo-thawed ETs; it is assumed that the patient is below 40 years of age [5]. There are many possible causes that may be responsible for the infertility of the couple. Uterine factors such as polyps or uterine abnormalities, infections, thrombophilia, and immunological factors or genetic factors are just a few examples. In this context, endometriosis, which is particularly frequently associated with an increased sterility rate, deserves special mention. The prevalence of endometriosis in female infertility patients, at 25%–50%, is significantly higher than in fertile women. It is assumed that 30%–50% of endometriosis patients are confronted with sterility [6]. Endometriosis remediation is associated with an increased pregnancy rate and should be performed prior to planned fertility treatment [7, 8].

### Endometrial scratching

Several approaches have been used to overcome the problem of implantation failure in the treatment of sterility or improve the chances of successful nidation. Scratching of the endometrium prior to ET is one method of enhancing the likelihood of implantation. Usually, in the luteal phase of the cycle preceding IVF, the endometrium is "scratched" with a small catheter, 3 mm in width, known as the Pipelle®. Usually, without hooking on the cervix, the catheter is pushed forward through the cervix to the fundus, and then retracted in circular movements in order to stimulate the endometrium (**Figure 17.1**). In case further diagnostic investigation is desired, such as the investigation of chronic endometritis or the presence of plasma or uterine killer cells, the Pipelle® can be used simultaneously to obtain a biopsy specimen of the endometrium. This is regarded as a low-risk procedure with a low rate of complications. Scratching can be performed on an outpatient basis without anesthesia and is associated with minor pain for the majority of patients.

As an alternative to the use of the Pipelle, scratching can also be performed in the course of a diagnostic hysteroscopy. In order to evaluate the uterine cavity and detect or rule out potential barriers to implantation, such as a septum, a polyp, or a myoma, it is usually sufficient to perform a mini-hysteroscopy. **Figure 17.1** shows the hysteroscopic view of an inconspicuous cavum. In this intervention, the gynecologist may perform an endoscopy of the uterine cavity without anesthesia, and usually even without hooking the cervix. The small optical instrument, measuring just 3 mm in diameter, serves the purpose of inspection as well as "scratching" or endometrial stimulation. After inspection and photographic documentation, when the instrument is withdrawn, a mucosal lesion is created usually on the posterior wall (**Figure 17.2a–c**).

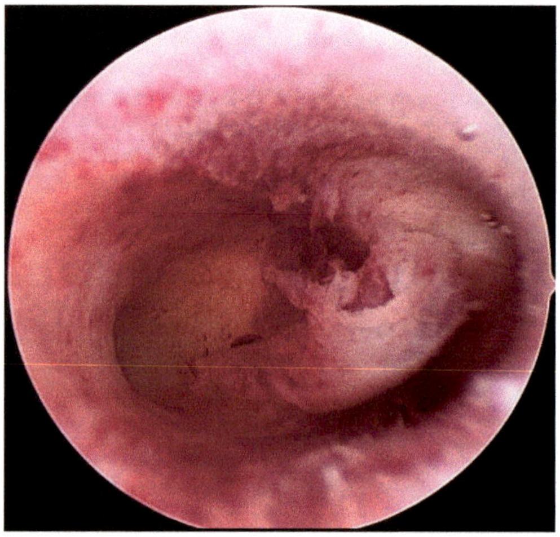

FIGURE 17.1 Hysteroscopy. Hysteroscopic view of an inconspicuous cavum uteri. In the middle of the picture the thrown up endometrium is shown and in the rear part the exit of the right tube can be seen.

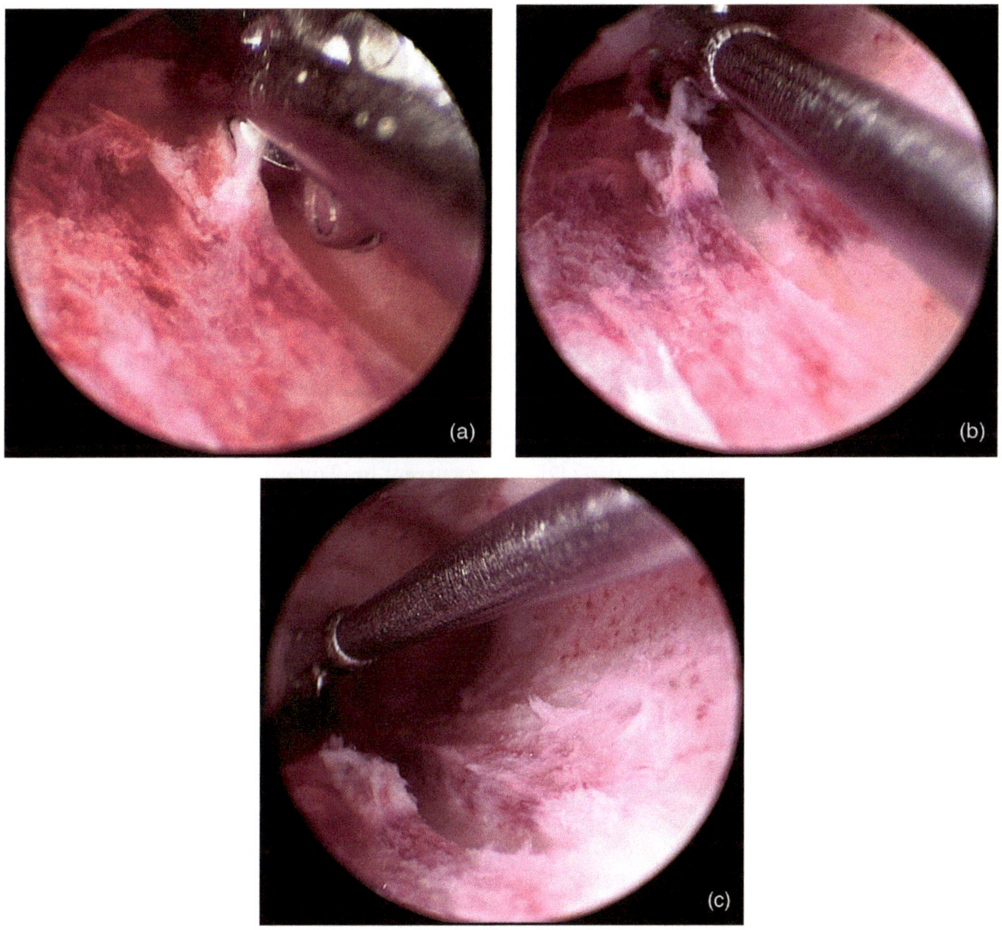


**FIGURE 17.2** (a–c) Endometrial scratching. For immunomodulatory stimulation, a mucosal lesion is created usually on the posterior wall with the hysteroscope.

First observations on scratching were made in 1907 by Loeb, who described the rapid proliferation of decidual cells after injury to the endometrium in the uterus of guinea pigs [9]. In 2003, Barash et al. first reported injury to the endometrium and its positive effect on implantation rates. They showed that a biopsy of the endometrium on day 8, 12, 21, and 26 of the menstrual cycle was associated with a higher pregnancy rate after IVF [10]. Endometrial injury resulted in the secretion of growth factors and cytokines during the healing process, which—according to the authors—exerts a positive effect on endometrial receptivity [10].

Three approaches have been used to enhance uterine receptivity by endometrial scratching and thus enhance pregnancy rates after IVF-ET:

1. Local stimulation of the endometrium induces decidualization, which in turn increases the likelihood of implantation of the transferred embryo [11].
2. The healing and repair process after successful scratching causes a significant increase in macrophages, dendritic cells, and proinflammatory cytokines, including the tumor necrosis factor alpha (TNF-α), the growth-regulated oncogene alpha (GRO-α), and the macrophage-inflammatory protein 1B (MIP-1B), which exert a positive effect on implantation [11, 12]. Especially TNF-α and MIP-1B were found in high concentrations during the implantation window, which underlines the inflammatory effect on the receptive endometrium [13].
3. Ovarian stimulation during IVF treatment is associated with high levels of estrogen, which causes an early increase in progesterone levels. Compared to the embryonic stage, the endometrium is already in an advanced stage of differentiation, which makes it difficult for implantation to take place [14–16]. Scratching during the preceding cycle may suppress proliferation and thus optimize synchronicity between the endometrium and the embryo to be transferred [11].

## Current data

A number of studies and overview articles have been focused on scratching and success rates of subsequent pregnancies.

### Studies on recurrent implantation failure

A meta-analysis and review in 2012 comprised 2,062 women from four randomized and three non-randomized controlled studies; one to six IVF attempts had been made prior to the study. A hysteroscopy in the early proliferative phase as well as endometrial scratching in the preceding cycle, interpreted as endometrial injury, were regarded as inclusion criteria. The evaluation revealed a 70% higher rate of clinical pregnancies in the intervention group compared to the control group [17]. Karimzadeh et al. (2009) [18] and Narvekar et al. (2010) [2], who were also included in the above mentioned meta-analysis, noted higher pregnancy rates after successful screening in their respective randomized controlled studies [2, 18].

Karimzadeh et al. included 58 patients in the treatment group and 57 patients in the control group. Implantation rates were 10.9% in women who underwent scratching and 3.38% in controls ($p = 0.039$); pregnancy rates were 27.1% and 8.9%, respectively ($p = 0.023$). No difference was noted in miscarriage rates ($p > 0.05$) [18]. Narvekar et al. included 49 patients in the treatment group and 51 women in the control group, both after recurrent implantation failure. Scratching was performed once in the follicular phase and a second time in the luteal phase, both in the cycle preceding IVF. It should be noted that in the control group, a hysteroscopy was performed on day 7 and 10 of the preceding cycle; the hysteroscopy might have caused mild mechanical stimulation and also effected an alteration of the endometrium [19]. Implantation, clinical pregnancy, and live birth rates were significantly higher in the intervention group than in controls (implantation rates 13.07% versus 7.1%; clinical pregnancy rates 32.7% versus 13.7%; $p = 0.01$; live birth rates 22.4% versus 9.8%; $p = 0.04$%) [2].

Shohayeb and El-Khayat [20] showed that scratching performed during hysteroscopy resulted in significantly higher implantation, pregnancy, and live birth rates compared to hysteroscopy without scratching. Two hundred patients with recurrent implantation failure were included in the study, and were assigned to the treatment and control groups in equal numbers. Group A received a hysteroscopy in the early follicular phase (day 4 and 7), with endometrial scratching of the fundus and the posterior wall, whereas Group B only underwent a diagnostic hysteroscopy [21]. Implantation rates were 12% in Group A and a mere 7% in Group B ($p = 0.015$). Clinical pregnancy rates were 32% in Group A and 18% in Group B ($p = 0.034$). Live birth rates were 28% in Group A and 14% in Group B ($p = 0.024$). Miscarriage rates did not differ significantly (12.5% in Group A and 22% in Group B; $p = 0.618$) [20].

In a randomized controlled study, Kumbak et al. [22] investigated the outcome of IVF after hysteroscopy and endometrial biopsy on day 21 of the cycle during the luteal phase. A sample was obtained with a small biopsy catheter and sent for histological investigation. Seventy patients in the treatment group were compared with 58 patients in the control group; the latter had received no intervention. Pregnancy rates were significantly higher in the treatment group (82% versus 73%; $p = 0.009$) than in controls. Given the same number of transferred embryos of category A, the implantation rates (38% versus 25%; $p = 0.04$) and pregnancy rates per embryo (67% versus 45%; $p = 0.01$) were significantly higher in the scratching group than in controls [22].

In two further randomized controlled studies, the authors registered no benefit from scratching [23, 24]. Baum et al. [23] performed a randomized double-blind study comprising 36 patients who had undergone at least three previous IVF attempts. The intervention group ($n = 18$) underwent scratching twice (day 9 and 12 and day 21 and 24), followed by IVF treatment. The special feature of the control group ($n = 18$) was that the patients underwent a placebo investigation during which the biopsy catheter was inserted into the cervix without contacting the endometrium. The study revealed lower implantation rates (2.08% versus 11.1%; $p = 0.1$), clinical pregnancy rates (0% versus 31.25%; $p < 0.05$), and live birth rates (0% versus 25%; $p = 0.1$) in the treatment group compared to controls.

A more recent randomized controlled study performed in 2015 by Gibreel et al. [24] also revealed no statistically significant improvement in live birth rates after scratching compared to controls. A subgroup analysis, however, showed a higher live birth rate in women, who had undergone two or more failed IVF attempts after scratching compared to those who had undergone only one IVF attempt [24].

A Cochrane analysis performed by Nastri et al. [25] in 2015 comprised 14 studies with a total of 1,063 patients in the treatment group and 1,065 patients in the control group. Endometrial scratching was performed between day 7 of the preceding cycle and day 7 of the ET cycle. The control group underwent no manipulation of the endometrium. A prerequisite was at least two previous ETs. Higher rates of pregnancies and live births were noted in the intervention group (RR 1.42; 95% CI 1.08–1.85, $p = 0.01$). A subgroup analysis which excluded all studies with a potential bias yielded an equally significant result. If 30% of women who underwent no scratching would have become pregnant, the intervention group would have achieved a pregnancy rate of 33%–48% [25]. Scratching, according to the authors, had no impact on miscarriage rates, potential bleeding, or multiple pregnancies [25].

In contrast to the above mentioned studies, the following authors investigated the impact of scratching in women without recurrent implantation failure.

### Studies on women without recurrent implantation failure

In a prospective randomized study comprising 121 women who had undergone IVF treatment, Zhou et al. [26] performed endometrial scratching in the intervention group ($n = 60$) when they noted irregular endometrial patters in the vaginal ultrasound investigation (atypical, no trilaminar pattern, echogenic lesions). Scratching was performed during ovarian stimulation in all cases, with the purpose of enhancing endometrial receptivity. The control group underwent no scratching. The treatment group revealed higher implantation rates (33.33% versus 17.78%), clinical pregnancy rates (48.33 versus 27.86%), and live birth rates per ET (41.67% versus 22.96%) after scratching [26].

In accordance with their study design, Nastri et al. [27] performed scratching with a Pipelle® 7–14 days prior to scheduled hormonal stimulation for an IVF cycle, while the women were taking an oral contraceptive. The authors registered higher pregnancy and live birth rates ($p = 0.01$) in the treatment group compared to the control group, with no impact on miscarriage rates ($p = 0.53$) [27].

Guven et al. [28] achieved similar results, although they performed scratching on day 3 of the transfer cycle rather than the preceding cycle. The authors registered higher pregnancy (48.2% versus 29%, $p = 0.025$) and live birth rates (33.9% versus 17.7%, $p = 0.035$) in the treatment group compared to controls [28].

In contrast to the majority of authors, who investigated the effect of scratching by local manipulation in the preceding cycle, Karimzade et al. [29] investigated the effect of scratching with the Novak curette on the day of follicle aspiration. One hundred and fifty-six patients were included in this prospective controlled study. However, this study revealed negative effects on implantation rates (7.9% versus 22.9%, $p = 0.002$) and the outcome of IVF (9.6% versus 29.1%, $p = 0.004$) after scratching compared to controls. It may be assumed that, since manipulation was performed shortly before ET, proinflammatory cytokines, macrophages, and dendritic cells could not be formed rapidly enough in adequate numbers. The receptivity of the endometrium was damaged rather than enhanced as a result thereof [29].

In their treatment group ($n = 50$), Safdarian et al. [30] performed scratching with a biopsy catheter on day 21 of the preceding cycle, and registered no statistically significant difference compared to controls ($n = 50$) in regard of implantation and pregnancy rates [30].

Yeung et al. [31] achieved similar results. In their randomized controlled study, the authors included 300 subfertile women, selected randomly, who were scheduled to undergo or had undergone IVF cycles. In the treatment group the authors performed scratching with a Pipelle® in the mid-luteal phase of the preceding cycle. Compared to controls, the authors registered no differences in regard of implantation, pregnancy, multiple pregnancy, or miscarriage rates. In a subgroup analysis of women who had undergone repeated IVF attempts, the pregnancy rate after scratching was lower than that in controls [31].

In a recent but retrospective case control study performed in May 2017 in Israel [32], 238 patients were included in the treatment group and 238 in the control group. Women in the treatment group underwent scratching for the first time. Scratching was performed once or twice in the proliferation phase as well as the luteal phase. The results in the scratching and control groups were similar in regard of implantation (28.06% versus 30.08%, p = 0.8), pregnancy (34.03% versus 40.33%, p = 0.18), and continued pregnancy rates (18.48% versus 28.99%, p = 0.33) [32].

At the ESHRE meeting, which was held from July 1–4, 2018, in Barcelona, Dr. Sarah Lensen from New Zealand presented the recent results of her work on the subject of scratching [33]. Her contribution received the Clinical Science Award for oral presentation. Data from this randomized multicenter study were collected between June 2014 and June 2017 at 13 centers in five countries. One thousand three hundred and sixty-four women (690 in the scratching arm versus 674 in the control group) who had undergone ET after IVF during the fresh embryo or cryo-thawed cycle were included in the study. The results revealed no increase in live birth rates after endometrial scratching: 26.1% (180/690) versus 26.1% (176/674) in controls, odds ratio 1.00 (0.78–1.27). Even a subgroup analysis in regard of recurrent implantation failure, fresh or cryo-thawed cycles, and the interval between scratching and ET yielded no specific group that would benefit from scratching. The authors concluded that endometrial scratching should not be offered or performed in the course of fertility treatment [33].

## Conclusion and practical significance

To estimate the final value or benefit of scratching in regard of implantation, pregnancy, and live birth rates, it is important to precisely define the respective patient population that would benefit from this intervention. Scratching is able to enhance the receptivity of the endometrium, but a number of other pathologies may be responsible for implantation failure. The present overview of studies shows that unselected subfertile women generally benefit less from endometrial scratching. In contrast, scratching appears to be a successful measure for enhancing the chances of implantation in women with recurrent implantation failure. However, recent data presented at the ESHRE 2018 in Barcelona contradict this thesis. Rather, these data have shown that endometrial scratching is not associated with a higher live birth rate even in women with recurrent implantation failure. Patients should be informed of these recent data.

Scratching is convenient, easy to perform, and associated with very little pain. Based on the existing body of data, as mentioned above, scratching could be offered to patients with recurrent implantation failure in order to try to enhance pregnancy and live birth rates, after the women have been informed in detail about the procedure. The patients should definitely be informed of the heterogeneous data on the subject, especially those presented at ESHRE 2018. Taking these latest data into account, endometrial scratching did not show any advantage in pregnancy and live birth rate, so it can be discussed that this method should not be offered any more.

## References


1. ESHRE, A., *Fact Sheet July*, 2014. https://http://www.eshre.eu/guidelines-and-legal/art-fact-sheet.aspx., Accessed 22 December 2015.
2. Narvekar, S.A., et al., *Does local endometrial injury in the nontransfer cycle improve the IVF-ET outcome in the subsequent cycle in patients with previous unsuccessful IVF? A randomized controlled pilot study*. J Hum Reprod Sci, 2010. **3**(1): p. 15–9.
3. Dekel, N., et al., *The role of inflammation for a successful implantation*. Am J Reprod Immunol, 2014. **72**(2): p. 141–7.
4. Tan, B.K., et al., *Investigation and current management of recurrent IVF treatment failure in the UK*. BJOG, 2005. **112**(6): p. 773–80.
5. Coughlan, C., et al., *Recurrent implantation failure: definition and management*. Reprod Biomed Online, 2014. **28**(1): p. 14–38.
6. Vercellini, P., et al., *Surgery for endometriosis-associated infertility: a pragmatic approach*. Hum Reprod, 2009. **24**(2): p. 254–69.
7. Alkatout, I., et al., *Combined surgical and hormone therapy for endometriosis is the most effective treatment: prospective, randomized, controlled trial*. J Minim Invasive Gynecol, 2013. **20**(4): p. 473–81.
8. Mettler, L., R. Ruprai, and I. Alkatout, *Impact of medical and surgical treatment of endometriosis on the cure of endometriosis and pain*. Biomed Res Int, 2014: p. 264653.
9. Loeb, L., *The experimental proof changes in the uterine decidua of guinea pig after mating*. Zentralbl Allg Pathol, 1907. **18**: p. 563–565.
10. Barash, A., et al., *Local injury to the endometrium doubles the incidence of successful pregnancies in patients undergoing in vitro fertilization*. Fertil Steril, 2003. **79**(6): p. 1317–22.
11. Li, R. and G. Hao, *Local injury to the endometrium: its effect on implantation*. Curr Opin Obstet Gynecol, 2009. **21**(3): p. 236–9.
12. Gnainsky, Y., et al., *Local injury of the endometrium induces an inflammatory response that promotes successful implantation*. Fertil Steril, 2010. **94**(6): p. 2030–6.
13. Haider, S. and M. Knofler, *Human tumour necrosis factor: physiological and pathological roles in placenta and endometrium*. Placenta, 2009. **30**(2): p. 111–23.
14. Lass, A., et al., *Histological evaluation of endometrium on the day of oocyte retrieval after gonadotrophin-releasing hormone agonist-follicle stimulating hormone ovulation induction for in-vitro fertilization*. Hum Reprod, 1998. **13**(11): p. 3203–5.
15. Ubaldi, F., et al., *Endometrial evaluation by aspiration biopsy on the day of oocyte retrieval in the embryo transfer cycles in patients with serum progesterone rise during the follicular phase*. Fertil Steril, 1997. **67**(3): p. 521–6.
16. Fatemi, H.M. and B. Popovic-Todorovic, *Implantation in assisted reproduction: a look at endometrial receptivity*. Reprod Biomed Online, 2013. **27**(5): p. 530–8.
17. Potdar, N., T. Gelbaya, and L.G. Nardo, *Endometrial injury to overcome recurrent embryo implantation failure: a systematic review and meta-analysis*. Reprod Biomed Online, 2012. **25**(6): p. 561–71.
18. Karimzadeh, M.A., M. Ayazi Rozbahani, and N. Tabibnejad, *Endometrial local injury improves the pregnancy rate among recurrent implantation failure patients undergoing in vitro fertilisation/intra cytoplasmic sperm injection: a randomised clinical trial*. Aust N Z J Obstet Gynaecol, 2009. **49**(6): p. 677–80.
19. Ko, J.K. and E.H. Ng, *Scratching and IVF: any role?* Curr Opin Obstet Gynecol, 2016. **28**(3): p. 178–83.
20. Shohayeb, A. and W. El-Khayat, *Does a single endometrial biopsy regimen (S-EBR) improve ICSI outcome in patients with repeated implantation failure? A randomised controlled trial*. Eur J Obstet Gynecol Reprod Biol, 2012. **164**(2): p. 176–9.
21. Singh, N., et al., *Does endometrial injury enhances implantation in recurrent in-vitro fertilization failures? A prospective randomized control study from tertiary care center*. J Hum Reprod Sci, 2015. **8**(4): p. 218–23.
22. Kumbak, B., et al., *Impact of luteal phase hysteroscopy and concurrent endometrial biopsy on subsequent IVF cycle outcome*. Arch Gynecol Obstet, 2014. **290**(2): p. 369–74.

23. Baum, M., et al., *Does local injury to the endometrium before IVF cycle really affect treatment outcome? Results of a randomized placebo controlled trial.* Gynecol Endocrinol, 2012. **28**(12): p. 933–6.
24. Gibreel, A., et al., *Endometrial scratching for women with previous IVF failure undergoing IVF treatment.* Gynecol Endocrinol, 2015. **31**(4): p. 313–6.
25. Nastri, C.O., et al., *Endometrial injury in women undergoing assisted reproductive techniques.* Cochrane Database Syst Rev, 2015(3): p. CD009517.
26. Zhou, L., et al., *Local injury to the endometrium in controlled ovarian hyperstimulation cycles improves implantation rates.* Fertil Steril, 2008. **89**(5): p. 1166–76.
27. Nastri, C.O., et al., *Endometrial scratching performed in the non-transfer cycle and outcome of assisted reproduction: a randomized controlled trial.* Ultrasound Obstet Gynecol, 2013. **42**(4): p. 375–82.
28. Guven, S., et al., *Endometrial injury may increase the clinical pregnancy rate in normoresponders undergoing long agonist protocol ICSI cycles with single embryo transfer.* Eur J Obstet Gynecol Reprod Biol, 2014. **173**: p. 58–62.
29. Karimzade, M.A., et al., *Local injury to the endometrium on the day of oocyte retrieval has a negative impact on implantation in assisted reproductive cycles: a randomized controlled trial.* Arch Gynecol Obstet, 2010. **281**(3): p. 499–503.
30. Safdarian, L., et al., *Local injury to the endometrium does not improve the implantation rate in good responder patients undergoing in-vitro fertilization.* Iran J Reprod Med, 2011. **9**(4): p. 285–8.
31. Yeung, T.W., et al., *The effect of endometrial injury on ongoing pregnancy rate in unselected subfertile women undergoing in vitro fertilization: a randomized controlled trial.* Hum Reprod, 2014. **29**(11): p. 2474–81.
32. Levin, D., et al., *The effect of endometrial injury on implantation and clinical pregnancy rates.* Gynecol Endocrinol, 2017: p. 1–4.
33. Lensen, S.O., et al. *Endometrial scratching by pipelle biopsy in IVF (the PIP study): A pragmatic randomised controlled trial.* ESHRE, Barcelona 2018, 34. annual conference, 2018. Abstract O-139.

# 18

## 3D ULTRASOUND IN THE DIAGNOSIS AND MANAGEMENT OF ROBERT'S UTERUS

*A Glimpse into a Rare Uterine Anomaly*

**Liselotte Mettler, Ibrahim Alkatout, Anupama Deenadayal-Mettler, Aarti Tolani, Rooma Sinha, and Mamata Deenadayal**

## Introduction and background

### Congenital uterine anomalies (CUAs)

Female genital malformations are defined as deviations from normal anatomy that could impair the reproductive potential of a woman or, in complex cases (such as obstructive anomalies), a woman's health. The malformations arise embryologically from the failure of Müllerian duct formation, canalization, fusion, or absorption. The anomalies are either isolated defects or occur in combination with conditions in various parts of the female genital tract. The latter results in so-called complex anomalies.

The overall prevalence of uterine anomalies is 0.5%. Awareness of these conditions is extremely important in order to avoid misdiagnosis and inappropriate management [3, 4].

Pelvic pain, prolonged or abnormal bleeding at the time of menarche, recurrent pregnancy loss, or preterm delivery are symptoms of CUAs. Some CUAs may be suspected because of associated findings on physical examination, such as a longitudinal vaginal septum. Others may be detected when imaging studies are performed to evaluate patients with severe menstrual pain, pain at intervals of 4 weeks without bleeding in young girls, infertility, symptoms related to non-reproductive organ systems, or trauma.

### Classification systems of congenital uterine anomalies

Classification systems are useful because they permit grouping of similar anomalies. Conclusions can be derived on the basis of several cases rather than individual case reports. The classification, diagnosis, and clinical manifestations of major congenital anomalies of the corpus (septate, unicornuate, bicornuate or didelphys uterus), along with their associated cervical and vaginal anomalies have been discussed in the past and were summarized in the American Fertility Society Classification of 1988, by Grimbizis et al. in 2013 and 2016, and by Di Spiezia Sardo et al. in 2015 [5–8]. A few comprehensive evaluations of CUAs have also been published.

### Robert's uterus and its incidence

The incidence of Robert's uterus is 5%. As the condition is rare, it is not as well characterized as other uterine anomalies. Moreover, the number of cases reported in the published literature is scarce. Knowledge of this condition is extremely important in order to avoid misdiagnosis and inappropriate management. A Robert's uterus identified early can be managed by minimally invasive procedures. Failure to identify the condition may lead to adnexal lesions or endometrioma [9–12].

### General characteristics, causes and symptoms of a Robert's uterus

A septate uterus with a non-communicating blind uterine horn, a contralateral unicornuate uterine cavity communicating with the cervix, and an external uterine fundus of normal shape is an extremely rare congenital Müllerian anomaly. This uterine malformation was first published by Robert in 1969/1970 [1, 2].

The origin of the defect may be a segmental agenesis of the isthmus with a persistent septum between the upper portions of the Müllerian ducts.

The first symptoms of this condition are usually experienced after menarche. The obstructed unicornuate cavity has a functional endometrium, due to which menstrual secretions are retained and cause hematometra or even a hematosalpinx. This is followed by cyclic dysmenorrhea. Reflux of the retained menstrual secretion into the peritoneal cavity may cause endometriosis. The second uterine cavity communicates with the single cervix and is responsible for menstrual flow.

### Diagnostic options

In accordance with the recommendations of the ESHRE/ESGE consensus, we performed a complete gynecological examination, two- and three-dimensional (2D and 3D) ultrasound exploration of the pelvis and kidneys, and magnetic resonance imaging (MRI). A hysterosalpingography or hysterosalpingo-contrast sonography was not performed because we believed the disadvantages of these procedures outweighed the advantages. A computed tomography is no longer used for the diagnosis of female genital abnormalities because of its poor depiction of female genital structures. The anatomy of the cervix, uterus, ovaries, and pelvic pathologies were evaluated during 2D ultrasound.

Ideally, a diagnostic method should provide objective and measurable information about the anatomy of (1) the vagina, (2) the cervix, (3) the uterine cavity, (4) the uterine wall, (5) external contours of the uterus, and (6) other intraperitoneal structures.

**Two-dimensional ultrasound** is able to provide reliable, objective and, most importantly, measurable information about the anatomy of the cervix, the uterine cavity, the uterine wall and the external contours of the uterus. 2D ultrasound also yields useful information about associated pelvic pathologies (such as ovarian pathologies, benign or malignant tumors, endometriosis), hydrosalpinges, and renal anomalies. It may also provide measurable information about obstructive parts of the female genital tract. Transperineal two-dimensional ultrasound (2D US) yields information about the vaginal cavity, especially in the presence of an imperforate hemivagina. The procedure is simple, economical, non-invasive, and widely available. It provides valuable additional information about potential intracavitary (major adhesions seen as "bridges" between walls, polyps, or myomas) or intramural pathologies (myomas, adenomyosis) in cases of infertile women.

As 2D US is a dynamic procedure, its diagnostic accuracy is highly dependent on proper execution of the method and the experience of the examiner. Acquisition of the required planes may be hindered by the patient's anatomy.

**Three-dimensional ultrasound** provides highly reliable, objective and, most importantly, measurable information about the anatomy of the cervix, the uterine cavity, the uterine wall, the external contours of the uterus, and pelvic pathologies. The coronal plane of the uterus yields a clear view of the cavity and the external profile of the uterine fundus. 3D volume images provide a reliable and objective rendition of the examined organs. The procedure is less dependent on the examiner, and thus overcomes the limitations of coronal images on 2D ultrasound. 3D ultrasonography also provides measurable information about obstructed portions of the female genital tract.

**Advantages of 3D:** The procedure is non-invasive and feasible. In this respect, it does not differ from conventional ultrasound. 3D ultrasound visualizes uterine anatomy in the sagittal, transverse, and coronal planes, independent of the examiner's skills. It provides precise and objective measurements of the dimensions of the uterus, which is very useful for differential diagnosis. The images are now routinely saved by the electronic mode for re-evaluation or off-line analysis. Subsequently the investigator is able to assess the uterus/uterine wall in different sections and select the plane of maximum interest in the coronal/sagittal or transverse sections for the purpose of measurement. 3D US provides more reliable information than 2D US in cases of infertile women.

Transperineal three-dimensional ultrasound (3D US) may offer the opportunity to view pelvic structures, including the vagina and the cervix.

**Disadvantages of 3D:** The equipment is not as widely available as 2D US. 3D US calls for experienced investigators with special training in 3D image acquisition and post-processing techniques. The investigation is associated with artifact relating to inappropriate volume acquisition and/or manipulation of the volume. It cannot provide very detailed or reliable data in cases of complex anomalies. 3D US without saline infusion or contrast medium cannot be used as a real-time tubal patency test in infertile patients.

Recommendations for its proper use: Start with a 2D evaluation of the uterus. The mid-cycle or the luteal phase is advantageous because it is the best time to view the endometrial wall and the outline of the cavity. Contrast medium may be used for the evaluation of the cavity and the tubes; in these cases the examination should be performed in the early follicular phase. The 3D images should be saved for off-line analysis. The reconstructed coronal plane of the uterus might show the cavity and the external uterine profile as well as the tubal angle and the junctional zone, in some cases the endometrium and cavity. For the acquisition of an isolated cervical volume without the uterus from the mid-sagittal plane, an axial plane of the cervix can be obtained in 80%, and a coronal plane in 20% of cases. In cases of uterine malformations, the extent of the cervix and the limits of the cervical canal can be studied better. Concomitant vaginal anomalies can be detected by transperineal acquisition of the pelvic floor volume after filling the vagina with gel or saline; an axial plane can be obtained from the mid-sagittal plane.

### Magnetic resonance imaging

**Diagnostic potential of the method:** It provides highly reliable and objective information about the anatomy of the vagina, cervix, uterine cavity, uterine wall, the external contour of the uterus and other peritoneal structures, with the exception of the tubes. It also yields reliable information about dilated or obstructed parts of the female genital tract.

**Advantages:** The procedure is non-invasive and devoid of radiation. It provides a reliable and objective representation of the examined organs in the sagittal, transverse and coronal planes (three dimensions). It can be used for the detection of complex and obstructive anomalies. The images are routinely saved for re-evaluation.

**Disadvantages:** The procedure is more expensive and less widely available than ultrasound. It is inappropriate for patients prone to claustrophobia or morbidly obese persons. Assessment of the results calls for experience and training. The required planes are non-flexible because the planes are predefined and independent of the examiner; this could potentially impair the diagnostic accuracy of the method if the examiner lacks experience. The procedure cannot be used as a tubal patency test in cases of infertile patients.

Recommendations for its proper use: Gynecologists should be trained in MRI and should work closely with the radiologist to review the images; the clinical background of the gynecologist complements the radiological interpretation of the images by the radiologist.

### Treatment

This anomaly may be suspected on 2D transabdominal or transvaginal ultrasound, but 3D ultrasound or MRI will be needed for its specific diagnosis. Once diagnosed, the patient may undergo the following surgical procedures:

1. *Laparoscopy*: Horn resection/endometrectomy by laparoscopy is the modern approach. If not available, the procedure can be safely performed by laparotomy.
2. *Hysteroscopy + Laparoscopy*: The two horns are unified surgically through the hysteroscope under laparoscopic control.
3. *In young girls*: minimally invasive hysteroscopic metroplasty guided by transrectal ultrasound in cases of a thick septum and no associated endometriosis.
4. *In cases of continuing pain and endometriosis*, a total laparoscopic hysterectomy (TLH) with bilateral tubectomy may be performed in women beyond the childbearing age.

## 3D Ultrasound and Robert's Uterus

### 3D ultrasound imaging

In the present study, we used an advanced 3D ultrasound imaging technique for the diagnosis, treatment and postoperative screening of Robert's uterus. Ultrasound imaging is superior to MRI screening; the latter is expensive and less widely available. To our knowledge, this is the first report of five cases of Robert's uterus from a single center within 12 months.

Three-dimensional ultrasound has unique advantages compared to 2D ultrasound, hysterosalpingography, or even MRI for the diagnosis of uterine malformations. Real-time 3D US has attracted much more attention in medical research because it provides interactive feedback, aids clinicians in the acquisition of high-quality images, and also yields timely spatial information of the scanned area. A number of publications have reported on real-time or near-real-time application of 3D US using volumetric probes or routine 2D probes.

Linear, tilted, or rotating freehand scanners are flexible and convenient; no cumbersome mechanisms are needed for their use. With a freehand scanner, the clinician is able to scan the organ of interest—such as the uterus—in arbitrary directions and positions, select optimal views, and accommodate the complexity of any anatomical surface. The positions and orientations of 2D B-scans are needed for the reconstruction of 3D images. Four approaches with different positional sensors have been proposed for tracking the US probe: the acoustic, optical, and articulated arm positioner, and magnetic field sensors [13]. We used the Voluson E10BT19 device transabdominally, combined with transvaginal ultrasound [14, 15].

This ultrasound system receives reflections from acoustic energy transmitted into the body, and performs various signal processing functions to produce an ultrasound image.

## Treatments used in five cases of Robert's uterus

Robert's uterus is a very rare type of Müllerian duct malformation and a Class V variant of a septate uterus according to the American Society of Reproductive Medicine (ASRM) classification. The ESHRE-ESGE classified it as a Class U2bC3V0 anomaly or a complete uterus with partial cervical aplasia. The treatment of this condition varies. Robert's uterus is also known as an asymmetric septate uterus with characteristics of a complete uterine septum, asymmetrically separating the endometrial cavity from the non-communicating hemi-uterus due to obstruction caused by the septum. With some exceptions, laparoscopy combined with hysteroscopy is the gold standard for confirming the diagnosis of Robert's uterus. The shape of the uterus might be normal on laparoscopy. There might be a normal external uterine fundal contour or a slight hollow/protrusion, with or without hematometra and hematosalpinx. On hysteroscopy the uterus has only one ostium of the fallopian tube.

We performed an endometrectomy under laparoscopic control with restitution of uterine integrity in a 13-year-old girl, one hysteroscopic septum resection, one laparoscopic uterine horn resection, and one hysterectomy. The fifth patient had recurrent abortions and was scheduled to undergo a hysteroscopic septum resection, but became pregnant again before the treatment could be performed.

## Results and types of surgical treatment

In the following, we report in detail five cases of Robert's uterus, their 3D US diagnosis, and their subsequent hysteroscopic and laparoscopic treatment (**Table 18.1**)

### *Case 1: Unmarried teenage girl with dysmenorrhea*

An unmarried 13-year-old girl reported with incapacitating dysmenorrhea starting 3 days after commencement of her menstrual cycle, associated with pain radiating to the back, vomiting and constipation.

As the transabdominal 2D ultrasound provided no clear information (**Figure 18.1a**) and the patient was not sexually active, we had to consider other imaging options such as MRI and rectal ultrasound imaging. The latter was explained to the patient and her parents, who then consented to the procedure. Transrectal ultrasound was performed with volume options, contrast imaging in the multiplanar mode, and the HD live rendering mode, which identified a blind uterine horn with unilateral hematometra and a contralateral unicornuate uterine cavity. Both kidneys were normal.

Transrectal ultrasound with a C1-5D probe also revealed a hematometra measuring 5 × 5 cm on the left side, and a right horn with an endometrium of 10 mm, type III (**Figure 18.1b**).

Transrectal ultrasound investigation with a RIC-9D probe, 3D rendering, and HD live confirmed the presence of hematometra in the left horn, a unicornuate-like right horn, and a septum of 1.49 cm thickness dividing the two cavities. The outer contour of the uterus was normal, thus confirming the diagnosis of Robert's uterus (**Figure 18.1c**).

The images were useful in counseling the patient about the surgical approach.

The exact anomaly was illustrated in a line drawing and enabled clear communication between the ultrasonographer, the surgeon and the patient (**Figure 18.1d**).

As the thickness of the septum between the two cavities was between 1.6 cm and 1.35 cm in the longitudinal aspect and was well vascularized (color score 2), we decided to perform a laparoscopic endometrectomy. An initial diagnostic hysteroscopy revealed a single right horn with a right ostium (**Figure 18.1e**). The laparoscopic view is shown in **Figure 18.1f**.

The treatment was performed as a laparoscopic procedure. An incision was made on the fundus (**Figure 18.1g**), and the endometrial cavity along with hematometra was identified (**Figure 18.1h**). The excision was performed with a margin of 2–3 mm of myometrium

**TABLE 18.1: Factors That Play a Role in Deciding the Treatment**

1. Age
2. Adenomyosis and endometriosis
3. Desire to retain childbearing ability
4. Ultrasound:
   a. Confirmation of Robert's uterus
   b. Thickness of the septum
   c. Vascularity of the septum
   d. Thickness of the uterine walls

| | Age | Key Information | Thickness of Septum | Vascularity Score | Associated Findings | Surgery |
|---|---|---|---|---|---|---|
| Case 1 | 13 years | Dysmenorrhea | 1.35 cm | 2 | | Endometrectomy of the blind cavity and closure of the cavity. |
| Case 2 | 25 years | Primary infertility, Dysmenorrhea | 4.1 mm | 1 | Adenomyosis, endometrioma | Hysteroscopic septal resection |
| Case 3 | 36 years | 2 full term LSCS, Dysmenorrhea | 2.7 cm | 2 | | Laparoscopic excision of the blind horn |
| Case 4 | 39 years | 2 live children | 100 cm | 2 | Adenomyosis, recurrent Grade 4 endometriosis | Hysterectomy with unilateral salpingo-oophorectomy (recurrent endometrioma) |
| Case 5 | 28 years | 3 abortions at 16 weeks | 3 mm | 1 | | Patient conceived during the investigations |

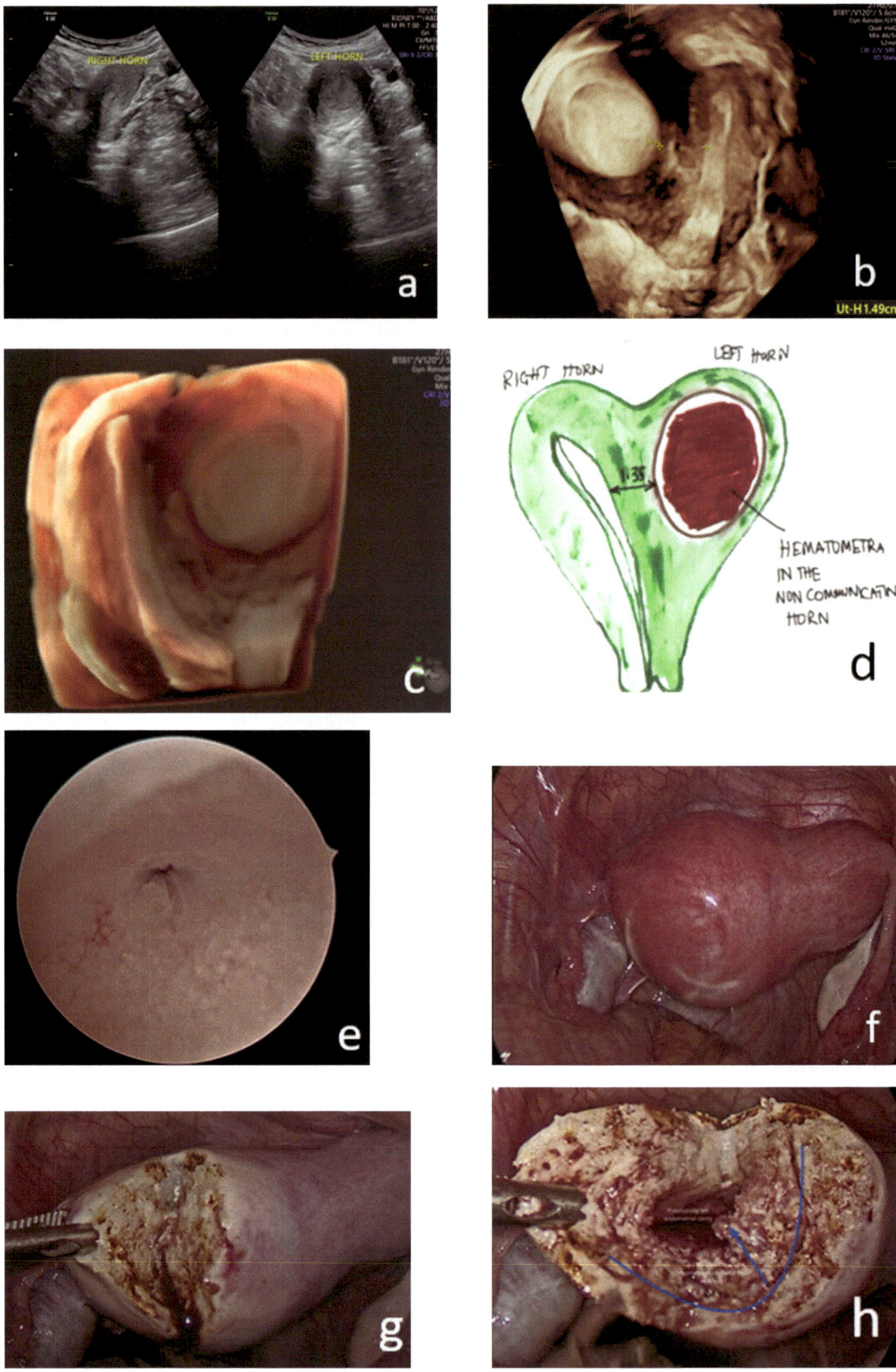


**FIGURE 18.1** (a) 2D ultrasound suggested a hematometra on the left side and a right uterine horn, with an endometrium of 10 mm, (b) transrectal ultrasound with a C1-5D probe confirmed a hematometra of 5 × 5 cm on the left side, and a right horn with an endometrium of 10 mm, (c) the transrectal scan with a RIC-9D probe, a 3D-rendered view and HD live confirmed the presence of a hematometra in the left horn, a unicornuate-like right horn and a septum of 1.49 cm dividing the two cavities, (d) explanatory line drawing of Robert's uterus, (e) only the right tubal ostium was seen on hysteroscopy, (f) laparoscopic view of the uterus, (g–h) surgical endometrectomy and (i) myometrial reconstruction of the right uterine horn.

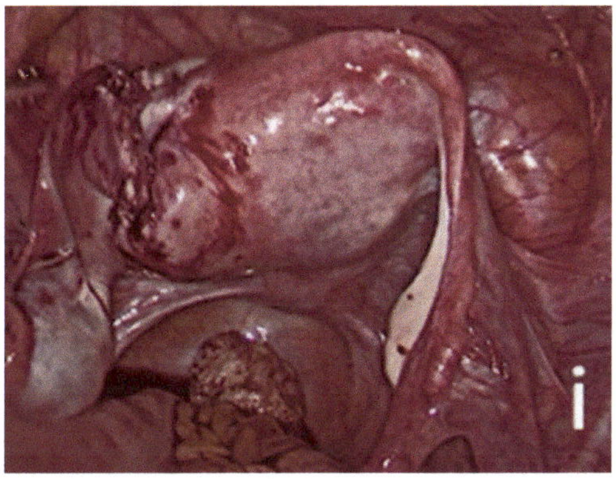

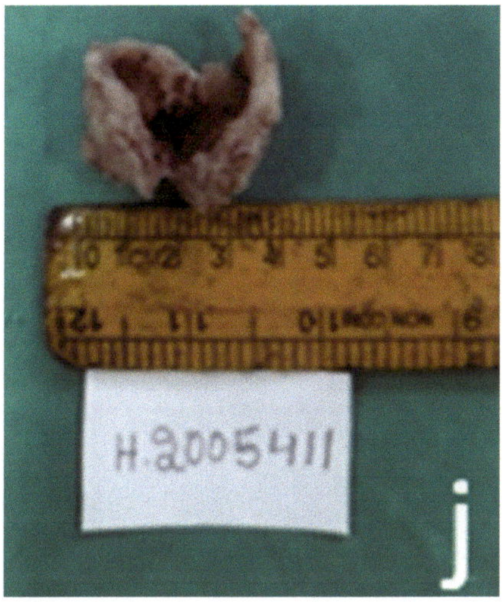


**FIGURE 18.1** (Continued) (j) Excised specimen.

on all sides. The myometrium was subsequently reconstructed on the left side of the uterus (**Figure 18.1i**). The excised specimen is shown in **Figure 18.1j**. We selected this procedure because the septum that separated the two cavities was thick; hysteroscopic resection would have been difficult in this setting. Excision of the functioning endometrial cavity relieved the patient of her intractable dysmenorrhea. The resultant single right horn of the uterus is expected to be sufficient for obstetric purposes in the future.

The procedure was selected because the patient was young and we wished to avoid an extensive operative hysteroscopy due to the risk of perforation and additional damage. Alternatively, we could have performed stepwise hysteroscopy-guided opening of the septum to release the hematometra and eventually transform both cavities into a single cavity.

### *Case 2: Primary infertility with endometriosis*

A 25-year-old patient with primary infertility and regular menstrual cycles presented with severe congestive dysmenorrhea, which persisted for 7 days after the end of her period.

A transverse 2D image by transvaginal ultrasound with a RIC5-9D volume probe revealed a hematometra in the left horn of the uterus. The right horn showed a unicornuate-like cavity and adenomyosis with myometrial cysts. The outer contour of the transverse section of the uterus appeared normal. The left ovary revealed an endometrioma of 3 cm adherent to the fundus of the uterus (**Figure 18.2a**).

The 3D rendered view demonstrated a 4.1-mm-thick septum with no vascularity (color score 1). The outer contour of the uterus appeared normal on the coronal section (**Figure 18.2b**). An MRI image confirmed the 3D-rendered image and provided no additional information (**Figure 18.2c**). The explanatory drawing served as a basis for explaining the surgical procedure (**Figure 18.2d**). On hysteroscopy, the right ostium was visualized with a complete septum towards the left aspect of the cavity (**Figure 18.2e**).

Under laparoscopic control, the septum was resected by hysteroscopy using a Collin's knife and bipolar current, midway between the fundus and the internal os, at a pre-determined depth of 48 mm. Thus, communication between the two endometrial cavities was established (**Figure 18.2f**). The septum was resected along its entire length and the two cavities were unified. Subsequently, the patient achieved complete relief from dysmenorrhea. Laparoscopy revealed a single fundus with evidence of endometriosis in the left adnexa (**Figure 18.2g**). The endometrioma was enucleated and extracted. A normal ovary was created with the use of bipolar energy for hemostasis.

### *Case 3: Woman with two live children and dysmenorrhea*

A 36-year-old patient with severe dysmenorrhea had conceived spontaneously on two occasions. She had delivered both children at full term by elective cesarean section because of breech presentation.

The patient was given analgesics for dysmenorrhea and was referred for identification of the cause of dysmenorrhea. 2D ultrasound revealed a normal right horn and hematometra in the left horn (**Figure 18.3a**).

As the patient wished to retain her childbearing ability, we performed a laparoscopic excision of the left horn with reconstruction of the uterus (**Figure 18.3b–d**).

### *Case 4: Woman with two live children, persistent congestive dysmenorrhea and recurrent endometriosis*

A 39-year-old patient, married for 19 years, reported with severe congestive dysmenorrhea since menarche. Details of her obstetric history included para 2, the last abortion in 2010, and grade 4 endometriosis for which she had been operated earlier. An endometrioma on the left side had been excised in 2011. The patient was referred for routine ultrasonography with severe dysmenorrhea and recurrent endometriosis on the left side. As shown in **Figure 18.4a**, 3D ultrasound revealed a normal serosa and myometrium, and adenomyosis of the right horn. The left part of the illustration shows the right horn of the uterus with adenomyosis of the anterior wall and an endometrium of 6 mm. The right side of the illustration shows the left horn of the uterus and an endometrium of 7 mm with a polyp. There was no communication between the left and right horn. An endometrioma of 6 cm was seen in the left ovary. The contours of the uterine fundus were normal on the 3D image (**Figure 18.4b**).

As the patient had completed her family, and due to adenomyosis with recurrent endometriosis, we performed an elective hysterectomy with left-sided salpingo-oophorectomy.

### *Case 5: Recurrent miscarriage and dysmenorrhea*

A 28-year-old patient with three abortions in the 16th week of gestation was sent for ultrasonography.

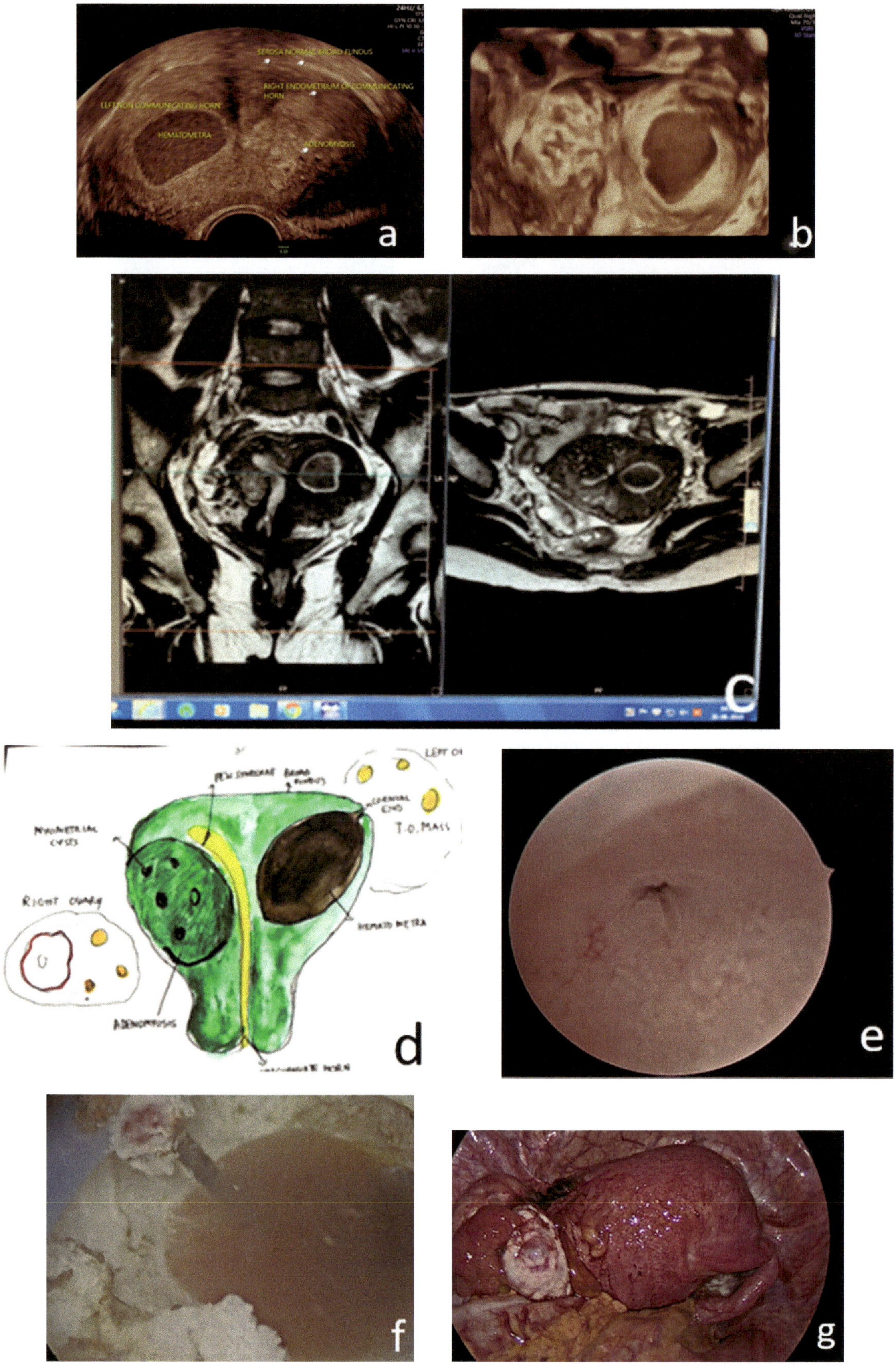


**FIGURE 18.2** (a) 2D ultrasound image with a transvaginal RIC 5-9D volume probe of the left horn hematometra and a right-sided unicornuate cavity, (b) 3D-rendered view showing a 4.1-mm thick septum and a normal outer contour of uterus, (c) MRI image, (d) explanatory drawing, (e) hysteroscopic view of the right tubal ostium, (f) situs after hysteroscopic septum resection, (g) laparoscopic view with a single fundus and endometrioma of the right ovary, which was resected.

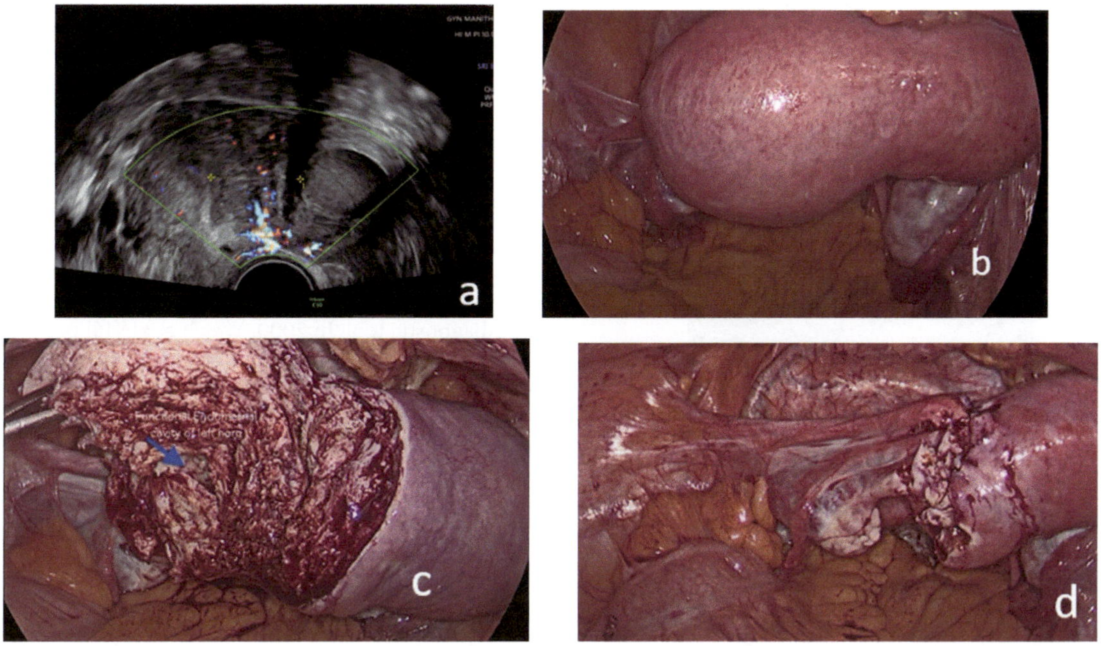


**FIGURE 18.3** (a) 2D ultrasound image with left-sided hematometra, (b) laparoscopic view of the uterus with the left-sided unconnected horn, and (c–d) laparoscopic excision of the left horn and uterine reconstruction.

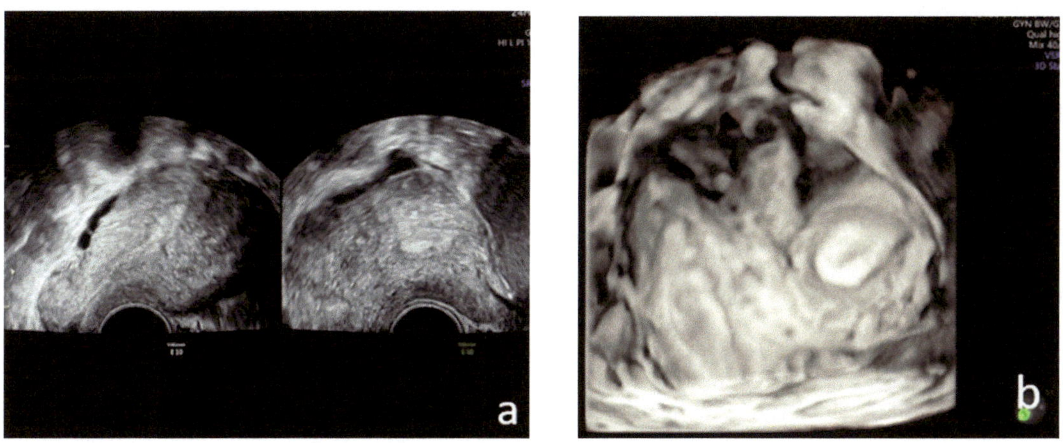


**FIGURE 18.4** (a) (left side of the picture) Right horn of the uterus with adenomyosis in the anterior wall and an endometrium of 6 mm. (right side of the picture) Left horn of the uterus and an endometrium of 7 mm with a polyp. No communication between the left and right horn. An endometrioma of 6 cm is seen in the left ovary. (b) 3D image showing normal uterine contours.

A small communicating uterine cavity was seen on the right side, and a blind uterine cavity on the left side. The external shape of the uterus was normal. **Figure 18.5a** shows the 3D-rendered ultrasonographic view. **Figure 18.5b** demonstrates a 3D HD live reconstruction.

While we were planning a hysteroscopic septum resection with unification of the two uterine cavities, the patient became pregnant again and is currently being monitored carefully (**Figure 18.5a, b**).

## Discussion

### Importance of diagnosing Robert's uterus

Robert's uterus is extremely difficult to diagnose preoperatively, and is therefore missed frequently. Diagnostic modalities may include ultrasound, hysterosalpingography (HSG), and MRI. 2D ultrasound is not very sensitive for the detection of Robert's uterus; the condition is frequently misdiagnosed as a unicornuate uterus with a non-communicating rudimentary horn, as in our above-mentioned case number one. While HSG may raise suspicion of a unicornuate uterus with a typical "banana" shape and only one fallopian tube, a septate uterus cannot be clearly visualized by HSG without imaging the external fundus. MRI is the best modality to demonstrate the uterine septum, the normal external fundal contour, hematometra and hematosalpinx, but is an expensive procedure. In cases of Robert's uterus, coronal T2-weighted MRI images are ideal for demonstrating the uterine septum dividing the endometrial cavity asymmetrically along with the blind-ending cavity and hematometra. T1-weighted images show the hematometra and hematosalpinx as a bright fluid in the endometrial cavity and in a dilated fallopian tube.

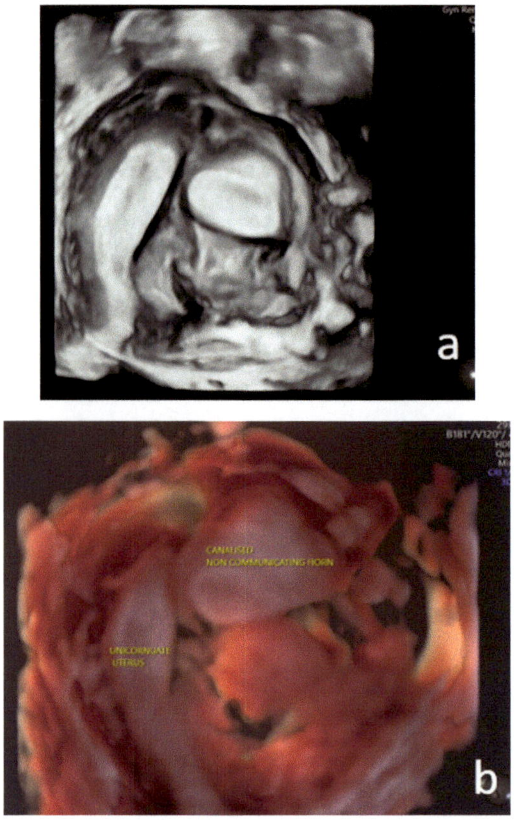


**FIGURE 18.5** (a) A small communicating uterine cavity on the right side and a blind uterine cavity on the left side in a 3D-rendered vaginal ultrasonic view and (b) 3D live reconstruction.

3D ultrasound is equivalent to MRI and even better in providing a correct diagnosis. Both diagnostic techniques require an experienced investigator.

3D ultrasound helps in the following six ways:

1. Identifies the non-communicating horn with hematometra.
2. Demonstrates the vascularity of the septum.
3. Provides measurement of the thickness of the septum.
4. Based on 3D ultrasound features, the clinician is able to establish the type of management (whether the hysteroscopic or laparoscopic approach, or combined surgery).
5. Enables the clinician to determine the mode of management, based on the thickness of intervening tissue and its vascularity.
6. Non-invasive identification of the postoperative outcome.

## Advantages of each classification, and advantages of diagnosis based on 3D ultrasound compared to MRI

Gynecological examination and two-dimensional ultrasound (2D US) are recommended for the evaluation of asymptomatic women. Three-dimensional (3D) US is recommended for the diagnosis of female genital anomalies in "symptomatic" patients belonging to high-risk groups, and anomalies suspected on routine investigation in asymptomatic women. MRI and endoscopic evaluation are recommended for patients with suspected complex anomalies or in cases of diagnostic dilemma. Adolescents with symptoms suggestive of a female genital anomaly should be thoroughly evaluated with 2D US, 3D US, MRI, and endoscopy [7].

With the use of modern 3D ultrasound technology, a well-trained and dedicated ultrasonographer or gynecologist will be able to establish Robert's uterus non-invasively and plan the correct surgical procedure accordingly. The high quality of tissue characterization by MRI makes it an excellent diagnostic modality to confirm the diagnosis of Robert's uterus and differentiate between septate and bicornuate uteri. Many studies have shown the efficacy of MRI as well as its ability to demonstrate the endometrial cavity and uterine contours in exquisite detail. However, 3D ultrasonography is an effective alternative because it provides images of very similar quality as MRI [4]. In addition, ultrasound is well tolerated by patients, economical, and easily available at many centers.

The repertoire of modern technologies includes 3D CT as a further diagnostic tool. In 2000, Welch et al. [16] proposed a real-time freehand 3D US system for image-guided surgery, which utilized a 5-MHz linear transducer and an optical positioner for location and orientation. At a rate at 15 frames per second, the system was able to dynamically reconstruct, update, and render 3D volumes. After performing volume measurement and visualization in real time, a magnetic field position sensor was added to the freehand US system. Optimized sequential algorithms permitted reslicing of the 3D US volume at 10 Hz. The real-time freehand 3D US system permits semi-automatic determination of the ROI using a 3.5-MHz concave probe and an electromagnetic position sensor. The system was capable of rapid predetermination of the reconstruction volume and assignment of the optimal viewing direction, which achieved accurate and fast reconstruction in real time. In the absence of a predefined route, the freehand scanner should be moved over the skin surfaces at the appropriate speed that avoids significant gaps. The Voluson E10BT19 system we used for our evaluation has all of these advantages.

A less than optimum ultrasound investigation may well cause the investigator to miss Robert's uterus.

## What surgical procedures are used today for the treatment of Robert's uterus?

Surgical correction is the sole effective treatment of Robert's uterus. The condition was managed via laparotomy in the early 1970s. Total horn resection or endometrectomy of the blinded cavity, abdominal metroplasty, or a combination of these procedures with hysteroscopy/laparoscopy were used. Irreversible surgeries (horn resection/endometrectomy of the blinded cavity) were performed to improve the shape and volume of the uterine cavity. A complete endometrectomy of the blind hemi-cavity is suitable only in patients with no communication between the blind cavity and the ipsilateral fallopian tube. A complete endometrectomy is believed to prevent the recurrence of hematometra. In 2011, Vural et al. [17] performed a hysterotomy incision and endometrectomy for Robert's uterus; the patient had a successful pregnancy and delivered a healthy infant by cesarean section in the 39th week of gestation. In 2017, Sardeshpande, Chipalkatti and Doctor [18] performed an endometrectomy of the blind cavity in a 15-year-old patient with recurrent abdominal cramps. In 2015, Li et al. [19] reported that excision of the septum and unification of the endometrial cavity by laparotomy or hysteroscopy proved to be the correct treatment for Robert's uterus. The authors performed a septum resection with hysteroscopy under ultrasonic surveillance. The patient became pregnant and delivered a healthy child. Hysteroscopic treatment of Robert's uterus using sonohysterography without laparoscopy or laparotomy has also been reported [20]. Under 3D sonohysterography the authors performed a hysteroscopic metroplasty guided by transrectal ultrasound, without laparotomy or laparoscopy. The outcome of the treatment was satisfactory. The patient's menstruation ceased to be painful and she had a normal uterine cavity of 3.6 cm after a communicating hemi cavity of 0.3 cm following two hysteroscopic procedures.

Our five patients were treated in accordance with the most modern standards. The entire range of treatment options were taken into account. In the fifth patient with recurrent abortions and no viable pregnancy, we planned the initiation of protective contraception to avoid the next abortion. However, the patient became pregnant again and is being monitored carefully.

## Conclusion

We discuss five cases of Robert's uterus as rare types of Müllerian duct anomalies. Our study underlined the value of 3D vaginal ultrasound technology in detecting this congenital uterine anomaly. The diagnosis of Robert's uterus remains a challenge for clinicians.

We found that, once the exact diagnosis of Robert's uterus has been established by 3D ultrasound, hysteroscopy in combination with laparoscopy is the gold standard for final confirmation of the diagnosis. As regards treatment, 3D ultrasound imaging combined with hysteroscopy is considered a practical and safe choice for asymmetric septal ablation. Laparoscopy, when used for monitoring purposes, provides additional information for guiding surgery. A simple hysteroscopic septum resection under laparoscopic control can be performed to unite the two uterine cavities when the septum is smaller than 1.0 cm. This was true of case number 2, in which the septum measured >5 mm. When the distance between the two uterine horns is larger than 1.5 cm, it would be advisable to perform a laparoscopic endometrectomy (as in case number 1) or a uterine horn resection by laparoscopy (as in case number 3). A tube connected to the uterine horn should also be resected but the ovaries must be preserved, provided the patient has no pathology at this site.

Our five cases compare well with the international literature and published classifications of uterine anomalies [6, 8, 21, 22].

A patient diagnosed with a Robert's uterus must be counseled about the possibility of pregnancy in the normal or non-communicating horn, recurrent endometriosis, adenomyosis, the advantages and disadvantages of complete horn removal, endometrectomy alone with fortification of the wall of the uterus, septal resection with unification of the uterus or non-interference, and the possibility of preterm or term delivery and recurrent abortions. Septal resection may involve surgery in several steps. Preliminary screening of a patient with recurrent pregnancy loss (RPL) or primary infertility should always include a 3D US investigation by an experienced investigator.

## References


1. Robert, H. G. (1969). Septate uterus with blind cavity without hematometra. CR Soc Fr Gynecol. 39: 767.
2. Robert, H. G. (1970). Asymmetrical bifidities with unilateral menstrual retention (apropos of 12 cases). Chirurgie. 96: 796.
3. Acien, P. M. and M. Sanchez-Ferrer (2004). "Complex malformations of the female genital tract. New types and revision of classification." Hum Reprod. **19**(10): 2377–2384.
4. Deutch, T. D. and A. Z. Abuhamad (2008). "The role of 3-dimensional ultrasonography and magnetic resonance imaging in the diagnosis of Müllerian duct anomalies: a review of the literature." J Ultrasound Med. **27**(3): 413–423.
5. The American Fertility Society classifications of adnexal adhesions, distal tubal occlusion, tubal occlusion secondary to tubal ligation, tubal pregnancies, mullerian anomalies and intrauterine adhesions (2016). 1988. Fertil Steril. **49**(6): 944–955. "Uterine septum: a guideline." Fertil Steril. **106**(3):530–540.
6. Grimbizis, G. F., S. Gordts, A. Di Spiezio Sardo, S. Brucker, C. De Angelis, M. Gergolet, T. C. Li, V. Tanos, H. Brolmann, L. Gianaroli and R. Campo (2013). "The ESHRE/ESGE consensus on the classification of female genital tract congenital anomalies." Hum Reprod. **28**(8): 2032–2044.
7. Grimbizis, G. F., A. Di Spiezio Sardo, S. H. Saravelos, S. Gordts, C. Exacoustos, D. Van Schoubroeck, C. Bermejo, N. N. Amso, G. Nargund, D. Timmermann, A. Athanasiadis, S. Brucker, C. De Angelis, M. Gergolet, T. C. Li, V. Tanos, B. Tarlatzis, R. Farquharson, L. Gianaroli and R. Campo (2016). "The Thessaloniki ESHRE/ESGE consensus on diagnosis of female genital anomalies." Gynecol Surg. **13**: 1–16
8. Di Spiezio Sardo, A., R. Campo, S. Gordts, M. Spinelli, C. Cosimato, V. Tanos, S. Brucker, T. C. Li, M. Gergolet, C. De Angelis, L. Gianaroli and G. Grimbizis (2015). "The comprehensiveness of the ESHRE/ESGE classification of female genital tract congenital anomalies: a systematic review of cases not classified by the AFS system." Human Reprod. **30**(5): 1046–1058.
9. Ludwin, A., I. Ludwin, K. Pitynski, P. Basta, A. Basta, T. Banas, R. Jach, M. Wiechec, R. Grabowska, K. Stangel-Wojcikiewicz, T. Milewicz and A. Nocun (2013). "Transrectal ultrasound-guided hysteroscopic myomectomy of submucosal myomas with a varying degree of myometrial penetration." J Minim Invasive Gynecol. **20**(5): 672–685.
10. Ludwin, A., I. Ludwin, K. Pityński, T. Banas and R. Jach (2014). "Role of morphologic characteristics of the uterine septum in the prediction and prevention of abnormal healing outcomes after hysteroscopic metroplasty." Human Reprod. **29**(7): 1420–1431.
11. Ludwin, A., W. P. Martins and I. Ludwin (2017). "Uterine cavity imaging, volume estimation and quantification of degree of deformity using automatic volume calculation: description of technique." Ultrasound Obstet Gynecol. **50**(1): 138–140.
12. Ludwin, A., W. P. Martins, C. O. Nastri, I. Ludwin, M. A. Coelho Neto, V. M. Leitao, M. Acien, J. L. Alcazar, B. Benacerraf, G. Condous, R. L. De Wilde, M. H. Emanuel, W. Gibbons, S. Guerriero, W. W. Hurd, D. Levine, S. Lindheim, A. Pellicer, F. Petraglia and E. Saridogan (2018). "Congenital uterine malformation by experts (CUME): better criteria for distinguishing between normal/arcuate and septate uterus?" Ultrasound Obstet Gynecol. **51**(1): 101–109.
13. Huang, Q. and Z. Zeng (2017). "A review on real-time 3D ultrasound imaging technology." BioMed Res Int. **2017**: 6027029–6027029.
14. Tolani, A., D. Kadambari, A. Deenadayal, S. Donthi, I. R. Yellenki and M. Deenadayal (2018). "Timely identification of pregnancy in non-communicating horn of unicornuate uterus by three-dimensional transvaginal ultrasonography." J Clin Imaging Sci. **8**: 39.
15. Jayaprakasan, K., L. Polanski and K. Ojha (2020). Gynecological Ultrasound Scanning: Tips and Tricks, Cambridge University Press.
16. Welch, J.N., J. A. Johnson, M. R. Bax, R. Badr, and R. Shahidi, "A real-time freehand 3D ultrasound system for image-guided surgery," in Proceedings of the IEEE Ultrasonics Symposium, pp. 1601–1604, October 2000. View at: Google Scholar
17. Vural, M., S. Yildiz, H. Cece, and H. Camuzcuoglu (2011). "Favourable pregnancy outcome after endometrectomy for a Robert's uterus." J Obstet Gynaecol. **31**(7): 668–669.
18. Sardeshpande, N., P. Chipalkatti and J. Doctor (2017). Roberts uterus: a rare congenital anomaly. **6**(12): 3.
19. Li, J., W. Yu, M. Wang and L.-M. Feng (2015). "Hysteroscopic treatment of Robert's uterus with laparoscopy." J Obstet Gynecol Res. **41**(9): 1491–1494
20. Ludwin, A., I. Ludwin and W. P. Martins (2016). "Robert's uterus: modern imaging techniques and ultrasound-guided hysteroscopic treatment without laparoscopy or laparotomy." Ultrasound Obstet Gynecol. **48**(4): 526–529.
21. Di Spiezio Sardo, A., P. Giampaolino, M. Scognamiglio, C. Varelli, G. Nazzaro, G. Mansueto, C. Nappi and G. F. Grimbizis (2016). An exceptional case of complete septate uterus with unilateral cervical aplasia (Class U2bC3V0/ESHRE/ESGE Classification) and isolated Mullerian remnants: combined hysteroscopic and laparoscopic treatment. J Minim Invasive Gynecol **23**(1): 16–17.
22. Ludwin, A. and I. Ludwin (2015). Comparison of the ESHRE-ESGE and ASRM classifications of Mullerian duct anomalies in everyday practice. Hum Reprod. **30**(3): 569–580.

# 19

## LAPAROSCOPIC ADNEXAL SURGERY FOR BENIGN CONDITIONS

**Liselotte Mettler, Ibrahim Alkatout, and Meenu Agarwal**

## Background

In adnexal surgery, we can look from various angles. In this chapter, we focus on ovarian endometriomas, on adnexal torsion and on the question of when are oophorectomy, salpingectomy and adnexectomy indicated at hysterectomies beyond the reproductive age.

## Endometriomas

### Surgical approach

The surgical removal of endometriomas in symptomatic patients is one of the standard therapeutic procedures for ovarian endometriosis recommended in national and international guidelines, such as those reported by Dunselman et al. [15]. The most frequent indications for surgery are cyst-related symptoms, especially pain. Despite a lack of extensive data from prospective randomized trials, there is clear evidence that surgical removal or even ablation of an endometriosis cyst leads to pain reduction [10, 18]. In addition, it has been shown that complete removal of endometriosis, including ovarian endometriosis, may lead to an increased fertility rate for up to 12 months after surgery. However, a recent Cochrane analysis comparing aspiration, cyst enucleation, and expectant management did not show a significant difference in pregnancy rates when these different strategies were followed by assisted reproductive technology (ART) [7].

Although the sensitivity and specificity of (transvaginal) ultrasound and tumor-marker analysis are both insufficient to classify an ovarian tumor as benign, premalignant, or even malignant, there are still morphologic criteria that can support the decision for surgical removal in order to achieve histopathologic certainty and avoid missing a malignancy.

Finally, ovarian endometriosis and other forms of deep-infiltrating endometriosis are associated with a 50% increase in the risk for developing ovarian cancer (OC). Thus, it may become important to reduce cancer risk by removing the endometriosis at a later time [17, 28, 40, 45, 46].

There is always a potential for recurrence, however, even after a complete second-line cyst enucleation. The recurrence risk increases over time, rising to as much as 37% in 5 years after surgery [24].

### Alternatives to surgical removal

There are compelling arguments for and against the surgical removal of endometriomas. The removal of an endometrioma, while reducing pain, may also compromise the integrity of primordial and antral follicles. Studies have shown that primordial follicles are lost and the density of cells is decreased in proximity to an endometrioma [30, 47, 48]. Some authors blame this on an increased oxidative stress outside the cyst and the presence of free iron inside the cyst [31, 47, 48]. Additionally, a focal inflammation may incite fibrosis in the cortex-specific stroma. The coexisting oxidative stress and inflammation may lead to the increased recruitment and atresia of follicles [25]. Ovulation may be impaired [6] and the response to stimulation reduced. Interestingly, Barri et al. reported a 12% pregnancy rate after spontaneous conception with endometrioma in situ, compared with a 54% pregnancy rate after surgical removal [5]. It is clear that the risk of adnexal torsion, cyst growth and rupture, and malignant progression tend to favor surgical removal [41].

Another important issue is "relapsed endometriosis." From a surgical standpoint, neither the stripping technique nor the ablative technique (opening and coagulating an endometriosis cyst without removing it) leads to a significantly different recurrence rate. In a study by Muzii et al. comparing the two techniques in 51 patients with bilateral endometriomas, the recurrence rate was 6% after stripping and 2% after coagulation. Thus, even if available data conflict in different studies, it may be preferable to perform an ablation in patients who desire future pregnancy [9, 10, 36]. But in infertile women with a recurrence of ovarian endometrioma, secondary surgery appears to impair the ovarian reserve and worsen reproductive performance. The pregnancy outcome in these cases may be better after direct ART, as shown by Park et al. [39].

Two parameters can pose major obstacles for endometriosis patients trying to conceive: the "ovarian reserve" and the quality of the germ cells. While the germ cells tend to undergo a more rapid ageing process than in women without endometriosis, the ovarian reserve is decreased even further due to the endometrioma-related effects noted above. The ovarian reserve can be measured (indirectly) in terms of the antral follicle count or the level of anti-Müllerian hormone (AMH). These different aspects—a decreased ovarian reserve in endometriosis patients in general, further impairment due to endometrioma formation, and damage from a surgical procedure such as stripping or coagulation—must be taken into account when counseling a patient about surgery for ovarian endometriosis [51].

Despite conflicting data in the literature, many studies have demonstrated that surgical excision can decrease the ovarian reserve. This may result from the removal of healthy ovarian tissue, damage due to coagulation, or local inflammation after surgery. Indeed, it has been shown that endometrioma removal is more likely to remove ovarian tissue than the removal of another benign cyst such as a dermoid or functional cyst [42]. This is particularly true in reoperations. Hormonal stimulation of an ovary appears to be more difficult after surgery. However, neither the pregnancy rate with IVF alone nor the sequence of surgery and IVF leads to a statistically significant difference [22].

### Techniques

In counseling a patient about surgery, it is essential to consider the motivation for surgery. We recommend a differentiated approach:

- For pain or other endometriosis-related symptoms: Surgical removal of the cyst (by stripping or coagulation).

- For infertility: Surgical removal before or after fertility treatment. We recommend surgery for patients with a unilateral endometrioma and no prior surgical treatment. For patients with recurrent endometrioma, we recommend direct fertility treatment without surgery.
- For patients with an OC risk (atypical endometriosis): Surgical removal of the cyst.

**Salpingoovariolysis**: Endometriosis causes dense adhesions to form between the ovary and its surroundings. Thus the ovary may be adherent to the pelvic sidewall, uterus, bowel, and even the contralateral ovary depending on size and bilaterality. In removing any cyst, it is important to free the ovary completely without damaging either the ovary or adjacent structures. If the bowel is adherent, gentle traction should be placed on the bowel to expose the plane of dissection between the bowel and ovary. The adhesions should be cut with scissors rather than an energy device to prevent thermal injury to the tissues. In the case of a "frozen pelvis," it may be helpful to open the retroperitoneal space at the level of the sacral promontory so that the ureter can be identified. Then the ureter is followed and the bowel, ureter, and ovary are separated from one another. The next step may be to detach the ovary from the uterus. This may require applying traction to the ovary with a grasper. The adhesion can then be identified and divided with scissors or an energy device (i.e., using monopolar or bipolar current or ultrasound). The last step is to free the ovary from the pelvic sidewall. The ovary is held anteriorly with a grasper, which may be held by the surgeon or by an assistant. The suction-irrigation device can then be used for blunt dissection, carefully freeing the ovary from the endometriosis-affected peritoneal tissue of the pelvic sidewall. The suction-irrigation tube is swiped between the ovary and pelvic wall in a parallel direction rather than perpendicular.

Frequently, the cyst will rupture at this stage, and the chocolate cyst can be confirmed. The fluid is evacuated and dissection is continued in the same fashion until the ovary is completely freed. Any bleeding sites can be carefully coagulated with bipolar current. In most cases, the anatomic structures of the ovarian ligament, infundibulopelvic ligament, fallopian tube (FT), ovary, and pelvic wall can be identified. Do not coagulate the pelvic wall before identifying the ureter! This is because the ureter is always close to the surgery site and is vulnerable to thermal injury.

**Ovarian cyst enucleation**: Most endometriomas will rupture during ovariolysis. If that occurs, the rupture site on the ovary can serve as the starting point for cyst enucleation. The opening should be enlarged along the ovarian axis or equatorially so that the ovary is divided into two equal parts.

It is important at this stage to identify the proper plane of dissection. This may be difficult because endometriomas adhere to the ovarian tissue. This is especially true for lesions with a fibroblastic rather than fibrocystic histology. All dissection should proceed very slowly and carefully so that normal ovarian tissue is damaged as little as possible. If the layers cannot be separated at one site, another should be tried. Always start the dissection at the easiest site, leaving the more difficult part for the end. The graspers should always be placed close to each other; otherwise, if the surgeon ends up pulling a long piece of tissue, the normal tissue may tear or the cyst itself may tear, and this will make the dissection more difficult. Coagulation should be used sparingly so that "safe" germ cells are spared. Most bleeders will stop by themselves; only heavier bleeders should be selectively cauterized. If the endometrioma measures 5 cm or less, the ovary will shrink after cyst enucleation and there is no need for reapproximating sutures. If the defect approaches the ovarian ligament, an (intracorporeal) suture may be used, taking care to avoid stitching the vessels (**Figures 19.1–19.7**).

**Ovariopexy**: In almost all cases of ovarian endometriosis, the ovary is involved by peritoneal endometriosis of the pelvic wall. This makes it necessary to remove the peritoneal and deep-infiltrating endometriosis involving adjacent tissues, i.e., the peritoneal tissue of the ovarian fossa and the uterosacral ligament. A temporary ovariopexy is helpful in exposing the field for this part of the procedure. There are many ways to fix the ovary temporarily. We prefer an extracorporeal suture on a straight needle introduced into the abdominal cavity under vision at a site lateral to the lower working portal. The needle is then passed through the ovary and returned through the abdominal wall. The suture is tied outside the abdomen. The ovary may be kept in that position for up to 1–2 days postoperatively to prevent immediate postoperative adhesions between the ovary and the pelvic wall or bowel. Alternatively, an assistant can lift the ovary with a grasper to expose the field for deperitonealization and ureterolysis.

**Deperitonealization of the ovarian fossa and ureterolysis**: The peritoneum adjacent to the ureter is often involved by endometriosis. Since deep-infiltrating endometriosis can lead to hydroureter and hydronephrosis, and because complete excision is the best way to prevent recurrence and yields the highest pregnancy rates, deperitonealization of the ovarian fossa and, if necessary, of the uterosacral ligament is recommended. To spare the ureter, the ureter should be identified and ureterolysis performed, carefully preserving the vessels and nerve fibers accompanying the ureter.

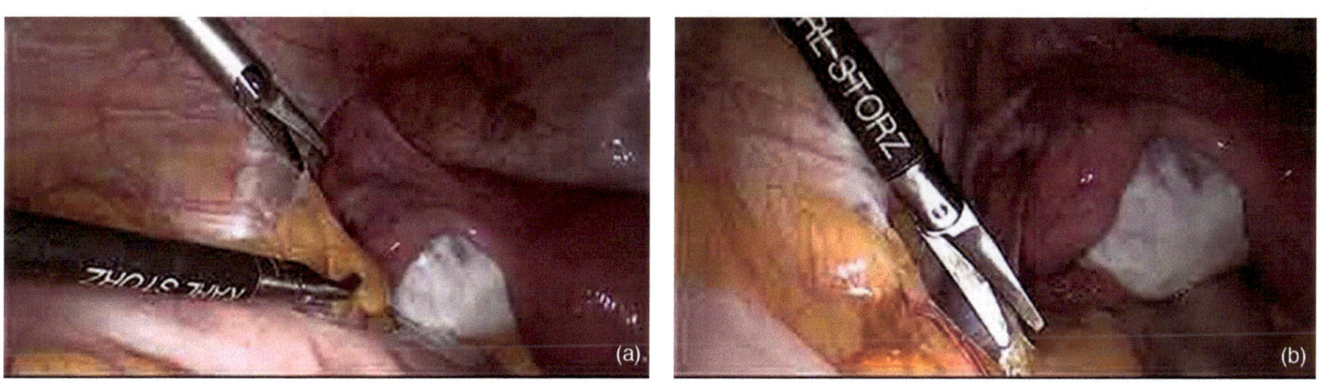


FIGURE 19.1 (a, b) Adhesiolysis. Gentle traction on the mesosigmoid exposes an avascular plane, which is cut with scissors (a). The adhesion is divided until the sigmoid colon is completely freed (b).

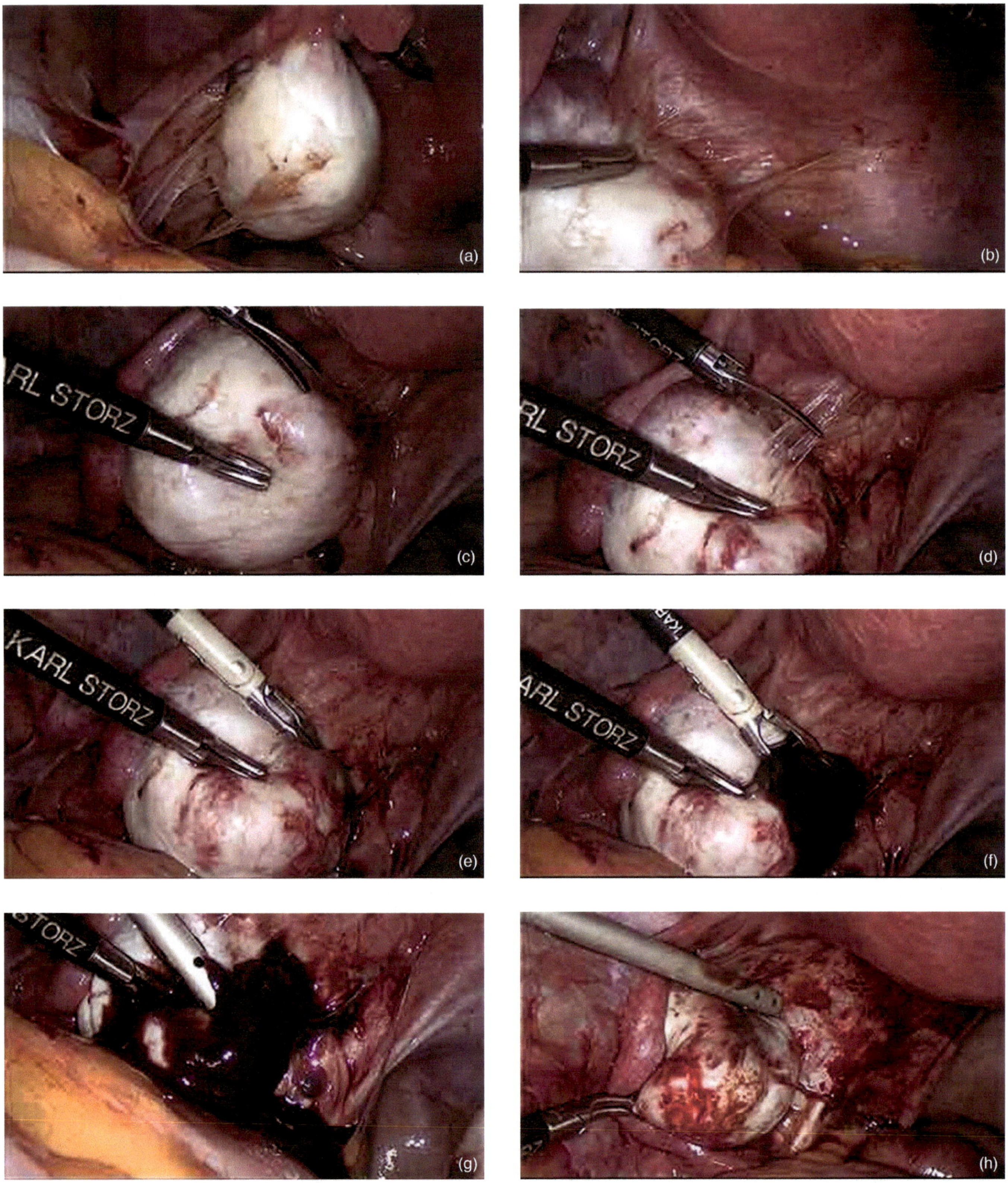


**FIGURE 19.2** (a–h) Ovariolysis. The uterus is anteverted, exposing adhesions between the ovary and pelvic wall (a). The ovary is freed by blunt dissection between the ovary and uterus (b). Indentation of the ovary exposes flimsy adhesions between the ovary and uterus close to the ovarian ligament (c, d). The ovary and uterus are gently forced apart, using a bipolar Maryland grasper without current (e). The cyst will often rupture during dissection, and a chocolate-like fluid is seen (f). The fluid is evacuated (g). Blunt dissection with the suction-irrigation tube is performed parallel to the cleavage line between the ovary and adjacent tissue of the pelvic wall (h).

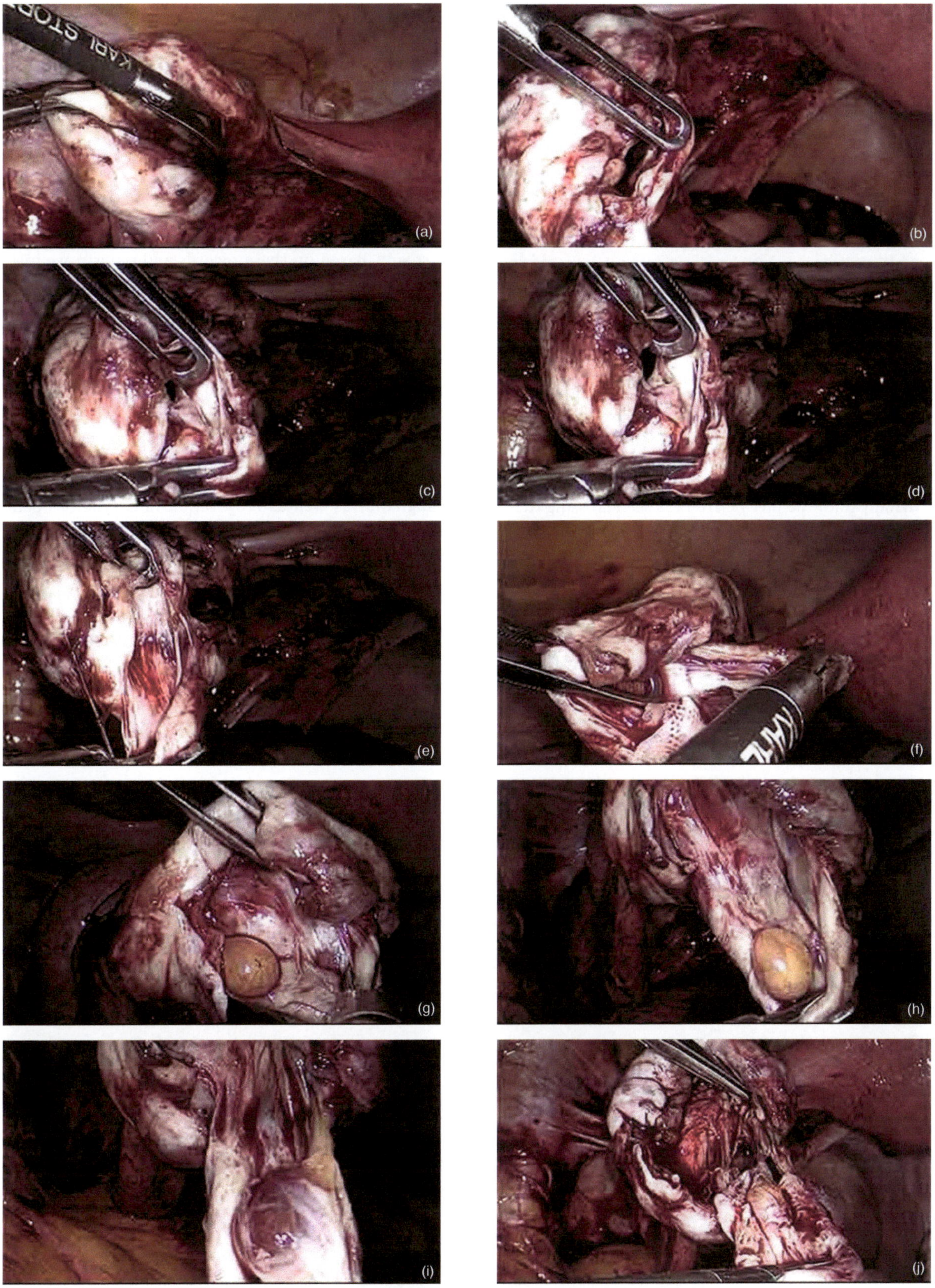


**FIGURE 19.3** (a–j) Cyst enucleation (stripping). The ovary is pulled anterolaterally. The rupture site is exposed and enlarged with scissors (a). Normal ovary and cyst are identified and grasped separately (b–d). The line (plane) between the ovary and cyst is visualized, and gentle traction is applied in perpendicular fashion to gradually separate the cyst from normal ovarian tissue. There should be little or no bleeding when this is done in the correct plane. The two graspers should be placed fairly close together for stripping the cyst (e). Even if the dissection is performed very carefully, normal tissue (e.g., a small functional cyst) is removed with the endometrioma. After the endometriosis cyst has been removed, bleeding vessels are sparingly coagulated (g–j).

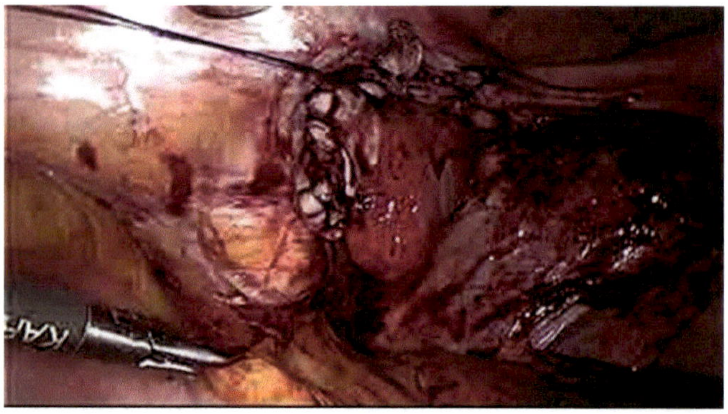

**FIGURE 19.4** Ovariopexy. An ovariopexy helps to expose the ovarian fossa.

The ureter should be visualized where it crosses the iliac vessels, approximately at the level of the sacral promontory. The retroperitoneal space is then opened parallel to the ureter. This can be accomplished by blunt dissection with a Maryland grasper. Look for unaffected peritoneum to start the dissection. The ureter is traced distally until the uterine artery is seen crossing the ureter medially to reach the uterus. It may even be necessary to dissect the ureter as far as the parametrial tissue. The peritoneum is stripped to ensure the removal of all endometriosis-affected tissue.

**Adhesion prophylaxis**: Surgeons may use any preferred barrier method to prevent adhesions, such as oxidized regenerated cellulose (Interceed), expanded polytetrafluoroethylene (Gore-Tex), or sodium hyaluronate with carboxymethylcellulose (Seprafilm). There is no clear evidence however that any barrier method can prevent adhesion formation or lead to improved pregnancy rates [2].

**Drain**: Since coagulation is used sparingly on the ovary, the cyst bed may still ooze at the end of the surgery. A drain should be inserted and remain in place until its output is less than 100 mL/24 h.

## Statistical analysis of endometrioma surgery

### *Material and methods*

From 1995 to 2004, we retrospectively analyzed 3,057 patient medical records and surgical reports at the Department of Obstetrics and Gynecology of Kiel University Hospital in Kiel, Germany. Based on these records and reports, we histologically verified 550 cases of ovarian endometriotic cysts that underwent conservative excision via laparoscopy or laparotomy. Data on general patient characteristics, endometrioma symptoms, and diagnostic and surgical findings were collected from clinical records and reviewed (**Figure 19.8**). Patient characteristics are summarized in **Table 19.1**. Letters were sent to the patients asking them to fill in and return a questionnaire. With a final return rate of 52.5%, there were 289 patients in the follow-up study. The questionnaire asked about the possible postoperative occurrence of another endometriosis cyst, timing of occurrence, possible malignancy as well as reoperation rate, type of operation, and recurrent pain symptoms (pain lasting >1 week, dysmenorrhea, and dyspareunia). Patients were surveyed about their preoperative and postoperative fertility, whether they had had a planned spontaneous pregnancy with or without complications, and in infertile patients, whether artificial insemination had been successful. The recurrence of ovarian endometrioma was defined as a positive response to the presence of an endometriosis cyst, as reported by the patient on the questionnaire. The average follow-up period was 12.9 years, with a range from 7.0 years to 16.9 years between surgery and follow-up.

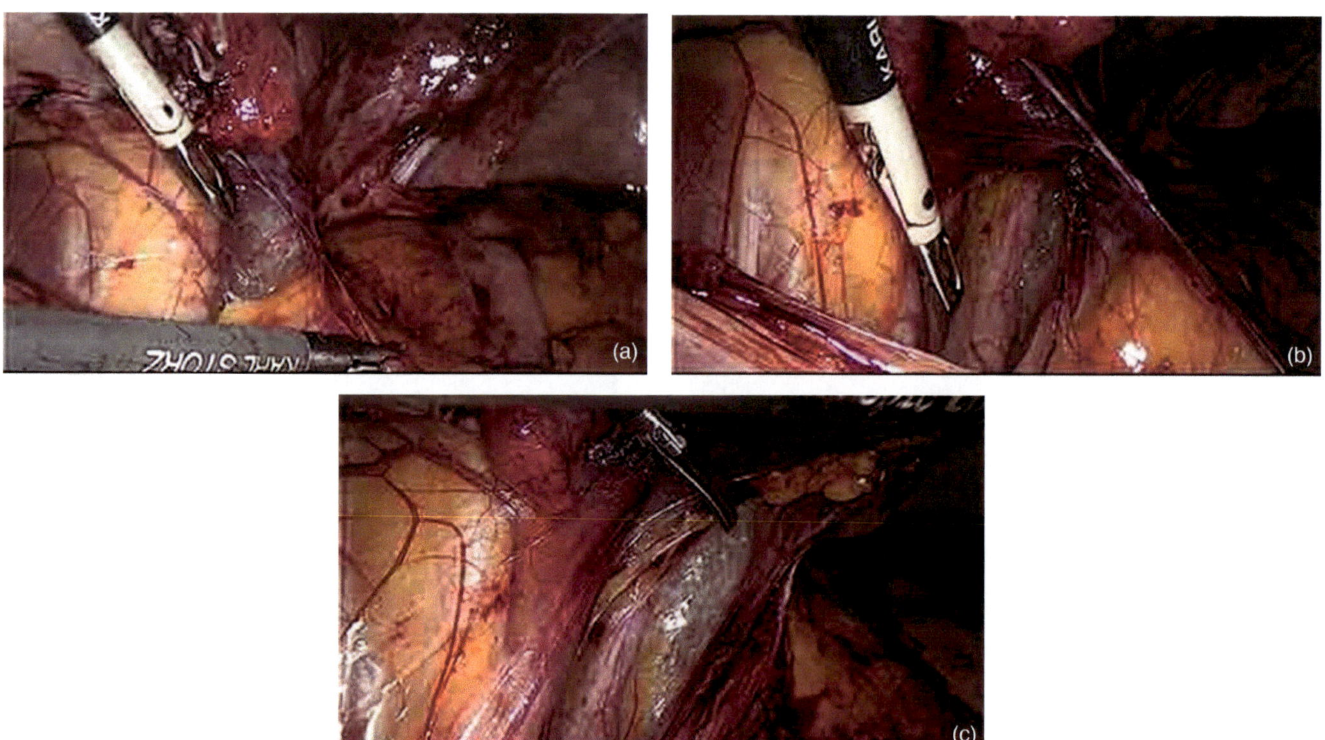


**FIGURE 19.5** (a–c) Ureterolysis. Gentle traction is placed on the sigmoid colon. The Maryland grasper is used for blunt dissection, identifying and exposing the ureter (a, b). Scissors are used to cut avascular fibers of connective tissue (c).

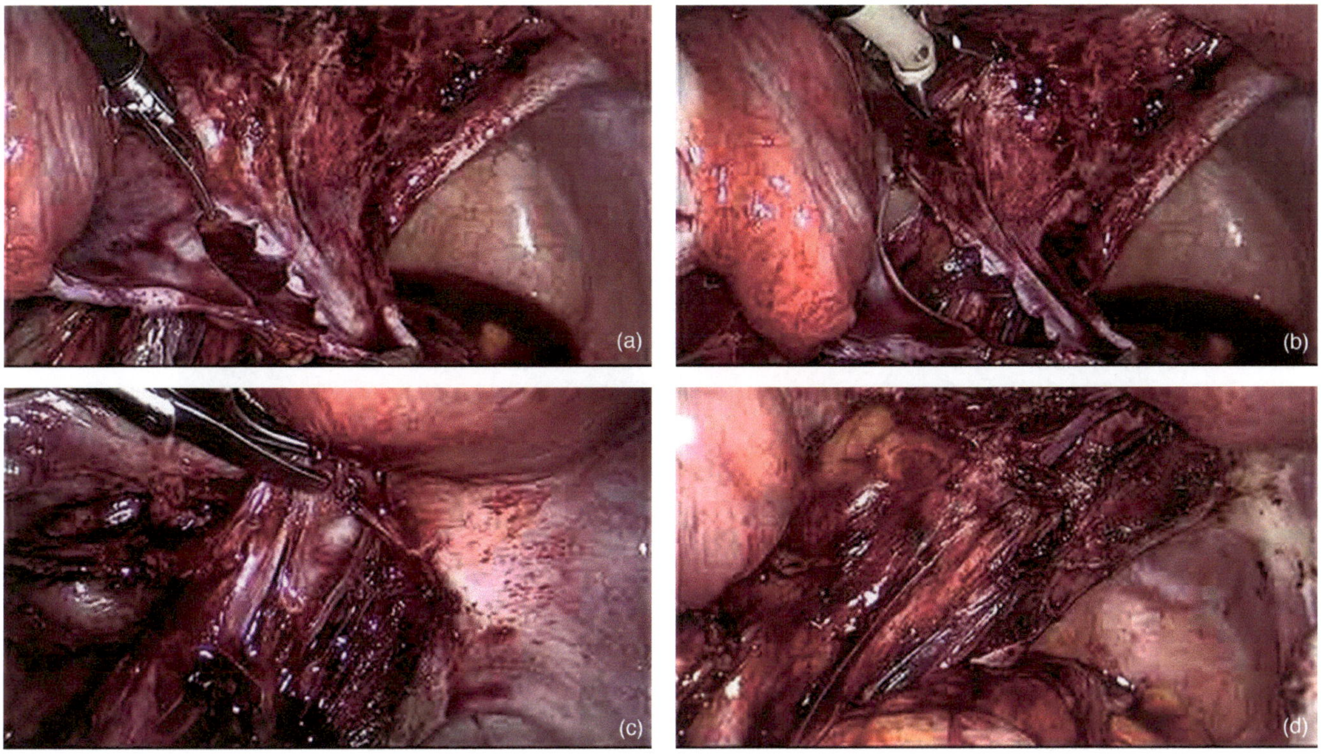


**FIGURE 19.6** (a–d) Deperitonealization of the ovarian fossa. While traction is placed on the peritoneum, the endometriosis-affected peritoneal tissue is excised with a scissor (a). The Maryland grasper may help to force apart healthy and affected peritoneal tissue (b). The peritoneum is excised with scissors close to the uterus (c). Final view after deperitonealization of the ovarian fossa (d).

Data for analysis were recorded using Microsoft Access software (Redmond, Washington). Statistical analysis was performed using Microsoft Excel and SPSS software (IBM Corporation, Armonk, New York). Patient identification numbers were assigned to ensure confidentiality. The percentage data are based primarily on total case numbers; but in the absence of information, the corrected probability is given. The chi-squared test was used in the analysis of categorical values. The statistical significance level was set at 5% ($P < 0.05$). The recurrence-free interval probabilities were estimated using the Kaplan-Meier method. The log-rank test (Mantel-Cox) was used to compare the survival times of two groups. Postmenopausal women were not considered in the postoperative analysis of dysmenorrhea [32].

### *Results*

At the time of surgery, the mean age of all endometrioma patients was 37.2 (±9.0) years. Their mean age at follow-up was 50.5 (±9.3) years (**Table 19.1**). Younger preoperative age, nulliparity, and prior laparoscopic surgery for ovarian endometrioma positively predicted the presence of pain and dysmenorrhea. Larger cyst size (> 8 cm) was also associated with occurrence of pain, while primary or secondary sterility was associated with a higher rate of dysmenorrhea.

Factors associated with recurrence of dysmenorrhea were younger age ($P < 0.01$), nulliparity ($P < 0.05$), and larger cyst size ($P < 0.05$). Prior laparoscopic surgery for ovarian endometrioma ($P < 0.05$) was the only significant risk factor relating to the recurrence of pain (**Table 19.2**).

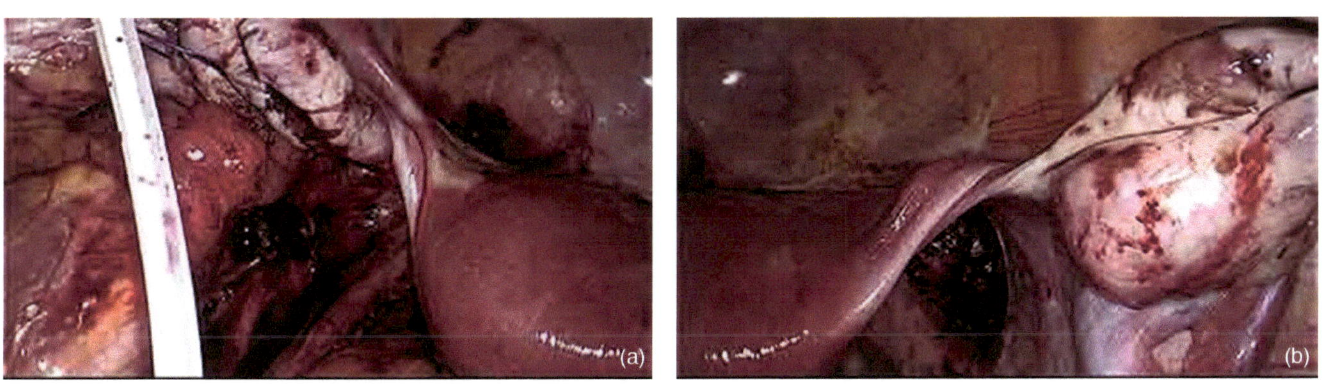


**FIGURE 19.7** (a, b) Final view at the conclusion of surgery. The ovariopexy remains in place for 2 days. The drain is removed as output diminishes.

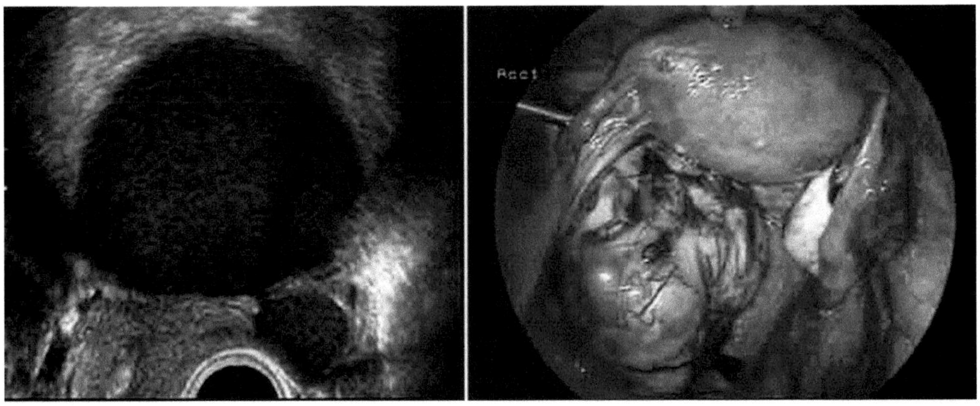

FIGURE 19.8 Transvaginal sonogram of a 6 cm (diameter) endometrioma of the left ovary and corresponding laparoscopic image.

TABLE 19.1: **Patient Characteristics (n = 550)**

| **Factors** | | **Number of Cases (%)** |
|---|---|---|
| **Age** (years) | | 37.2 ± 9.0[b] |
| **BMI** ($kg/m^2$) | < 19 | 43 (7.8) |
| 19–24 | | 344 (62.5) |
| 25–30 | | 123 (22.4) |
| > 30 | | 40 (7.3) |
| Sterility | Primary | 261 (47.5) |
| | Secondary | 52 (9.5) |
| Parity | ≥ 1 | 194 (35.3) |
| Abortion or miscarriage | ≥ 1 | 72 (13.1) |
| Pain | | 338 (61.5) |
| Dysmenorrhea | | 214 (38.9) |
| Recurrence of previous endometrioma | | 153 (27.8) |
| Previous laparoscopic surgery of endometrioma | | 226 (41.1) |
| Presence of uterine myoma | | 105 (19.1) |
| **CA-125**[a] (U/mL) | increased (> 35 U/mL) | 147 (47.6) |
| Cyst size (cm) | 2–4 | 316 (57.5) |
| | 5–8 | 209 (38.0) |
| | > 8 | 25 (4.5) |
| **Cyst rupture** | Preoperative | 23 (4.2) |
| Intraoperative | | 281 (51.1) |
| Follow-up patient characteristics (n = 289) | | |
| **Age** (years) | | 50.5 ± 9.3[b] |
| Postoperative medical treatment | | 162 (56.1) |
| Postoperative pain | | 96 (33.2) |
| Postoperative dysmenorrhea | | 93 (34.8) |
| Recurrence of first diagnosed ovarian endometrioma | | 47 (23.9) |
| Reoperation rate of first diagnosed ovarian endometrioma | | 32 (68.1) |
| Postoperative pregnancy desire | | 111 (38.4) |
| Postoperative pregnancy | | 60 (54.1) |

[a] The sum does not add up to the total because of missing values or because of a new subtotal.
[b] Mean ± SD.

There were 179 patients initially diagnosed with endometriomas at the time of surgery. Forty-seven of these patients (23.9%) had a recurrent ovarian endometrioma in the follow-up period; and 68.1% of the same subset of patients (32 of 47) had undergone a reoperation in the follow-up period (**Table 19.1**). Of those 32 patients, 17 (53.1%) required one reoperation, 9 (28.1%) required two reoperations, and 6 (18.8%) required three or more reoperations due to new endometriosis cysts. The probability of a recurrence-free interval was 76.1% for all primarily diagnosed endometriomas over our study period.

**TABLE 19.2: Analysis of Factors Related to the Occurrence and Recurrence of Pain and Dysmenorrhea**

| | Preoperative | Postoperative | Preoperative | Postoperative |
|---|---|---|---|---|
| | Pain | | Dysmenorrhea | |
| Factors | *P*-value (n = 550) | *P*-value (n = 289) | *P*-value (n = 550) | *P*-value (n = 267) |
| Younger age (years) | < 0.01 | NS | < 0.01 | < 0.01 |
| BMI (kg/m$^2$) | NS | NS | NS | NS |
| Sterility | NS | NS | < 0.01 | NS |
| Nulliparity | < 0.05 | NS | < 0.05 | < 0.05 |
| Abortion/miscarriage | NS | NS | NS | NS |
| Previous laparoscopy of endometrioma | < 0.01 | < 0.05 | < 0.05 | NS |
| Lager cyst size (> 8 cm) | < 0.05 | NS | NS | < 0.05 |
| Cyst rupture | NS | NS | NS | NS |

NS: not significant.
From Maul et al., 2014 [32].

Patients with preoperative pain showed a significantly higher recurrence rate (log-rank test P = 0.013). The Kaplan-Meier graph shows that patients without preoperative pain had a significantly higher recurrence-free interval of 84.7% when compared with patients who had a history of preoperative pain. The latter group was only 69.4% recurrence-free by the end of the follow-up period (**Figure 19.9**). Another statistically significant risk factor for endometrioma recurrence was preoperative dysmenorrhea (log-rank test P = 0.013). The Kaplan-Meier curve (**Figure 19.10**) shows that women without preoperative dysmenorrhea have a recurrence-free interval of 81.4% compared with a recurrence-free interval of only 66.2% in women with preoperative dysmenorrhea.

Other risk factors that were not significant but showed an association with a higher recurrence rate were larger cyst size (> 8 cm: recurrence rate of 33.3% [5 of 15] versus 16.3% [15 of 92] for cyst size 5–8 cm and 16.8% [24 of 143] for cyst size < 5 cm), younger age at surgery (< 25 years: 6.4% [3 of 47] in the recurrence cohort versus 2.8% [8 of 289] in the follow-up cohort), and preoperative cyst rupture (recurrence rate of 28.6% [2 of 7] versus 20.5%).

As for the efficacy of endometrioma surgery, laparoscopy yielded the best results in terms of freedom from symptoms in the postoperative period: 49.0% of the patients were symptom-free after laparoscopic surgery compared with only 33.3% after laparotomy. Only 43.7% of patients were asymptomatic following conversion from laparoscopy to laparotomy.

Postoperative medical treatment was given in 56.1% of the cases (162 of 289). Additional postoperative hormone therapy (gonadotropin-releasing hormone agonist, oral contraceptive, medroxyprogesterone acetate, or danazol) led to a higher recurrence of endometrioma, with a recurrence-free interval rate of only 70.5% versus 82.6% in patients who did not receive hormonal therapy (log-rank test P = 0.050) (**Figure 19.11**). The recurrence rates in both groups increased steadily with time from diagnostic surgery. When combined surgical and hormonal treatment was compared with surgical treatment alone, the following differences were found: postoperative pain in 36.4% versus 29.1%, dysmenorrhea in 37.8% versus 26.0%, and dyspareunia in 19.1% versus 18.1%.

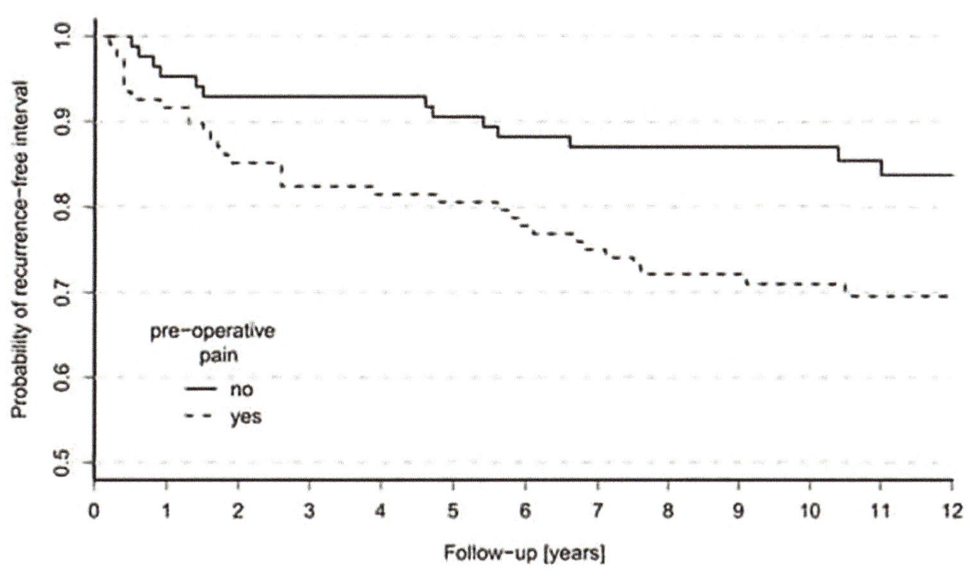


**FIGURE 19.9** Probability of recurrence-free interval within the follow-up period in patients with and without preoperative pain. (Courtesy of Maul et al., 2014 [32].)

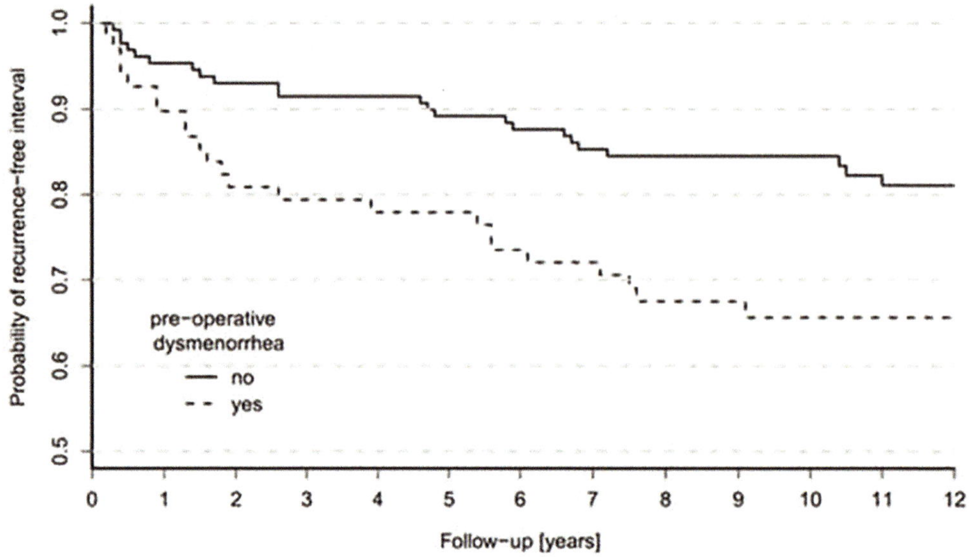


**FIGURE 19.10** Probability of recurrence-free interval within the follow-up period in patients with and without preoperative dysmenorrhea. (Courtesy of Maul et al., 2014 [32].)

111 of 289 patients expressed a desire to become pregnant in the postoperative period (38.4%). Combined surgical and hormonal treatment was given to 61 of 111 patients (55.0%), whereas surgery alone was performed in 50 of 111 patients (45.0%). Among these patients, the postoperative spontaneous pregnancy rate was 54.1% (60 of 111). Of the 60 patients, who conceived, 46 of 111 (41.4%) had received surgery plus medical treatment and 14 of 111 (12.6%) had surgery alone. A statistically significant difference ($P < 0.001$) was noted between combined surgical and hormonal therapy and surgery alone.

## Evaluation of our retrospective cohort study

Preoperative risk factors found to have significant predictive value for pain and dysmenorrhea were younger age at surgery, prior laparoscopic surgery for ovarian endometrioma, and nulliparity. Pain complaints appeared to be significantly associated with larger cyst size (> 8 cm), while primary or secondary sterility was associated with a higher rate of dysmenorrhea. As for recurrent symptoms, younger age, nulliparity, and larger cyst diameter significantly influenced the recurrence of dysmenorrhea, while only prior laparoscopic surgery for ovarian endometrioma was found to be a significant risk factor for the recurrence of pain, as reported by Busacca et al. and Porpora et al. [11, 32, 43].

In agreement with Vercellini et al., a lower incidence of dysmenorrhea in older patients is attributable to postmenopausal changes [54]. Other studies have suggested that adhesions have causal importance in pain associated with endometriosis, whereas no significant correlation has been found between cyst diameter and pain symptoms [16, 21]. Like earlier studies that described pregnancy as a protective factor against pain associated with endometriosis, more recent studies have also identified nulliparity as having predictive value for pain symptoms [26, 43].

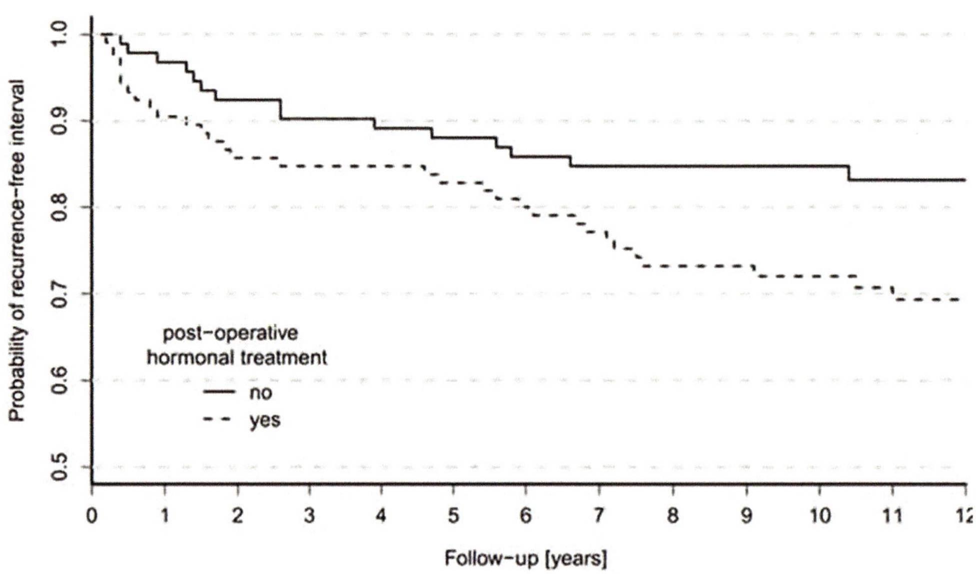


**FIGURE 19.11** Probability of recurrence-free interval within the follow-up period in patients with and without postoperative hormonal treatment. (Courtesy of Maul et al. (2014) [32].)

Many studies have analyzed the recurrence rate of endometriomas after laparoscopic surgery and found a recurrence rate between 11.0% and 30.4% after 2 or more years of observation [26, 54]. As recurrence is among the most significant challenges of endometriosis, reoperation is often considered the best treatment option at present, although the extent and duration of benefits from second-line surgery remain unclear [53]. In the present follow-up, a reoperation rate of 68.1% was noted in 32 of 47 patients with recurrent endometrioma who had ovarian endometriomas initially diagnosed at surgery. These observations agree with those of Cheong et al., but not with the lower reoperation rates reported by other authors [1, 13, 53].

A history of preoperative pain or preoperative dysmenorrhea was shown to be a significant factor associated with higher recurrence rates, which agrees with a study by Renner et al. [44]. Our study found significantly lower recurrence-free intervals for those preoperative complaints. In the present study, larger cyst size (as also reported by Kikuchi et al. and Koga et al.), younger age at surgery, and preoperative cyst rupture appeared to increase the risk for recurrence of ovarian endometrioma [23, 26].

Laparoscopy yielded the best results regarding the efficacy of endometrioma surgery. Efficacy was assessed in terms of uneventful postoperative course and pain reduction. In fact, because of its good tolerance, low morbidity, and low total cost of treatment, laparoscopy with sampling for histologic analysis has become the gold standard for the evaluation of endometriosis patients with persistent complaints [35, 43].

The impact of postoperative hormone therapy on ovarian endometriosis is not yet fully understood. To determine the effect of additional postoperative medical treatment in the present follow-up, patients on hormonal therapy (56.1%) were compared with patients not receiving hormones (43.9%). Our findings were consistent with previous observations that patients do not significantly benefit from additional postoperative hormone therapy (gonadotropin-releasing hormone agonist, oral contraceptive, medroxyprogesterone acetate, or danazol) in terms of reduced risk of disease and pain recurrence [8, 43, 50, 52, 53]. We observed even lower probabilities for a recurrence-free interval based on an average follow-up of 12.9 years in patients receiving hormone therapy versus those who received surgical treatment only. A retrospective study found that previous medical treatment of endometriosis was a significant risk factor (P = .009) for higher recurrence [26]. Yap et al. found a significant improvement in recurrence rates after postoperative hormone therapy, noting also that there were no recorded beneficial effects on pain and pregnancy rates relative to surgery alone [56].

Among the 111 patients who wished to conceive, the postoperative spontaneous pregnancy rate was 54.1%, which corresponds to fertility rates reported by Vercellini et al. and Jones and Sutton [20, 54]. As this study analyzes only the outcomes of total endometrioma excision, we were unable to draw comparisons with other surgical techniques such as fenestration or ablation [3, 18]. This study indicates that additional medical treatment positively impacts the postoperative spontaneous pregnancy rate, which is in line with previous observations [4, 34]. This contrasts with other studies, however, which did not observe a hormonal impact on fertility rates after surgery [12, 29]. Further studies are needed to determine the most effective treatment for ovarian endometrioma.

One limitation of this study is that its study model, a retrospective cohort study, does not provide the same level of evidence or validity as a prospective randomized controlled study. The definition of "recurrence" varies in the literature. Some studies define recurrence as a typical morphologic change depicted in a vaginal sonogram, while others define it as a recurring or worsening subjective perception of pain. Although the general definition of "recurrent endometriosis" remains to be determined, our definition represents a limitation because it is based on a questionnaire.

Biases in this study include differences in surgeons' experience, the low return rate of questionnaires, and developments in the field of hormonal therapy over the period of data collection and observation. (For example, danazol, despite its interesting immunosuppressive effects, has been superseded by drugs with fewer side effects, such as GnRH analogues and progestin-only pills.)

## Adnexal torsion and treatment by laparoscopy

### *Background*

The condition is more common in premenarcheal females (children or premenarcheal adolescents), in whom torsion involving previously normal adnexa may constitute up to 15%–50% of adnexal torsion cases. It is difficult to diagnose because, although adnexal torsion may present in the form of acute pelvic pain, the symptoms can sometimes be deceptive. When the lesions are asymptomatic, the diagnosis may be made only during the surgical procedure. Doppler evaluation in cases of ovarian torsion can be a useful tool, but it was found to be normal in 60% of these cases. The absence of Doppler flow was predictive of surgically confirmed cases of ovarian torsion, demonstrating the low sensitivity but high pecificity of Doppler studies in the diagnosis of torsion [57]

In the past, adnexal torsion was treated by salpingo-oophorectomy without untwisting the adnexa to avoid potential thromboembolism from ovarian vein thrombosis. However, a significant association between thromboembolism and untwisting an ischemic pedicle has never been established. Recently, a review of literature concluded that the risk of pulmonary embolism after adnexal torsion was 0.2% and was not increased when the adnexa was untwisted. Over 400 cases managed with untwisting the adnexa have been reported, with no embolic phenomena.

The conservative management of torsion with untwisting (detorsion) of the FT and ovary has proved to be safe and effective in multiple case series in the late 1980s and early 1990s. This type of management, first proposed by Way in 1946, is highly desirable since torsion occurs most often in women of reproductive age, and ovarian conservation is preferable in this age group.

Progress made in operative laparoscopy now suggests that treatment of adnexal torsion can be carried out laparoscopically, which is the procedure of choice. Laparoscopic management of adnexal torsion has been shown to be feasible and preferable to laparotomy. The advantages of laparoscopy include short hospital stay and recovery time, in addition to the fact that conservative procedures, such as detorsion and ovarian cystectomy, can be done laparoscopically.

### *Material and results*

The laparoscopic management of 33 patients with adnexal torsion was retrospectively evaluated over an 11-year period. All patients underwent a clinical examination, ultrasound scanning, routine blood count, electrolyte analysis, urine analysis, and coagulation profile. In patients diagnosed to have an adnexal cyst, tumormarkers, namely CA125 and CEA, were measured. Other imaging techniques, such as MRI, were done in selected cases according to sonographic findings. Presence of any predisposing factors such as adhesions, neoplasm, and pregnancy were noted.

Data regarding patient's demographics, intraoperative findings, and the operation performed were obtained from the clinical records. Cases were included in the analysis only if there was evidence of torsion of the ovary, FT, or entire adnexa at the time of definitive surgical evaluation. The final pathological diagnosis was also documented.

The mean age of the 33 patients treated for adnexal torsion was 34.9 years (range 14–68 years). Of the 33 patients, 4 patients (12%) were in the premenarcheal age group, 23 patients (70%) were in the reproductive age group, and 6 patients (18%) were postmenopausal. Four out of 23 patients in the reproductive age group (17%) were pregnant at the time of the operative intervention. One of them had a singleton pregnancy of 10 weeks' gestation and two patients had triplets (IVF/ICSI cycle) of 7 and 14 weeks' gestation, respectively. Both of them had multiple ovarian cysts because of ovarian hyper-stimulation syndrome (OHSS). One patient had a cornual interstitial ectopic pregnancy of 6 weeks gestation as well as a dermoid cyst on the same side.

All 33 patients had a unilateral torsion. The torsion was more common on the right side (61%, n = 20) than on the left side (39%, n = 13). Fourteen patients (43%) had only an ovarian torsion, 10 patients (30%) only a tubal torsion and 9 patients (27%) had a torsion of the entire adnexa. Multiple predisposing conditions were found in association with torsion. The most common association was adnexal cyst in 24 patients (72%), adhesions in 10 cases (30%), pregnancy in 4 cases (12%), long tube in 3 cases (9%), OHSS in 3 cases (9%), endometriosis in 2 cases (6%), and pelvic inflammatory disease (PID) in only 1 case (3%). More than one predisposing factor exists in some patients. There was no identifiable cause in 10 cases (30%).

The size of the adnexal mass was documented in 26 cases (79%). Measurements were considered accurate only if the specimen was removed intact and measured at pathological examination. The diameter of the cyst ranged from 3 to 15 cm, with a median size of 8 cm. There were nine tumors (35%) which measured less than 5 cm in size and seven tumors (27%) which measured more than 10 cm. The majority of them, 10 tumors (38%), measured between 5 and 10 cm in size.

The categorization of the operations ranged from a conservative procedure, such as laparoscopic detorsion, to an aggressive procedure, such as adnexectomy. There was no conversion to laparotomy. In 17 cases (52%), the adnexa were preserved by performing detorsion. In two cases (6%) detorsion alone was performed, in 13 cases (40%) detorsion and cyst enucleation, and in another two cases (6%) detorsion and cyst aspiration were performed.

Following detorsion, we waited for about 30 minutes, if allowed by the operation conditions, for recovery. Meanwhile the operative field was continuously irrigated with warm saline in order to observe any sign of reperfusion. After torsion, the enlarged and blood-filled tube, ovary, or whole adnexa, with a variable diameter, is usually dark blue to black and partly necrotic. After detorsion, the according organ is left atraumatically to wait for any signs of reperfusion. This is a slight change of color toward the pinkish appearance; however, if reperfusion did not occur, the ovary, tube, or both were resected, and occurred in 16 patients (48%). Unilateral salpingectomy was performed in 5 patients (15%) and unilateral adnexectomy in 11 patients (33%), 6 of them (37%) were postmenopausal. The mean operating time was 69.2 minutes (range 40–120 minutes). No patient had serious complications, such as thromboembolic events, blood transfusion, febrile morbidity, or reoperation. The average duration of stay in the hospital was 2.5 days (range 1–3 days).

The histopathological reports revealed functional or developmental adnexal cyst in 15 cases (45%), dermoid cyst in 4 cases (12%), endometrioma in 2 cases (6%), serous cystadenoma in 3 cases (9%), ovarian fibroma in only 1 case (3%), hydrosalpinx in 3 cases (9%), and normal adnexa in 1 case (3%). All removed tubes and ovaries showed focal necrosis next to hemorrhage in submucosal as well as orthotopic normal ovarian cortical tissue. There was no histopathological specimen in four patients (4%), who underwent adnexal sparing procedures.

### *Evaluation of adnexal torsion*

Despite recent progress with the color Doppler techniques [8], preoperative diagnosis is often difficult, and adnexal torsion can be confused with many other gynecological conditions. The surgical evaluation of these patients should be performed by laparoscopy, thereby avoiding unnecessary laparotomies.

Adnexal torsion is a rare condition which predominantly occurs in the reproductive age group, although it has also been reported in a premenarcheal girl. Unilateral torsion associated with an adnexal mass is seen more commonly, although cases of torsion of normal adnexa have been reported. The mechanism of adnexal torsion is not known conclusively; however, various theories, such as the presence of a long tube, sudden valsalva maneuver, pelvic congestion, and autonomic dysfunction of tubal peristalysis have been suggested [14]. Factors that could possibly influence the occurrence of FT torsion are divided into two types: internal and external. Taken together, the existing reports indicate that the mechanism underlying tubal torsion is apparently a sequential mechanical event.

In our study, the most common predisposing factor was adnexal cyst in 24 patients (72%). Ten patients (30%) had no individual predisposing factors; however, an equal number of patients (30%) had adhesions which may promote torsion. These results correspond with current literature. Four patients (12%) were pregnant. The presence of long tube, OHSS, endometriosis, and PID were all associated with less than 10% of cases.

Adnexal torsion was more common on the right side (61%) than on the left (39%), which may be attributed to the protective effect of the sigmoid colon on the left side and subclinical appendicial infection on the right side, as confirmed, for example, by Nichols. In the present study, we encountered isolated ovarian torsion in 14 (43%), entire adnexal torsion in 9 (27%), and isolated FT torsion in 10 (30%) patients. However, isolated FT torsion has been reported as sporadic cases by many authors.

The most common pathological diagnosis in our series was benign ovarian neoplasm (24%). Half of them were dermoid cyst, functional ovarian cyst (21%), paraovarian and paratubal cyst (24%), endometrioma (6%), hydrosalpinx (9%), and normal adnexa (3%). There was no case of malignancy in our series. Many studies report organic ovarian pathologies to be the most common pathological finding. Altogether, extrinsic and intrinsic causes of tubal torsion exist.

Historically, the treatment of choice for adnexal torsion has been laparotomy and unilateral salpingo-oophrectomy. Although there has been concern about the significant risk of thromboembolic events by detorsion, various reports, starting from as early as 1946 by S. Way, have suggested the safety of ovarian conservation by detorsion. Laparoscopy has been shown to be a favorable option in patients with torsion. There has been a trend toward increased use of laparoscopy and adnexal sparing procedures in many centers because of its obvious benefits regarding safety, reliability, and preserving fertility.

For the whole of our series, we were able to use laparoscopic surgery to treat 100% of cases (33 patients), because there was no suspicion of neoplastic pathology during the diagnostic part of the laparoscopy. Seventeen cases of adnexal torsion (52% of patients) benefited from conservative laparoscopic treatment. These patients underwent detorsion only, with or without cyst aspiration or enucleation. The majority of these were young women desiring fertility. In 48% of cases, detorsion followed by salpingectomy or adnexectomy was performed. More than half of the patients having an adnexectomy were postmenopausal. In the recent literature, the rate of conservative laparoscopic treatment varies from 35% to 93% [57].

Laparoscopy in early pregnancy provides a better chance for successful continuation of pregnancy. In our study, there were four pregnant women at the time of conservative laparoscopic surgery. One of the pregnant women, who underwent laparoscopic detorsion and cyst aspiration during the 10th week of gestation, has an ongoing pregnancy of 30 weeks' gestation. Two women of 7 and 14 weeks gestation, respectively, with triplets after IVF, miscarried at 20 and 22 weeks, respectively, due to cervical incompetence. The last one had an interstitial ectopic pregnancy. Laparoscopy in pregnancy, especially in later pregnancy, is technically difficult owing to the increased risk of perforation and bleeding. Postoperatively, there is an increased risk of miscarriage or preterm delivery

## Tubectomies, oophorectomies/ adnexectomies at necessary hysterectomies beyond the reproductive age

With many indicated hysterectomies at the age beyond 45 years, we have to decide on concomitant adnexectomies, tubectomies, or oophorectomy. As oophorectomy is associated with decreased long-term health outcomes, ovarian conservation should be considered in many woman having pelvic surgery. Adnexectomy or salpingo-oophorectomy may be the procedure of choice for "ovarian/tubal" cancer prophylaxis or after numerous previous surgical interventions on the adnexas. Oophorectomy is indicated for women with an adnexal mass that is suspicious for malignancy or for a mass that increases in size or complexity when monitored with serial sonography. Adnexal torsion can usually be treated with detorsion rather than adnexectomy. Oophorectomy decreases the likelihood of repeat surgery in women with severe symptomatic endometriosis, but ovarian conservation should be considered in those women who are younger than age 40, since conservation avoids early surgical menopause.

Tubectomy or salpingectomy with hysterectomies, however, is considered today as good standard care at hysterectomies for adnexal cancer prevention.

### *Details on tubectomy*

Prophylactic bilateral salpingectomy (PBS) without ovariectomy has been proposed as a new preventive approach to reduce the risk of sporadic neoplasia in women at average risk of OC, without exposing these patients to the adverse effects of iatrogenic premature menopause [57].

Even if opinions vary regarding short- and long-term outcomes of PBS, consistent preliminary data demonstrated its safety, both in terms of ovarian reserve preservation and surgical complication. Moreover, several authors have shown a significant reduction in OC risk among women with previous bilateral salpingectomy compared to tubal preservation or unilateral salpingectomy.

A 2011 position paper by the Society of Gynecologic Oncology of Canada [3] encouraged physicians to discuss the risks and benefits of PBS at the time of hysterectomy or tubal ligation with women at average risk for OC, and this recommendation was confirmed in 2015 by the American College of Obstetricians and Gynecologists.

The advantage of PBS has been estimated also in terms of cost-effectiveness. A recent analysis on PBS (elective salpingectomy at hysterectomy or instead of tubal ligation) showed that salpingectomy with hysterectomy for benign conditions will reduce OC risk at acceptable cost and is a cost-effective alternative to tubal ligation for sterilization.

### *Salpingectomy/permanent contraception*

Surgical sterilization is the most used method worldwide involving 8.1% of the 15- to 49-year-old married women in developed countries and 22.3% of women of reproductive age in less-developed countries

Surgical sterilization is often achieved by resection (i.e., during a Caesarean section) or laparoscopic coagulation of the isthmic portion of the FT. The remnant segment of the transected tube, however, frequently exhibits histological modifications that led to unsuccessful micro-reanastomotic procedures; the most successful contraception, moreover, is recognized to be obtained by total salpingectomy.

For those women (1%–2%) who revise the previous decision for sterilization for any reason, it was demonstrated that the best method to obtain a pregnancy would be IVF, so that bilateral salpingectomy doesn't have any disadvantages in this population of women, while tubal preservation with subsequent tubal disease definitively impair the implantation of transferred embryos.

Hysteroscopic sterilization was recently introduced as an attempt to provide a less invasive but similarly effective alternative to the abdominal approach. Current methodologies, unfortunately, have limitations that make the procedure less promising than expected.

Considering the new theory on Ovarian Cancer (OC) pathogenesis, even if also tubal ligation seems to reduce the risk of Epithelial Ovarian Cancer (EOC) of 33% both in no-BRCA1 and BRCA1 carriers, recent data demonstrated that excisional tubal sterilization confers greater risk reduction (64%) than other methods [19], thus representing the more advisable sterilization procedure to be adopted in the clinical practice.

Bilateral salpingectomy, indeed, would offer to those women requesting for permanent contraception not only the absolute prevention of intrauterine pregnancies and the almost complete elimination of tubal pregnancies, but also protection against EOCs, further providing the chance to assess, along the years, the efficacy of this risk-reducing procedure With increasing reports on adnexal malignancies after the reproductive age the question whether to leave tubes and ovaries inside at hysterectomies became more and more important.

### *Single center study on tubectomies and partly ovarectomies*

Out of 1,014 laparoscopic hysterectomies performed between 2010 and 2018 at the Department of Obstetrics & Gynecology at the University in Kiel, Germany, 378 Subtotal Laparoscopic Hysterectomies (SLHs) and Total Laparoscopic Hysterectomies (TLHs), partially performed by conventional laparoscopic and partially by robotic-assisted laparoscopic surgery, resulted to be in females beyond the age of 50 years.

In the 212 SLHs and 166 TLHs performed in females after the age of 50 years who were premenopausal or after the menopause, all FTs were resected while only in 146 patients' bilateral ovarectomy was also performed.

### *Patients and results*

Neither intraoperatively nor in the consecutive 6 years was any tubal or ovarian malignancy detected at a retrospective evaluation of this patient collective.

#### Salpingectomies

While bilateral tubectomy at hysterectomy is an accepted fact to prevent adenocarcinomas of tubes and ovaries, the question of ovarectomies before the age of 65 is discussable. As ovaries also possess functions other than oestrogen and progesterone production, their resection has to be considered individually in cases of normally looking ovaries. In our 232 patients, the ovaries remained at hysterectomy—all patients had no family history of cancer—and in the whole observation period of six years no genital malignancies occurred.

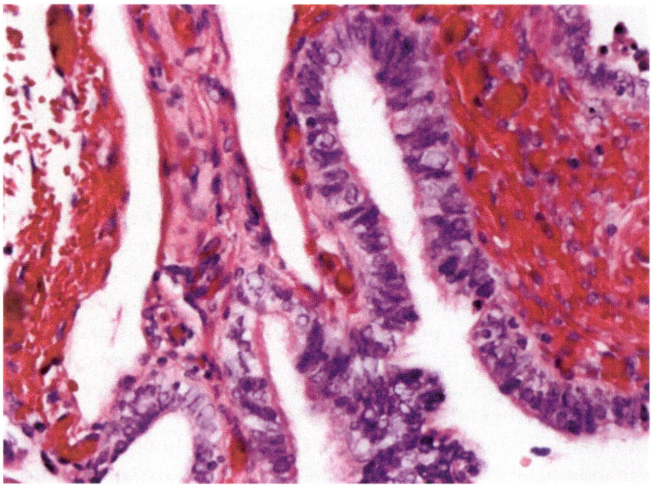

**FIGURE 19.12** Histologic view of a serous tubal intraepithelial cancer (STIC).

Recently, the origin of "EOC" has been questioned. The ovary contains no epithelial cells, and metaplasia of surface mullerian cells to epithelial cells has been hypothesized to explain the types of EOC: serous, mucinous, and endometriod. The origin of EOC in the FTs is subjected at present to many studies and supports the resection of the FTs at hysterectomy as a required medical performance beyond the reproductive age.

The new proposed theory shifts the early events of carcinogenesis to the FT instead of the ovary [20], suggesting that type II tumors derive from the epithelium of the FT, whereas clear cell and endometrioid tumors derive from endometrial tissue that migrate to the ovary by retrograde menstruation [21]. These observations have been mainly collected from women carrying BRCA1/2 mutations and undergoing prophylactic salpingo-oophorectomy, in which most of the incidentally diagnosed in situ carcinomas or serous tubal intraepithelial cancer (STIC) was detected not in the ovary but in the fimbrial end of the FT [22–24, 33] (**Figure 19.12**).

### *Ovariectomies/Adnexectomies*

While together with ovariectomies, both tubes are often also resected, a tubectomy is a must with any indicated ovariectomy in nonmalignant cases [26–27].

In order to prevent the subsequent development of OC, prophylactic ovariectomy was first proposed in the 1970s. This proposal led to approximately 250,000 U.S. females having normal ovaries removed at the time of hysterectomy for benign disease every year in the United States.

However, endocrine studies first performed in the 1970s, and subsequently confirmed, showed that the ovaries continue to produce androgens which are converted to estrone throughout a woman's lifetime.

In 2013, an analysis of the Nurses' Health Study cohort examined health outcomes after 28 years of follow-up for 16,873 (56.3%) women who had a hysterectomy with bilateral oophorectomy for benign disease and 13,113 (43.7%) women who had a hysterectomy with ovarian conservat. Although oophorectomy was associated with a much lower mortality from OC, less than 1% of the women with ovarian conservation died of OC. In contrast, more women who had bilateral oophorectomy died from lung cancer (HR = 1.32), colorectal cancer (HR = 1.56), total cancers (HR = 1.18), and coronary heart disease (HR = 1.26) when compared with women who had ovarian conservation. Importantly, at no age was oophorectomy associated with an increased survival.

Studies from the Mayo Clinic had similar findings; women who had bilateral oophorectomy before age 45 had a 44% increased risk of cardiovascular mortality [28]. Rocca et al. showed higher risks of anxiety/depression, dementia/cognitive impairment, and Parkinsonism in women who had their ovaries removed [29]. In addition, after oophorectomy about 90% of premenopausal women will have vasomotor symptoms and many women will also experience mood changes, a decline in well-being, a decrease in sexual desire, sleep disturbances, and headaches.

Additionally, vaginal dryness, painful intercourse, bladder dysfunction, and symptoms of depression may occur.

In both the NHS and Mayo studies, these detrimental effects on health outcomes were not seen in women who took estrogen following oophorectomy. Therefore, some gynecologists have suggested that oophorectomy be performed at the time of hysterectomy for benign disease and these women be given prescriptions for menopausal hormone therapy and statins to ward off harmful cardiovascular effects. But studies show that within 5 years of a first prescription, only 17% of women continue to take estrogen and fewer than 18% are still taking statins [57].

Recently, the origin of "EOC" has been questioned. Interestingly, the ovary contains no epithelial cells and metaplasia of surface mullerian cells to epithelial cells has been hypothesized to explain the types of EOC: serous, mucinous, and endometriod. With careful pathologic analysis of ovaries and tubes removed from BRCA positive women, precursor lesions called STIC have been found in the FTs, but no such precursor lesions have been found in the ovary. STIC lesions have the same p53 mutations as found in high-grade serous "ovarian" cancers. The more indolent and treatable Stage I low-grade cancers, found rarely inside the ovary, do not have these p53 mutations. Astonishingly, the deadly form of OC does not come from the ovary. Most aggressive "ovarian" cancers are, in fact, tubal cancers.

Bilateral salpingectomy has been proposed as an alternative to oophorectomy, as it removes the source of aggressive cancers but conserves functioning ovaries. Interestingly, a recent study found that women having hysterectomy and salpingectomy had similar sonographically measured antral follicle counts, mean ovarian diameters, and similar blood levels of AMH and FSH. Therefore, it appears that the ovaries function normally after salpingectomy.

### *Adnexal torsion*

As previously discussed in this paper in premenopausal women, detorsion of the adnexa even in apparently severely injured ovaries can be accomplished with good recovery of ovarian follicles and hormonal function. The not infrequent black-blue appearance of a torsed adnexa results from venous and lymphatic stasis, but some blood supply continues from the ovarian or uterine artery. Some studies suggest that time from the onset of pain to detorsion best predicts viability of the ovary. One study found evidence of necrosis on microscopy only after 48 hours following the onset of pelvic pain. Eighteen young women, ages 23–35, undergoing in vitro fertilization and ovarian stimulation, were studied with sonography following detorsion of the adnexa. There was no difference in mean antral follicle counts when the detorsed ovary was compared with the contra-lateral ovary at 6 months following surgery.

Oophorectomy is indicated when the mass is considered suspicious for a neoplastic lesion. Criteria for suspicious lesions include a high initial morphology index, increasing size, or complexity on serial sonography over a 6–12-week time period, or an elevated CA-125 in a postmenopausal woman.

It is well known that most ovarian tumors, even those with morphologic complexity, resolve over time. However, tumors that have an increase in MI over time should be considered for surgical exploration, oophorectomy, frozen section, and surgical staging if malignancy is found.

### Association of oophorectomy to breast and colon cancer

Women with BRCA1 have 40% risk of having OC in their lifetime and BRCA 2 confers a 20% lifetime risk. Women with a BRCA1 mutation have an increased risk of ovarian/tubal cancer as early as age 35, and 2%–3% of these women will develop OC by age 40. The risk of women with the BRCA2 mutation developing ovarian/tubal cancer occurs about one decade later [38]. Women with Lynch Syndrome, especially those with the MSH2 gene, have a lifetime risk of OC of 33% and they also have a 40%–60% risk of developing endometrial cancer.

In a BRCA positive woman, oophorectomy, or more correctly, adnexectomy, reduces the risks of ovarian/tubal cancer to less than 3%. Current recommendations suggest adnexectomy at the completion of child bearing or: for BRCA1, before age 35–40; for BRCA2, before age 50; for Lynch Syndrome, adnexectomy and hysterectomy before age 40.

### Large ovarian masses, endometriosis, and oophorectomy

For women with severe, symptomatic endometriosis unresponsive to conservative management, bilateral oophorectomy concurrent with hysterectomy may decrease recurrent or persistent symptoms and the need for reoperation. One study of women with symptomatic endometriosis compared outcomes between women who had a hysterectomy with ovarian conservation and women who had hysterectomy with concurrent bilateral oophorectomy. In the women who had ovarian conservation, 18/29 (62%) had recurrent pain and 9/29 (31%) required reoperation. In the group of women who had both ovaries removed, 11/109 (10%) had recurrent pain and 4/109 (4%) required reoperation.

Another study of women with endometriosis found that of the 47 women who had a hysterectomy with ovarian conservation, 9 (19%) required further surgery over the 7 years of follow-up [42]. Of the 50 women who had hysterectomy with bilateral oophorectomy, only 4 (8%) required reoperation. Preservation of both ovaries doubled the risk of reoperation regardless of the patient's age. Nevertheless, given the problems associated with early menopause, the authors recommended that for women younger than 40 years, hysterectomy with ovarian conservation should be considered. In patients with endometriosis and ovarian cysts (**Figure 19.2**), partial ovarian resection or ovarectomy depends on symptoms as abdominal pain, dysmenorrhea, and dyspareunia as well as on the stage of endometriosis. Beyond the reproductive age, an adnexectomy may be preferable.

Some women may be symptomatic from larger cysts, or they may not be comfortable with or available for close follow-up. For these women, surgery may be indicated. There is some evidence for removal of endometriomas that ovarian function decreases after removal of cysts > 4 cm when compared with cystectomy for cysts smaller than 4 cm. However, a review of the literature found no studies showing loss of ovarian function related to the size of cyst removed. It may be prudent to conserve ovarian tissue even in large cysts clearly thought to be benign [57].

## Summary

### Endometriomas

Endometriosis cysts of the ovary occur in up to 44% of all endometriosis patients. Half of those patients suffer from bilateral endometriomas. Surgical treatments, which usually involve enucleating (stripping) or coagulating the cyst, have become the first-line option because it has been shown that the complete removal of endometriosis is most effective in alleviating symptoms and improving pregnancy rates. Apart from endometriosis-related symptoms, endometriosis cysts may impair fertility. However, the removal of endometriosis cysts is a controversial issue, as other studies have shown that any kind of manipulation may worsen the outcome of fertility treatment by decreasing the ovarian reserve. Translational research has revealed that endometriosis is associated with endometriod, clear-cell, and low-grade serous OC. However, ovarian endometriosis is frequently removed upon identification of symptoms together with unwanted childlessness. This chapter provides an introduction to the controversial debate and explores the indications and techniques of surgical treatment.

### Adnexal torsion

Conservative treatment should be considered in women within the reproductive age still desiring fertility. Only beyond the reproductive age should adnexectomy at all be considered and really only in cases with extreme pathology on the adnexa. Difinitlyl laparoscopy is the primary therapeutic option in patients with adnexal torsion.

### Tubectomies, oophorectomies, and adnectomies

Tubectomy and oophorectomy at the time of hysterectomies are being reconsidered. While oophorectomy decreases definitely, in the long-term health outcome of females the ovarian conservation is advised till the age of 65 years. Adnexal torsion can usually be treated better by detorsion than by adnexectomy. However, in cases of endometriosidoes decrease necessary repeat surgeries.

Bilateral tubectomy should be performed in cases of hysterectomy at any age, carefully and not compromising the vascular supply of the ovaries. In addition, tubectomy definitely serves for permanent contraception. Living in the time of successful uterine transplantations, even tubectomy might be reconsidered in a different way in the medical literature.

## References

1. Abbott JA, Hawe J, Clayton RD, Garry R. The effects and effectiveness of laparoscopic excision of endometriosis: a prospective study with 2-5 year follow-up. Hum Reprod 2003;18(9):1922–7.
2. Ahmad G, O'Flynn H, Hindocha A, Watson A. Barrier agents for adhesion prevention after gynaecological surgery. Cochrane Database Syst Rev 2015;4:CD000475. doi:10.1002/14651858.CD000475.pub3.
3. Alborzi S, Momtahan M, Parsanezhad ME, Dehbashi S, Zolghadri J. A prospective, randomized study comparing laparoscopic ovarian cystectomy versus fenestration and coagulation in patients with endometriomas. Fertil Steril 2004;82(6):1633–7. doi:10.1016/j.fertnstert.2004.04.067.
4. Alkatout I, Mettler L, Beteta C, Hedderich J, Jonat W, Schollmeyer T et al. Combined surgical and hormone therapy for endometriosis is the most effective treatment: prospective, randomized, controlled trial. J Minim Invasive Gynecol 2013;20(4):473–81. doi:10.1016/j.jmig.2013.01.019.
5. Barri PN, Coroleu B, Tur R, Barri-Soldevila PN, Rodriguez I. Endometriosis-associated infertility: surgery and IVF, a comprehensive therapeutic approach. Reprod Biomed Online 2010;21(2):179–85. doi:10.1016/j.rbmo.2010.04.026.

6. Benaglia L, Somigliana E, Vercellini P, Abbiati A, Ragni G, Fedele L. Endometriotic ovarian cysts negatively affect the rate of spontaneous ovulation. Hum Reprod 2009;24(9):2183–6. doi:10.1093/humrep/dep202.
7. Benschop L, Farquhar C, van der Poel N, Heineman MJ. Interventions for women with endometrioma prior to assisted reproductive technology. Cochrane Database Syst Rev 2010(11):CD008571. doi:10.1002/14651858.CD008571.pub2.
8. Bianchi S, Busacca M, Agnoli B, Candiani M, Calia C, Vignali M. Effects of 3 month therapy with danazol after laparoscopic surgery for stage III/IV endometriosis: a randomized study. Hum Reprod 1999;14(5):1335–7.
9. Brosens IA, Puttemans PJ, Deprest J. The endoscopic localization of endometrial implants in the ovarian chocolate cyst. Fertil Steril 1994;61(6):1034–8.
10. Brown J, Farquhar C. Endometriosis: an overview of Cochrane Reviews. Cochrane Database Syst Rev 2014;3:CD009590. doi:10.1002/14651858.CD009590.pub2.
11. Busacca M, Marana R, Caruana P, Candiani M, Muzii L, Calia C et al. Recurrence of ovarian endometrioma after laparoscopic excision. Am J Obstet Gynecol 1999;180(3 Pt 1):519–23.
12. Busacca M, Somigliana E, Bianchi S, Marinis S de, Calia C, Candiani M et al. Postoperative GnRH analogue treatment after conservative surgery for symptomatic endometriosis stage III-IV: a randomized controlled trial. Hum Reprod 2001;16(11):2399–402.
13. Cheong Y, Tay P, Luk F, Gan HC, Li TC, Cooke I. Laparoscopic surgery for endometriosis: How often do we need to re-operate? J Obstet Gynaecol 2008;28(1):82–5. doi:10.1080/01443610701811761.
14. Donnez J, Nisolle M, Gillet N, Smets M, Bassil S, Casanas-Roux F. Large ovarian endometriomas. Hum Reprod 1996;11(3):641–6.
15. Dunselman GA, Vermeulen N, Becker C, Calhaz-Jorge C, D'Hooghe T, Bie B de et al. ESHRE guideline: management of women with endometriosis. Hum Reprod 2014;29(3):400–12. doi:10.1093/humrep/det457.
16. Fauconnier A, Chapron C, Dubuisson JB, Vieira M, Dousset B, Breart G. Relation between pain symptoms and the anatomic location of deep-infiltrating endometriosis. Fertil Steril 2002;78(4):719–26.
17. Forte A, Cipollaro M, Galderisi U. Genetic, epigenetic and stem cell alterations in endometriosis: new insights and potential therapeutic perspectives. Clin Sci (Lond) 2014;126(2):123–38. doi:10.1042/CS20130099.
18. Hart RJ, Hickey M, Maouris P, Buckett W. Excisional surgery versus ablative surgery for ovarian endometriomata. Cochrane Database Syst Rev 2008(2):CD004992. doi:10.1002/14651858.CD004992.pub3.
19. Hughesdon PE. The structure of endometrial cysts of the ovary. J Obstet Gynaecol Br Emp 1957;64(4):481–7.
20. Jones KD, Sutton CJ. Pregnancy rates following ablative laparoscopic surgery for endometriomas. Hum Reprod 2002;17(3):782–5.
21. Kaya H, Sezik M, Ozkaya O, Sahiner H, Ozbasar D. Does the diameter of an endometrioma predict the extent of pelvic adhesions associated with endometriosis? J Reprod Med 2005;50(3):198–202.
22. Keyhan S, Hughes C, Price T, Muasher S. An update on surgical versus expectant management of ovarian endometriomas in infertile women. Biomed Res Int 2015;2015:204792. doi:10.1155/2015/204792.
23. Kikuchi I, Takeuchi H, Kitade M, Shimanuki H, Kumakiri J, Kinoshita K. Recurrence rate of endometriomas following a laparoscopic cystectomy. Acta Obstet Gynecol Scand 2006;85(9):1120–4. doi:10.1080/00016340600627154.
24. Kim ML, Kim JM, Seong SJ, Lee SY, Han M, Cho YJ. Recurrence of ovarian endometrioma after second-line, conservative, laparoscopic cyst enucleation. Am J Obstet Gynecol 2014;210(3):216.e1–6. doi:10.1016/j.ajog.2013.11.007.
25. Kitajima M, Dolmans MM, Donnez O, Masuzaki H, Soares M, Donnez J. Enhanced follicular recruitment and atresia in cortex derived from ovaries with endometriomas. Fertil Steril 2014;101(4):1031–7. doi:10.1016/j.fertnstert.2013.12.049.
26. Koga K, Takemura Y, Osuga Y, Yoshino O, Hirota Y, Hirata T et al. Recurrence of ovarian endometrioma after laparoscopic excision. Hum Reprod 2006;21(8):2171–4. doi:10.1093/humrep/del125.
27. Kurman RJ (ed.). WHO classification of tumours of female reproductive organs. 4th ed. Lyon: Internat. Agency for Research on Cancer; 2014. (ISBN No. 978-92-832-2435-8).
28. La Brinton, Sakoda LC, Sherman ME, Frederiksen K, Kjaer SK, Graubard BI, et al. Relationship of benign gynecologic diseases to subsequent risk of ovarian and uterine tumors. Cancer Epidemiol Biomarkers Prev 2005;14(12):2929–35. doi:10.1158/1055-9965.EPI-05-0394.
29. Loverro G, Carriero C, Rossi AC, Putignano G, Nicolardi V, Selvaggi L. A randomized study comparing triptorelin or expectant management following conservative laparoscopic surgery for symptomatic stage III-IV endometriosis. Eur J Obstet Gynecol Reprod Biol 2008;136(2):194–8. doi:10.1016/j.ejogrb.2006.10.034.
30. Maneschi F, Marasa L, Incandela S, Mazzarese M, Zupi E. Ovarian cortex surrounding benign neoplasms: a histologic study. Am J Obstet Gynecol 1993;169(2 Pt 1):388–93.
31. Matsuzaki S, Houlle C, Darcha C, Pouly JL, Mage G, Canis M. Analysis of risk factors for the removal of normal ovarian tissue during laparoscopic cystectomy for ovarian endometriosis. Hum Reprod 2009;24(6):1402–6. doi:10.1093/humrep/dep043.
32. Maul LV, Morrision JE, Schollmeyer T, Alkatout I, Mettler L. Surgical therapy of ovarian endometrioma: recurrence and pregnancy rates. JSLS 2014;18(3). doi:10.4293/JSLS.2014.00223.
33. Meinhold-Heerlein I, Fotopoulou C, Harter P, Kurzeder C, Mustea A, Wimberger P, et al. Statement by the Kommission Ovar of the AGO: The New FIGO and WHO Classifications of Ovarian, Fallopian Tube and Primary Peritoneal Cancer. Geburtshilfe Frauenheilkd 2015;75(10):1021–7. doi:10.1055/s-0035-1558079.
34. Mettler L. Pathogenesis, diagnosis and treatment of genital endometriosis. Acta Obstet Gynecol Scand Suppl 1989;150:31–7.
35. Mettler L, Schollmeyer T, Lehmann-Willenbrock E, Schuppler U, Schmutzler A, Shukla D et al. Accuracy of laparoscopic diagnosis of endometriosis. JSLS 2003;7(1):15–8.
36. Muzii L, Achilli C, Bergamini V, Candiani M, Garavaglia E, Lazzeri L et al. Comparison between the stripping technique and the combined excisional/ablative technique for the treatment of bilateral ovarian endometriomas: a multicentre RCT. Hum Reprod 2016;31(2):339–44. doi:10.1093/humrep/dev313.
37. Nezhat F, Nezhat C, Allan CJ, Metzger DA, Sears DL. Clinical and histologic classification of endometriomas. Implications for a mechanism of pathogenesis. J Reprod Med 1992;37(9):771–6.
38. Nisolle M, Donnez J. Peritoneal endometriosis, ovarian endometriosis, and adenomyotic nodules of the rectovaginal septum are three different entities. Fertil Steril 1997;68(4):585–96.
39. Park H, Kim CH, Kim EY, Moon JW, Kim SH, Chae HD, et al. Effect of second-line surgery on in vitro fertilization outcome in infertile women with ovarian endometrioma recurrence after primary conservative surgery for moderate to severe endometriosis. Obstet Gynecol Sci 2015;58(6):481–6. doi:10.5468/ogs.2015.58.6.481.
40. Pavone ME, Lyttle BM. Endometriosis and ovarian cancer: links, risks, and challenges faced. Int J Womens Health 2015;7:663–72. doi:10.2147/IJWH.S66824.
41. Pearce CL, Templeman C, Rossing MA, Lee A, Am Near, Webb PM, et al. Association between endometriosis and risk of histological subtypes of ovarian cancer: a pooled analysis of case-control studies. Lancet Oncol 2012;13(4):385–94. doi:10.1016/S1470-2045(11)70404-1.
42. Perlman S, Kjer JJ. Ovarian damage due to cyst removal: a comparison of endometriomas and dermoid cysts. Acta Obstet Gynecol Scand 2016;95(3):285–90. doi:10.1111/aogs.12841.
43. Porpora MG, Pallante D, Ferro A, Crisafi B, Bellati F, Benedetti PP. Pain and ovarian endometrioma recurrence after laparoscopic treatment of endometriosis: a long-term prospective study. Fertil Steril 2010;93(3):716–21. doi:10.1016/j.fertnstert.2008.10.018.
44. Renner SP, Rix S, Boosz A, Lermann JH, Strissel PL, Thiel FC, et al. Preoperative pain and recurrence risk in patients with peritoneal endometriosis. Gynecol Endocrinol 2010;26(3):230–5. doi:10.1080/09513590903159623.

45. Rossing MA, Cushing-Haugen KL, Wicklund KG, Doherty JA, Weiss NS. Risk of epithelial ovarian cancer in relation to benign ovarian conditions and ovarian surgery. Cancer Causes Control 2008;19(10):1357–64. doi:10.1007/s10552-008-9207-9.
46. Sainz de la Cuesta R, Eichhorn JH, Rice LW, Fuller AF JR, Nikrui N, Goff BA. Histologic transformation of benign endometriosis to early epithelial ovarian cancer. Gynecol Oncol 1996;60(2):238–44.
47. Sanchez AM, Papaleo E, Corti L, Santambrogio P, Levi S, Vigano P, et al. Iron availability is increased in individual human ovarian follicles in close proximity to an endometrioma compared with distal ones. Hum Reprod 2014;29(3):577–83. doi:10.1093/humrep/det466.
48. Sanchez AM, Vigano P, Somigliana E, Panina-Bordignon P, Vercellini P, Candiani M. The distinguishing cellular and molecular features of the endometriotic ovarian cyst: from pathophysiology to the potential endometrioma-mediated damage to the ovary. Hum Reprod Update 2014;20(2):217–30. doi:10.1093/humupd/dmt053.
49. Schmidt D, Ulrich U. Endometriosis-related ovarian tumors. Pathologe 2014;35(4):348–54. doi:10.1007/s00292-014-1949-4.
50. Sesti F, Capozzolo T, Pietropolli A, Marziali M, Bollea, Piccione E. Recurrence rate of endometrioma after laparoscopic cystectomy: a comparative randomized trial between postoperative hormonal suppression treatment or dietary therapy vs. placebo. Eur J Obstet Gynecol Reprod Biol 2009;147(1):72–7. doi:10.1016/j.ejogrb.2009.07.003.
51. Seyhan A, Ata B, Uncu G. The impact of endometriosis and its treatment on ovarian reserve. Semin Reprod Med 2015;33(6):422–8. doi:10.1055/s-0035-1567820.
52. Tsai YL, Hwang JL, Loo TC, Cheng WC, Chuang J, Seow KM. Short-term postoperative GnRH analogue or danazol treatment after conservative surgery for stage III or IV endometriosis before ovarian stimulation: a prospective, randomized study. J Reprod Med 2004;49(12):955–9.
53. Vercellini P, Barbara G, Abbiati A, Somigliana E, Vigano P, Fedele L. Repetitive surgery for recurrent symptomatic endometriosis: what to do? Eur J Obstet Gynecol Reprod Biol 2009;146(1):15–21. doi:10.1016/j.ejogrb.2009.05.007.
54. Vercellini P, Fedele L, Aimi G, Giorgi O de, Consonni D, Crosignani PG. Reproductive performance, pain recurrence and disease relapse after conservative surgical treatment for endometriosis: the predictive value of the current classification system. Hum Reprod 2006;21(10):2679–85. doi:10.1093/humrep/del230.
55. Vercellini P, Vigano P, Somigliana E, Fedele L. Endometriosis: pathogenesis and treatment. Nat Rev Endocrinol 2014;10(5):261–75. doi:10.1038/nrendo.2013.255.
56. Yap C, Furness S, Farquhar C. Pre and post operative medical therapy for endometriosis surgery. Cochrane Database Syst Rev 2004(3):CD003678. doi:10.1002/14651858.CD003678.pub2.
57. Alkatout I, Mettler L. Practical Manual for Laparoscopic and Hysteroscopic. Surgery 3rd edition. 2019; Jaypee Brothers Medical Publishers, New Delhi, London, Panama, 798 pages.

# 20

## SUBTLE FALLOPIAN TUBE PATHOLOGY

### *Diagnosis and Surgical Treatment*

**Rubin Raju, Omar M. Abuzeid, and Mostafa I. Abuzeid**

## Introduction

The fallopian tubes, also known as the oviducts, are embryologic derivatives of the paramesonephric ducts. The paramesonephric ducts develop from the coelomic epithelium during the 5th and 6th week of development [1]. The fallopian tubes arise from the cranial portion of the paramesonephric ducts, with the cranial openings of the paramesonephric ducts into the coelomic cavity forming the fimbrial ends of the fallopian tubes, and the caudal portions fusing to for the uterovaginal canal [2, 3]. In the absence of the Müllerian inhibitory substance, a glycoprotein secreted by the Sertoli cells in the developing testes, the paramesonephric ducts develop into the fallopian tubes, uterus, and upper two-third of the vaginal canal. The formation of the paramesonephric ducts is dependent on *Wnt* signaling, which is involved in maintaining the expression of a sequence of *Hox* family of homeobox genes spread out through the female genital tract. The Hoxa-9 genes are expressed in the fallopian tubes [2]. Initially, at around 8 weeks, the tubes are narrow with a circular tubular epithelium. As gestation progresses, the mucosa becomes highly folded, especially in the infundibular and ampullary regions. The mesenchymal tissue around the epithelium differentiates into a stromal layer and a smooth muscular layer called the muscularis [3].

The fallopian tube is divided into four anatomical segments: intramural, isthmus, ampulla, and infundibulum. The fallopian tubes play an essential role in sperm transport, oocyte capture and transport, fertilization, and early embryo development. Therefore, the normal functioning of the fallopian tube is crucial for spontaneous human fertility [4]. The fimbriae help with ovum pickup during ovulation and transport of the ovum into the ampullary region of the fallopian tube, where fertilization with the sperm takes place. The cilia and smooth muscle of the fallopian tube then aids with the transport of the embryo into the uterus, where implantation normally takes place. It is not surprising that subtle variations in tubal anatomy may impact the fertility potential.

The aim of this chapter is to discuss the various congenital tubal and para-tubal pathology, its consequences, diagnosis, and surgical treatment. The second purpose of this chapter is to review the association between early stage of endometriosis and subtle fimbrial pathology. The various types of such pathology, their diagnosis, surgical management, and the reproductive outcome after laparoscopic correction are also discussed.

## Congenital tubal and para-tubal pathology

Congenital disorders of the fallopian tube include aplasia, hypoplasia, para-tubal cysts, congenital accessory tubal ostia, accessory fallopian tubes, congenital tubal diverticula, and congenital hydrosalpinx [1]. *Aplasia/hypoplasia of the fallopian tubes* results in total absence of the fallopian tube as a result of failure of development of the cranial portion of the paramesonephric ducts (Müllerian ducts), and can be associated with other congenital Müllerian anomalies and ovarian agenesis (**Figure 20.1**) [5, 6]. The exact incidence of aplasia or hypoplasia of the fallopian tube is unknown. Congenital absence of the fimbria and part of the distal portion of the fallopian tube has been associated with *congenital hydrosalpinx* (**Figure 20.2a–d**) [7]. *Congenital absence of other parts of the fallopian tube* can also occur [8]. In such cases, the proximal segment of the isthmic portion of the fallopian tube near the cornual region may be absent (**Figure 20.3a,b**). In other cases, other parts of the fallopian tube may be absent (**Figure 20.4**).

*Para-tubal cysts*, also known as Hydatid cysts of Morgagni, are remnants of paramesonephric (Müllerian) or mesonephric (Wolffian) ducts [9–11]. They represent 4.7%–20% of all adnexal masses in women [12]. It is not uncommon to have normal cysts around 5 mm in diameter to be attached to the fimbrial end of the fallopian tubes called appendix vesiculosa. These are sometimes referred to as Hydatid cysts of Morgagni by some authors, whereas other authors refer to only the larger cysts as Hydatid cysts of Morgagni (**Figure 20.5**) [1]. In addition, Hydatid cysts of Morgagni can be pedunculated (**Figure 20.6a,b**) or sessile in nature (**Figure 20.7a,b**). Furthermore, Hydatid cysts of Morgagni can be multiple in nature (**Figure 20.8**). *Congenital accessory tubal ostia* are normal variants of fallopian tube with an ectopic fimbrial opening at a distance from the normal fallopian tube fimbrial opening (**Figure 20.9**) [13]. They are often missed during laparoscopy. The prevalence of accessory tubal ostia is thought to be between 1.9% and 10% [14]. They are thought to occur from bifurcation of the distal end of the Müllerian ducts [13]. *Accessory fallopian tubes* are also congenital in origin. They are nonpatent cylindrical structures attached to the ampullary part of a normal fallopian tube. The prevalence of accessory fallopian tubes is thought to be around 4%–10%, and is often missed by surgeons [15]. *Congenital tubal diverticula* are rare (**Figure 20.10**). It was first described by Troell S in 1970 as a thin-walled pouch, with the wall made of the three layers of the fallopian tube (i.e., serosa,

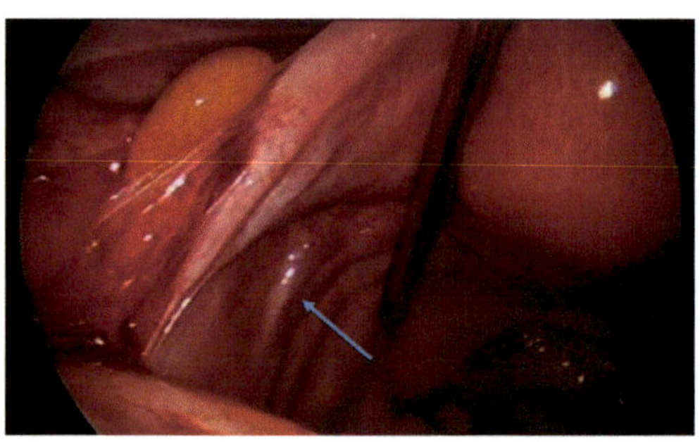

**FIGURE 20.1** Aplasia of the left ovary and partial aplasia of the distal two-thirds of the left fallopian tube (blue arrow).

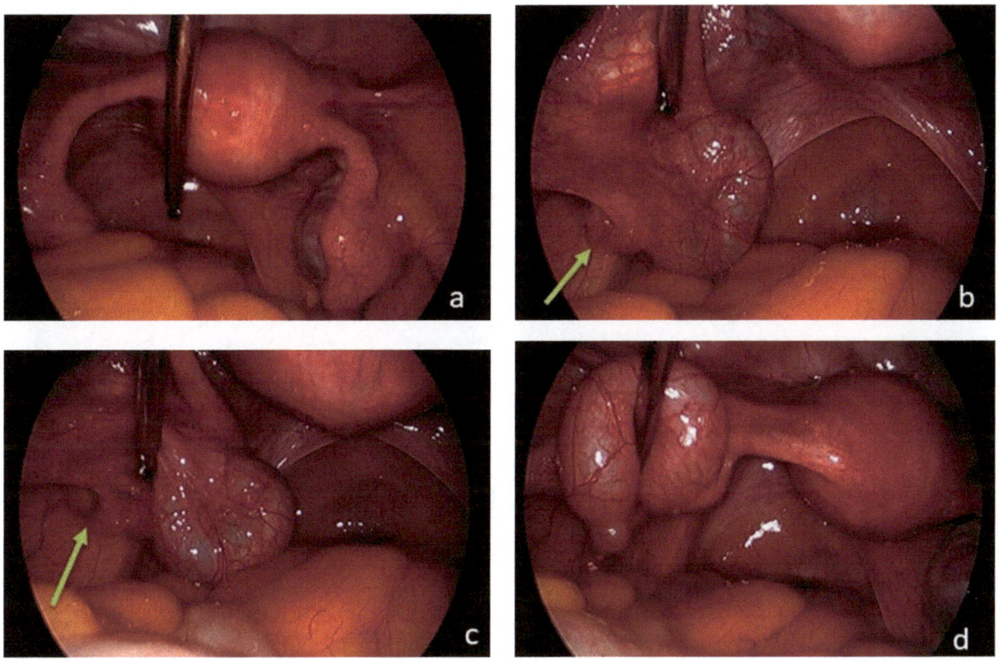


FIGURE 20.2 (a–d) Left congenital hydrosalpinx. A small noncommunicating rudimentary fimbria is seen in (b) and (c) (green arrow).

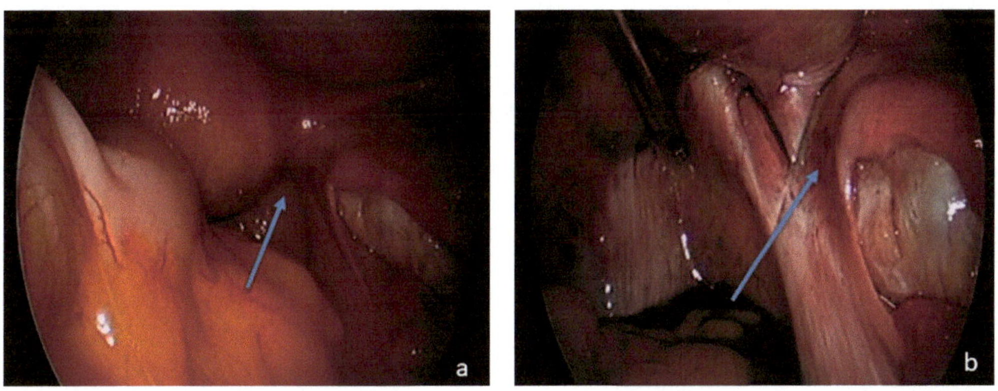


FIGURE 20.3 (a) Congenital absence of the proximal segment of the isthmic portion of the left tube (blue arrow); (b) in close-up.

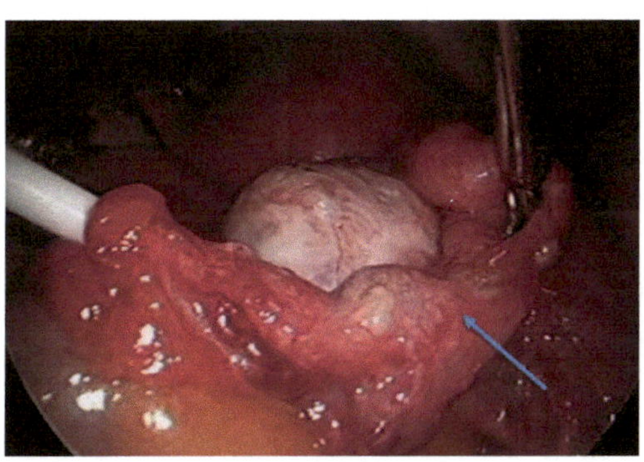

FIGURE 20.4 Congenital absence of the mid-segment of the ampullary portion of the right fallopian rube (blue arrow).

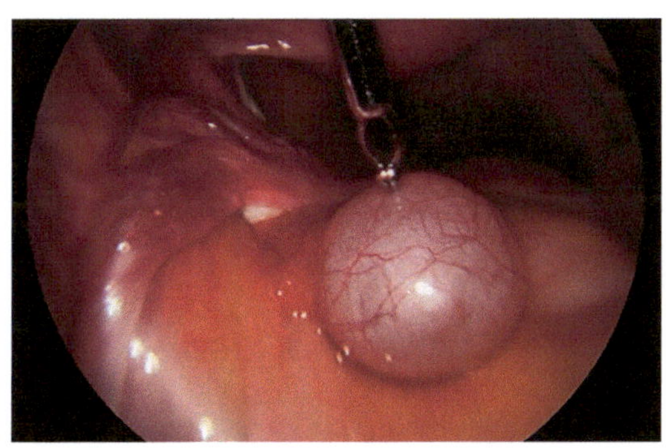

FIGURE 20.5 A large pedunculated hydratid cyst of Morgagni.

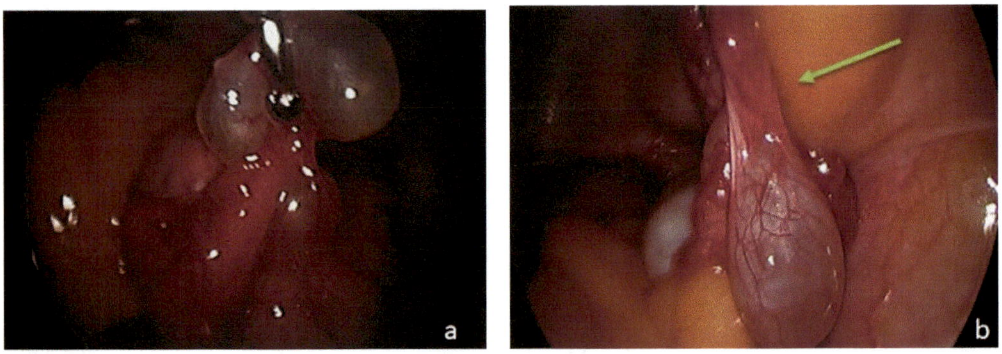


**FIGURE 20.6** (a) A small pedunculated hydratid cyst of Morgagni; (b) a large pedunculated hydratid cyst of Morgagni with a wide pedicle (green arrow).

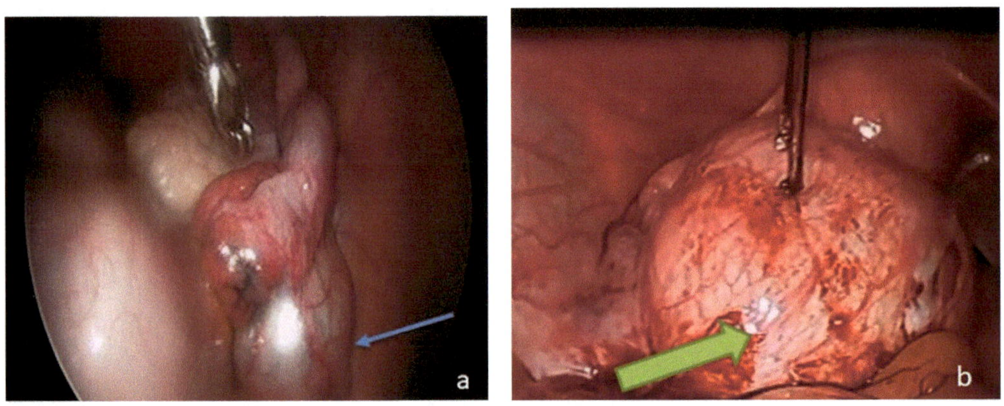


**FIGURE 20.7** (a) A large sessile (blue arrow); (b) a very large (8 cm) sessile hydratid cyst of Morgagni (green arrow).

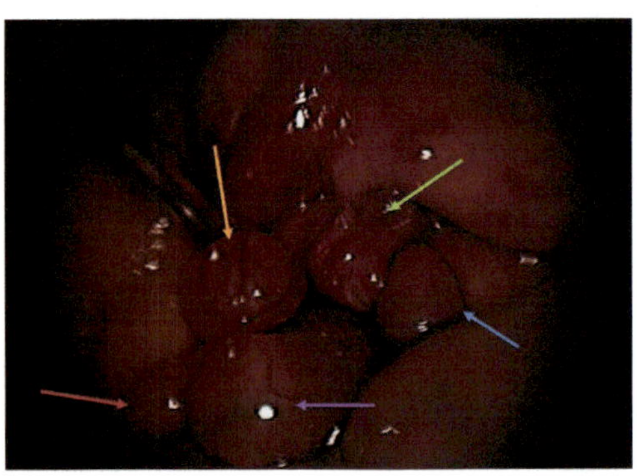

**FIGURE 20.8** Multiple small cysts of Morgagni (arrows).

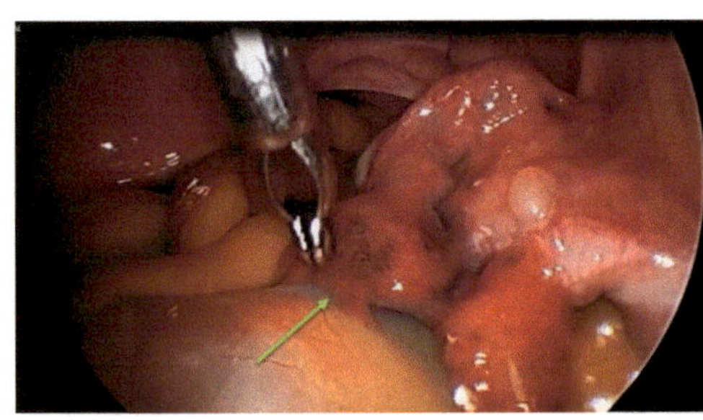

**FIGURE 20.9** A right accessory tubal ostium about 1.5 cm from the fimbria (green arrow).

muscularis, and mucosal layers) [16]. However, the term *congenital tubal sacculation*, or tubal hernia, was used to describe a sort of ampullary hernia, which is different from tubal diverticulum in the fact that it is characterized by muscularis hypoplasia. The authors of this chapter believe that based on appearance at the time of laparoscopy, it is difficult to differentiate between the two pathologies clinically. Therefore, in this chapter, the term tubal diverticulum will be used to describe any thin-walled pouch on the surface of the fallopian tube seen at the time of laparoscopy. In turn, the tubal diverticulum we are describing in this chapter could actually be a tubal sacculation. Tubal diverticula can be large (**Figure 20.11a–d**), and occasionally they can be located away from the fimbria (**Figure 20.12a–c**).

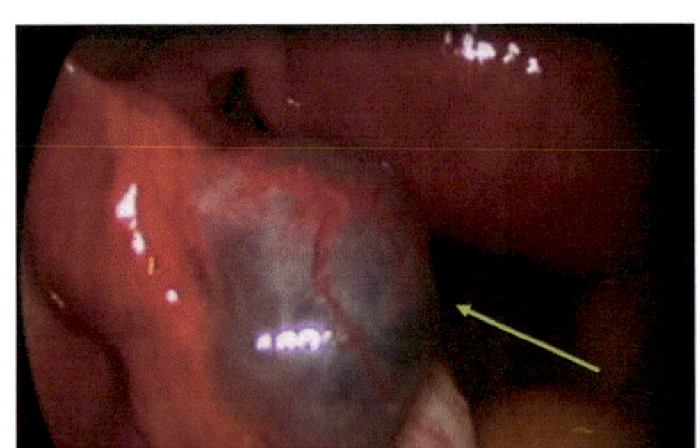

**FIGURE 20.10** A right congenital tubal diverticulum very near to the fimbria (green arrow).

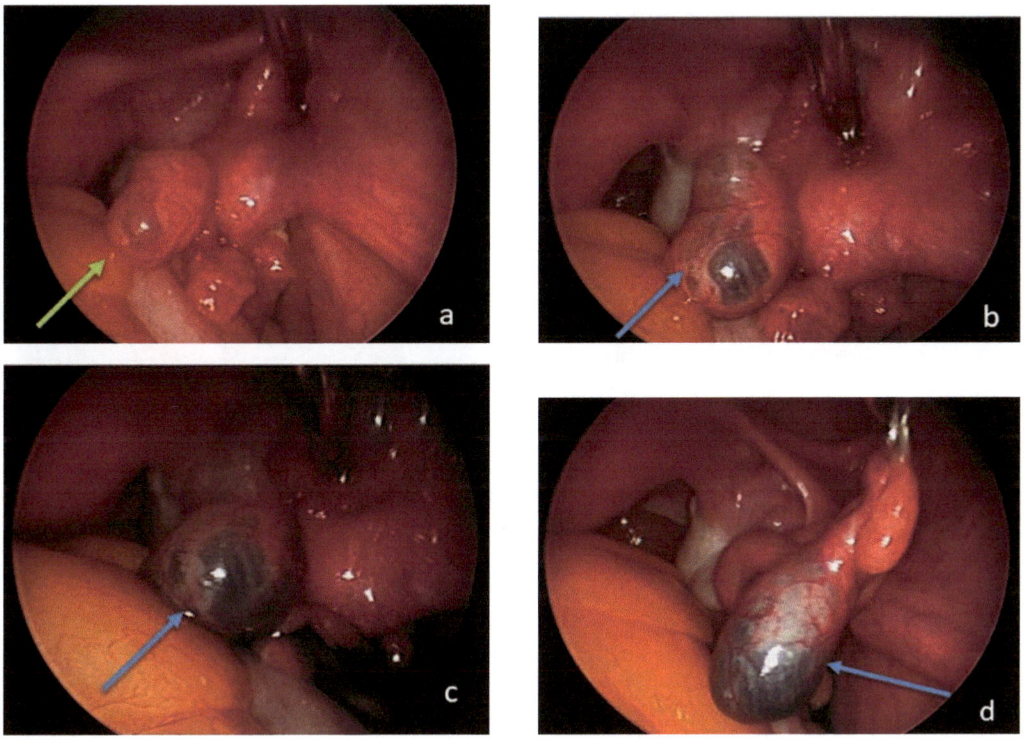


FIGURE 20.11 A large tubal diverticulum near to the fimbria; (a) there is a very thin serosal wall (green arrow); (b, c, d) distension of the tubal diverticulum during tubal perfusion (blue arrows).

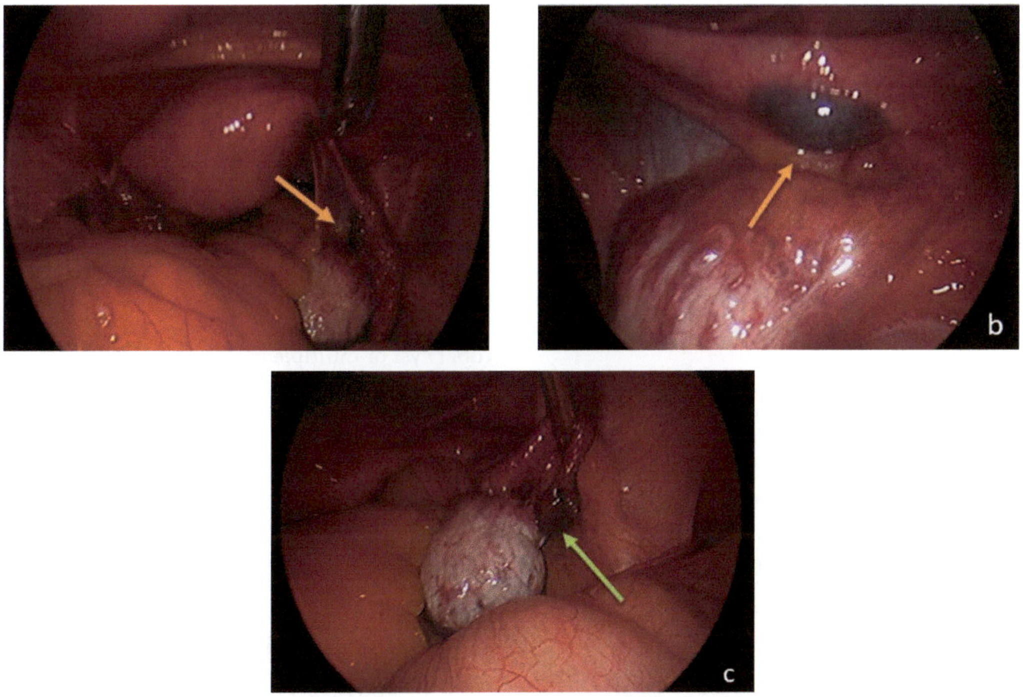


FIGURE 20.12 (a) A small right tubal diverticulum in a rare location (mid-portion of the tube near the mesosalpinx) away from the fimbria (orange arrow) during tubal perfusion; (b) close-up of the small diverticulum (orange arrow); (c) tubal patency in the same patient (green arrow).

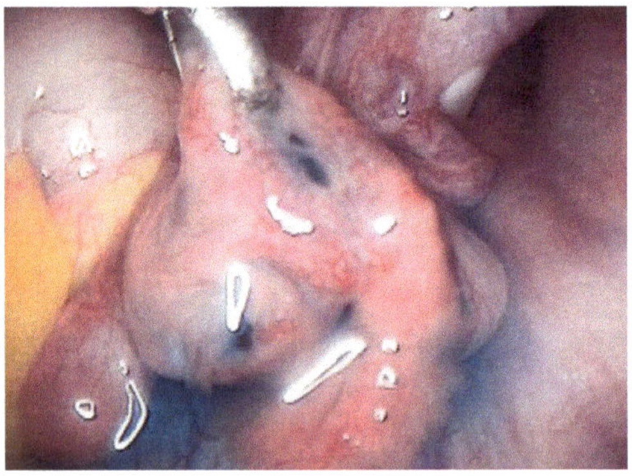

FIGURE 20.13 Fimbrial agglutination with one or more adhesive bridges of fimbria across the ostium. (From Abuzeid MI, et al., 2007 [17]. With permission.)

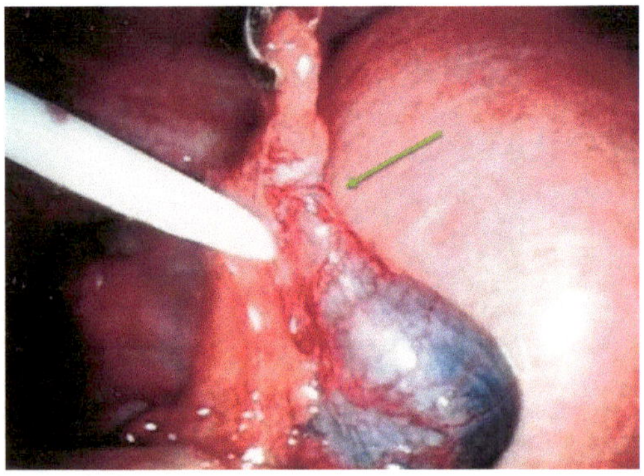

FIGURE 20.15 Fimbrial phimosis with narrowing of the fimbriated end. There is a concentric stricture of the fallopian tube at its distal end noted at the ampullary fimbrial junction (green arrow), leading to ballooning of the distal end of the tube. (From Abuzeid MI, et al., 2007 [17]. With permission.)

## Subtle distal tubal pathology and early endometriosis

Subtle distal tubal pathology has been associated with early stages of endometriosis [17]. Fimbrial end pathology can be divided into: (1) Fimbrial agglutination, (2) Fimbrial blunting, and (3) Fimbrial phimosis. Fimbrial agglutination occurs when fimbriae adhere to each other across the fimbrial ostium (**Figure 20.13**). Fimbrial blunting, however, occurs when adjacent fimbriae adhere to each other in a side to side manner (**Figure 20.14**). Last, when fimbrial adhesions lead to narrowing of the fimbriated end, it is referred to as fimbrial phimosis (**Figures 20.15** and **20.16**) [18].

The presence of fimbrial agglutination, blunting, and phimosis is not always associated with endometriosis. Such pathology can also be seen in infertile women with past history of pelvic inflammatory disease, abdominal or pelvic surgery, appendicitis, and bowel inflammatory diseases. In 2007, our group published the first report on the association between subtle fimbrial pathology and early stages of endometriosis [17]. In this report, we discuss the prevalence of such pathology in early stages of endometriosis and their possible effects on reproductive potential [17]. The data in this report suggest that the incidence of such subtle fimbrial pathology is greater in infertile women with early stage endometriosis than those without endometriosis (**Figure 20.17**) [17].

It is however rare to see complete tubal occlusion in early stages of endometriosis [4]. Apart from these fimbrial pathology, Cohen BM (1980 and 1987) reported that elongated fimbria ovarica (the fimbria that reaches the ovarian surface), with marked displacement of the fimbrial ostium from the surface of the ovary, is commonly seen in early stages of endometriosis as well [11, 19].

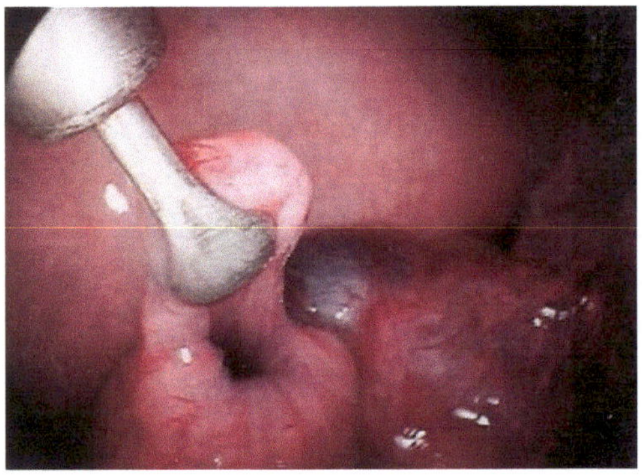

FIGURE 20.14 Fimbrial blunting with fimbrial adherence side by side, giving rise to a mitten rather than a glove appearance of the fimbriated end. (From Abuzeid MI, et al., 2007 [17]. With permission.)

## Clinical presentation and diagnosis

### Clinical presentation

Congenital tubal and para-tubal conditions are often associated with female infertility. Depending upon their severity, they may affect the normal function of the fallopian tube and be one of the causes of infertility. They may also be an incidental finding in workup for other gynecologic conditions. Aplasia/hypoplasia of the fallopian tube is usually an incident finding on laparoscopy or laparotomy, and can be associated with Müllerian anomalies and ovarian agenesis [20]. Congenital hydrosalpinx can present in the pediatric and reproductive age group with symptoms of abdominal or pelvic pain, especially in the presence of torsion of the fallopian tube [21]. Para-tubal cysts are mostly asymptomatic and incidentally found on radiologic studies, such as transvaginal 2D ultrasound scan (TV 2D US) or during laparoscopy/laparotomy [12]. A large para-tubal can sometimes be mistaken for a hydrosalpinx on TV 2D US. They may also be present with pelvic pain or pressure [22]. A solitary large para-tubal cyst or multiple para-tubal cysts can exert a mechanical effect on the ipsilateral fallopian tube and, in turn, cause infertility. In theory, solitary large para-tubal cyst or multiple para-tubal cysts may pull the fimbria down away from the ovary and, in turn, this may reduce ovum pickup

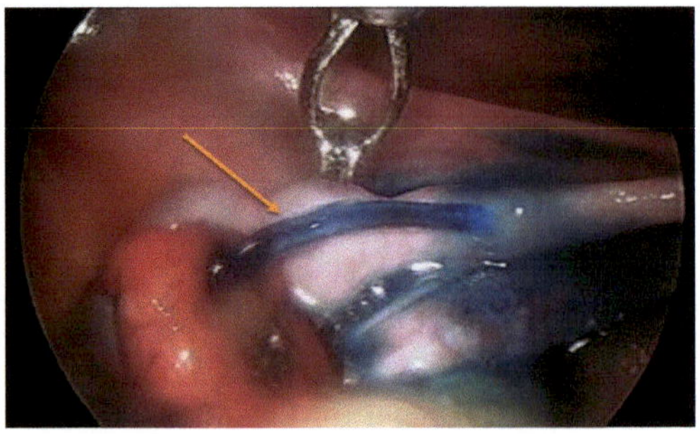

FIGURE 20.16 A unique phenomenon of a narrow stream of blue dye through the fimbria during tubal perfusion, seen in some patient with severe fimbria phimosis (orange arrow).

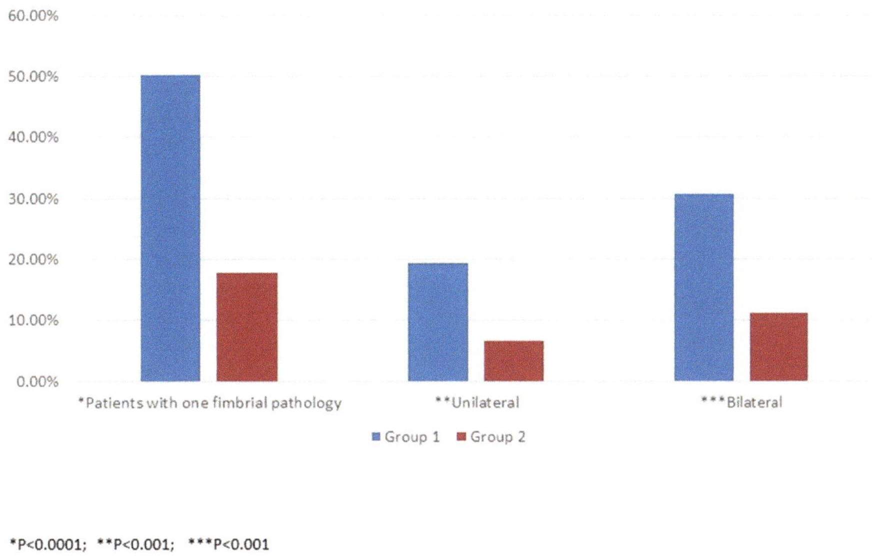


**FIGURE 20.17** Incidence of fimbrial pathology in patients with early stage endometriosis (Group 1) and controls (Group 2). (From Abuzeid MI, et al., 2007 [17]. With permission.)

mechanism (**Figure 20.18**). Such lesions may also interfere with ovum pick by other unknown mechanisms. These cysts can also cause torsion of ipsilateral fallopian tube (**Figure 20.19**) [21, 23]. Congenital accessory tubal ostia and accessory fallopian tubes are mainly incidentally findings noted on laparoscopy or laparotomy. If they are present within 1–2 cm of the primary fimbrial ostium, they may affect ovum pickup and transport. They are often associated with infertility and seen on laparoscopy for early stages of endometriosis [13]. Similarly, congenital tubal diverticulum is also incidentally found on laparoscopy for infertility and endometriosis. Patients with tubal diverticula may also present acutely with a ruptured ectopic pregnancy, as tubal diverticula increases the risk of ectopic implantation [24]. The authors of this chapter have noticed an association between congenital accessory tubal ostia and congenital tubal diverticulum and early stages of endometriosis (unpublished data). Fimbrial agglutination, blunting, and phimosis are often suspected during hysterosalpingogram (HSG) or on laparoscopy during the workup of infertility and endometriosis. They are often seen in association with early stage of endometriosis and can lead to infertility by affecting normal ovum pickup [17].

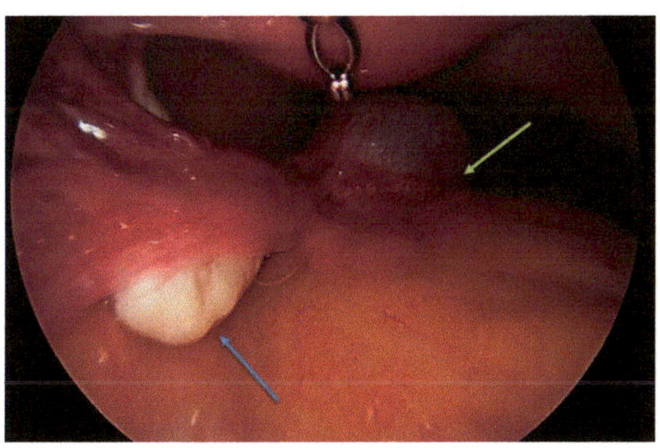

**FIGURE 20.18** A large left hydratid cyst of Morgagni (green arrow) pulling the fimbria away from the left ovary (blue arrow).

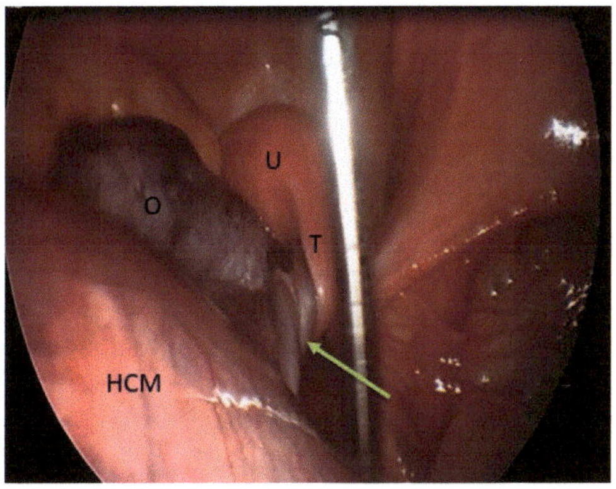


**FIGURE 20.19** Right adnexal torsion (green arrow) due to a huge hydratid cyst of Morgagni (15 cm): U, uterus; O, right ovary; T, right fallopian tube; HCM, hydratid cyst of Morgagni.

## History

As noted, most often patients are asymptomatic and the diagnosis is made incidentally on radiological imaging or at the time of laparoscopy for the evaluation of various gynecological conditions, including endometriosis and infertility. Once distal tubal pathology is suspected, a thorough history should be obtained from the patient, including menstrual history, history of dysmenorrheal, dyspareunia, and pelvic pain. In addition, any history of infertility, sexually transmitted diseases, pelvic inflammatory disease, appendicitis, bowel inflammatory disease, and previous surgical procedures should be reviewed.

## Physical examination

A general physical exam, including a Tanner staging, to evaluate the presence of secondary sexual characteristics should be performed. A routine pelvic exam, including a bimanual exam, to evaluate the uterus (presence, size, shape, position, tenderness, and mobility) and the adnexa (masses or tenderness) should be performed. A rectovaginal exam can be performed to evaluate the presence of cul-de-sac tenderness or nodularity that can be seen in patients with endometriosis.

### Investigations

The workup for infertility includes TV 2D US and HSG. A TV 2D US may suggest the presence of hydrosalpinx, moderate to large para-tubal cysts, adenomyosis, an endometrioma, and ovaries behind the uterus (suggestive of possible pelvic adhesions). A HSG can be used to evaluate tubal patency, tubal blockage (secondary to absent segment or congenital hydrosalpinx), and also other possible subtle tubal pathology. HSG can be helpful in suspecting tubal diverticulum [25]. The phenomena of loculation of the radio opaque dye around the tube may suggest peri-tubal adhesions irrespective of etiology (**Figure 20.20a,b**) [26]. One needs to be aware that such phenomena can also occur as a result of slow passage of the dye from the distal end of the fallopian tube as a result of subtle fimbrial pathology such as phimosis and agglutination. Tubal diverticula can also be suspected on HSG by observing the phenomenon of localization of the radio opaque dye around the distal end of the tubes. However, an incorrect diagnosis of distal tubal occlusion can be mistakenly made on HSG in the presence dilatation of the ampullary portion as a result of tubal diverticula. Dispersion of the radio opaque dye on delayed films in patients with tubal diverticulum may help in differentiating this pathology from patients with partial hydrosalpnix [1]. Localization of the radio opaque dye around the distal end of the tubes can also occur as a result of accessory tubal ostium and para-tubal cysts. This is especially the case in the absence of obesity or polycystic ovarian syndrome (PCOS) with enlarged ovaries [26]. In obese patients and in those with PCOS, the phenomena of localization of the radio opaque dye can be due to physiologic reasons such as pressure by the momentum or the enlarged ovaries on the distal end of the fallopian tube. However, one needs to be aware of other possible causes of such phenomena. Such causes may include early termination of the study by the radiologist or gynecologist performing the procedure once some of the radio opaque dye is seen dispersing from the tube or because of marked discomfort to the patient for fear of vasovagal attack. Another potential cause of false positive diagnosis of distal fimbrial pathology of the fallopian tube or peri-tubal adhesions is technical difficulty during the procedure. Such technical difficulty can be due to problematic cervical canal, retroverted uterus, acutely anteflexed uterus, uterus being tilted to one side, and stenotic or patulous cervix. Most of the technical difficulty that occur during HSG usually happens when the procedure is performed using a disposable HSG catheter. Such technical difficulty may be due to failure or difficulty in insertion of the disposable HSG catheter as a result of problematic cervix, cervical stenosis, obesity, or high position of the cervix in the vagina [27]. A technical difficulty can also be due to incorrect positioning of the balloon in the lower portion of the cervical canal, which may be associated with leakage of the radio opaque dye leak into the vagina leading to lack of proper pressure buildup in the uterus and, in turn, failure of proper filling of the tube or minimal spillage of the dye from the end of the tube [26]. In such situations, the use of Kahn's/acorn tipped cannula (Novo Surgical Inc. Oak Brook, IL, USA) can prevent inaccurate assessment and unnecessary interventions [28].

*Saline sonohysterosalpingography* (also known as the bubble study) can be used to assess tubal patency, but it is not useful to screen for pelvic adhesions and subtle fimbrial pathology. *Diagnostic laparoscopy* and *tubal perfusion* still remain as the goal standard test to diagnosis of tubal, para-tubal, and subtle distal tubal pathology. Tubal perfusion is performed using diluted indigo carmine dye. It is important to be aware of the various tubal, para-tubal, and subtle distal tubal pathologies, in order to be able to identify them at the time of laparoscopy. When performing a diagnostic laparoscopy, it is preferred to do at least a three-portal entry laparoscopy to be able to adequately evaluate the distal ends of the tubes [17, 18, 29]. Guan and Watrelot (2019) pointed out that careful observation of the drainage of the blue dye not only from the fimbria, but also from the entire tube is required, in order to avoid overlooking tiny fallopian tube lesions [1].

During laparoscopy, surgical correction in the form of tubal reconstruction can also be simultaneously performed by an experienced surgeon. It is thus prudent that diagnostic laparoscopy be performed by a trained surgeon comfortable with not only identifying such pathology, but also in performing reconstructive tubal surgery. This eliminates the need for having a secondary surgical procedure to address the identified pathology.

## Treatment

### Congenital tubal and para-tubal pathology

#### *Aplasia/hypoplasia of the fallopian tube*

In patients with aplasia/hypoplasia of the fallopian tube noted during an infertility workup, the normal appearance and functioning of the contralateral fallopian tube should be evaluated using HSG, or at the time of laparoscopy using tubal perfusion. The presence of tubal aplasia/hypoplasia may be associated with absent ovary on the same side (**Figure 20.1**). In the presence of normal functioning

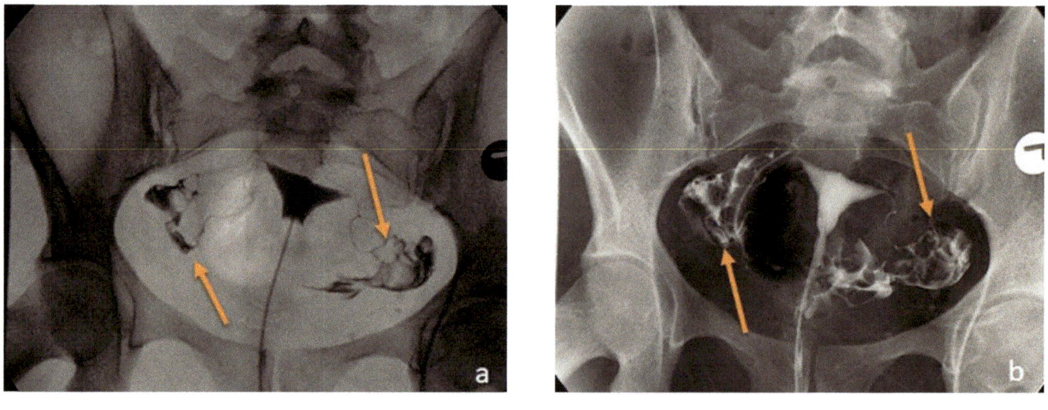


**FIGURE 20.20** (a) HSG illustrating the phenomenon of localization of radio opaque dye around the distal ends of the fallopian tubes (orange arrows); (b) HSG illustrating normal dispersion of radio opaque dye.

and appearance of the contralateral fallopian tube, expectant management is sufficient. If the ipsilateral ovary is also absent, the function of the remaining ovary should be assessed by antral follicle count (AFC), Anti-Müllerian Hormone (AMH), and day 2–3 Follicle-Stimulating Hormone (FSH). Assisted Reproductive Technology (ART) should be offered if the status of the remaining fallopian tube is suboptimal and/or in the presence of diminished ovarian reserve if the ipsilateral ovary is absent.

### *Congenital hydrosalpinx*

In the setting of a congenital hydrosalpinx, if mild and tubal structure is not compromised, a distal neosalpingostomy can be performed (**Figure 20.21a–f**). This can be done using the same technique of distal neosalpingostomy of a hydrosalpinx due to endometriosis, as described before [30]. Following distal salpingostomy, in order to keep the new ostium adequately open and prevent tubal occlusion, it is imperative to evert the edges of the new ostium well. This can be done either by suturing the edges of the new ostium to the surrounding tubal serosa using 6-0 Vicryl sutures (intracorporeal knot) and microsurgical principles and instruments with 3 mm needle holders (Koh Micro Instruments, Karl Storz Endoscopy, Culver City, CA, USA). Alternatively, one can perform the flowering technique of Bruhat by everting the edges of the new ostium using Argon Beam Coagulator (Birtcher Medical System, Irvine, CA, USA) (**Figure 20.21a–f**) [4]. As this condition is very rare, there is no data in the literature to assess the reproductive outcome after this type of surgery. If the hydrosalpinx is large and/or there is a concern about the functioning of the fallopian tube (secondary to marked atrophy of the endosalpnix), a total salpingectomy should be performed. This is especially the case if one is planning to proceed with in vitro fertilization (IVF) and embryo transfer (ET), as the fluid from the hydrosalpinx

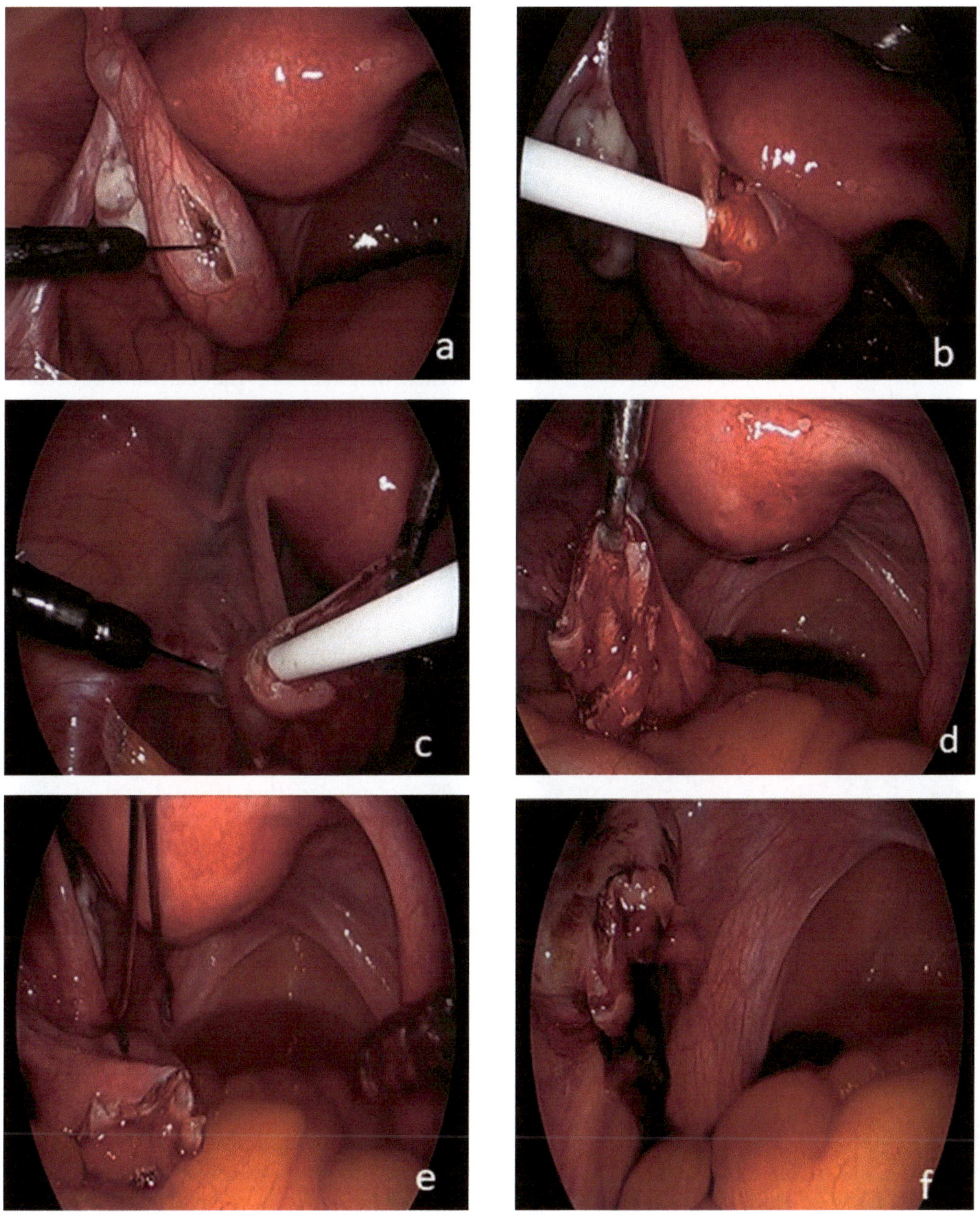


FIGURE 20.21 (a–f) The stages of left neosalpingostomy for congenital hydrosalpinx.

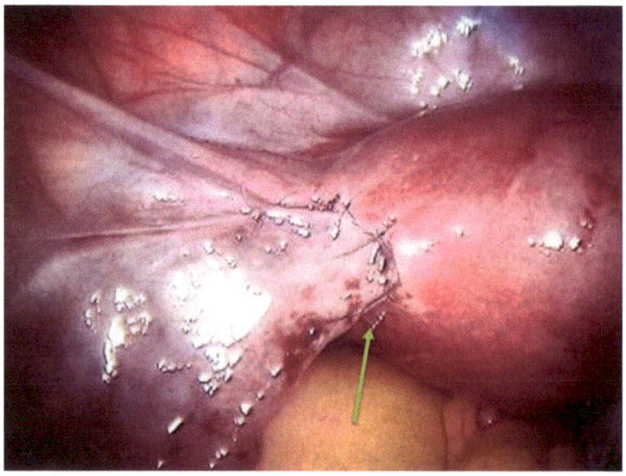

**FIGURE 20.22** End result after laparoscopic isthmo-cornual anastomosis (green arrow).

can be toxic to the embryo and it can simply cause mechanical flushing of the embryo after ET. Salpingectomy should also be performed to reduce risk of ectopic pregnancy after IVF-ET.

### *Congenital absence of other parts of the fallopian tube*

The absence of a small segment of the fallopian tube, irrespective of its location, can be surgically corrected by performing end to end anastomosis via laparotomy and micro-tubal surgery using the same principles, described decades ago, for reversal of tubal ligation [31]. During the last 25 years, few publications described performing the same procedures via operative laparoscopy and da Vinci robotic-assisted operative laparoscopy with equivalent results to laparotomy and micro-tubal surgery [31, 32]. In cases of congenital absence of the proximal segment of the isthmic portion of the fallopian tube near the cornual region, as illustrated in **Figure 20.4**, isthmic cornual anastomosis can be attempted, providing the remaining portion of the fallopian tube appears to be normal, healthy, and patent as demonstrated during the anastomosis procedure. **Figure 20.22** illustrates the end result of a laparoscopic isthmo-cornual anastomosis during reversal of tubal ligation. **Figure 20.23** illustrates the end result of a laparoscopic isthmo-isthmic anastomosis during reversal of tubal ligation. These procedures should only be performed by an experienced

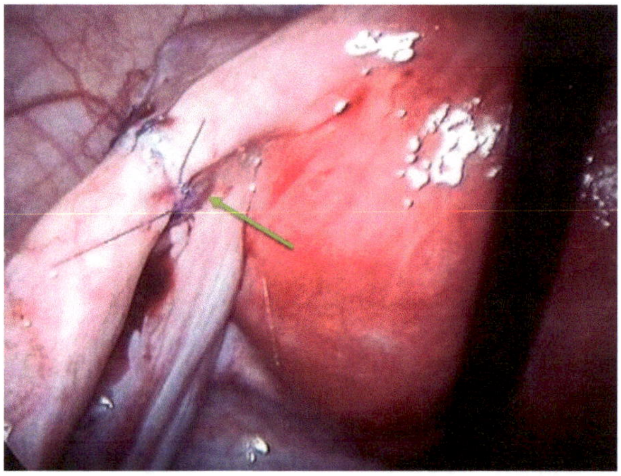

**FIGURE 20.23** End result after laparoscopic isthmo-cornual anastomosis (green arrow).

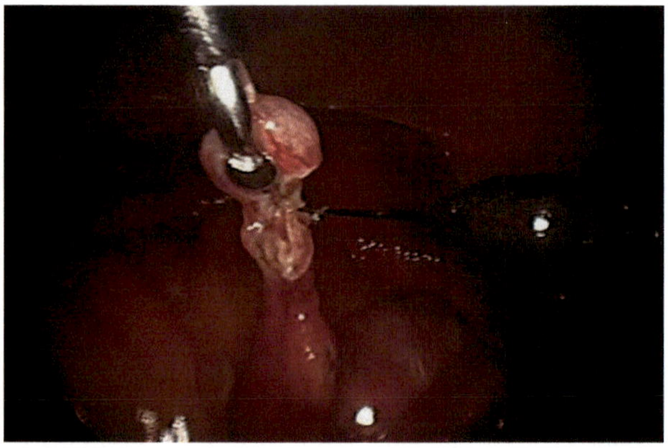

**FIGURE 20.24** Excision of a small right pedunculated hydratid cyst of Morgagni.

reproductive surgeon with formal training in micro-tubal surgery. Unfortunately, in the era of IVF-ET, such training is dwindling, and there are only a few programs that provide adequate training and experience to perform such surgery. However, it is important to emphasize that if the contralateral fallopian tube is patent and healthy, there is no need for surgical correction. One may use fertility medications to boost the chances of conceiving. However, if the contralateral tube is diseased, blocked, or absent, surgical treatment versus IVF-ET should be considered.

### *Para-tubal cyst*

A solitary large para-tubal cyst or multiple para-tubal cysts can mechanically affect the functioning of the tube. In theory, due to their weight or size, they can kink or occlude the lumen of the ipsilateral fallopian tube. In addition, as mentioned earlier, a large or multiple para-tubal cyst may pull the fimbria down away from the ovary, and in turn, this may reduce ovum pickup mechanism [9, 33]. We therefore recommend surgical management of solitary large or multiple para-tubal cysts. Depending on the location, size, and type (pedunculated or sessile), they can be excised or marsupialized (**Figures 20.24, 20.25a–d, 20.26a–e, 20.27**) [23, 34]. In addition, Rasheed SM and Abdelmonem AM (2010) suggested that Hydatid cyst of Morgagni is a possible underestimated cause of unexplained infertility [35]. The authors also reported a high spontaneous pregnancy rate after laparoscopic excision of such cysts [35]. This was especially the case with bilateral and/or fimbrial Hydatid cysts of Morgagni [35]. Furthermore, in a three-case report, Abd-El-Maeboud KH (1997) concluded that Hydatid cyst of Morgagni may reduce ovum pickup after ovulation resulting in infertility, and that laparoscopic surgical correction can enhance the chance of spontaneous pregnancy [33]. Tubal or adnexal torsion is a complication of a large para-tubal cyst (**Figure 20.19**). This can be corrected surgically once the diagnosis is made at the time of laparoscopy. The procedure, which include diagnosis, detorsion, and excision of the large para-tubal cyst, should be done by an experienced reproductive surgeon. Every effort should be made to preserve the fallopian tube if the patient desires future fertility. Otherwise, detorsion followed by salpingectomy and removal of the large para-tubal cyst should be performed.

### *Congenital accessory ostium*

Congenital accessory ostia can theoretically affect ovum pickup and transport. Although several studies reported on the presence of accessory tubal ostia during laparoscopy in infertility patients, their association with infertility remains controversial.

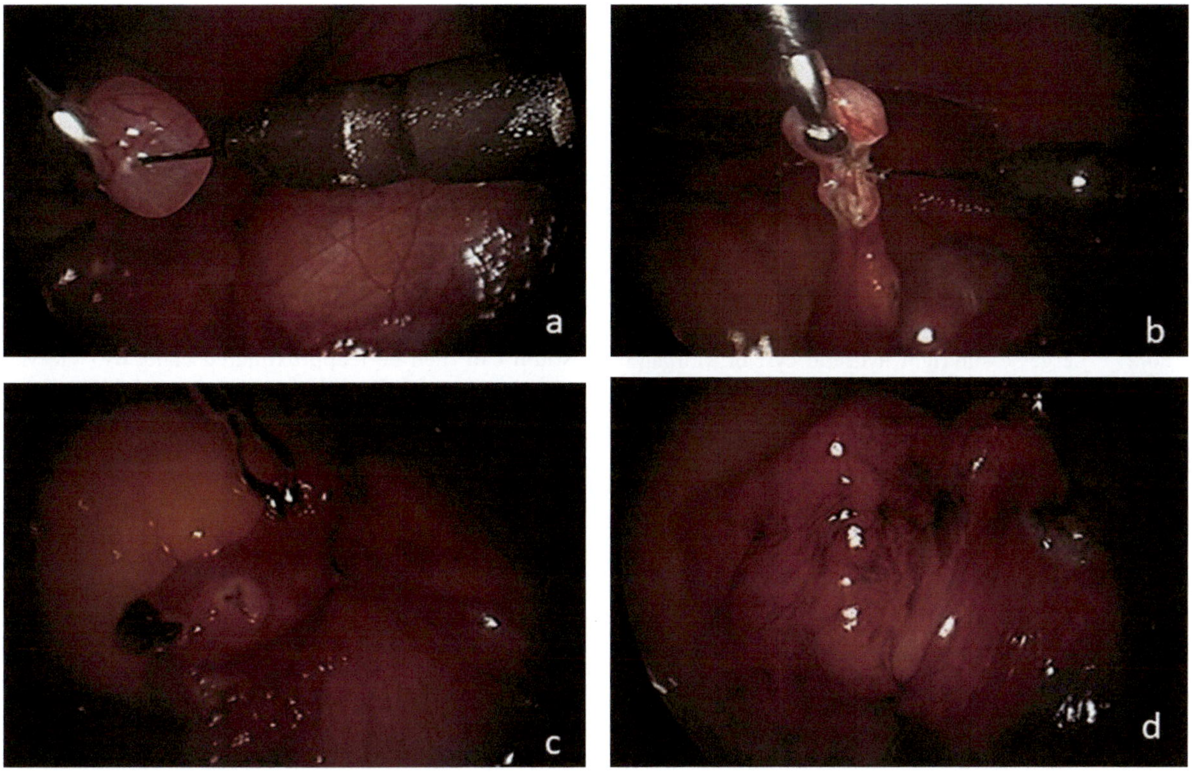


**FIGURE 20.25** (a, b) Excision of multiple left pedunculated hydatid cysts of Morgagni; (c, d) end result.

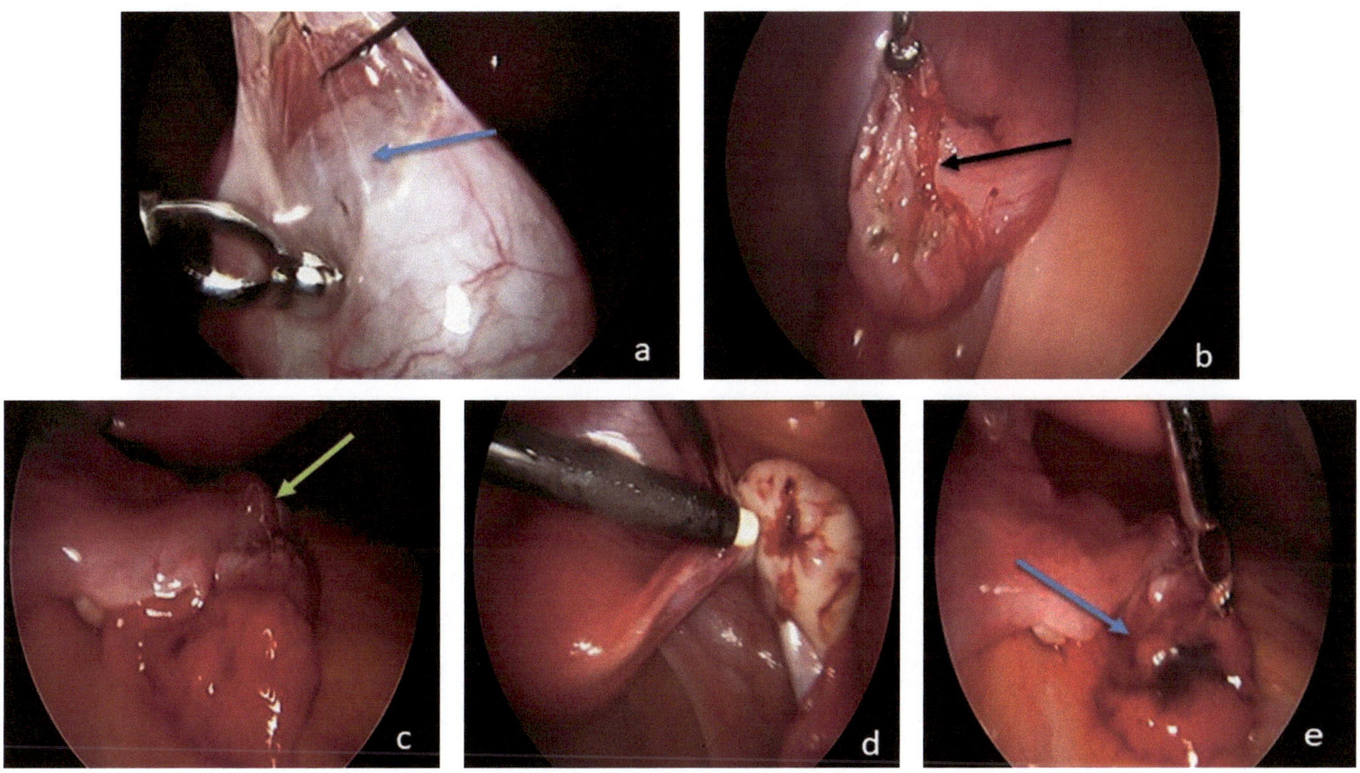


**FIGURE 20.26** (a) Large sessile left hydratid cyst of Morgagni (blue arrow); (b) repair of the defect in the right mesosalpinx (black arrow) with (c) 4-0 Vicryl (green arrow) in a patient with endometriosis on the right ovary; (d) the left tube is left patent at the end of the procedure.

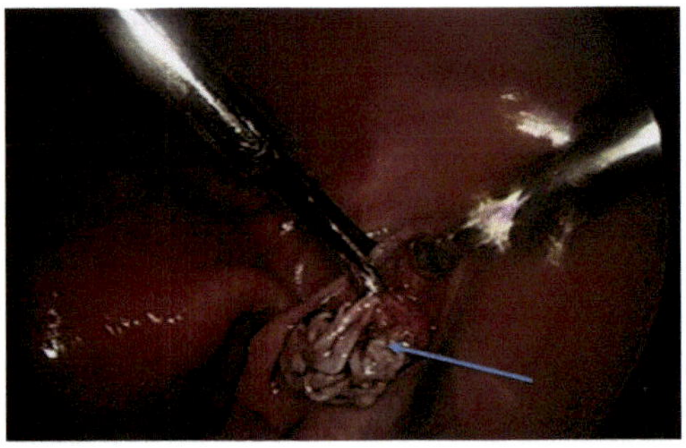

FIGURE 20.27 Large sessile right hydratid cyst of Morgagni being dissected from the mesosalpinx (blue arrow).

Yablonski et al. (1990) reported a higher incidence of accessory tubal ostia in infertile patients [36]. In addition, accessory tubal ostia may be associated with endometriosis and ectopic pregnancy [14, 37]. Surgical treatment of such lesions has been associated with improvement in fertility outcomes.

If the accessory ostium is present within 1–2 cm of the primary fallopian tube ostium, one can join the two ostia together [14, 38]. By passing a laparoscopic Teflon probe (Elmed, Chicago, IL, USA) through one opening and out through the other, then the intervening bridge of tissue along the antimesenteric border can be divided by using a monopolar micro diathermy needle tip (Elmed, Chicago, IL, USA) (**Figure 20.28a,b**). The most common technique is to pass the laparoscopic Teflon probe through the fimbrial opening and out through the accessory tubal ostium after grasping and lifting the fimbria with an atraumatic grasping forceps (Ubef, Vernon Hills, IL, USA) [17]. Careful hemostasis should be achieved and the cut edges should be everted to prevent reapproximation using microsurgical technique with 6-0 Vicryl or the flowering technique of Bruhat, as mentioned earlier (**Figure 20.28c,d**) [4]. If an accessory tubal ostium is present, away from the primary fimbrial ostium (>2 cm), in theory this pathology can also be surgically corrected. The edges of the accessory tubal ostium can be refreshed using a monopolar micro diathermy needle tip. Then, care should be taken to achieve careful homeostasis. Thereafter, the margins of the accessory tubal ostium can then be reapproximated using 6-0 Vicryl. Another laparoscopic surgical technique to close such type of accessory ostium was proposed by Zheng et al. (2015) [14]. Zheng et al. (2015) used this technique if the accessory ostium was at least 1 cm from the fimbria [14]. These investigators used a monofilament purse-string suture at the base of the accessory ostium with a 5-0 absorbable thread to close the accessory ostium [14]. Thereafter, they removed the accessory ostium by resection or electrocoagulation [14]. However, such procedures should be considered experimental and should only be done by an experienced reproductive surgeon. Otherwise, it is better to avoid this kind of surgery as one may do more harm than good. If an accessory fallopian tube is present, it can be excised, and careful homeostasis should be achieved using a micro diathermy monopolar needle tip. Prior to the era of operative laparoscopy, Cohen B (1987) proposed closure of accessory ostium using microsurgery

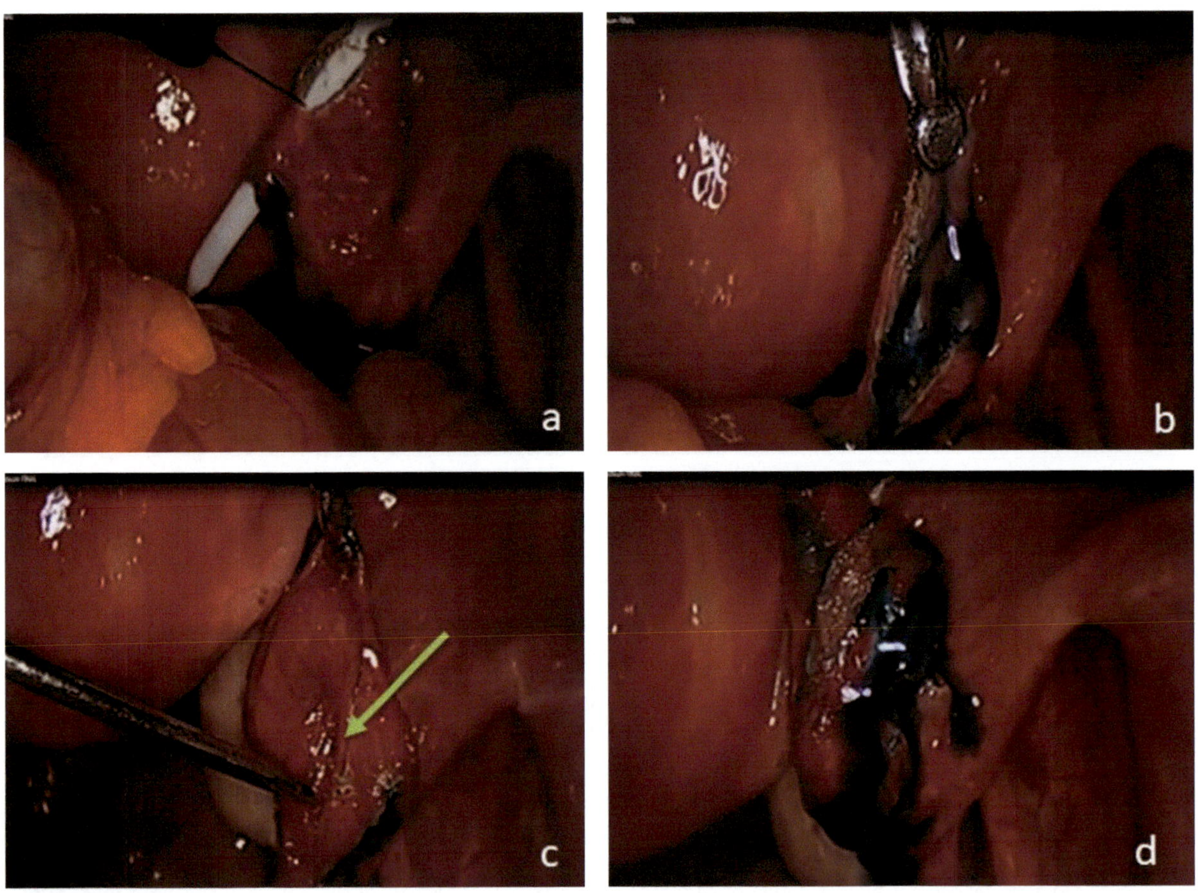


FIGURE 20.28 (a, b) Connecting a congenital accessory tubal ostium to the fimbria; (c) a $CO_2$ laser (green arrow) is used to achieve the flowering technique of Bruhart; (d) end result of surgery.

during laparotomy [11]. It is worth noting that Zheng et al. (2015) reported higher incidence of accessory ostium in patients with endometriosis. The authors also reported that laparoscopic surgical correction of accessory ostium together with conservative surgery for endometriosis improved reproductive outcome [14]. Other investigators also reported an association between accessory ostium and endometriosis [13].

### *Accessory fallopian tubes*

Accessory fallopian tubes may cause infertility, ectopic pregnancy, cystic swelling, and torsion. If accessory fallopian tube is found during laparoscopy, especially in infertility patients, it is recommended to do surgical excision. This may improve fertility potential and will decrease potential complications such as ectopic pregnancy and torsion.

### *Congenital tubal diverticulum*

The association between tubal sacculation and infertility is not well defined. Some reports suggest an improvement in fertility outcomes after surgical correction [39]. In addition, the role of tubal diverticulum in infertility remains unclear with some investigators suggesting an association, while others did not find such association [16, 36, 40]. Han et al. (2014) reported that tubal diverticulum was more prevalent in patients with endometriosis than in infertile patients [41].

In addition, the authors reported an improvement in fertility potential after surgical correction of tubal diverticula [41].

If congenital tubal diverticulum is present within 1–2 cm of the fallopian tube fimbrial opening, this can be opened and incorporated into the fimbrial opening [42]. A laparoscopic Teflon probe can be passed through the fimbrial opening into the diverticulum sac after grasping and lifting the fimbria with an atraumatic grasping forceps (**Figure 20.29a,b**). The intervening bridge is then incised using a monopolar micro diathermy needle tip along the antimesenteric border (cutting current is 20 Watt), and hemostasis is achieved along the cut edges using a monopolar micro diathermy needle tip (coagulation current is 20–30 Watt). The edges of the new ostium should be everted using flowering technique of Bruhat, as described before (**Figure 20.29c,d**) [4].

If the tubal diverticulum is present more than 2 cm from the fallopian tube fimbria, this, in theory, can be surgically corrected to reduce the possible risk of ectopic pregnancy. The diverticulum can be excised by placing a fine ligature at the base of the diverticulum using a fine Vicryl endo loop. After placing the ligature, the tubal diverticulum can then be safely excised. Alternatively, a 6-0 Vicryl suture can be placed in the seromuscular layer at the base of the diverticulum in a purse string manner and then tied. The tubal diverticulum can then be safely excised. The later procedure should be considered experimental and should only be done by an experienced reproductive surgeon who should avoid injury to the endosalpnix and, in turn, iatrogenic tubal damage. Otherwise, it is better to avoid this kind of surgery as one may do more harm than good.

## Subtle fimbrial pathology in early stage endometriosis

*Fimbrial agglutination* can obstruct or narrow the primary fimbrial opening and compromise the fimbrial functioning (**Figure 20.13**). Surgical fimbrial reconstruction (fimbrioplasty) can be performed via laparoscopy by grasping the fimbria with an atraumatic grasping forceps, then passing a laparoscopic Teflon probe underneath the adhered opposing fimbriae (**Figure 20.30a–d**). This should be followed by making an incision

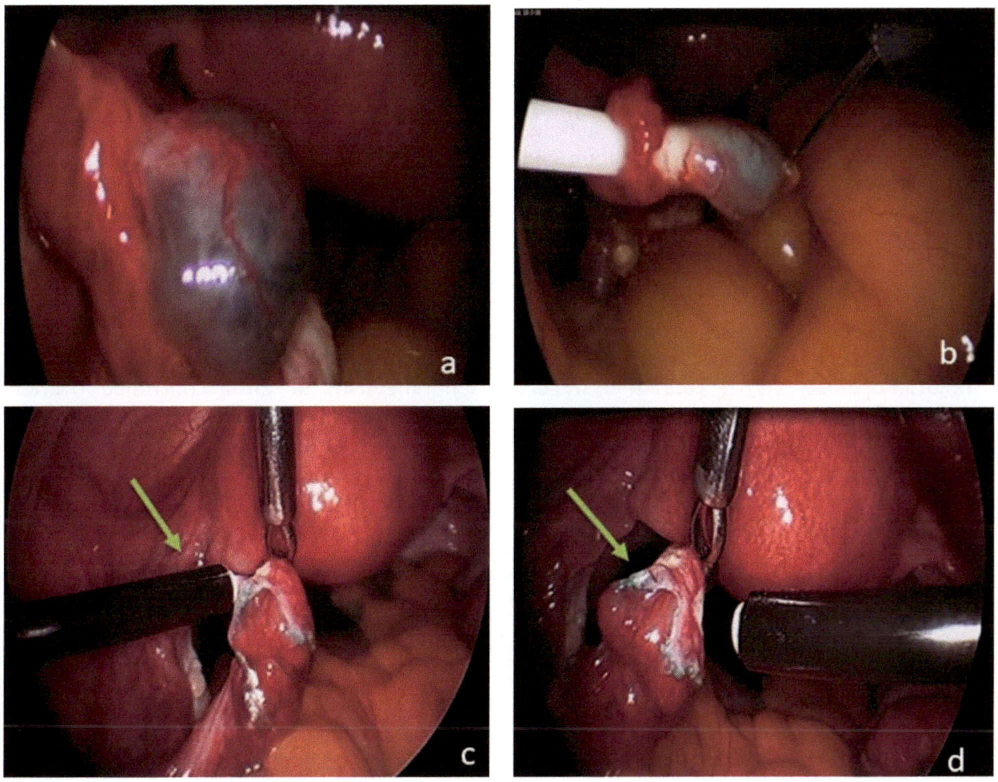


**FIGURE 20.29** (a, b) Connecting a congenital tubal diverticulum to the fimbria; (c, d) An argon beam coagulator is used to achieve the flowering technique of Bruhart.

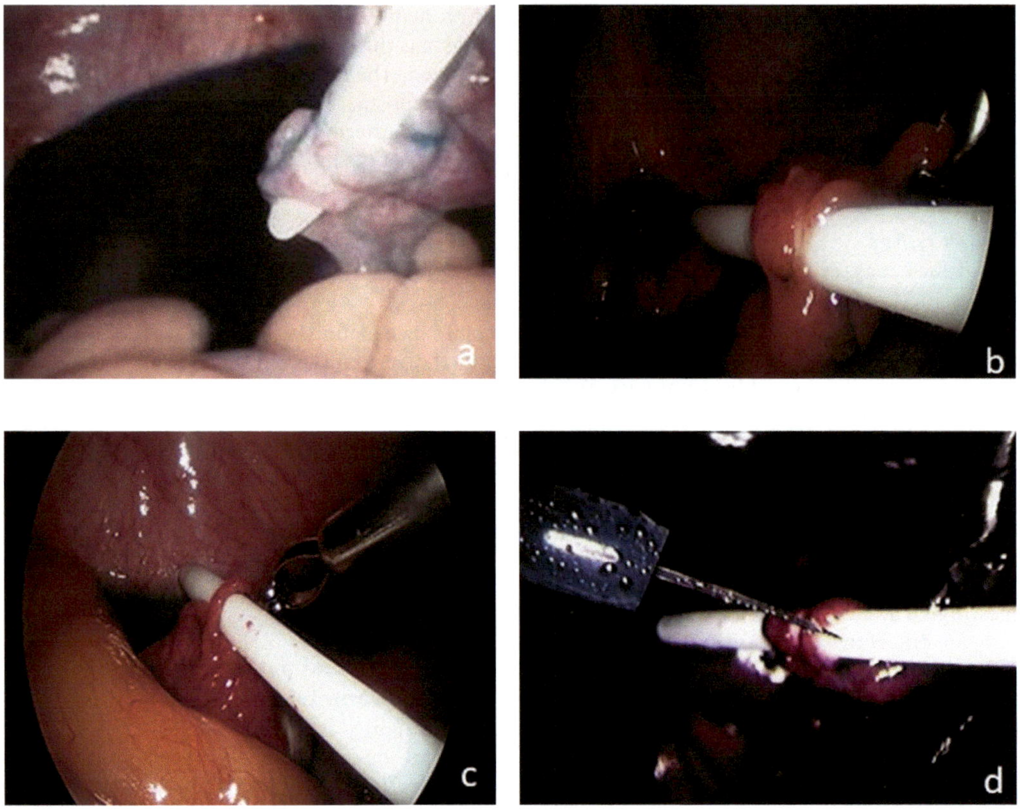

FIGURE 20.30 (a–c) Fimbrial agglutinations of the fimbria being lifted by Teflon probe; (d) A monopolar microdiathermy needle tip used to divide the band of agglutination.

along the intervening bridge using a monopolar micro diathermy needle tip (cutting current of 20 watts) (**Figure 20.30d**). *Fimbrial phimosis* can also be surgically managed by passing a laparoscopic Teflon probe through the fimbrial opening, and making a 1–2 cm incision along the antimesenteric border using a monopolar micro diathermy needle tip (cutting current of 20-30 watts) (**Figure 20.31a,b**). Hemostasis is then achieved using the monopolar micro diathermy needle tip (coagulation current of 20–30 watts), and the cut edges are then everted to using the microsurgery technique or flowering technique of Bruhat, described earlier (**Figure 20.31a–d,e**) [4, 18]. In some cases, the phimosis is so severe that one may not be able to pass the laparoscopic Teflon probe through the fimbrial opening (**Figure 20.32a–e**). In such cases, we modified the technique described above in the following manner. First, the tube is distended with diluted indigo Carmine dye, which allowed us to make an incision along the antimesenteric border of the tube (without injury to the endosalpnix near the mesenteric side) using the monopolar micro diathermy needle tip (cutting current of 20–30 watts) (**Figure 20.32f**). The laparoscopic Teflon probe is then introduced through the new ostium in a retrograde fashion and is advanced through the fimbrial ostium (**Figure 20.32g,h**). The remaining bridge of tissue is then divided, homeostasis is ensured, and edges of the new ostium is everted, as described before (**Figure 20.32h,i**). All through the procedure, irrigation and suction should be performed using heparinized Lactated Ringer's solution (5000 IU/1L of Lactated Ringer's solution). The principles of microsurgery in terms of tissue handling, use of microsurgical instruments should always be followed [4, 18]. Such procedures should only be performed by an experienced reproductive surgeon, preferably at the same time of making the diagnosis. Therefore, proper planning is important to avoid additional surgeries.

The reproductive outcome after laparoscopic fimbrioplasty in patients with endometriosis was published by our group in 2009 [4]. In this study, we compared the effectiveness of two surgical techniques (suturing versus flowering of Bruhat) after laparoscopic fimbrioplasty for treatment of distal tubal pathology in infertile women with endometriosis (154 patients). This was a historical cohort study with 12 months of follow-up comparing pregnancy, delivery, and cumulative conception rates achieved spontaneously, or after controlled ovarian hyperstimulation (COS) with intrauterine insemination (IUI). The pregnancy outcome in patients with endometriosis who conceived spontaneously after unilateral or bilateral laparoscopic fimbrioplasty is illustrated in **Figure 20.33**. The pregnancy outcome in patients with endometriosis who conceived with COS+IUI after unilateral or bilateral laparoscopic fimbrioplasty is shown in **Figure 20.34**. **Figure 20.35** illustrates the cumulative conception rates in patients with endometriosis who conceived after all methods (spontaneously and COS+IUI) following unilateral or bilateral laparoscopic fimbrioplasty. Our results are similar to what has been published in the literature by other investigators [43–45]. Published data in the literature reported an intrauterine pregnancy rate that varied between 35% and 69% [43–45]. It is worth to note that most of this data were published before 2000 and all the studies are retrospective in nature.

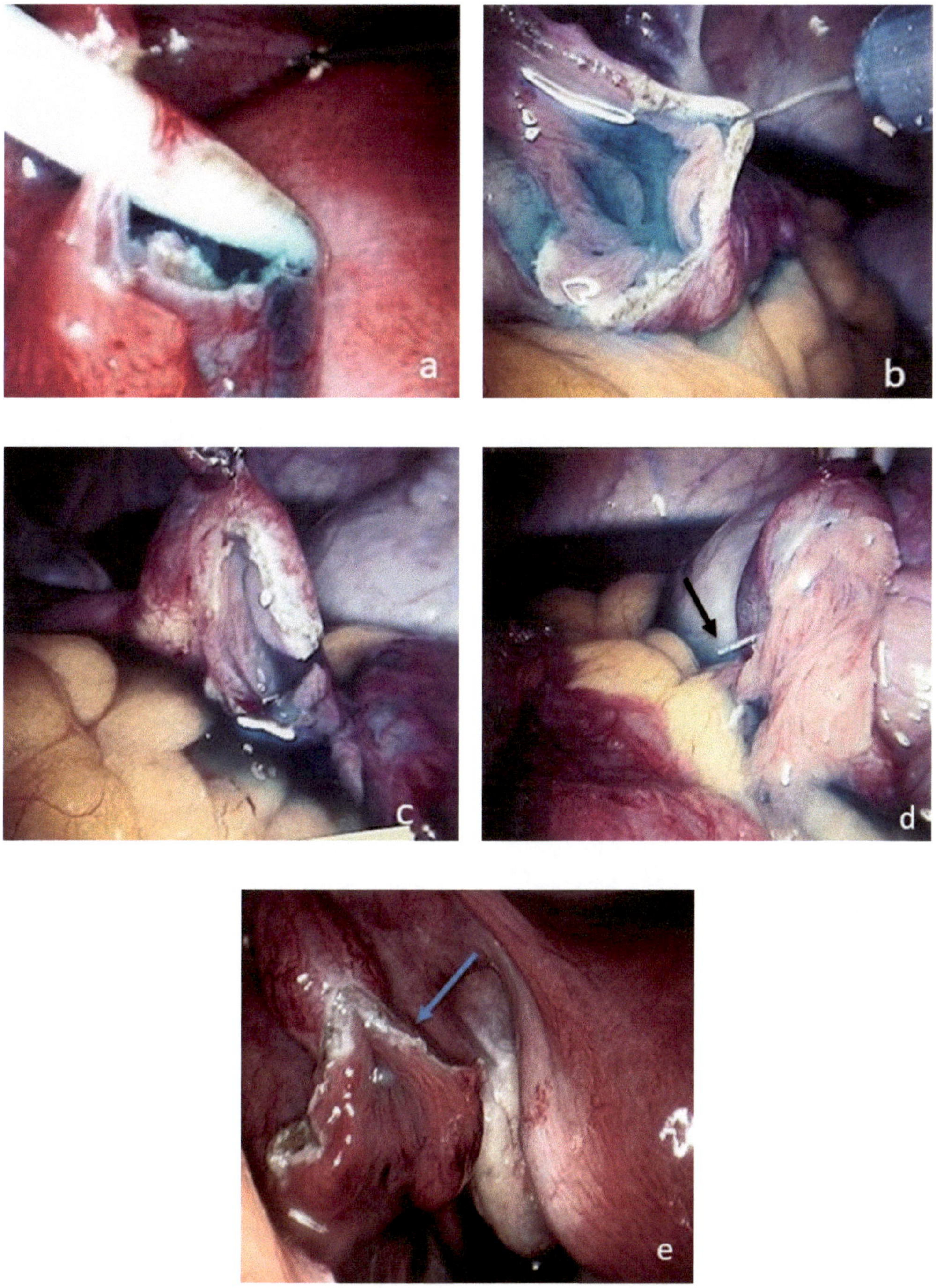


**FIGURE 20.31** (a, b) Fimbroplasty for fimbrial phimosis; (c) the new ostium; (d) after eversion of the edges using 6-0 Vicryl sutures (black arrow); (e) end result after using the flowering technique of Bruhart to evert the edges of a new ostium after fimbrioplasty (blue arrow).

## Summary

Although this chapter discuses the diagnosis and surgical management of specific pathologies that may affect the function of the fallopian tube, such management comes under the heading of tubal surgery. Therefore, we would like to briefly discuss the various opinions on the place of tubal surgery in infertility treatment in the era of ART. It is well acknowledged by many infertility specialists that there has been a decline in the use of infertility surgery and a similar decline in the number of skilled reproductive surgeons. This, together with the high success rate with IVF-ET, has led some authorities to declare that infertility surgery is dead and what was left is to write its obituary [46]. The same group also suggested that the role for surgery in infertile patients with endometriosis continued to diminish [46]. However, other authorities indicated that infertility surgery still

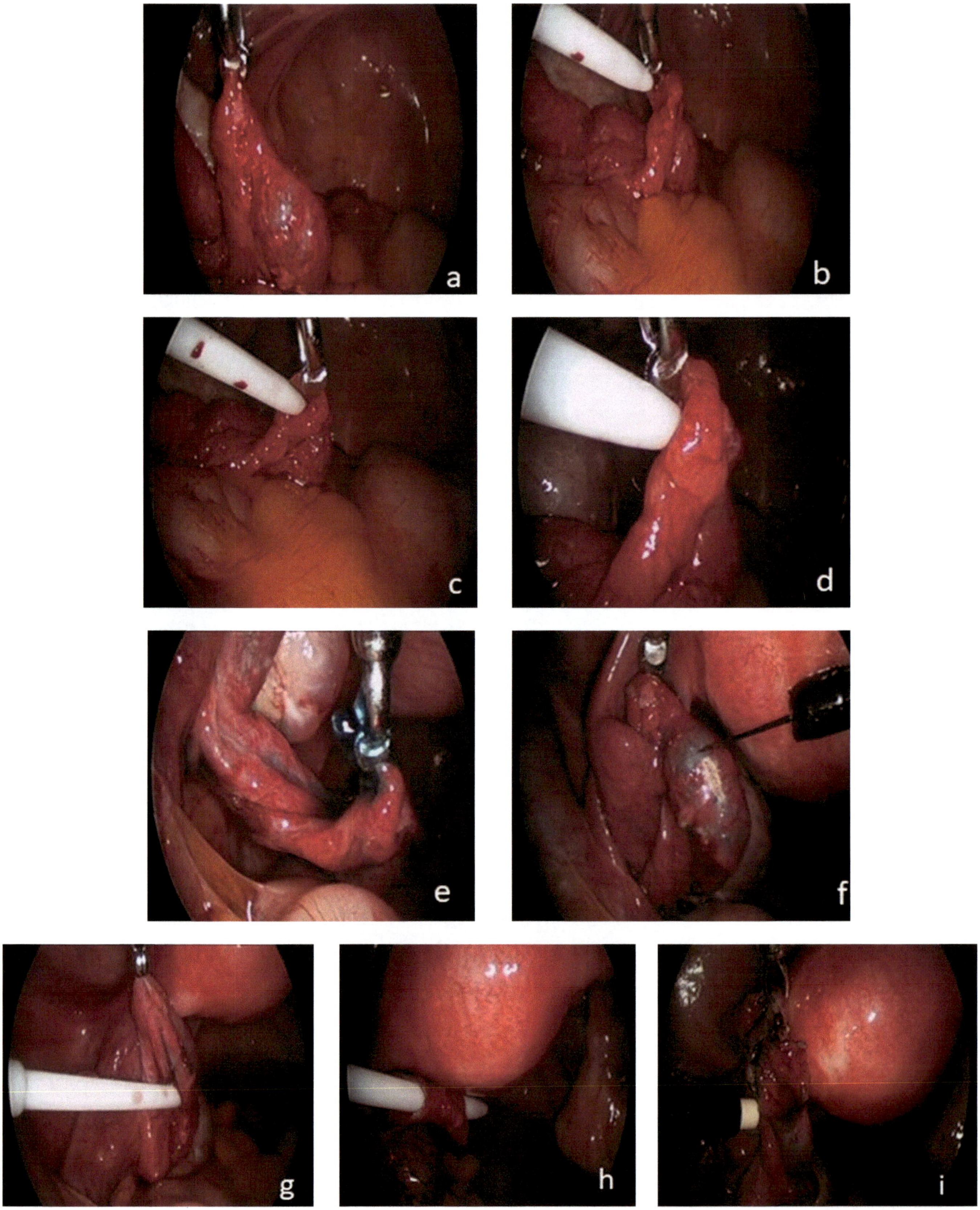

FIGURE 20.32 (a–e) Severe fimbrial phimosis, with failure to pass the Teflon probe through the fimbria; (f) making a small incision along the antimesentric border of the distended ampullary portion of the tube near the fimbria during tubal perfusion; (g) through which the Teflon probe was introduced; (h) and passed through the fimbria; (h) end result after the remaining bridge of tissue was divided and the edges of the new ostium everted.

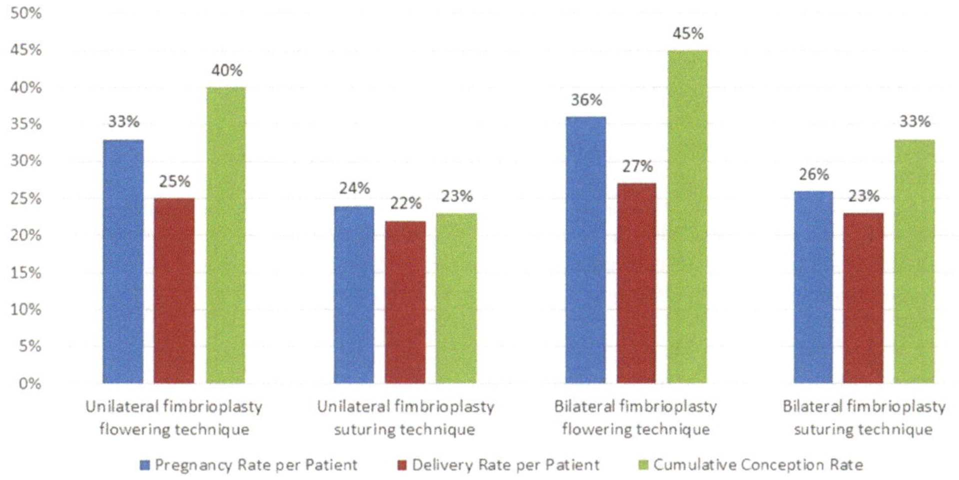


**FIGURE 20.33** Pregnancy outcome in patients with endometriosis who conceived spontaneously after unilateral or bilateral fimbrioplasty.

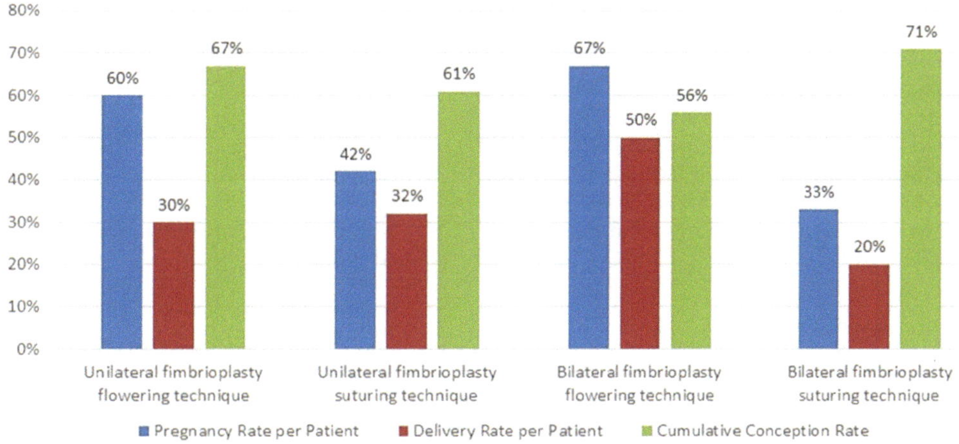


**FIGURE 20.34** Pregnancy outcome in patients with endometriosis who conceived with COS+IUI after unilateral or bilateral fimbrioplasty.

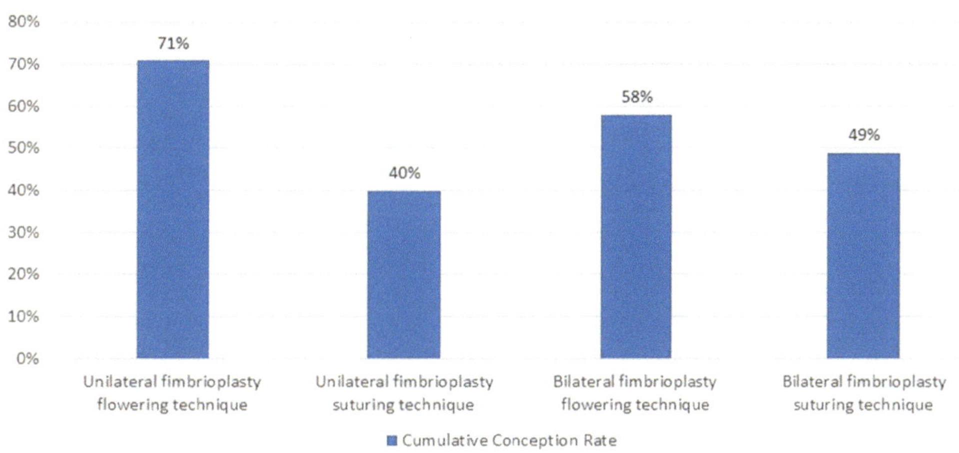


**FIGURE 20.35** Cumulative conception rates in patients with endometriosis who conceived after all methods (spontaneously and COS+IUI) following unilateral or bilateral fimbrioplasty.

plays an important role in infertility treatment, especially in view of the advances in endoscopic instruments [47]. The authors of this report suggested (rightly so) that this is the case in view of the limitations of access to IVT-ET treatment due to its high cost [47]. They also pointed out that IVF-ET treatment may not be acceptable to some couples for religious reasons [47]. In addition, they indicated that some patients give up on fertility treatment after one failed IVF-ET cycle [47]. The stand of the American Society of Reproductive Medicine on the role of tubal surgery in the era of ART is that "the evidence is fair to recommend laparoscopic fimbrioplasty or neosalpingostomy for the treatment of mild hydrosalpinxes in young women with no other significant infertility factors" [48]. In a recent report by Goldberg et al. (2019), they suggested that "appropriately selected patients can benefit from a cost-effective, minimally invasive outpatient procedure and avoid the need for IVF. Many patients would prefer this if given the option" [49].

## Conclusion

The authors of this chapter believe that reproductive surgery continues to play an important role in infertility treatment when performed by an experienced endoscopic surgeon for the appropriate indications. Although some authorities believe that IVF-ET and tubal surgery are complementary and not competitive in the management of infertile couple, others believe that surgical management should only be reserved to cases in which IVF-ET was not initially effective [46, 50]. However, Watrelot A and Chauvin G (2011) suggested that tubal surgery should be used as a first treatment option in favorable cases [47]. This should be followed by IVF-ET treatment when surgery fails, after some time, depending on the patient's age [47].

## References


1. Guan J and Watrelot A. Fallopian tube subtle pathology. Best Pract Res Clin Obstet Gynaecol. 2019;59:25–40.
2. Bruce M and Carlson P. Urogenital System. Human Embryology and Development Biology. 6th ed. St. Louis, Missouri: Elsevier; 2019. p. 358–90.
3. Laurence S. and Baskin P. Embryology of the Genitourinary Tract. In: Partin AW, editor. Campbell-Walsh Urology. 12th ed. Philadelphia, PA: Elsevier 2021. p. 305–40.e4.
4. Mitwally MF, Abuzeid O, Mohammed A, Diamond M, and Abuzeid M. Suturing versus flowering technique of Bruhat after fimbrioplasty for endometriosis-related infertility. Gynecol Surg. 2009;6:147–52.
5. Suh BY and Kalan MJ. Septate uterus with left fallopian tube hypoplasia and ipsilateral ovarian agenesis. J Assist Reprod Genet. 2008;25(11–12):567–9.
6. Uckuyu A, Ozcimen EE, and Sevinc Ciftci FC. Unilateral congenital ovarian and partial tubal absence: report of four cases with review of the literature. Fertil Steril. 2009;91(3):936.e5–8.
7. Dahan MH, Burney R, and Lathi R. Congenital interruption of the ampullary portion of the fallopian tube. Fertil Steril. 2006; 85(6):1820–1.
8. Shrotri T and Ahuja M. Bilateral absence of fallopian tube segments: an uncommon condition. Int J Reprod Contracept Obstet Gynecol. 2019 Jan;8(1):335–7
9. Cebesoy FB, Kutlar I, Dikensoy E, Yazicioglu C, and Lalayci H. Morgagni hydatids: a new factor in infertility? Arch Gynecol Obstet. 2010;281(6):1015–7.
10. Vang R and Wheeler JE. Diseases of the fallopian tube and paratubal region. In: Kurman RJ, Ellenson LH, Ronnett BM, editors. Blaustein's Pathology of the Female Genital Tract. 6th ed. New York: Springer; 2011. p. 529.
11. Cohen BM. Microsurgical reconstruction of congenital tubal anomalies. Microsurgery. 1987;8(2):68–77.
12. Atileh LIA, Dahbour D, Hammo H, and Abdullattif M. Laparoscopic removal of a 40-cm paratubal cyst in a morbidly obese patient. Gynecol Minim Invasive Ther. 2020;9(1):39–41.
13. Pereira N and Kligman I. Clinical implications of accessory fallopian tube ostium in endometriosis and primary infertility. Women's Health. 2016;12:404–6.
14. Zheng X, Han H, and Guan J. Clinical features of fallopian tube accessory ostium and outcomes after laparoscopic treatment. Int J Gynaecol Obstet. 2015;129(3):260–3.
15. Beyth Y and Kopolovic J. Accessory tubes: a possible contributing factor in infertility. Fertil Steril. 1982;38(3):382–3.
16. Troell S. Diverticula of the walls of the fallopian tubes. Acta Obstet Gynecol Scand. 1970;49:17–20.
17. Abuzeid MI, Mitwally MF, Ahmed AI, Formentini E, Ashraf M, Abuzeid OM, et al. The prevalence of fimbrial pathology in patients with early stages of endometriosis. J Minim Invasive Gynecol. 2007; 14(1):49–53.
18. Abuzeid O and Abuzeid MA. Laparoscopic management of subtle fimbrial pathology secondary to endometriosis In: Botros Rizk MM, editor. Standard Operational Procedures in Reproductive Medicine: Laboratory and Clinical Practice. Boca Raton, Florida: Taylor and Francis; 2017. p. 110–1.
19. Cohen BM. Surgical repair of abnormal fimbrial gonadal relationships in the human female. J Reprod Med. 1980;25(1):33–7.
20. Chen B, Yang C, Sahebally Z, and Jin H. Unilateral ovarian and fallopian tube agenesis in an infertile patient with a normal uterus. Exp Ther Med. 2014;8(3):831–5.
21. Casey RK, Damle LF, and Gomez-Lobo V. Isolated fallopian tube torsion in pediatric and adolescent females: a retrospective review of 15 cases at a single institution. J Pediatr Adolesc Gynecol. 2013; 26(3):189–92.
22. Sarah K. and Dotters-Katz. Paratubal/Paraovarian masses: a study of surgical and non-surgical outcomes. Med J Obstet Gynecol. 2014; 2:1–4.
23. Abuzeid O, Raju R, Hebert J, and Abuzeid M. Laparoscopic management of a large paratubal cyst. J Minim Invasive Gynecol. Nov 2016;23(7):S152.
24. Madanes A, Homer M, Turksoy RN, and Farber M. A single diverticulum of the fallopian tube. Fertil Steril. 1982;37(1):121–2.
25. Hertzanu Y, Ferteira M, and Blumenthal NJ. A solitary diverticulum of the fallopian tube. Aust N Z J Obstet Gynaecol. 1983; 23(3):186–7.
26. Abuzeid O, Yip M, Hebert J, and Abuzeid M. Laparoscopy is the gold standard for the diagnosis of subtle fimbrial pathology, peritubal and periovarian adhesions. J Minim Invasive Gynecol. Nov 2016; 23(7):S239–40.
27. Sanya R, Raju R, Abuzeid O, Khalid N, Hebert J, and Abuzeid M. Perfecting hysterosalpingography: limitations. J Minim Invasive Gynecol. Nov 2016;23(7):S80.
28. Fahmi I, Abuzeid MI, and Badawy SZA. Hysterosalpingography. In: Botros R, editor. Standard Operational Procedures in Reproductive Medicine Laboratory and Clinical Practice. CRC Francis & Taylor Group, 2017, Section 2, Chapter 50, p. 124–6.
29. Abuzeid M, Mitwally MF, Abuzeid OM, and Diamond MP. Detection and surgical correction of fimbrial pathology in patients with early stages of endometriosis. Fertil Steril. 2005; 84:Supplement 1:S478.
30. Abuzeid M, Sakhel K, Alwan R, Ahmed A, Ashraf M, Mitwally M, and Diamond MP. Unilateral versus bilateral adnexal disease in stage III and stage IV endometriosis does not affect pregnancy outcome after operative laparoscopy. Gynecol Surg. 2009;6(1):39
31. Cha SH, Lee MH, Kim JH, Lee CN, Yoon TK, and Cha KY. Fertility outcome after tubal anastomosis by laparoscopy and laparotomy. J Am Assoc Gynecol Laparosc. 2001;8:348–52. doi: 10.1016/S1074-3804(05)60329-5
32. Falcone T, Goldberg JM, Harout Margossian H, and Stevens L. Robotic-assisted laparoscopic microsurgical tubal anastomosis: a human pilot study Fertil Steril. 2000;73(5):140–2

33. Abd-el-Maeboud KH. Hydatid cyst of Morgagni: any impact on fertility? J Obstet Gynaecol Res. 1997;23(5):427–31.
34. Darwish AM, Amin AF, MD, and Mohammad SA. Laparoscopic management of paratubal and paraovarian cysts. J Soc Laparoscopic Surg. 2003;7:101–6.
35. Rasheed SM and Abdelmonem AM. Hydatid of Morgagni: a possible underestimated cause of unexplained infertility. Eur J Obstet Gynecol Reprod Biol. 2011;158(1):62–6.
36. Yablonski M, Sarge T, and Wild RA. Subtle variations in tubal anatomy in infertile women. Fertil Steril. 1990;54:455e8
37. Novak E, Novak ER, and Woodruff JD. Novak's Gynecologic and Obstetric Pathology: With Clinical and Endocrine Relations. 8th ed. Philadelphia: Saunders; 1979.
38. Abuzeid O, Raju R, Hebert J, and Abuzeid M. Surgical management of accessory tubal ostium. J Minim Invasive Gynecol. Nov 2016; 23(7):S130.
39. Benmokhtar S, Chauvin G, Chaibi R, and Watrelot A. Operative fertiloscopy results. About 67 cases. Gynecol Obstet Fertil. 2012; 40:204–7.
40. Roland M and Leistan M. Tuboplasty in 130 patients. Obstet Gynecol. 1972:3957–64.
41. Han H, Guan J, Wang Y, Zhang Q, and Shen H. Diagnosis and treatment of tubal diverticula: report of 13 cases. J Minim Invasive Gynecol. 2014;21(1):142–6.
42. Rubin Raju, Omar Abuzeid, John Hebert, and Mostafa Abuzeid. Surgical management of solitary tubal diverticula. J Minim Invasive Gynecol. Nov 2016;23(7):S121.
43. Dubuisson JB, de Jolinière JB, Aubriot FX, Darai E, Foulot H, and Mandelbrot L. Terminal tuboplasties by laparoscopy: 65 consecutive cases. Fertil. Steril. 1990;54(3):401–3
44. Lavergne N, Krimly A, Roge P, and Erny R. 1996. Results and indications of laparoscopic tubal tuboplasty. Contracept Fertil Steril. 1996;24:41–8.
45. Saleh WA and Dlugi AM. 1997. Pregnancy outcome after laparoscopic fimbrioplasty in non occlusive distal tubal disease. Fertil Steril. 1997;67:474–80.
46. Feinberg EC, Levens ED, and DeCherney AH. Infertility surgery is dead: only the obituary remains? Fertil Steril. 2008; 89(1):232–6
47. Watrelot A and Chauvin G. Current practice in tubal surgery and adhesion management: a review. Reproductive BioMedicine Online 2011;23:53–62.
48. The Practice Committee of the American Society for Reproductive Medicine. Committee opinion: role of tubal surgery in the era of assisted reproductive technology. Fertil Steril. 20121;97(3):539–45
49. Goldberg JM, Falcone T, and Diamond MP. Current controversies in tubal disease, endometriosis, and pelvic adhesion. Fertil Steril. 2019;112(3):417–25.
50. Bosteels J, Van Herendael B, Weyers S, and D'Hooghe T. The position of diagnostic laparoscopy in current fertility practice. J Reprod Med. 2009;54:126–32.

# 21

## ECTOPIC PREGNANCY

### *Focusing the Incidence after Assisted Reproductive Technologies*

**Liselotte Mettler, Ibrahim Alkatout, Vishvanath C. Karande, Rupinder Kaur Ruprai, and Meenu Agarwal**

### Introduction and reality of ectopic pregnancies

Usually the oocyte and the sperm meet in the ampullary part of the fallopian tube and fertilization takes place there. The growing embryo, morula, moves slowly toward the uterine cavity, rotating within the Fallopian tube, while differentiating into embryoblast and trophoblast. Implantation in the uterine cavity usually takes place after 5 or 6 days. Implantation of the zygote outside the uterine cavity occurs in about 2% of all pregnancies. Pregnancies outside the uterine cavity have been described for the last hundreds of years. Today, intraoperatively at laparoscopy, the product of conception and its surroundings, can be removed safely and submitted for histological examination (**Figures 21.1–21.3**).

The rate of ectopic pregnancies (EPs) has increased from 0.5% in 1970 to 2% today. Although the incidence is low, the prevalence of EP in all women presenting with first-trimester bleeding, lower abdominal pain, or a combination of the two to an emergency department is between 6% and 16%. These numbers justify a more intensive diagnosis due to the persistent suspicion of EP and a threshold for operative investigation [1].

The incidence of EP after Assisted Reproductive Technology (ART) is increased approximately 2.5–5-fold compared with natural conceptions, although this rate has been declining in recent years. EPs account for 31.9 pregnancy-related deaths per 100,000 pregnancies in the United States [2]. Primary risk factors for EP include smoking, intrauterine devices, previous EP, pelvic inflammatory disease, and tubal factors [3] as well as in the last 30 years ART techniques [4]. Studies have shown that the use of assisted hatching, higher transfer volume, deep fundal transfer, the day of embryo transfer (ET), changes in endometrial receptivity, and multiple ETs increase the incidence of EP [5, 6].

Women of the same age may possess different responses to ovarian stimulation, leading to a variation in the reproductive potential. Women of reproductive age with regular menses who respond poorly to ovarian stimulation or fecundity compared with others of the same age are defined as having decreased ovarian reserve (DOR) [7]. The prevalence of DOR is approximately 10% among infertile women and leads many

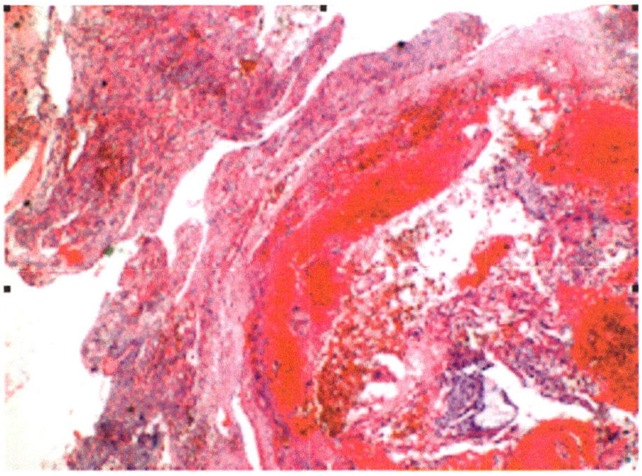

FIGURE 21.1 Gestational material being in organization next to hemorrhage and fibrin exudation as well as regressive altered villi.

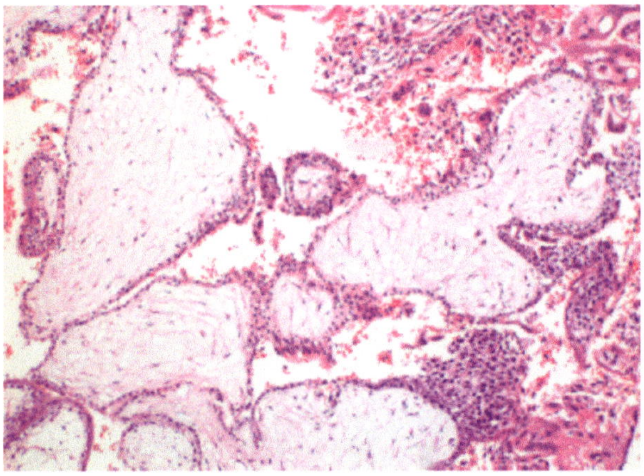

FIGURE 21.2 Trophoblastic giant cells next to regressive altered villous stroma, trophoblast, and decidual stroma.

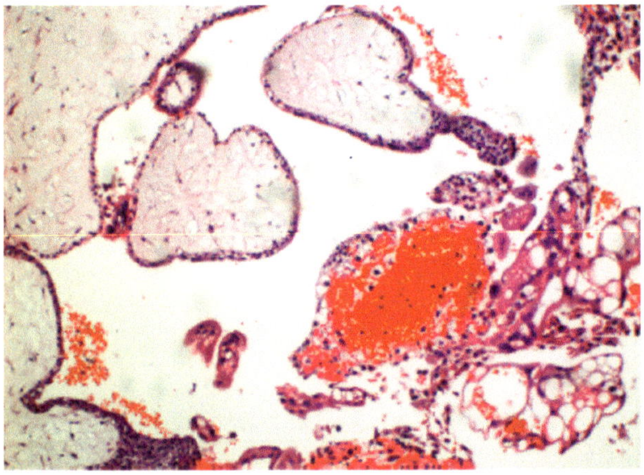

FIGURE 21.3 Regressive altered villous stroma, trophoblast, hemorrhage and fibrin, trophoblastic giant cells.

**TABLE 21.1: Major Contributing Factors (Risk Factors) for Ectopic Pregnancy**

| |
|---|
| Previous tubal surgery |
| History of ectopic pregnancy |
| Sexually transmitted disease |
| Pelvic inflammatory disease |
| *In utero* diethylstilbestrol exposure |
| History of infertility |
| Anatomical uterine/tubal abnormality |
| Previous tubal ligation |
| Previous or current IUD use |
| Assisted reproductive technologies |
| Current smoking |
| Nonwhite (all races other than white) |
| Age between 35 and 44 (compared to those from 15 to 24) |
| Induced abortion |
| T-shaped uterus |
| Myomata |
| Progestin-only contraceptives |

to seek ART. Several methods are available for detecting DOR. Follicle-stimulating hormone (FSH) is secreted by the anterior pituitary gland and promotes follicle development. Serum FSH levels increase with age, and an early follicular phase serum FSH level >10 IU/L is a predictor of DOR. In addition, Anti-Müllerian Hormone (AMH), the antral follicle count, ovarian volume, and the clomiphene citrate challenge test are also used to predict the ovarian reserve [8]. Women with DOR display decreased fertilization rates and increased blastocyst aneuploidy and miscarriage rates [9, 10].

Recent efforts have been made to predict the occurrence of EP prior to an IVF cycle, without defining a clear algorithm yet [11–12]. To explore the issue, EP rates between patients with DOR and those with normal ovarian reserve (NOR) following IVF-ET were compared and an increased incidence of EPs after *in vitro* fertilization in women with DOR was detected [13]. Major contributing factors for an EP are detailed in **Table 21.1**.

## Types of ectopic pregnancies

The majority of EPs are located in the fallopian tube (approximately 97%): ampulla, isthmus, and fimbria, in descending order. This might be accounted for by the narrowing of the tubal diameter from ampullary to isthmic region and the fact that fertilization begins in the ampulla. However, the ampullary region is the most distal place where ascending infections can cause phymosis and therefore either infertility or an increased risk for motility disorder. EP is often mentioned synonymously with tubal pregnancy due to the location of majority of the cases. Nevertheless, one must be aware of the unusual sites of EPs. About 3% are located in the rudimental uterine horn, ovary, abdominal cavity, broad ligament, cervix, and vagina or are simultaneously intra- and extrauterine [2].

Two hundred years ago, the mortality rate of EPs was over 60%. Today, it has decreased to 9% of pregnancy-related mortality and less than 1% of overall mortality in women. Despite a fivefold increase in the incidence of EP from 1970 to 1992, its mortality could be reduced by more than 90%. Until 1970, over 80% of EPs were not diagnosed before rupture, leading to a high rate of morbidity and mortality. Owing to the advances made in transvaginal ultrasound and radio immunoassays for serum β-hCG levels and an increased vigilance by clinicians with more experience of diagnostic laparoscopy, more than 80% of EPs are now diagnosed intact. This allows a more conservative management and is responsible for the decline from 35.5 deaths to 3.8 per 1,000 ectopics. The decrease of mortality is due to early diagnosis before the occurrence of hemoperitoneum and/or hypovolemic shock [2, 3].

Nevertheless, as ruptured EPs are responsible for 10%–15% of all pregnancy-related deaths, further improvement of earlier diagnosis is desirable. Earlier diagnosis is made by sensitive and specific radioimmunoassay for human chorionic gonadotropin (β-hCG), high-resolution transvaginal ultrasonography (TVS), and most importantly, laparoscopy. Before the improvement of these diagnostic methods, a majority of EPs were only detected after rupture and a life-threatening emergency [1, 4].

The great advances in diagnostic methods and the decrease of their side effects over the last 35 years has enabled the diagnosis of mildly symptomatic or even asymptomatic patients with EP. As a consequence, more than 80% of women with an EP are treated correctly before tubal rupture or severe intra-abdominal bleeding in most of the developed countries where the above-mentioned capabilities are available. The gain in knowledge and the advancing operative experience of EPs lead to a high rate of fertility-preserving operating methods. Despite all diagnostic and therapeutical progress and the decline in the invasiveness of laparoscopic procedures, in 50% of all women with EP presenting to an emergency department, the condition is not detected at the initial medical assessment [1, 5].

### Etiology and risk factors

The incidence of EPs is independent of maternal age and ethnic origin. Moreover, there is no accumulation at a certain place outside theuterus [1]. Theoretically, anything that impedes migration of the conceptus to the uterine cavity may predispose woman to develop an ectopic gestation. These may be intrinsic anatomic defects in the tubal epithelium, hormonal factors that interfere with normal transport of the conceptus, or pathologic conditions that affect normal tubal functioning. The hormonal interference is explained by the different effect that estrogen and gestagen show on the growth and the motility of the epithelial cilia. A disbalance of the hormonal concentration can lead to a longer stay of the developing morula in the fallopian tube. Other maternal reasons can be explained by a dysfunction of the epithelial cilia that can be caused by smoking [4, 6, 7].

### Diagnostics

1. **Preoperative assessment:** The aim of professional and target-aiming diagnostics is the early diagnosis and adequate treatment of an EP as well as minimizing the number of unnecessary laparoscopies. The suspicion of an extrauterine gravidity has to be excluded if a woman of reproductive age presents with abdominal pain and vaginal bleeding approximately 5–7 weeks after her last period and has a positive pregnancy test. Although these symptoms are common in women with early physiologic intrauterine pregnancy (IUP), extrauterine pregnancy, and women who may miscarry, they are nonspecific with a negative pregnancy test [8].

After a positive pregnancy test, additional unspecific parameter are a normal or slightly enlarged uterus, vaginal bleeding or spotting, pelvic pain triggered by manipulation of the cervix and a palpable adnexal mass. Although these parameters increase the risk of a prevalent EP and significant abdominal tenderness, guarding and rebound tenderness together with hypotension or syncopes can suggest a ruptured EP, these clinical parameters remain unspecific. Consequently, no clinical examination alone can reliably exclude EP. Apart from mimicking the symptoms of other gynecological and even nongynecological diseases, EPs come in many variations often causing no pain at vaginal examination. Severe pain can also be experienced in a normal pregnancy. Usually the earliest appearance of symptoms occurs in the 6th week after the last period. Patients with EP can show all symptoms of a normal early pregnancy, such as interruption of the normal menstrual period, nausea, vomiting, breast fullness, and fatigue. Beyond that, typical symptoms of EPs are lower abdominal pain and abnormal uterine bleeding, ranging from spotting to severe bleeding. Muscular defense and peritonism are indicative of intraperitoneal blood flowing. Severe hemorrhage leading to hypovolemia can cause syncope or tachycardia. There may be tenderness on cervical motion. On examination, the uterus is enlarged and soft in consistency. In some cases, an adnexal mass can be palpated [1]. Lower abdominal pain is caused by the distension of the peritoneum due to the swelling of the affected tube or free blood in the abdominal cavity.

Usually the pain is alternating and spasmodic, followed by intervals free of complaints. In general, the intensity and frequency of pain increases [4]. Another leading symptom is vaginal bleeding. An extrauterine gravidity can be associated with a complete amenorrhea, recurrent or persistent bleedings, or even a normal menstrual cycle. As most extrauterine gravidities produce only decreased β-hCG, the uterus is not able to sustain the decidually transformed endometrium. Therefore, it often comes to breakthrough bleedings appearing asspotting [4]. Hence, additional diagnostic tests are necessary to exclude an EP. These include repeated monitoring of β-hCG serum level, transvaginal ultrasonography, and in some cases, even diagnostic curettage or measurement of serum progesterone level. The two diagnostic parameters that have to be monitored are β-hCG serum levels and repeated transvaginal ultrasonography.

2. **β-hCG serum levels:** The first diagnostic step is the assurance of an existing pregnancy, which can be detected about 10 days following ovulation or ET, 5 days after induced ovulation in ART, using a sensitive β-hCG serum array. β-hCG is a glycoprotein produced by the syncytiotrophoblast starting with secretion on day 5 to day 8. A serum array detects levels as low as 5 mIU/mL, while the detection limit in urine is 20–50 mIU/mL. After diagnosis of an existing pregnancy, β-hCG level can be used as a follow-up titer and its change can be recognized and monitored. The β-hCG levels double every 1.5 days in the first 5 weeks of a regular gestation. After 7 weeks, the sequence for double titers is 3.5 days. In comparison, only 30% of EPs show a normal β-hCG course. In 70% of EPs β-hCG levels rise more slowly and reach a plateau or even show a decrease in serum levels.

An abnormal β-hCG pattern is highly suspicious for an ectopic gestation or a no longer intact gestation. Besides the unconventional rise of β-hCG level compared to normal pregnancies, ectopic pregnancy can be differentiated from a spontaneous abortion by a slower decrease of serum titer. Therefore, ectopic pregnancies and intrauterine pregnancies have a considerable overlap. Accordingly, a single measurement is insufficient and only a serial measurement can give the necessary additional information for the location of gestational sac. Although ectopic pregnancies can have normal as well as rising, falling or plateau β-hCG levels, the serial measurements of β-hCG levels are most useful to confirm or to prove false the fetal viability instead of giving straight evidence for an ectopic pregnancy. Taken together, an extrauterine pregnancy often presents with β-hCG levels below the expected value and the increase is delayed. The trend can be stagnating or decreasing [7, 9–11].

3. **Ultrasound imaging:** The development of transvaginal ultrasonography has enormously improved identification and visualization of both normally developing embryos and abnormalities. With a gestational age of about 5 weeks, a normally developing gestational sac can be visualized showing an ovoid collection of fluid clinging to the endometrium stripe as well as a yolk sac of 8 mm or more in diameter. However, a pseudo-gestational sac can mimic a gestational sac at an early stage. The pseudo-gestational sac is often situated in the center of uterine cavity. Its margin is homogenous and round, but it is difficult to define its boundary to the outside tissue. By contrast, a physiologic gestational sac is asymmetric and contains two concentric rings, separated by a thin echogenic layer. At a gestational age of 6–6.5 weeks, the embryonic structures measure 4–5 mm and cardiac activity might already be detected.

The threshold value of β-hCG serum reliably showing sonographic signs of an intrauterine growing pregnancy lies between 1,000 and 2,000 mIU/mL, depending on the ultrasound unit and the experience of the examiner. Even though β-hCG levels of women with EP are often less than 2,000 mIU/mL at presentation, an empty uterus does not allow a clear differentiation between an early undetected (IUC) and an EP. The regular or irregular increase of β-hCG level is the assisting factor interpreting the ultrasound signals; but again, β-hCG levels alone do not allow discrimination between a regular, an irregular, and an EP. The identification of an intrauterine gestational sac plus a yolk sac or additional embryonic signs minimizes the doubt of an EP. However, it is important to consider the rare possibility of a heterotopic pregnancy whose total number is growing with the increase of assisted reproduction.

Verifying an EP by the means of an ultrasound scan is burdened with a high false-negative rate. The infrequent identification of an extrauterine gestational sac containing a yolk sac and possibly an embryo with cardiac activity confirms the suspected diagnosis. Supporting the diagnosis of an extrauterine gestation is an empty uterus, a cystic, or solid extrauterine mass adjacent to the fallopian tube or the ovary (including the tubal ring sign, representing a tubal gestational sac), and echogenic or sonolucent free fluid in the cul-de-sac (**Figures 21.5** and **21.6**). The combination of transvaginal ultrasonography and serial quantitative β-hCG serum levels detects with a sensitivity of 96% and a specificity of 97% in an EP, and remains the gold standard as well as the most cost-effective strategy for diagnosing EP. A positive fetal heartbeat is often absent because extrauterine pregnancies seldom develop vitally and only display an agglomeration of trophoblast tissue and a surrounding hematoma [8, 12, 13].

4. **Progesterone serum level:** Progesterone levels can be useful in the substantiation of a suspected EP and in the identification of women at risk for EP. However, the progesterone serum level only has a sensitivity of 15% to detect pregnancy failure. As a stable marker in the first trimester, a serum level above 22 ng/mL speaks for a viable IUC, whereas levels under 5 ng/mL are indicative of a nonviable pregnancy. Nevertheless, the progesterone level cannot

**TABLE 21.2: The Three Pillars That Substantiate an Early Suspicion of Ectopic Pregnancy**

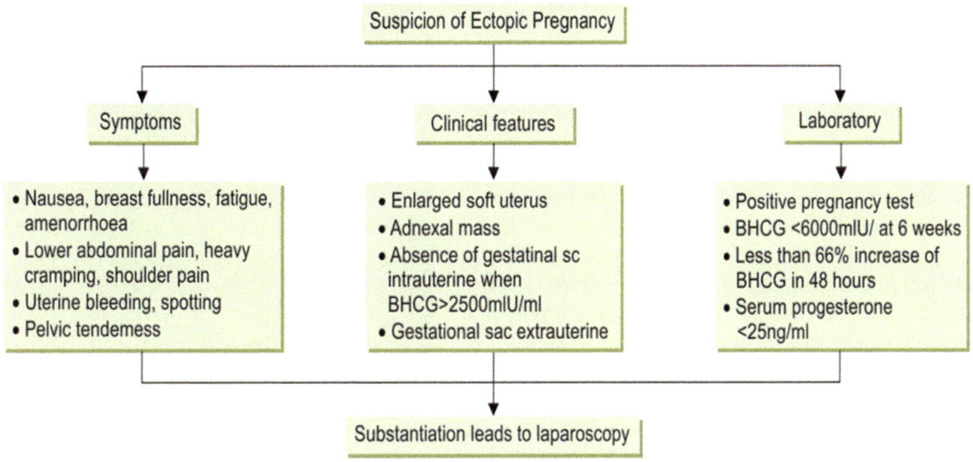


positively differentiate between EP and IUC. Furthermore, values in between the limiting values are more common and they make the progesterone serum level inconclusive. In conclusion, progesterone as a supplemental factor for identifying EPs has not proved itself and can therefore be disregarded [2, 8, 14].

5. **Hysteroscopy and uterine diagnostic curettage**: Uterine diagnostic curettage under vision can detect gestational material in the form of chorionic villi. If they are not detected, the suspicion of an EP is hardened. Nevertheless, hysteroscopy and a diagnostic curettage could abort an early and desired physiological pregnancy, and therefore its indication is really not given but has to be mentioned as it is practiced by some of us around the world. Diagnostic curettage provides additional information when β-hCG levels are falling or when β-hCG levels are elevated and there is no ultrasound confirmation of an IUC [8].
6. **Puncture of the pouch of Douglas** has become obsolete. Before the establishment of ultrasonography and β-hCG blood examination, the puncture of blood in the pouch of Douglas was an additional indicator leading to the clinical but indefinite diagnosis of extra-uterine gravidity [4]. Diagnosis of EP can be challenging, as its symptoms are often similar to normal early pregnancies or early miscarriages, and therefore confusing. Women suffering from EP can present with one-sided pelvic pain and variable bleeding. However, 20% of women with first trimester bleeding deliver a healthy baby even though bleeding might be the only sign of an EP. The awareness of the eventuality of an EP is most crucial for early detection. Doubling of the β-hCG serum levels every 2–3 days should be registered in a normal gestation. Nevertheless, about 10% of normal pregnancies vary in this regime as well as up to 60% of EPs demonstrate and imitate this doubling time. Transvaginal sonography has a reliable, sensitive predictive value if β-hCG levels are higher than 1,000 mIU/mL. The detection rate is then 98%, depending on the quality of the ultrasound unit and the experience of the examiner. An additional sign of an EP that might assist in an early diagnosis once an extrauterine pregnancy is suspected is culdocentesis. This used to be a more prognostic feature in times when β-hCG monitoring and transvaginal ultrasound scan were not available, presenting nonclotting blood after aspiration of the free fluid in the pouch of Douglas [2].

In summary, the straightforward diagnosis of EP is based on three pillars: symptoms that can be determined during physical examination, clinical features that appear in ultrasound scan, and laboratory tests that can substantiate a primary suspicion (**Table 21.2**). Pregnancy

After the suspicion of EP has hardened, the next steps should be routine. If the necessary clinical and laboratory investigations are carried out and the diagnosis of EP is made early, the risk for severe hemorrhage and rupture is minimal (**Table 21.3**).

**TABLE 21.3: Diagnostic and Operative Processing in Case of Potential Ectopic Pregnancy**

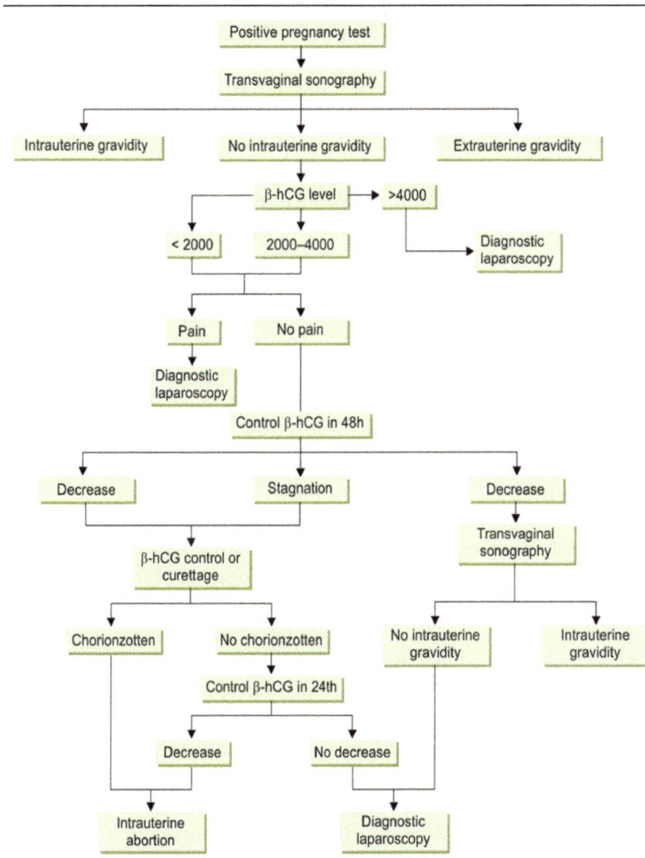

## Treatment

In view of the high incidence of EPs among pregnant women with first trimester bleeding, further investigation must be undertaken to exclude an EP. Once an EP has been confirmed, a treatment plan has to be created. The treatment decision includes operative management and medical treatment as well as the option not to treat and follow up with clinical and laboratory tests. It is known that many early EPs result in spontaneous abortion and reabsorption and this might make aggressive treatment unnecessary. Medical treatment with methotrexate is restricted to a few limited indications.

There is no general policy of treating suspected EPs, and each patient requires individual assessment particularly within an ART treatment circle. The indication for a primary laparotomy is given for patients with circulatory instability and a massive hemoperitoneum when the medical team is not trained for immediate and emergency laparoscopy or contraindications for laparoscopy exist. The other indication for primary laparotomy can be an isthmic location with a high intramural proportion and a severe risk for uncontrollable intraoperative bleeding. In all other circumstances, the operative management should be laparoscopy.

## Surgical treatment of tubal pregnancy

Several different conservative techniques have been developed to preserve tubal function. These include salpingotomy, partial salpingectomy followed by anastomosis, salpingectomy, and extirpation of the tubal pregnancy through the fimbrial end by milking it from the distant ampulla. Independent of the type of surgery, the existence of tubal abnormalities on the contralateral site predispose the patient to recurrence [7].

### *Salpingostomy, meaning the ostium is incised*

Before incising the fallopian tube, one has to recall that the tube is composed of the tunica mucosa and two muscular layers. The inner layer is oriented in a circular fashion and the outer layer is oriented in a longitudinal fashion to the axis of the tube. The surrounding blood vessels originate from uterine and ovarian blood supply and often lay in the thick longitudinal muscle layer. This branching is located in the mesosalpinx between the fallopian tube and the ovary. The lumen of the fallopian tube is paved with ciliated secretory cells that might be damaged after an ascending infection, previous EP, or any other circumstances, which might disrupt morula transport.

Preservation of the tube should be attempted in all patients without contraindications or explicit wish for salpingectomy. By preserving the tube, fertility can be maintained. Precondition for a tubal-preserving procedure is hemodynamic stability and evidence that the tube is not ruptured. The EP should be less than 5 cm in diameter, the gestational sac must be located in the ampulla, infundibulum or isthmic portion of the tube, and there should be no pathology of the contralateral tube (**Figure 21.4**).

Nevertheless, the majority of EPs located in infundibulum have to be operated either by salpingectomy or by segmental tubectomy and secondary reanastomosis after a certain interval [3, 4]. Whenever feasible, salpingostomy is preferred to salpingectomy. However, approximately 8% of patients have persistent EP after salpingostomy.

After careful inspection and identification of tubal pregnancy, the tubal part is mobilized with one or two forceps. Before preparation of the tube and the EP vasopressin, 20 IU diluted in 100 mL of normal saline is injected into the mesosalpinx. A syringe with a 22-gauge injection needle can be placed either through one of the working trocars under sight or the outer sheath of a Veress needle can be placed directly through the abdominal wall under sight, lateral to the deep inferior epigastric vessels. Alternatively,

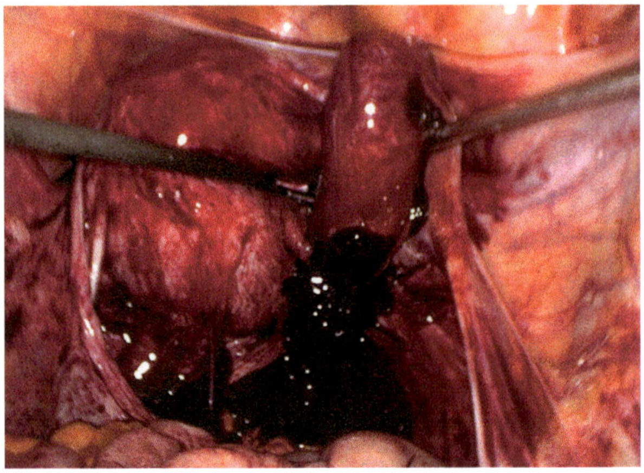

FIGURE 21.4 Tubal pregnancy already protruding out of the fimbrial end into the abdominal cavity.

vasopressin is inserted by a 22-gauge spinal needle through the sheath. Close attention must be given because of the good vascularization of the mesosalpinx and risk of laceration. After gently grasping the serosa, 10–20 mL of the solution is injected and controlled by a visible swelling of mesosalpinx just below the EP and over the antimesenteric surface of tubal segment containing gestational products. Hemostatic effect lasts for about two hours permitting a safer preparation.

Vasopressin must not be allowed to infiltrate into a blood vessel, as this can lead to acute arterial hypertension, bradycardia, and even death [3, 7]. Besides, the better operative management vasopressin has a positive side effect on prognosis. As trophoblast has a high cell division, its metabolic rate is equivalently high. The iatrogenic anoxia reduces the oxygen supply for about two hours and thereby reduces the persistence risk by a factor of 5. The use of vasopressin is contraindicated in patients with chronic vascular diseases (e.g., ischemic heart disease) [3].

*Salpingotomy* = Evacuation after incision by Aqua dissection or Aspiration, Luxation, and Preparation, meaning a new opening = ostium is created.

*Incision and evacuation*: A unipolar needle electrocautery (cutting current of 10 W), scissors, or a knife electrode is introduced through the 6 mm port. Alternatively, a $CO_2$ laser with a power density of 10,000 W/cm$^2$ can be used. A 1–2 cm longitudinal incision is made on the most distended part of the antimesenteric tubal wall, which is often of bluish discoloration, using a cutting or blended current (20 or 70 W). Usually, it is possible to identify the different tubal wall layers: serosa, muscularis externa and interna, and the mucosa. It is important to cut through all layers for the whole length of the incision.

If the product of conception cannot be identified after the primary incision, it is necessary to advance deeper as the muscularis externa and interna and/or the mucosa might be still intact. Once the lumen is open, the friable gestational sac bulges out of the wound and can be evacuated by aspiration [16]. If the product of conception is surrounded by coagel clotting, it must be extracted through tubal incision with alternating pressurized suction and irrigation or with the aid of grasping or biopsy forceps. The site of implantation is then irrigated extensively.

The irrigation fluid must drain from both sites—salpingotomy and fimbrial end [3]. Using a high-pressure irrigating solution, forceful irrigation in the salpingotomy can dislodge the gestation from its implantation. Combining hydro dissection and gentle blunt dissection with a suction irrigator, product remnants are removed from the tube. If possible, this technique is preferable to extraction in pieces as products of conception can then adhere to the implantation site by a ligamentous structure containing blood vessels. Minimal bleeding from the tubal bed is normal and ceases in most cases spontaneously [2]. To remove the product of gestation, it can be cut and taken out in small pieces; but generally, it is safer to extract the material with a spoon after dilating one of the working trocars to 11 mm. In most cases it is advisable to use an endobag for safe extraction of the gestational product. Suturing of the salpingostomy incision is controversial. Usually, the incision does not require suturing. The tubal incision is supposed to heal by secondary intention. Only if the defect is very wide and its edges do not come together spontaneously or the mucosa everts might suturing be recommended. In earlier years, we always closed third defect by sutures, but had to learn that if diligent suturing is not giving the patient a better chance of healing, it is tubal defect.

If the defect has to be closed, a continual suture or single knots approximating the edges with single 4-0 resorbable sutures excepting the mucosa are made. The follow-up and prognosis for recurrent extrauterine gravidities are not improved after suturing [2, 3, 22]. Oozing from the tube is common and usually ceases spontaneously. Slight bleeding from mucosal bed or from incisions of the tubal walls can be treated conservatively in a majority of cases. Bleeding can appear from the incision margins or the site of implantation. The bleeding situation can best be observed by inspection of the tube "underwater." The first hemostatic option should be a hemostatic tamponade applied with grasping forceps. Compression of bleeding location for 5 minutes is sufficient in most cases. Alternatively, for conservative bleeding management, adnexa can be elevated out of pelvis for an indirect compression of the vessels of mesosalpinx. Continuous bleeding points can be detected and coagulated with bipolar coagulation in a tissue-saving method. Stronger venous or even arterial bleeding can be controlled effectively and safe by using electrocoagulation with bipolar forceps, particularly if combined with continuous irrigation, especially in the muscle layer. A superficial eschar, not involving the tubal mucosa, heals normally.

With uncontrolled bleeding and bleeding that cannot be localized, meso-salpingeal vessels can be coagulated selectively until bleeding stops. Ultima ratio is the tubectomy [1, 3, 7]. Before terminating the operation, another "underwater" examination is done by the introduction of 500–1000 mL of saline solution or Adept. The abdominal cavity and the pelvic organs are once again inspected carefully [22].

### *Partial salpingectomy*

If salpingotomy cannot resolve the problem, partial salpingectomy can be tried before salpingectomy is performed. Indications for a partial salpingectomy are tubal rupture, pregnancy located in the isthmus, or a recurrent tubal pregnancy. In most cases of isthmic pregnancy linear salpingostomy is unsuccessful, as these gestations grow through lumen of the tube and into tunica muscularis; therefore, segmental resection is recommended.

After evacuation of hemoperitoneum and possibly infiltration of vasopressin in the corresponding mesosalpinx, coagulation of the tubal part is done by bipolar forceps on both ends of the affected part, including the corresponding mesosalpinx. The proximal and distal boundaries of affected tubal segment are grasped with forceps and thoroughly coagulated from antimesenteric surface to mesosalpinx. The segment is then cut with little risk for bleeding. After resecting the affected part of the tube, mesosalpinx is cauterized stepwise. Particular attention is given to arcuate anastomosing branches of the ovarian and uterine vessels. In the next step, mesosalpinx is cut. The tubal segment is taken out after dilation of one of the working trocars to 11 mm. If the piece is too big or unstable, the use of an endobag should be preferred. Hemostasis is achieved by bipolar coagulation of any bleeding parts. If the surgeon is experienced in such procedures, partial salpingectomy can be completed by reanastomosis. Otherwise, the reanastomosis is postponed to a later date.

### *Salpingectomy*

Salpingectomy, where the tube is removed from its anatomical attachments, is the alternative procedure to salpingostomy. This may be a safer method for persistent bleeding or tubal rupture. The indications for salpingectomy include no desire for future pregnancies, recurrent tubal pregnancies, and the occurrence of extrauterine pregnancy after a failed sterilization or a previously reconstructed tube. Other indications for salpingectomy are made intraoperatively, for example, severe adhesions, hydrosalpinx, tubal rupture, persistent bleeding after a safe tubal procedure, or if the tubal pregnancy is over 5 cm in diameter. After evacuation of hematoperitoneum, the proximal isthmus of the tube and mesosalpinx are coagulated and dissected and excised stepwise, beginning with the proximal isthmic portion and progressing to fimbriated end of the tube. The tube is immobilized with one or two grasping forceps. Coagulation of the intramural tubal segment to be excised is performed with bipolar cautery and cut either with laser, electrocautery, or scissors.

Alternative methods include stapling devices, harmonic energy, or endoloops. After preparation of the tube containing gestational sac, the tube is removed from peritoneal cavity in an endobag through one of the instrument trocars that has been dilated to 10 mm. Afterward, a final inspection is made to coagulate any bleeding caused by grasping the tube and the mesosalpinx and to make sure that the product of conception has not slipped out of the tube unnoticed [22].

### *Extirpation of tubal pregnancy through the fimbrial end*

If the product of conception is located at the outer region of fallopian tube or fimbrial end, it can be removed by grasping tubal segment and stepwise milking the gestational product out of fimbriae of the tube (**Figure 21.5a,b**)

Nevertheless, this operation technique is only feasible if the total extraction of the EP is assured. The product of conception is gently pushed until it is extruded. The stepwise movements begin in the proximal part and gently push the product into abdominal cavity. Alternatively, small EPs located at the very outside of fimbriae can be extracted by aspiration.

Then, however, there is no histologic confirmation of an EP. After removal of trophoblast, suction tip should be placed in the tubal end and the tube cleaned by suction and irrigation. Remnants are washed out of the tube without damage to the tubal wall. Although this type of operation is gentle and organ saving, it has a higher rate of incomplete removal and therefore a higher risk of recurrence and of trophoblast residuals. This is because many EPs are not implanted in the intraluminal tubal portion and therefore cannot be completely removed in a gentle way without severe damage to the tubal wall. In addition, an eventual extraluminal pregnancy, implanted between serosa and tunica muscularis, would be treated more mildly by salpingostomy. Therefore, the indication for this operative technique should be made reluctantly. For cases of intraluminal EPs that are not yet visible and where it is postulated that the tubal wall has not yet been invaded, irrigation and suction of the tube might dislodge and expel the product of conception into peritoneal cavity and thereby avoid an

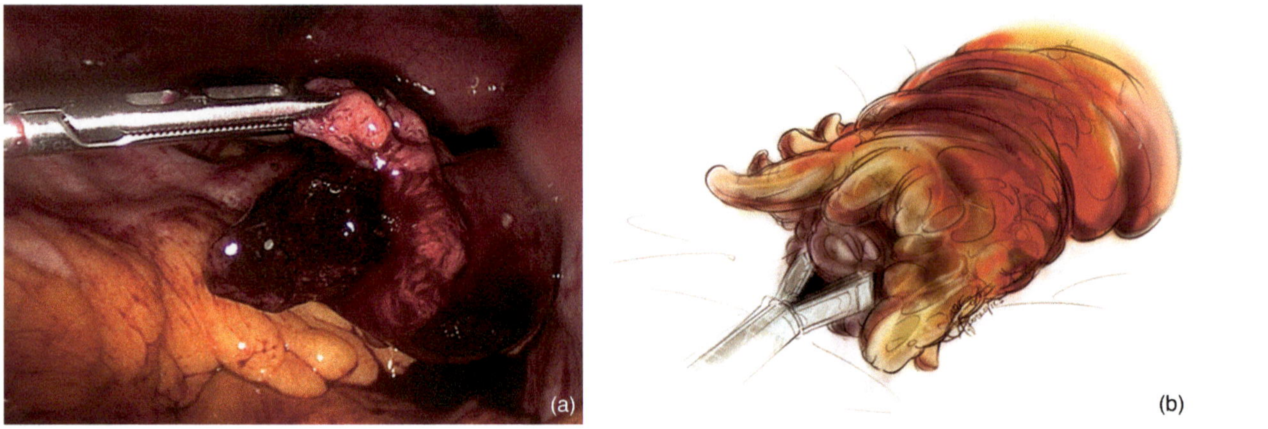

FIGURE 21.5 Protruding EP of the fimbrial end with the option of extirpation without incising the tube (a). Schematic drawing of the Protruding EP out of the fimbrial end with the option of extirpation without incising the tube (b).

incision of the tubal wall. Postoperative examination of β-hCG levels below the detectable limit must be carried out twice [4].

## Surgical technique for nontubal ectopic pregnancy

### *Ovarian pregnancy*

Localization of primary ovarian gravidity can be separated into a superficial and an intrafollicular type due to their pathogenesis. Ninety percent of ovarian gravidities are located intrafollicularly. The unusual site and rarity of ovarian pregnancies lead to a more complex clinical course, beginning with the difficulty in making an early and accurate diagnosis, an inconsistent therapeutic approach, leading to an unpredictable outcome and a life-threatening status if the ovary ruptures.

1. *Superficial pattern:* The implantation takes place in an ovarian focus of endometriosis.
2. *Intrafollicular pattern:*
   - *Primary:* Insemination of an ovum that has not yet ovulated.
   - *Secondary:* After regular ovulation implantation of the inseminated ovum in the follicle or corpus luteum.

The exact etiology is still unclear. It is postulated that the superficial form is correlated to extra genital endometriosis. The presumption is that fertilization occurs extraovarian and abundant granulosa cells of the zygote adhere to the ruptured follicle. The intrafollicular pattern allows the division into two subunits. The subcortical or cortical place of development is associated with insemination in an unruptured follicle and is called primary, whereas juxta follicular or secondary implantation postulates that inseminated ovum after regular ovulation is placed in deeper parts of the ovary in a second step.

Preoperative diagnosis of ovarian pregnancy is difficult as the clinical findings are similar to those of tubal pregnancy, hemorrhagic ovarian cyst, endometrioma, and other pelvic diseases. The defined diagnosis of an ovarian gravity is still bound to the four anatomical and histopathological criteria suggested by Spiegelberg in 1878:

1. The fallopian tube and the infundibulum with its fimbriae of the affected site are intact. There is no connection between the fallopian tube and the ovary.
2. The gestation should occupy the normal position of ovary.
3. The gestation should be connected to uterus by uterine ligament.
4. Ovarian tissue must be present in the specimen attached to gestation sac.

The Spiegelberg criteria can be extended to include the follow-up of the serum β-hCG levels. Criteria number 4 is no longer compulsory in view of the improved operative methods. The traditional operative treatment for ovarian pregnancies has been oophorectomy. However, the desire to maintain reproductive capability and improvements in laparoscopy has more recently led to the ovarian-preserving operational technique.

The first operative steps are the same as for tubal pregnancy. Once the EP has been localized and bleeding is under control, an operative plan has to be decided upon. This is either oophorectomy, wedge resection (in both cases by laparotomy or by laparoscopy), or laparoscopic enucleation of the ovarian pregnancy (**Figure 21.6**). Laparoscopic enucleation of the gestational product is the gentlest type of operation for ovarian pregnancy. By enucleating gestational sac bluntly from ovary, the surrounding ovarian tissue is protected to the greatest possible extent. Careful surgical extraction of the trophoblast tissue from the place of nidation under optical magnification is an essential precondition (**Figure 21.6A**).

Gestational sac is enucleated with no more than the outer margins of the functional ovary. In the overview, hemorrhage from the ruptured EP was identified. In the background, a soft, slightly enlarged uterus was found. The left and right fallopian tubes were normal without dilation or bleeding from fimbrial end; however, the left ovary was enlarged to approximately 6.5–7.0 cm in diameter with a central bleeding defect. The right ovary showed a fresh corpus luteum cyst without bleeding. Manipulation of the left ovary led to bleeding and rupture of the cyst, and for management after suction (**Figure 21.6B**) 10 mL of diluted POR 8â solution (5 IU ornipressin in 100 mL saline) was injected into the infundibulo-pelvic ligament to achieve vasoconstriction (**Figure 21.6C**). The product of conception was bluntly prepared and enucleated from the orthotopic ovarian tissue (**Figure 21.6D,E**) and removed from left ovary using microscissors and spoon forceps (**Figure 21.6F**). After complete separation of the trophoblast from the left ovary, it could be easily removed from abdominal cavity through a 20 mm trocar in the midline using the 10 mm spoon forceps. Adequate hemostasis on the ovarian tissue was maintained with the use of endocoagulation.

Histopathological examination of the tissues removed from the left ovary showed signs of diffuse bleeding alongside chorion villi,

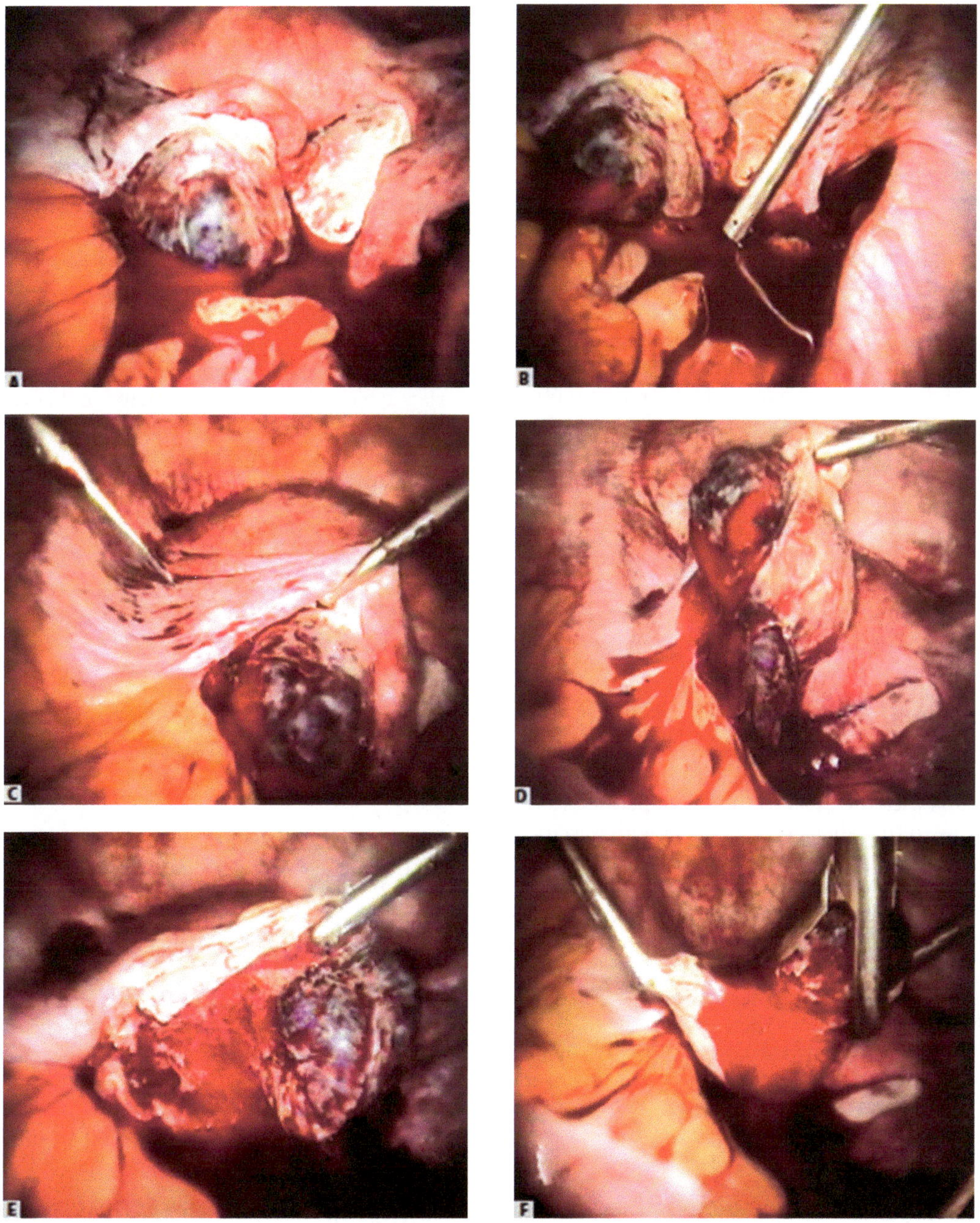

**FIGURE 21.6** (A–F): (A) Overview after creating a pneumoperitoneum for diagnostic laparoscopy. Bleeding from the ruptured EP of the left ovary. In the background, the slightly enlarged uterus and the right ovary with the corpus luteum cyst; (B) suction of the blood out of the cul-de-sac; (C) preparation of the left ovary and injection of ornipressin into the infundibulo-pelvic ligament; (D) blunt preparation and enucleation of the gestational sac from the orthotopic ovarian tissue; (E) Removal of the product of conception by enucleation. Healthy ovarian tissue can be seen on the left; (F) removal after complete separation of the trophoblast from the ovary.

decidual cells, and decidual changed stroma with normal ovarian cortical tissue in the outer margins. The problem of leaving behind the remaining trophoblast material or disseminated trophoblast tissue is mentioned in context with tubal pregnancy.

After performing laparoscopic enucleation technique, an adequate follow-up of the β-hCG serum level decrease is a necessary part of the postoperative monitoring regime. Operative laparoscopy has the benefit of reduced morbidity, reduced hospitalization, and rapid recovery of the patient. Because it has the advantage of reducing postoperative adhesions compared to laparotomy, it is the preferable technique for treatment of ovarian gestation after laparoscopic diagnosis, especially for women who wish to preserve their fertility potential. With more extensive use of pelviscopy to evaluate abnormal quantitative β-hCG values, intact ovarian pregnancy can be diagnosed at an early stage and hemorrhage or hypovolemic shock can be avoided [20].

### *Extraluminal ectopic pregnancy*

EP is defined as extraluminal when the gestational product is situated between muscularis externa and serosa. Etiology is a fast-growing tubal pregnancy with early infiltration of the tubal wall. Incision with monopolar needle or hook over the point of maximum distention results in the product of conception slipping out without the need of a long incision. Irrigation of the wound does not lead to liquid flowing out of the fimbrial end as there is no connection to the tubal lumina and its opening should be avoided if possible. β-hCG has to be controlled.

### *Ectopic abdominal pregnancy*

Ectopic abdominal pregnancy can either be primary or secondary if a tubal pregnancy ruptures and implants abdominally. This rare localization occurs in only about 1% of all EPs. Nevertheless, it has a high morbidity and mortality rate and makes detection by ultrasound or magnetic resonance imaging (MRI) necessary. Laparoscopic removal is possible if the tumor is detected early and does not involve vessels that can cause uncontrollable bleeding. Due to comparatively few symptoms, abdominal gravidity is often recognized very late. The usual clinical features, such as persistent diffuse abdominal pain, nausea, and vomiting, often appear at a late stadium, and sometimes only painful fetal movements in the upper abdomen are recognized. Treatment of an advanced abdominal pregnancy is associated with an enormous risk for life-threatening maternal bleeding. Removal of placenta is dependent on its localization as it can be implanted on any organ in the abdominal cavity. Sometimes, placenta is better left intra-abdominally to be calcified and reabsorbed or embolized by an interventional radiologist prior to removal at a second intervention. Its management is strictly by laparotomy. It has not occurred or been described after IVF/ICSI and ET.

### *Interstitial or cornual pregnancy/ rudimental uterine horn*

The intramural or interstitial part of the fallopian tube is about 1 cm long and begins with the tubal ostium, then permeates the myometrium leading to the fallopian tube. This highly vascularized area has to be passed by the sperm on its way to fertilization and backward by the embryo before nidation takes place in the uterine cavity. Anatomy of this area makes conservative operating procedures difficult. This rare type of tubal pregnancy occurs in 1 of 5,000 live births (2%–4% of all EPs) and has an increased risk of traumatic rupture with hemorrhagic shock and maternal death. Its mortality rate is about 2%. This is due to the high vascularity of this area where the uterine and ovarian vessels join together. This localization is a great challenge even for experienced surgeons. The classical treatment methods are laparotomy, uterine horn resection, or even hysterectomy. Laparotomy can be necessary if expert laparoscopic knowledge is not available.

Intramural or interstitial pregnancy lies deep in the myometrium, and therefore has to be treated conservatively or by laparoscopy with the possibility to convert quickly to laparotomy in combination with hysteroscopy. Cornual pregnancy, by contrast, implants in the same anatomical area of the tube but opens to the uterine cavity. Therefore, the operative method of choice can be hysteroscopy. True cornual gestations can be respected by hysteroscopy using electrosurgery. Alternatively, laparoscopy can be combined with a hysteroscopic approach. If the overlying myometrium is thick and intact, removal can be completely performed by hysteroscopy. To avoid uterine perforation, larger pregnancies can be removed by curettage under laparoscopic guidance. Intraoperatively, it has to be decided whether the overlaying myometrium is thin enough to respect the gestational product by laparoscopy [2].

In most cases, the corresponding part has to be resected. A major part of the tube can be saved in this way, but end-to-end anastomosis has only a low success rate as the interstitial part is completely destroyed. If pregnancy has eroded through myometrium, depending on the experience of the surgeon, it may be better to perform laparotomy to evacuate pregnancy. No matter what solution is taken, it should always be possible to perform an immediate laparotomy [3, 7]. Vasopressin is used in the same way and in the same concentration as for tubal pregnancy at any other site. The thinnest interstitial portion has to be coagulated properly with bipolar forceps before the lumen is incised. Once the lumen is open, the gestational product is removed in the same way as for tubal pregnancy at a more distal location.

Hemostasis is performed with bipolar forceps and the uterus has to be reconstructed. Reconstruction can be performed by extracorporeal or intracorporeal knotting techniques. The best anatomic reconstructing effect is given by inverted single knots in one layer [24]. Resection of the cornu is done step by step using bipolar coagulation. Severe bleeding can lead to coagulation of the ascending branch of the uterine artery as well as the utero-ovarian arteries [3]. The risk of acute and severe bleeding leads to preoperative preparation of several blood units of packed red blood cells. Prior consent of the patient should be obtained for a possible laparotomy.

### *Intraligamental gravidity*

This entity is very rare and occurs in about 1 of 250 EPs. For intraligamental development, the gestational sac must split the oviduct precisely between the leaves of the broad ligament. Amnion, at least, must remain intact to permit the fetus to continue to develop in its extraperitoneal sac. Rupture must occur early enough so that the villi are capable of expanding their areas of nidation. Anatomically intraligamental gravidity is bordered anteriorly and posteriorly by the two leaves of the broad ligament.

### *Cervical and vaginal pregnancy*

The criteria for a cervical pregnancy have been described by Rubin in 1911:

- Cervical glands must be present opposite the placental attachment.
- The attachment of placenta to cervix must be intimate.
- Placenta must be below the peritoneal reflection of the anterior and posterior surfaces of uterus.
- Fetal elements must not be within the uterine cavity [26].

Cervical and vaginal pregnancies are threatening localizations for the patient.

### *Simultaneous intra- and extrauterine pregnancies*

The incidence of a simultaneous intra- and extrauterine gravidity has become a remarkable differential diagnosis with the increase of ART methods. Having detected an intrauterine gravidity, a simultaneous extrauterine pregnancy is not usually expected. In a majority of the cases, simultaneous pregnancy is an incidental finding. Persistent abdominal pain or other clinical features alongside an irregular rise in the β-hCG level can lead to this infrequent diagnosis. Once a simultaneous pregnancy has been discovered, the operative method of choice is laparoscopic salpingectomy. Alternative methods to preserve the fallopian tube do not allow postoperative β-hCG measurements due to the existing intrauterine gestation and therefore cannot be used as a therapeutic option.

### *Medical treatment*

The predominant drug is methotrexate, but other systemic drugs can also be used to treat EP, for example, actinomycin D, prostaglandins, and RU486. In view of the uncertainty of treatment success and possible adverse side effects, the indication for a conservative treatment has to be weighed up carefully.

Methotrexate is a well-studied folic acid antagonist. It deactivates dihydrofolate reductase that can inhibit the synthesis of deoxyribonucleic and ribonucleic acid. Methotrexate can therefore disrupt the rapidly dividing trophoblastic cells. The expected time to resolution of the EP is 3–7 weeks after methotrexate application. The selective use of methotrexate can be as effective as surgery, although adverse side effects are possible such as bone marrow suppression, elevated liver enzymes, rash, alopecia, stomatitis, nausea, diarrhea, and to a lesser extent pleuritis, dermatitis, conjunctivitis, gastritis, and enteritis. The success rate of methotrexate is up to 94%. Nevertheless, this depends on the β-hCG level. The lower the serum level at the beginning of the therapy, the higher the success rate.

The use of medical treatment for extrauterine pregnancy is only indicated if the invasiveness of treatment can be diminished (**Table 21.3**). The indication for methotrexate treatment has to be recommended carefully and reserved for special situations. The use of methotrexate to destroy an EP has been advocated for women with an atypical localization in the cervix, interstitially, cornual, or in the abdominal cavity, an incomplete resolution of surgically treated ectopic gestation, residual trophoblast tissue, or persisting low β-hCG levels after curettage with no evidence of trophoblast material in the histological examination. Furthermore, patients with a high operative risk and contraindications to anesthesia, for example, after induced ovarian hyperstimulation syndrome and patients who are expected to have extensive intraperitoneal abdominal adhesions might be optimal candidates for a preliminary medical treatment if they are hemodynamically stable.

The use of methotrexate for the treatment of extrauterine pregnancy can only be considered if the diameter of the tumor is less than 4 cm, there is no sonographic evidence of fetal cardiac activity, and the β-hCG level is below 5000 mIU/mL. Methotrexate can be given locally or systemically by intramuscular injection of 1 mg/kg or 50 mg/m$^2$. Patients with a hematocrit below 35% should take 325 mg ferrous sulfate twice daily. Before recruiting patients for a conservative treatment method, the absence of fetal cardiac activity must be confirmed and the patients have to agree to comply with the follow-up requirements. If the β-hCG level does not decline over 15% after 7 days, a second dose of methotrexate has to be given. The weekly follow-up includes monitoring of the β-hCG decrease and transvaginal ultrasonography. If clinical symptoms persist or ultrasonography reveals more than 100 mL of free fluid in the cul-de-sac, a laparoscopy has to be performed. During and after methotrexate therapy, reliable contraception is necessary (**Table 21.4**) [2, 4, 8, 17, 21, 30].

## IVF and ectopic pregnancies—final evaluation

It remains a reality that the first IVF pregnancy, reported in 1976, was in fact an EP. Since these early IVF days, there have been numerous reports of both ectopic and heterotopic pregnancies occurring after IVF [1]. With an empty cavity in vaginal ultrasound and positive β-hCG values, it is today self-understood after an ET to diagnose EP early and nearly always prior to any rupture.

EP's are reported to complicate 2%–11% of all IVF pregnancies and are usually due to reverse migration of embryos into the tube. The etiology is multi-factorial, with destruction of the anatomy of the tube as the main factor. The stimulation protocol used for IVF does not contribute to the incidence of EP; however, the transfer of multiple embryos does. Since blastocyst single ET and the freeze-all project caught more ground, the rate of EP in ART has decreased. The technique of ET may contribute to extrauterine implantation by forcing the embryos through the tubal ostia by hydrostatic pressure. The volume of transfer medium should be as small as possible and the injection has to be very gentle, avoiding excessive force during ET. The transabdominal ultrasound guidance for ET helps to place the embryo in distance to the uterine wall. Deep fundal transfer may increase incidence of EP. Even tubal stump pregnancies after bilateral salpingectomy occur; however, they are mostly due to an incomplete tubal resection at the corneal ends in a previous tubectomy. A conic incision into the utero-tubal junctions and suturing is therefore recommended at salpingectomy [1].

Tubal factor infertility now accounts for an estimated 14% of all infertility and is usually the result of infection with Chlamydia trachomatis, the leading cause of bacterial sexually transmitted disease worldwide. Consequently, the implementation of national programs aiming to reduce the incidence of tubal infertility, such as the UK's National Chlamydia Screening Program, should be further reinforced. Campaigns for the widespread use of single ET in IVF would certainly lower the risk of EP even further by minimizing the number of multiple pregnancies. However, due to laws in different countries, this cannot always be applied. A recent analysis of national IVF data in the United States found that the rate of EP was 1.6% when one embryo was transferred, and 1.7%, 2.2%, and 2.5% when two, three, four, or more embryos were transferred [17–25].

TABLE 21.4: **Algorithm of Methotrexate Therapy**

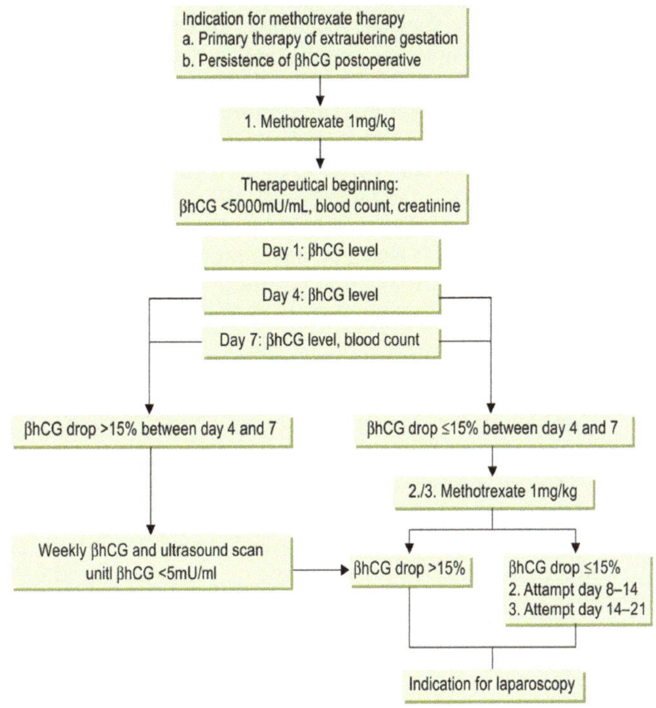


### *Serum β-hCG levels and ultrasound screening*

Early normal IUPs are associated with a doubling of β-hCG concentrations every 1.4–2.1 days [18]. An EP produces less β-hCG than a normal IUP, resulting in the prolongation of the β-hCG doubling time [3]. However, 15% of normal pregnancies will have an abnormal doubling time and 13% of EP's will have a normal doubling time [4]. A discriminatory zone has been described, whereby a β-hCG titer of 1000–1500 mIU/mL will be associated with the presence of an intrauterine sac on transvaginal ultrasound (6000–6500 mIU/mL for transabdominal ultrasound) in most cases of IUCs [18].

EP can be distinguished from miscarriage on the basis of falling β-hCG levels over a 48-hour period. If the half-life of β-hCG was less than 1.4 days, then a complete miscarriage would be likely, and the patient would be best managed expectantly. If the half-life was more than 7 days, then an ectopic is likely [19, 20]. In IVF patients, a serum β-hCG level more than 295 mIU/mL on day 16 post-ET was reported to give a 90% chance of an IUP [1]. Early diagnosis of EP following IVF with ultrasound is complicated by the presence of enlarged ovaries and fluid in the pelvis, as described in the case history. It is therefore usually a diagnosis of exclusion which is based on the finding of an empty uterus along with abnormally rising β-hCG titers.

In advanced cases of EP, there are three sonographic features as seen by a vaginal transducer:

1. The demonstration of a live embryo within a gestational sac in the adnexa. It typically appears as an intact, well-defined tubal ring (the "doughnut" or "bagel" sign) in which the yolk sac and/or the embryonic pole, with or without cardiac activity, are seen within a sonolucent sac.
2. A poorly defined tubal ring, possibly containing echogenic structures. If there is fluid in the cul-de-sac, it could indicate a tubal pregnancy that is aborting.
3. Varying amounts of fluid in the cul-de-sac indicating a ruptured tubal pregnancy.

A pseudo-gestational sac in the uterus can complicate the diagnosis of an EP. Color Doppler may have a role in the diagnosis of EP. The presence of a vascular ring outside the uterine cavity ("ring of fire") can be useful to diagnose an EP [21, 22].

## Summary

### *Laparoscopy*

In some cases, the diagnosis of EP is not clear-cut and laparoscopy is necessary to visualize the pelvis and establish the diagnosis, for example, in cases where there is high suspicion of EP (significant symptoms and signs) but still a possibility of a viable IUP (normally rising β-hCG but before an IUP could be seen on ultrasound). However, a few points are worth keeping in mind if laparoscopy is being performed in such cases. First, if there is still a possibility of a viable IUP, uterine instrumentation should be avoided. Second, it has to be remembered that following IVF, the ovaries are often cystic and enlarged and actually might look pathological to the inexperienced eye. Extra care must be taken to avoid ovarian injury during abdominal entry with a Veress needle or trocar. Also, unnecessary ovarian surgery by a well-intended but an inexperienced surgeon must be avoided. Finally, it is well recognized that early laparoscopy has a 1% false negative rate in EP; that is when the laparoscopy is clear, but the patient actually has an EP, too small to distend the tube and be visible on laparoscopy.

### *Conservative treatment of ectopic pregnancy*

The majority of EP's after IVF are diagnosed early and are unruptured, and therefore amenable to a conservative medical approach like the *Methotrexate treatment.* Methotrexate inhibits the synthesis of purines and pyrimidines, thus interfering with DNA synthesis and the multiplication of cells. *An IUP must be ruled out prior to administering methotrexate.*

Selection criteria for patients suitable for methotrexate treatment include hemodynamically stable patients with unruptured EP with the mass measuring ≤4 cm in diameter by ultrasound. Patients with larger masses, cardiac activity within the adnexal mass, or evidence of acute intra-abdominal bleeding are ineligible for methotrexate therapy. Methotrexate has been used in single (50 mg/m$^2$ of body surface area) (4) or multiple intramuscular doses (methotrexate 0.5–1.0 mg/kg body weight every other day for 5–7 days alternated with four doses of folic acid 0.1 mg/kg orally). Instillation of methotrexate directly into the EP under sonographic guidance has met with some success, but is not commonly used [18].

Transient pelvic pain frequently occurs 3–7 days after the start of methotrexate therapy. This pain is presumably due to tubal abortion and normally lasts 4–12 hours. It can be clinically challenging to differentiate between the transient abdominal pain of successful therapy from that of a rupturing EP. Surgical intervention is necessary if the pain is associated with tachycardia, hypotension, or a falling hematocrit. The β-hCG level is measured at baseline, and again on days 4 and 7, and weekly thereafter till negative. The β-hCG level may rise initially on day 4 compared to baseline. The day 7 β-hCG level, however, should show a drop of at least 15% compared to the day 4 level. If the level does not drop, a second dose of methotrexate can be administered. On average, it takes 4–6 weeks for the β-hCG levels to become negative following methotrexate treatment. A success rate of 90%–95% has been reported with a tubal rupture rate of 3%–4%.

### *Surgical treatment of EP*

Surgical treatment, usually via laparoscopy, is indicated in EP patients where methotrexate treatment is unsuitable or unsuccessful. Surgical treatment is also indicated where the diagnosis has been made by laparoscopy or when there is imminent or actual rupture of EP. Salpingotomy should be considered as the surgical treatment of choice when managing EP in the presence of contralateral tubal disease and the desire for future fertility. However, in the presence of a healthy contralateral tube, it is debatable whether to perform salpingotomy or salpingectomy. Salpingotomy may be associated with a higher subsequent IUP rate, but exposes the patient to a small risk of tubal bleeding in the immediate postoperative period and the potential need for further treatment for persistent trophoblast. Salpingotomy is also associated with a higher rate of recurrent EP.

## Pregnancies of unknown location

A patient found to have a negative TVUS, with serum β-hCG more than the discriminatory zone or a gestational age by last menstrual period of more than 5 weeks, is described as having a pregnancy of unknown location (PUL).

Approximately 30% of patients with PUL will have an ongoing IUP, whereas most (50%–70%) will be diagnosed with failing pregnancy (IUP or EP) with spontaneously declining β-hCG levels [26]. The remainder of patients will have a persistently elevated β-hCG level in the absence of TVUS findings, or confirmed EP by either TVUS or surgery. Studies have not, however, specifically examined outcomes of PUL resulting from IVF, which confers both a higher baseline risk of EP (2%) more than the general population (1%) [27].

Identification of subsequent decline in β-hCG level of 15% or more is consistent with a failed IUP, and although dilatation and suction curettage (D&C) is considered the gold standard [28], usually no further treatment is indicated [29–31].

## Pregnancies in C-section scars

### *C-section pregnancies (CSP)*

Diagnosis and treatment of ectopic cesarean scar pregnancy has become a challenge for our present field of obstetrics. With an increase in the number of pregnancies concluded with a cesarean section and with the development of transvaginal ultrasonography, the frequency of cesarean scar pregnancy diagnoses has increased as well. The most effective CSP treatment is simultaneous application of two to three techniques. The combination of local MTX with simultaneous gestational sac aspiration under ultrasound or hysteroscopy guidance seems optimal and minimally invasive. In the second stage, the remaining gestational tissues can be removed hysteroscopically in combination with vascular coagulation of the implantation site.

In more advanced cases (CSP exceeding 3 cm), local methotrexate administration should be considered, followed by laparoscopic or laparotomic CSP wedge resection with subsequent surgical correction of the cesarean section scar.

Promising results in CSP treatment have been obtained with an innovative HIFU technique that utilizes high-intensity focused ultrasound [32–34].

## Prevention of EP

The only real way to prevent EP is by reducing the incidence of tubal disease. This would include the early diagnosis and prompt treatment of PID. In IVF, modification of ET technique (such as reducing the volume of media used to load the catheter and avoidance of high fundal transfers) may reduce the incidence of EP based on theoretical grounds. However, the occurrence of EP following IVF should not be taken as an indication for a suboptimal transfer technique. In the early days of IVF, it was originally thought that the risk of tubal EP could be eliminated by removing the Fallopian tubes. However, this was later disproven by the case reports of tubal EP occurring following bilateral total salpingectomy. The EP could still implant in the interstitial part of the tube (that traverses the uterine wall), which is not removed during total salpingectomy. Therefore, pre-IVF salpingectomy without excision of the intramural tubal part for the prevention of EP is no longer recommended.

## Management options for ectopic pregnancy after IVF/ICSI and ET

- Early pregnancy monitoring with serial β-hCG levels and ultrasound scan avoid rupture of an EP.
- Ovarian enlargement due to controlled ovarian stimulation and presence of fluid in the cul-de-sac after IVF and make it difficult to visualize an EP on ultrasound, but the empty cavity is mostly a good sign.
- Intramuscular methotrexate remains equally important as laparoscopic treatment.
- Both IUP and heterotopic pregnancy must be ruled out prior to administration of methotrexate.
- Laparoscopy should always be performed in cases of uncertain diagnosis and where methotrexate treatment is unsuitable or unsuccessful.
- In the presence of hemodynamic instability, EP should be managed by the most expedient method, which may be laparoscopy or laparotomy, depending on the available surgical team!!!!!!

## References


1. Alkatout I and Mettler L. Ectopic Pregnancy: In Practical Manual of Laparoscopic and Hysteroscopic Surgery., Jaypee Brothers. Panama, London, New Delhi, 2019; 235–256
2. Tsakiridis, Ioannis PhD*; Giouleka, Sonia MSc†; Mamopoulos, Apostolos PhD‡; Athanasiadis, Apostolos PhD‡; Dagklis, Themistoklis PhD§ Diagnosis and Management of Ectopic Pregnancy: A Comparative Review of Major National Guidelines, Obstetrical & Gynecological Survey: October 2020 - Volume 75 - Issue 10 - p 611–623 doi: 10.1097/OGX.0000000000000832.
3. Kashanian M, Baradaran HR, Mousavi SS, Sheikhansari N, BorarPour F. Risk factors in ectopic pregnancy and differences between adults and adolescents, is consanguinity important? J Obstet Gynaecol. 2016; 1–5.
4. Weiss A, Beck-Fruchter R, Golan J, Lavee M, Geslevich Y, Shalev E. Ectopic pregnancy risk factors for ART patients undergoing the GnRH antagonist protocol: a retrospective study. Reprod Biol Endocrinol. 2016; 14:12.
5. Londra L, Moreau C, Strobino D, Bhasin A, Zhao Y. Is the type of gonadotropin-releasing hormone suppression protocol for ovarian hyperstimulation associated with ectopic pregnancy in fresh autologous cycles for *in vitro* fertilization? Fertil Steril. 2016; 106: 666–672.
6. Decleer W, Osmanagaoglu K, Meganck G, Devroey P. Slightly lower incidence of ectopic pregnancies in frozen embryo transfer cycles versus fresh *in vitro* fertilization-embryo transfer cycles: a retrospective cohort study. Fertil Steril. 2014; 101:162–165.
7. Testing and interpreting measures of ovarian reserve: a committee opinion. Fertil Steril. 2015; 103:e9–e17.
8. Lin S, Li R, Chi H, Huang S, Zhang H, Zheng X, Liu P, Qiao J. Effect of ABO blood type on ovarian reserve in Chinese women. Fertil Steril. 2014; 102:1729–1732.e1722.
9. Levi AJ, Raynault MF, Bergh PA, Drews MR, Miller BT, Scott RT, Jr. Reproductive outcome in patients with diminished ovarian reserve. Fertil Steril. 2001; 76:666–669.
10. Haadsma ML, Mooij TM, Groen H, Burger CW, Lambalk CB, Broekmans FJ, van Leeuwen FE, Bouman K, Hoek A. A reduced size of the ovarian follicle pool is associated with an increased risk of a trisomic pregnancy in IVF-treated women. Hum Reprod. 2010; 25:552–558.
11. Sisti G, Kanninen TT, Di Tommaso M, Witkin SS, Spandorfer SD. Autophagy induction by sera from women undergoing an *in vitro* fertilization cycle varies with subsequent outcome. J Reprod Immunol. 2016; 117:1–3.
12. Ramer I, Kanninen TT, Sisti G, Witkin SS, Spandorfer SD. The serum brain-derived neurotrophic factor concentration prior to initiation of an *in vitro* fertilization cycle predicts outcome. J Reprod Immunol. 2016; 116:46–49.
13. Lin S, Yang R, Chi H, Lian Y, Wang J, Huang S, Lu C, Liu P, Qiao J. Increased incidence of ectopic pregnancy after *in vitro* fertilization in women with decreased ovarian reserve. Oncotarget. 2017; 8:14570–14575. https://doi.org/10.18632/oncotarget.14679
14. Abusheikha N, Salha O, Brinsden P. Extra-uterine pregnancy following assisted conception treatment. Hum Reprod Update. 2000; 6:80–92.
15. Perkins KM, Boulet SL, Kissin DM, et al. Risk of ectopic pregnancy associated with assisted reproductive technology in the United States, 2001-2011. Obstet Gynecol. 2015; 125:70–78.
16. Alkatout I, Stuhlmann-Laeisz C, Mettler L, Organ preserving management of ovarian pregnancies by laparoscopic approach. Fertil Steril. 2011; 95(8):2467–2470.
17. Kader N, Caldwell B, Romero R. A method of screening for ectopic pregnancy and its indications. Obstet Gynecol 1981; 58:162–165.
18. Check J, Weiss R, Lurie D. Analysis of serum human chorionic gonadotropin levels in normal singleton, multiple and abnormal pregnancies. Hum Reprod. 1992; 7:1176–1180.
19. Ling F, Stovall T. Update on the diagnosis and management of ectopic pregnancy. Adv Obstet Gynaecol 1994; 1:55–83.
20. Kadar N, Romero R. Further observations on serial hCG patterns in ectopic pregnancies and abortions. Fertil Steril. 1988; 50: 367–370.
21. Tanaka T, Hayashi H, Kutsuzawa T. Treatment of interstitial ectopic pregnancy with methotrexate: report of a successful case. Fertil Steril. 1982; 37:851–852.
22. Feichtinger W, Kemeter P. Conservative treatment of ectopic pregnancy by transvaginal aspiration under sonographic control and methotrexate injection. Lancet. 1987; 1:381–382.
23. Royal College of Obstetricians and Gynaecologists. The management of tubal pregnancy. Guideline No. 21. London: RCOG Press; 2004.

24. Steptoe PC, Edwards RG. Reimplantation of a human embryo with subsequent tubal pregnancy. Lancet. 1976; 1:880–882.
25. Sharif K, Kaufmann S, Sharma V. Heterotopic pregnancy obtained after in-vitro fertilization and embryo transfer following bilateral total salpingectomy. Hum Reprod. 1994; 9:1966–1967.
26. Kirk E, Condous G, Bourne T. Pregnancies of unknown location. Best Pract Res Clin Obstet Gynaecol. 2009; 23:493–499.
27. Chung K, Sammel MD, Coutifaris C, Chalian R, Lin K, Castelbaum AJ, et al. Defining the rise of serum HCG in viable pregnancies achieved through use of IVF. Humanit Rep. 2006; 21:823–828.
28. Ailawadi M, Lorch SA, Barnhart KT. Cost-effectiveness of presumptively medically treating women at risk for ectopic pregnancy compared with first performing a dilatation and curettage. Fertil Steril. 2005; 83:376–382.
29. Barnhart KT. Clinical practice. Ectopic pregnancy. N Engl J Med. 2009; 361:379–387.
30. Kulp AJ, Appleby DH, Sammel MD, Barnhart KT. Utility of dilation and curettage in the diagnosis of pregnancy of unknown location. Am J Obstet Gynecol. 2011; 204:130.e1–e6.
31. Li YY, Yin ZY, Li S, Xu H, Zhang XP, Cheng H, Du L, Zhou XY, Zhang B. Comparison of transvaginal surgery and methotrexate/mifepristone-combined transcervical resection in the treatment of cesarean scar pregnancy. Eur Rev Med Pharmacol Sci. 2017; 21, 2957–2963
32. Koplay M, Dogan NU, Sivri M, Erdogan H, Dogan S, Celik C. Hindawi Publishing Corporation: Case Reports in Surgery. Volume 2016, Article ID 7460687, 4 pages
33. Giampaolino P, De Rosa N, Morra I, Bertrando A, Di Spiezio Sardo A, Zizolfi B, Ferrara C, Della Corte L, Bifulco G. Management of cesarean scar pregnancy: a single-institution retrospective review. Biomed Res Int. 2018; 2018:6486407.
34. Stovall TG, Ling FW. Ectopic pregnancy. Diagnostic and therapeutic algorithms minimizing surgical intervention. J Reprod Med. 1993; 38:807–812.

# 22

## ROBOTIC TUBAL REANASTOMOSIS

**Arwa Salehjawich and Ibrahim Alkatout**

### Robotic tubal reanastomosis after sterilization

A number of actions in life are intended to be permanent and cannot be undone; this is not always the case with regard to tubal sterilization.

The number of women using contraception is rising every year. Currently, about 63% of women aged 15–49 years—in all, 739 million women worldwide—use some form of contraception (United Nations, 2011). Providing effective and affordable contraception for all fertile women is one of the goals of the United Nations. Free access to contraception enables couples to make responsible decisions concerning reproduction, and improves maternal and infant health by preventing unintentional or closely spaced pregnancies (The Millennium Development Goals Report, 2012).

The most common method of contraception for women is sterilization. It accounts for 30% of all contraception use in women, which corresponds to 200 million women worldwide (United Nations, 2011). It is estimated that 5%–20% of sterilized women regret their decision later in life, and only 1%–2% request a reversal of sterilization (Van Voorhis, 2000). Regret is more likely to occur in the presence of the following factors: sterilization at a younger age or shortly after giving birth, a new relationship, and a low socioeconomic status (Hillis et al., 1999). The most common reason for a reversal of sterilization is the desire to enter a relationship with a new partner. In rare circumstances, the death of a child may encourage a woman to request a reversal of tubal sterilization.

Procedures for the reversal of sterilization were developed in the last few decades. The first procedure was performed in the early 1970s by laparotomy (Williams, 1973; Siegler and Perez, 1975). This surgical approach involves a midline abdominal incision through which the fallopian tubes can be accessed. Next, the occluded ends of the tubes are excised and methylene blue is instilled to test the degree of patency. An anastomosis is then performed with sutures, and is usually supplemented by the use of a splint (Siegler and Perez, 1975).

While the technical principles have remained largely unchanged, the subsequent introduction of a microscopic camera during surgery allowed for much greater accuracy (Diamond, 1977; Gomel, 1977; Wiegerinck et al., 2005). This made it possible to perform detailed anastomoses of various types. The two-layer technique was used most frequently, wherein the muscular and serosal layer are sutured separately with varying numbers of stitches. Some authors have described the use of a splint to bridge the lumen of the proximal and distal parts of the fallopian tube; the splint is then removed in the ensuing hours (Gordts et al., 2009; Berger et al., 2016).

The laparoscopic approach was implemented during the same period of time (Diamond, 1977; Gomel, 2007). Similar to laparotomic microsurgical procedures, the two-layer technique was used. Other techniques include single-layer, 1-stitch, 2-stitch, 3-stitch, 4-quadrant sutures, or sero-muscular fixation with microstaplers and biological glue (Wiegerinck et al., 2005; Tan and Loh, 2010; Schepens et al., 2011). Most laparoscopic procedures involve the use of a supplementary splint.

These techniques have been deployed for several years. In the meantime, other surgical solutions aimed at improving the quality of anastomosis were sought. This resulted in the first reported robotic tubal reanastomosis with the ZEUS robotic system in 1998, using a two-layer closure procedure. A patent anastomosis was achieved by this technique (Falcone et al., 2000).

Women who wish to conceive again have two options: reversal of sterilization or IVF. Prior to obtaining informed consent, patients must be informed about pregnancy rates after these two options. Before the 1960s, female sterilization was generally performed only for medical indications such as a further pregnancy being a risk to the mother's health. The changing cultural atmosphere in the 1960s encouraged women to reduce the size of their families. This marked the beginning of the sexual revolution, which enabled women to use safe and reversible contraception.

The development of surgical procedures in the same decade resulted in safe and less invasive female sterilization procedures. Insurance companies began to cover female sterilization procedures, making the procedure accessible and feasible to millions of women who were previously unable to afford the surgery.

We now have access to a 3D system that marks the beginning of an entirely new dimension in tubal reconstructive surgery.

The robotic camera allows for low power magnification to increase the accuracy of suture placement, helps delineate tissue planes, and improves the surgeon's approximation of the tubes, which is a critical aspect of successful reanastomosis. Pregnancy rates after robotic reanastomosis have been reported to be as high as 80%. In comparison with a large abdominal incision, minimally invasive surgery is associated with less pain, lower infection rates, and quicker recovery times.

The anatomy of the human being has not changed. However, technical advances in operating materials and methods call for improvements in surgical procedures as well as better management of complications. A fundamental distinction between any operating method and laparoscopy is that, for the latter, the initial entry is usually performed in a blind fashion. Blind entry may result in vessel or organ damage, especially in patients who have undergone previous surgery. One of the difficulties associated with the entry is that the damage might not be identified immediately and may then require major abdominal repair. Furthermore, improved surgical instruments and techniques have enabled surgeons to perform even major operations by the laparoscopic approach. This is associated with renewed learning curves and a high rate of complications due to vascular, bowel, uterine, or bladder damage. The improvement of surgical techniques must be accompanied by advancements in the management of complications.

Regardless of the approach, the type of tubal ligation is the most important determinant of success. Falope rings and Filshie clips provide the best chances of successful reversal. The Pomeroy method of tubal ligation has been associated with varied results;

its success depends on the location of ligation and whether equal diameters of tubes are available for reanastomosis.

While several factors affect the success of reanastomosis, women who have undergone tubal ligation and now desire children have a number of options. These include the robotic approach, which has become an integral part of minimally invasive surgery. Women must be counseled comprehensively about alternative contraception before undergoing surgical sterilization [1–5].

## Anatomy of the fallopian tube

### Structure and function (Figure 22.1)

The fallopian tubes originate at the uterine horns, extend laterally within the superior edge of the mesosalpinx of the broad ligament, and terminate close to the ipsilateral ovary. They are 11–12 cm in length, and the diameter of their lumen is less than 1 mm. The fallopian tube consists of four anatomical regions: uterine, isthmus, ampulla, and infundibulum. Lateral to the isthmus is the ampulla, which is the most common site of fertilization. In addition to providing a space for fertilization to occur, the fallopian tubes function as a passage for the ovum or gamete from the ovary to the uterus.

### Embryology

The paramesonephric ducts, otherwise known as the Müllerian ducts, form in female embryos at around week 5 or 6 due to the absence of the anti-Müllerian hormone (AMH). As a result of estrogen stimulation, the cranial ends of these ducts eventually form the fallopian tubes.

### Blood supply and lymphatics

Arterial supply to the fallopian tubes arises from anastomoses between the ovarian and tubal branches of the ovarian artery and the ascending branches of the uterine artery. On either side, the ovarian arteries branch off from the inferior abdominal aorta, just inferior to the renal artery. The uterine arteries stem from the internal iliac arteries; the ascending branches travel superiorly toward the uterine horns while the descending branches travel inferiorly toward the superior vagina. The ovarian arteries supply the lateral fallopian tube, while the ascending branches of the uterine artery supply the medial fallopian tube. However, anastomoses between the two generally ensure that neither of these will cause ischemia in any portion of the tube.

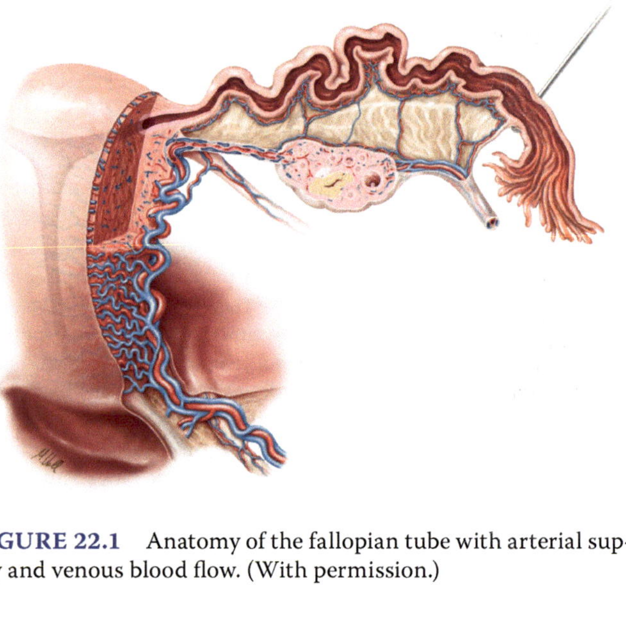

FIGURE 22.1 Anatomy of the fallopian tube with arterial supply and venous blood flow. (With permission.)

Venous blood flows from the fallopian tubes to the tubal branches of the uterine and ovarian veins, in a similar manner as arterial supply. The inferior vena cava (IVC) receives blood from the right ovarian vein, while the left renal vein receives blood from the left ovarian vein. The uterine veins drain into the internal iliac veins, which then drain into the IVC.

Lymph drainage of the fallopian tubes is similar to that of the ovaries. Lymphatic fluid flows from the fallopian tubes to both, the para-aortic (lumbar) lymph nodes and the pelvic lymph nodes.

### Nerves

Afferent fibers for the fallopian tubes travel along the same pathway as sympathetic efferent innervation, which originates from T11, T12, and L1. By contrast, minor parasympathetic innervation is shared between vagal fibers of the ovarian plexus for the lateral portion of the fallopian tube, and is provided medially from the pelvic splanchnic nerve from S1, S2, and S3. The most medial isthmus is most densely innervated. Both innervation and muscles become sparser from the proximal to the distal aspect of the fallopian tube.

### Muscles

The muscular layer of the fallopian tubes is covered by the inner mucosa (which contains longitudinal cilia extending into the lumen) and the outermost serosa. This layer is also known as the muscularis mucosa; it comprises an inner circular layer and an outer longitudinal layer.

Contractions of this muscular layer work in coordination with ciliary movements and tubal secretory fluids transport the ovum or gamete along the length of the fallopian tube. Short and frequent contractions help mix tubal fluid, while continuous tonic contractions assist anterograde transport of the ovum or gamete and also allow the admission of an embryo across the utero-tubal junction at the most optimal time during the menstrual cycle [6, 7].

## Family planning

The history of contraception is a long one, dating back to ancient times. Voluntary control of fertility is especially important in modern society. A woman who expects to have no more than one or two children spends most of her reproductive years trying to avoid pregnancy. Effective control of reproduction is an essential part of a woman's ability to accomplish her personal goals. From a larger perspective, the rapid growth of the human population in the present century threatens the survival of all.

From the individual as well as global point of view, reproductive health requires the effective prevention of pregnancy as well as sexually transmitted diseases (STD).

The most commonly used methods of contraception in Western countries, in the order of their frequency, are sterilization, oral contraceptives, and condoms. Condoms and other barriers reduce the risks of STDs and cervical cancer.

The two most commonly used intrauterine devices (IUDs) are the copper T380A ParaGard and the levonorgestrel T Mirena. These are as effective as tubal sterilization and associated with a long-term risk of pelvic infection no greater than that in the general population (**Table 22.1**).

The combined estrogen-progestin oral contraceptive, patch, and vaginal ring all provide excellent contraception when used correctly, but also increase the risk of venous thrombosis and thromboembolism.

TABLE 22.1: **Methods of Family Planning and Percentage of Women Who became Pregnant Accidentally during the First Year of Use**

| | Women Who became Pregnant Accidentally within the First Year of Use (%) | | Women Continuing Use at 1 Year (%) |
|---|---|---|---|
| **Method** | **Typical Use** | **Perfect Use** | |
| No method | 85 | 85 | |
| Spermicides | 29 | 18 | 42 |
| Periodic abstinence | 25 | | 67 |
| Calendar | | 9 | |
| Ovulation method | | 3 | |
| Symptothermal | | 2 | |
| Postovulation | | 1 | |
| Withdrawal | 27 | 4 | 43 |
| Cap | | | |
| Parous women | 32 | 20 | 46 |
| Nulliparous | 16 | 9 | 57 |
| Diaphragm | 16 | 6 | 75 |
| Condom | | | |
| Female | 21 | 5 | 49 |
| Male | 15 | 2 | 53 |
| Combined pill and progestin-only pill | 8 | 0.3 | 68 |
| Patch | 8 | 0.3 | 68 |
| Novaring | 8 | 0.3 | 68 |
| Intrauterine device | | | |
| Copper T380A | 0.8 | 0.6 | 78 |
| Levonorgestrel T | 0.1 | 0.1 | 81 |
| Depoprovera | 3 | 0.3 | 70 |
| Female sterilization | 0.5 | 0.5 | 100 |
| Male sterilization | 0.15 | 0.10 | 100 |

*Source:* From data in Hatcher RA, Stewart F, Trussell J, Kowal D, Guest F, Stewart GK, Cates W. 1990. *Contraceptive Technology 1990–1992.* Irvington Publishers, Incorporated.

The current low-dose combinations of estrogen and progestin do not increase the risk of heart attack among nonsmokers younger than 35 years of age who have no other risk of vascular disease.

Oral contraceptives do not increase the risk of breast cancer.

The use of injected progestin and implanted hormonal contraceptives results in very low pregnancy rates while dispensing with the risk of thrombosis associated with estrogen.

The benefits of hormonal contraceptives include a lower risk of endometrial and ovarian cancer. Levonorgestrel 1.5 mg Plan B and ulipristal acetate are the most effective hormonal means of achieving emergency contraception. Their efficacy is greatest within 24 hours of intercourse, but is still high at day 5. The copper T380A IUD inserted 5 days after intercourse is even more effective than hormonal methods.

Long-acting reversible contraceptive LARC methods include injectable progestins, subdermal progestin implants, and copper- or levonorgestrel-7-releasing IUDs. These are among the safest methods and associated with pregnancy rates similar to those after sterilization (**Table 22.2**).

Safe long-term contraception is achieved with laparoscopy and bipolar electrocautery applied at three adjacent sites on each tube, the Silastic band, or the Filshie clip.

Hysteroscopic sterilization techniques provide highly effective and permanent contraception for women, while dispensing with the use of general anesthesia or an abdominal incision.

Vasectomy provides highly effective low-cost sterilization for men, and is associated with neither heart disease nor prostate cancer.

Abortion mortality rates fell rapidly after its legalization. Currently, the overall mortality risk is less than 1 per 100,000, which is well below the maternal mortality rate of 12.7 per 100,000 live births (**Table 22.3**).

The risk of abortion mortality increases with gestational age, and is estimated at 0.1 per 100,000 at 8 weeks or less. Even at 16–20 weeks, abortion is safer than the continuation of pregnancy [7–9].

## Reasons for performing sterilization

The most common reason of undergoing surgical sterilization is the desire for no further children. However, social and economic factors, health issues, situational factors (such as age or financial considerations), and encouragement by the family or physician may also play a role. Some women may undertake the step for several reasons.

The majority of tubal sterilizations are performed simply because a woman desires no further children. However, women who wish to undergo the procedure for other reasons are more likely to regret the step later [10].

**TABLE 22.2: Overview of Contraceptive Methods**

| Method | Advantage | Disadvantage | Risks | Non-Contraceptive Benefits |
|---|---|---|---|---|
| Coitus interruptus | Available, free | Depends on male control | Pregnancy | Reduces risk of HIV |
| Lactation | Available, free | Duration of effect is unreliable | Pregnancy | Reduces breast cancer |
| Periodic abstinence | Available, free | Complex method, motivation is essential | Pregnancy | None |
| Condom | Available, no prescription needed | Motivation is essential, must be used each time, depends on the man | Pregnancy | Proven to reduce STDs and cervical cancer |
| Spermicide and sponge | Available, no prescription needed | Must be used each time | Pregnancy | None |
| Diaphragm, cap | Nonhormonal | Must be used each time, fitting required | Pregnancy, cystitis | Proven to reduce STDs and cervical cancer |
| ParaGard IUD | Highest efficiency, unrelated to coitus | Initial cost, skilled insertion, pain, and bleeding | Initial mild risk of PID and septic abortion if pregnancy occurs | None |
| Merina IUD | Highest efficiency, unrelated to coitus | Initial cost, skilled insertion, amenorrhea for some women | Initial mild risk of PID and septic abortion if pregnancy occurs | Reduces menstrual bleeding, can be used to treat menorrhagia |
| Oral contraception, patch, Novaring | High efficacy | Must be taken daily, costs | Thrombosis, risk of MI and stroke for older smokers | Can be used to treat symptoms of endometriosis and benign ovarian cyst |
| Emergency contraception (levonorgestrel, ulipristal) | Moderate efficacy | Frequent use disrupts menses | None | Unknown |

*Source:* From data in Berek JS, *Berek and Novak's Gynecology*, 15th edition, LWW 2011.

## Poststerilization regret and symptoms of depression

Poststerilization regret is usually assessed by asking persons whether they desire (more) children, whether they would like to have the procedure reversed, or by studying women who report for sterilization reversal or in vitro fertilization (IVF). In a non-representative prospective study, it was found that 20.3% of those who were 30 years of age or younger and 5.9% of those over the age of 30 years at the time of sterilization expressed regret within 14 years of their tubal sterilization (Hillis et al., 1999). Black and Hispanic women are more likely to undergo tubal sterilization and ask for reversal of the procedure than white women (Borrero et al., 2008). Sterilization regret is also more common among women with a few children at the time of sterilization (Kariminia et al., 2002), and women who experience a change in their marital status with a simultaneous desire to have children with a new partner (Karaminia et al., 2002; Moseman et al., 2006).

The psychological impact of sterilization regret has been addressed in a small number of studies. In a small prospective study conducted in Istanbul, Kelekci et al. (2005) registered a significant association between dissatisfaction after sterilization and a higher rate of self-reported depression. Research conducted outside the field of sterilization identifies reproductive problems as one of the most serious life stressors for a woman (Amir, Horesh & Lin-Stein, 1999). Relinquishing the intention to bear children is associated with significantly greater distress for women (White & McQuillan, 2006). Thus, women who regret sterilization may experience significantly greater stress due to the psychological consequences of sterilization compared to women who do not regret sterilization. Analogous to women who remain involuntarily childless due to infertility (McQuillan et al., 2012; McQuillan, Greil, and Torres-Stone, 2007), sterilization—if regretted—may prevent a woman's achievement of her identity as a mother and the accomplishment of her life goals.

Women will be more likely to report regret after sterilization when they did not undergo the procedure simply because they did not want (further) children. Women who express regret report greater depressive symptoms than women who do not. Being unmarried at the time of sterilization is an important risk factor for poststerilization regret, and was much more common among women than men. In addition to contributing to the predominance of female versus male sterilization, this pattern highlights the importance of educating women about the permanency of sterilization and the advantages of using long-acting reversible contraceptive methods.

A clinical study showed that about 70% of laparoscopic sterilizations could be carried out during a one-day admission; 25% of the women complained of long-term sequelae and 1% of the sterilizations were failures [2, 10].

**TABLE 22.3: Estimated Numbers and Rates of Safe and Unsafe Abortions Worldwide**

| | Number of Abortions (millions) | | | Abortion Rate* | | |
|---|---|---|---|---|---|---|
| | Total | Safe | Unsafe | Total | Safe | Unsafe |
| World | 41.6 | 21.9 | 19.7 | 29 | 15 | 14 |
| Developed countries | 6.6 | 6.1 | 0.5 | 26 | 24 | 2 |
| Developing countries | 35.0 | 15.8 | 19.2 | 29 | 13 | 16 |

*Abortions per 1,000 women aged 15–44 years.

*Source:* From data in Sedgh G, Singh S, Hussain R. Intended and unintended pregnancies worldwide in 2012 and recent trends. *Studies in Family Planning*. September 2014;45(3):301–14.

## Types of sterilization

The most common method of birth control among women between the ages of 35 and 44 years is surgical sterilization. A distinction is made between two categories of sterilization: a puerperal sterilization at the time of cesarean section or sterilization performed several days after vaginal delivery. A non-puerperal sterilization or interval sterilization is not related to the delivery.

Sterilization is achieved by occlusion or division of the fallopian tube. This can be performed by the laparoscopic or hysteroscopic approach, or by performing a mini-laparotomy.

Commonly used laparotomic procedures are the Parkland, the Pomeroy, and the modified Pomeroy technique. Sterilization can be performed during a laparoscopy by unipolar or bipolar electrocoagulation, by using the Falope ring, the Hulka clip, or the Filshie clip. Transcervical hysteroscopy may be performed with the aid of the Essure and Adiana systems, both of which are approved by the FDA.

Reversal of sterilization is more effective after mechanical occlusion than electrocoagulation because the latter causes more damage to tissue. Sterilization with the hysteroscopic Essure or Adiana system is irreversible.

### Methods of sterilization

- *Pomeroy technique*: A loop of the tube is excised after ligating its base with a single absorbable suture. A modification of the procedure is excision of a mid-portion of the tube after ligation of the segment with two absorbable sutures.
- *Irving technique*: A mid-portion of the tube is excised and each stump is sutured to the uterus, creating a blind loop.
- *Uchida technique*: A saline-epinephrine solution is injected into the subserosal area of the tube, causing the muscular tube to separate from the serosa. The ballooned serosa is incised and the muscular tube withdrawn. A section of the tube measuring about 5 cm is then excised and the proximal end ligated.
- *Bipolar electrocoagulation technique*: The tube is grasped with bipolar forceps and a radiofrequency electric current is applied at three adjacent areas, coagulating about 3 cm of the tube.
- *Hulka clip*: This is placed across the mid-isthmus while ensuring that the applicator is at right angles to the tube, and also ensuring the entire thickness of the tube is grasped before the clip is closed.
- *Filshie clip*: This is placed at right angles to the mid-isthmus. The anvil of the posterior jaw must be visualized through the mesosalpinx prior to closure in order to ensure that the entire thickness of the tube is grasped [9, 11–13].

## Sterilization and vasectomy

Vasectomy is a very effective and reversible method of birth control; pregnancy rates after reversal are about 50%. The longer the interval after vasectomy, the poorer is the outcome in terms of pregnancy.

A study among 540 eligible women at risk for pregnancy showed that six pregnancies occurred 6–72 weeks after vasectomy. The cumulative probability of failure per 1,000 procedures (95% confidence interval) was 9.4 (1.2, 17.5) at 1 year after vasectomy and 11.3 (2.3, 20.3) after 2, 3, and 5 years.

The cumulative probability of a woman expressing regret within 5 years after her husband's vasectomy was 6.1%, which was similar to the 5-year cumulative probability of regret in women after tubal sterilization (7.0%). Women who reported substantial conflict with their husbands before vasectomy were more than 25 times more likely to request a reversal of the vasectomy than women who had no such conflict. Similarly, women who reported substantial conflict with their husbands or partners before tubal sterilization were more than three times as likely to regret their decision and more than five times likely to request a reversal than women who reported no such conflict.

Couples considering vasectomy should be counseled about the low, yet real, risk of pregnancy after the procedure, and the fact that men are not sterile immediately after vasectomy. The vasectomies were carried out on an outpatient basis. Postoperative symptoms were minimal, and a failure rate of 0.5% failures was registered. Female sterilization was at least four times more expensive than vasectomy. The authors of these reports conclude that vasectomy should be given preference over female sterilization, and that both men and their wives should be counseled preoperatively [14–16].

## Index of sterilization

Many centers used the following formula (endorsed by the American College of Obstetricians and Gynecologists until 1969): age multiplied by parity must be greater than or equal to 120 before elective sterilization may be considered.

## Sterilization reversal versus IVF

IVF is an alternative for women who wish to conceive after tubal sterilization. While tubal anastomosis restores tubal function, IVF replaces it. Based on fertility outcomes and cost-effectiveness, surgical reversal was given preference over IVF for patients younger than 37 years, and the opposite was suggested to women over 37 years of age (Boeckxstaens et al., 2007).

In women younger than 40 years of age, tubal anastomosis appears to be more cost-effective than IVF, while the opposite is true for those over 40 years of age [1].

## Prognostic factors for reversal of sterilization

Prognostic factors must be taken into account before performing surgical sterilization.

### Age

Many studies described age as the most important factor. Age is inversely correlated with pregnancy rates.

### Body mass index

The data reported so far in regard of body mass index (BMI) have been inconclusive. BMI was found to influence pregnancy rates in one study, whereas another reported no impact of BMI on pregnancy rates.

### Postoperative tubal length

The authors of four studies registered no impact of tubal length in terms of prognosis. However, one study revealed a higher pregnancy rate for longer tubes; the length of the tube was 6.7 cm in the pregnant group versus 6.5 cm in the nonpregnant group ($P < 0.05$).

### Method of sterilization

Refer to the section entitled Types of Sterilization.

### Time from sterilization to reversal

Four studies addressed the period between sterilization and sterilization reversal. Three of these (Kim et al., 1997; Boeckxstaens et al., 2007; Schepens et al., 2011) mention no correlation between the duration of the interval and pregnancy rates. Just one study reported a pregnancy rate of 91% at 1–5 years after sterilization versus 72% at 11–15 years after sterilization (P = 0.0006) (Hanafi, 2003).

### Type of anastomosis

The effect of the location of anastomosis on fertility outcomes was analyzed in four studies (Kim et al., 1997; Yoon et al., 1999; Gordts et al., 2009; Schepens et al., 2011), none of which identified an association between the two.

### Ectopic pregnancies

Little is known about prognostic factors for ectopic pregnancies. No correlation has been observed between potential sites for creating an anastomosis and percentages of ectopic pregnancies (cornual–isthmic 4.0%, cornual–ampullary 4.5%, isthmic–isthmic 2.0%, isthmic–ampullary 5.0%, ampullary–ampullary 2.3%) (Kim et al., 1997). Another study reported inconclusive ectopic pregnancy rates relative to the method of sterilization; the small sample size in the Pomeroy sterilization cohort did not permit an expressive statistical analysis (11% Falope ring reversal, 0% clip sterilization group, 13% coagulation, and 33% Pomeroy sterilization) (Gordts et al., 2009) [1].

## Description of the procedure

### Docking and instrumentation

The robotic tower (**Figure 22.2**) is moved carefully under the control of the main operator to the operating table and positioned between the patient's feet in preparation for docking. The two robotic arms are attached to the lateral right and left trocars. Occasionally, a third arm is used. The robotic instruments (**Figure 22.3**) are then introduced. An EndoWrist PK grasper (Intuitive Inc., Sunnyvale, CA) is loaded in the left robotic arm. An EndoWrist monopolar hook (Intuitive Inc., Sunnyvale, CA) is used in the right robotic arm. The latter is replaced by an EndoWrist monopolar scissors (Intuitive Inc., Sunnyvale, CA), if needed. An EndoWrist Prograsper (Intuitive Inc., Sunnyvale, CA) is placed in the fourth robotic arm when it is used. For tubal anastomosis, the monopolar hook is replaced by an EndoWrist needle holder to enable intracorporeal stitching (Intuitive Inc., Sunnyvale, CA). No cautery is used on the muscularis-mucosal layer.

The assistant helps in performing irrigation, suction, tissue retraction, and the introduction and retrieval of sutures for tubal anastomosis via the accessory port.

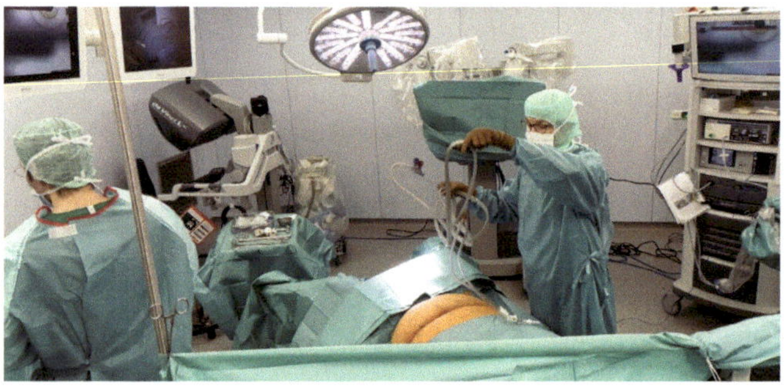

FIGURE 22.2 Operating room with robotic tower, da Vinci console, patient in Trendelenburg position.

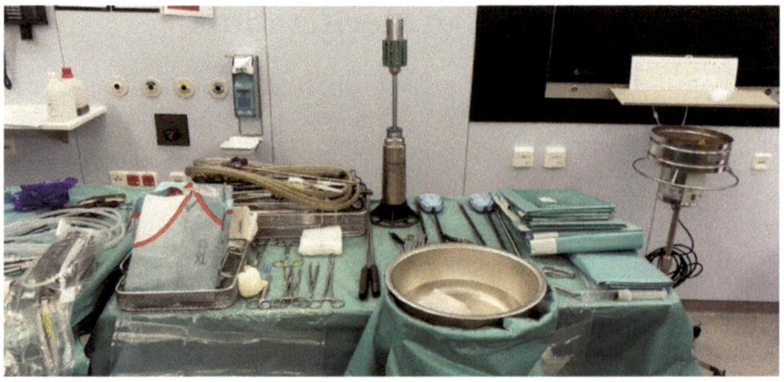

FIGURE 22.3 Operation settings and instruments.

### Surgical technique

Approaching the proximal and distal ends of the fallopian tube (**Figure 22.4**).

Injection of indigo carmine dye transcervically enables the surgeon to identify the proximal portion of the tube and rule out any obstruction of the proximal tube. A probe (Karl Storz Inc., Germany) is introduced through the fimbriated end of the distal portion, and indigo carmine is injected to identify the distal site of the anastomosis. Using the monopolar cautery, the serosal covering of the proximal and distal anastomosis site is incised. Microscissors are then used to cut the muscularis-mucosal portion of the tube and open its proximal and distal ends (**Figure 22.5**).

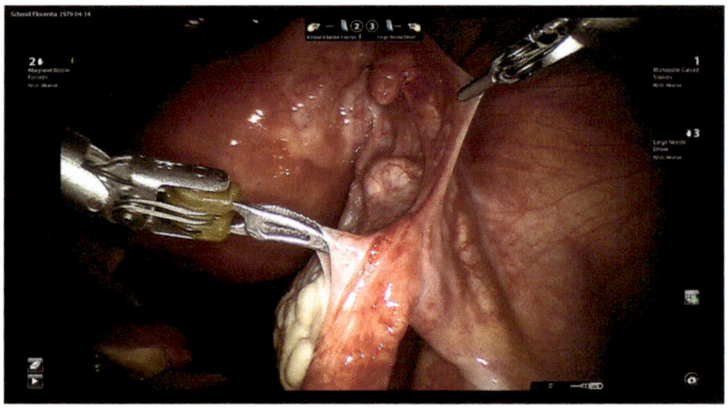

FIGURE 22.4 Exposing the distal and proximal ends of the fallopian tube.

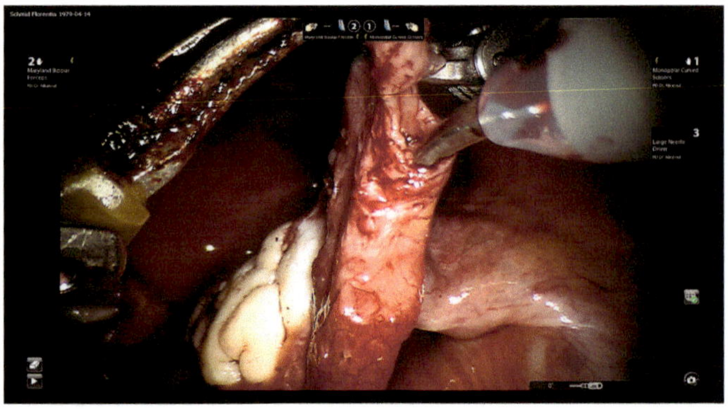

FIGURE 22.5 Opening the proximal and distal ends of the tube.

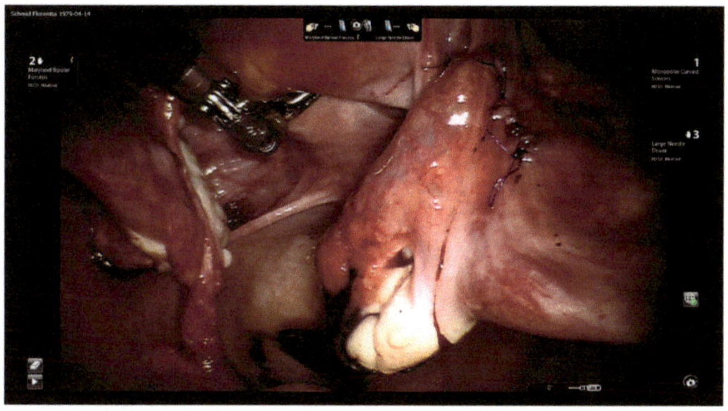

FIGURE 22.6 Suturing of the mucosal and muscular layers of the tubal segments with interrupted 5-0 PDS.

Reconstruction of the mesosalpinx: The mesosalpinx is approximated using a series of 6-0 vicryl stitches to bridge the gap between the two ends of the fallopian tube and facilitate subsequent suturing with fine sutures. This step brings the tubal segments close and prevents tension on the anastomosis. In the event of a major difference in size between the proximal and distal anastomosis site, a stent is placed to facilitate suturing of the two ends. Typically, we use the inner plastic component of the Novy cannula (COOK Medical Inc., Bloomington, IN, USA). This or a similar canula is commonly used to cannulate the tube hysteroscopically. A 9 cm length of this flexible tube is cut and introduced through a port. It is inserted through each anastomosis site for bridging.

Tubal reanastomosis: The mucosal and muscular layers of the tubal segments are sutured with 4–6 interrupted 5-0 Vicryl sutures or PDS (**Figure 22.6**). Excessive force may easily shift the needle or damage the suture.

The first suture is placed in 6 o'clock position and is performed as a sero-muscular knot, leaving out the mucosa. The suture is placed in such a way that the knot lies on the outside of the lumen, and is tied by the intracorporeal knotting technique. The second and third sutures are placed on 3 o'clock and 9 o'clock position, but not tied. The fourth suture is placed in 12 o'clock position. Then the 3 o'clock and 9 o'clock sutures are knotted. Proper suturing will avoid misalignment or rotation of the distal tubal segment along its longitudinal axis. The serosa is then closed separately with running 7-0 Vicryl sutures. Chromotubation is performed to document tubal patency and assess the immediate success of the procedure (**Figure 22.7**).

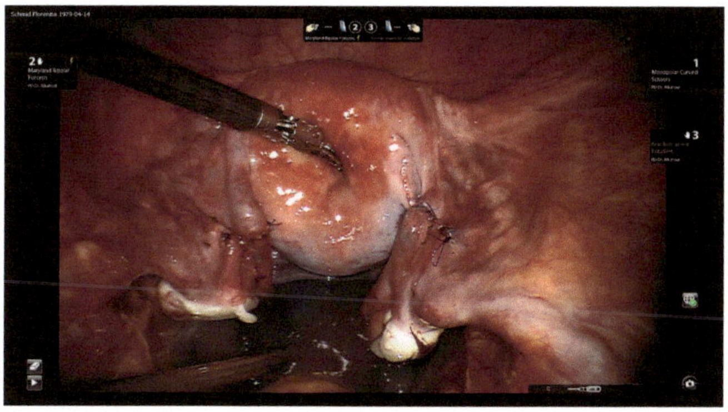

FIGURE 22.7 Closing the serosa with running 7-0 vicryl sutures. Evaluating tubal patency by chromotubation.

In addition to mini-laparotomy and traditional laparoscopic tubal anastomosis, robotic technology is an alternative approach for performing tubal anastomosis [3, 5, 17, 18].

## Reasons for the robotic approach

Robotic surgery is becoming increasingly popular because of its numerous advantages: reduced blood loss, reduced postoperative pain, shorter hospital stays, and better visualization of fine structures. Robots are being used in urological, cardiac, thoracic, orthopedic, gynecological, and general surgery. The use of robotic surgery in gynecology was approved by the US Food and Drug Administration in 2005.

Currently, robotic surgery is used for a variety of indications in the treatment of benign and malignant gynecological diseases. Interdisciplinary cooperation over large geographical distances has been rendered possible by telemedicine, and will ensure comprehensive patient care in the future by highly specialized surgery teams. In addition, the second operation console and the operation simulator constitute a new dimension in advanced surgical training. The disadvantages of robotic surgery remain the high cost of its acquisition and maintenance as well as the laborious training of medical personnel for its competent use.

Gynecological operations being performed by the use of robotic technology at the present time include myomectomy, total and supracervical hysterectomy, ovarian cystectomy, sacral colpopexy, tubal reanastomosis, lymph node dissection, surgery of retroperitoneal ectopic pregnancy, the Moskowitz procedure, and endometriosis surgery.

Limitations for the anesthetist include difficult intraoperative access to the patient, the steep Trendelenburg position, the long duration of surgery, and the impact of a pneumoperitoneum.

Robotic gynecological surgery can be performed safely, provided the surgeon takes the physiological effects of the steep Trendelenburg position and a pneumoperitoneum into account. In patients with cardiorespiratory problems, the benefits of the surgical procedure should be weighed against its risks.

With regard to microscopic tubal anastomoses, the mean operating time for robotic anastomoses was significantly longer than that for open anastomoses, although the duration of hospital stays was significantly shorter (robot 4 hours; open 34.7 hours). Patients who had undergone a robotic anastomosis could return earlier to their activities of daily living (robot 11.1 days; open 28.1 days). Although this was a small series, similar pregnancy rates were observed in both groups (robot 62.5%; open 50%). However, abnormal pregnancies were more common in the robotic group (ectopic: robot 4, open 1; spontaneous pregnancy loss: robot 2, open 1). Costs per delivery were similar in the two groups.

Robotic technology was used for sterilization reversal in four studies. Three of these were retrospective in nature (Goldberg and Falcone, 2003; Rodgers et al., 2007; Caillet et al., 2010) and one was a prospective cohort study (Dharia Patel et al., 2008). Pregnancy rates after robotic laparoscopic surgery ranged between 50% and 70%; the pooled pregnancy rate was 65% (95% CI: 59%–72%). Ectopic pregnancy rates were only mentioned in two studies (11% and 22%, respectively). Pooled together, these two studies yielded an ectopic pregnancy rate of 15%. The two-layer technique was used in three studies [3, 19].

## Pregnancy rates in the first 12 months after tubal anastomoses

In one study, the authors registered a pregnancy rate of 44.3% in the first 12 months following microtubal reanastomosis (MTR). The study also revealed higher pregnancy rates with the use of Hulka clips (Hulka-Clemens, Richard Wolf, Rosemont, Illinois) or Filshie clips (CooperSurgical, Lake Forest, California) for performing tubal occlusion and when MTR was performed bilaterally. No significant difference was observed in pregnancy rates following MTR (44.3%) versus IVF (38%). However, a statistically significant difference was noted in live birth rates after MTR (19%) versus IVF (31%) ($p = 0.007$). Rates of ectopic pregnancy and spontaneous abortion (SAB) after MTR were 10% and 15.7%, respectively [20].

## Future perspectives, tubal grafting

Of the various techniques of sterilization reversal after salpingectomy, tubal grafting or implantation could be a promising method. However, extensive studies will be needed to prove the efficacy of the method before it can be implemented in the clinical setting. Moreover, its political and cultural acceptance also needs to be resolved.

## Conclusion

The pace of human life is changing rapidly, in addition to novel options being created by the evolution of technology. The challenges of modern life and the waning resources of our planet have changed human conceptions about the family. Families, in general, are planned more wisely in Western communities. Sterilization surgery is becoming the most common and effective method of family planning in the last few years, and has been accompanied by advances in sterilization reversal through tubal reanastomosis. Sterilization reversal has significantly enhanced the flexibility of family planning. Age and the duration of the poststerilization interval are probably the two most important factors underlying the success of reversal surgery. The robotic approach of reversal surgery, which we consider superior to all others, could be the third most important factor. Family planning is a very sensitive and crucial issue with enormous psychological and economic impact in Western countries as well as developing countries. Therefore, comprehensive counseling by an experienced team is mandatory before a patient undergoes sterilization surgery or its reversal.

## References

1. Van Seeters JA, Chua SJ, Mol BW, Koks CA. Tubal anastomosis after previous sterilization: a systematic review. Human Reproduction Update. 2017 Feb 22;23(3):358–70.
2. Alkatout I. Communicative and ethical aspects of physician-patient relationship in extreme situations. Wiener Medizinische Wochenschrift (1946). 2015 Dec;165(23-24):4918.
3. Alkatout I, Mettler L, Maass N, Ackermann J. Robotic surgery in gynecology. Journal of the Turkish German Gynecological Association. 2016;17(4):224.
4. Alkatout I, Mettler L, Maass N, Noé GK, Elessawy M. Abdominal anatomy in the context of port placement and trocars. Journal of the Turkish German Gynecological Association. 2015;16(4):241.
5. Alkatout I. Complications of laparoscopy in connection with entry techniques. Journal of Gynecologic Surgery. 2017 Jun 1;33(3):81–91.
6. Han J, Sadiq NM. Anatomy, Abdomen and Pelvis, Fallopian Tube.
7. Cates Jr W, Stone KM. Family planning, sexually transmitted diseases and contraceptive choice: a literature update–Part I. Family Planning Perspectives. 1992 Mar 1:75–84.
8. Mosher WD, Jones J. Use of contraception in the United States: 1982-2008. Vital and health statistics. Series 23, Data from the National Survey of Family Growth. 2010 Aug(29):1–44.
9. Burkman RT. Berek & Novak's gynecology. JAMA. 2012 Aug 1;308(5):516–7.
10. Shreffler KM, Greil AL, McQuillan J, Gallus KL. Reasons for tubal sterilisation, regret and depressive symptoms. Journal of Reproductive and Infant Psychology. 2016 May 26;34(3):304–13.
11. Uchida H. Uchida tubal sterilization. American Journal of Obstetrics and Gynecology. 1975 Jan 15;121(2):153–8.
12. Filshie GM, Casey D, Pogmore JR, Dutton AG, Symonds EM, Peake AB. The titanium/silicone rubber clip for female sterilization. BJOG: An International Journal of Obstetrics & Gynaecology. 1981 Jun;88(6):655–62.
13. Penfield AJ. The Filshie clip for female sterilization: a review of world experience. American Journal of Obstetrics and Gynecology. 2000 Mar 1;182(3):485–9.
14. Kjersgaard AG, Thranov I, Rasmussen OV, Hertz J. Male or female sterilization: a comparative study. Fertility and Sterility. 1989 Mar 1;51(3):439–43.
15. Jamieson DJ, Costello C, Trussell J, Hillis SD, Marchbanks PA, Peterson HB. The risk of pregnancy after vasectomy. Obstetrics & Gynecology. 2004 May 1;103(5):848–50.
16. Jamieson DJ, Kaufman SC, Costello C, Hillis SD, Marchbanks PA, Peterson HB, US Collaborative Review of Sterilization Working Group. A comparison of women's regret after vasectomy versus tubal sterilization. Obstetrics & Gynecology. 2002 Jun 1;99(6):1073–9.
17. Bedaiwy MA, Barakat EM, Falcone T. Robotic tubal anastomosis: technical aspects. Journal of the Society of Laparoendoscopic Surgeons. 2011 Jan;15(1):10.
18. Alkatout I. An atraumatic retractor for interdisciplinary use in conventional laparoscopy and robotic surgery. Minimally Invasive Therapy & Allied Technologies. 2018 Sep 3;27(5):265–71.
19. Patel SP, Steinkampf MP, Whitten SJ, Malizia BA. Robotic tubal anastomosis: surgical technique and cost effectiveness. Fertility and Sterility. 2008 Oct 1;90(4):1175–9.
20. Hirth R, Zbella E, Sanchez M, Prieto J. Microtubal reanastomosis: success rates as compared to in vitro fertilization. The Journal of Reproductive Medicine. 2010;55(3-4):161–5.

# 23

# MANAGEMENT OF OVARIAN MALDESCENT

**Stephanie Leiva, Andrea Pacheco Arias, and Mostafa I. Abuzeid**

## Introduction

Undescended ovaries (also known as ectopic or maldescent ovaries) are rarely encountered and frequently associated with urogenital anomalies [1]. Clinical presentation can vary or mimic other conditions and pathologies, therefore diagnoses can be challenging and should always be considered in clinician's differential. The most common setting, where ectopic ovaries are diagnosed, is during infertility workup [1]. This is most likely due to its strong association with Müllerian anomalies [2]. The pathology of undescended ovaries is a rare condition where ovaries may be found outside the ovarian fossa, usually along the migration pathway dependent on the gubernaculum [3]. The most common ectopic site is above the level of the common iliac vessels at the pelvic brim (**Figures 23.1, 23.2A–C, 23.3A–C**) [4]. Other less common locations for ectopic ovaries have been described in the literature in the adult and pediatric population. Some of these sites include: right upper quadrant or subhepatic, labia majora, inguinal canal, and sigmoid colon [5–9]. The most common presenting symptom of such rare locations of the ovary is pain. Of the disclosed pathology, some show normal ovarian tissue, other reveal cyclical ovarian changes, or signs of ovarian torsion.

A variety of nomenclature has been used for undescended or ectopic ovary [10]. Lachmann and Bermann (1991) proposed a modification of the terminology used to describe ectopic ovaries. They suggested to do away with the term supernumerary (a third ovary completely separated from the ovary) and the term accessory ovary (excess ovarian tissue connected to the ovary) [10]. Instead, they suggested the use of the term ectopic ovary, which they divided into three categories: (i) post-surgical implant, (ii) post-inflammatory implant, and (iii) true embryologic [10].

The purpose of this chapter is to review the pathogenesis and diagnosis of this rare malformation, and to discuss its implication on the management of infertile female. This chapter will focus on ectopic locations above the pelvic brim.

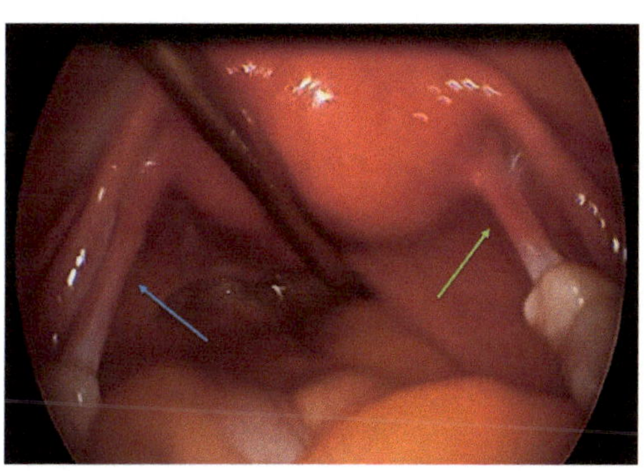

**FIGURE 23.1** Elongation of both ovarian ligaments—more on the right (blue arrow) than on the left (green arrow)—in a patient with bilateral maldescent ovaries.

## Embryology and anatomy

A review of the embryology is critical for a complete understanding and management of this pathology. Development of the gonads starts around the 5th week after conception. It begins as a group of proliferating cells at the medial side of the urogenital ridge near the kidneys in the upper abdomen [11]. A string of mesenchymal tissue called the gubernaculum plays an important role for the normal ovarian descent around week 12 of gestation [12–16]. This is orchestrated by complex chemotactic

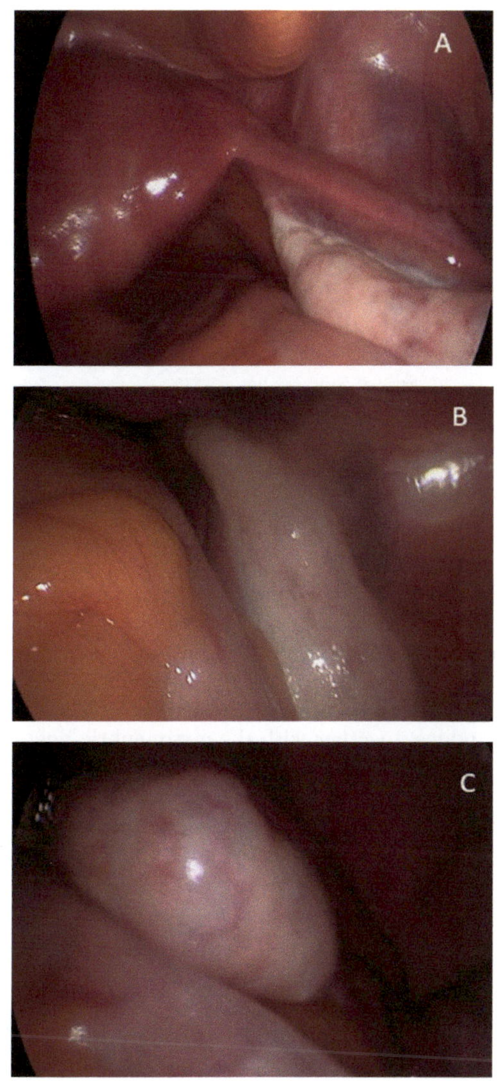


**FIGURE 23.2** Right maldescent ovary in the same patient in **Figure 23.1**.

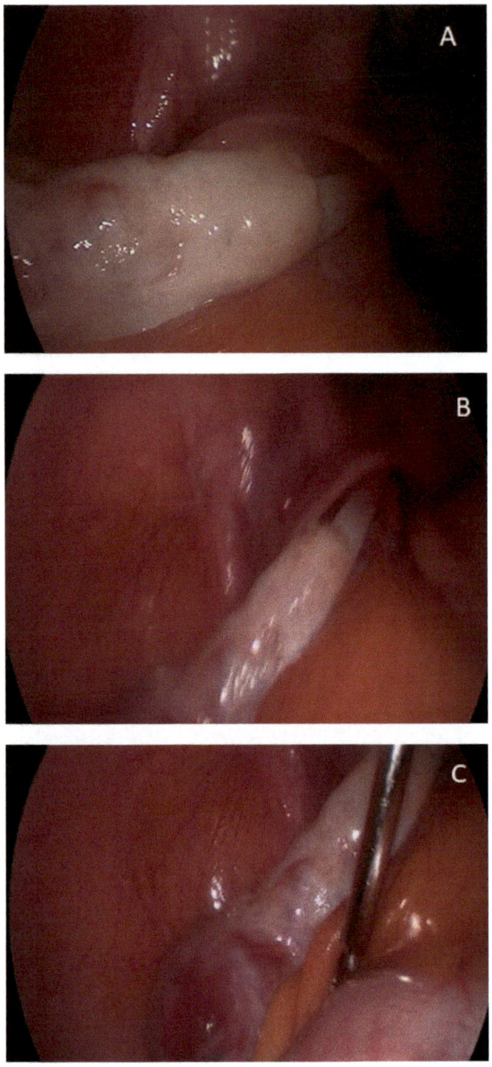


FIGURE 23.3 Left maldescent ovary in the same patient in **Figures 23.1** and **23.2**.

mechanisms in which the gubernaculum brings the ovaries to their permanent anatomical position [17]. Ultimately, the normal positioned ovaries lie below the pelvic brim, on the ovarian fossa, between the utero-ovarian and infundibulopelvic ligaments [18, 19]. Finally, the gubernaculum which fixed and fused with the Müllerian ducts and attaches to the lower pole of the ovaries, allow or induce, together with the mesonephric ducts, the adequate development and formation of the uterus [20]. The gubernaculum later becomes the utero-ovarian and round ligaments [21]. To date, the insult causing undescended ovaries is unknown. The pathogenesis of this rare entity is believed to be either lack of caudal descent or gonadal growth restriction [19]. Due to its close association with Müllerian anomalies, a multifactorial process could also explain a lack of descent [12–16].

## Incidence and associated pathology

Review of the literature has exhibited inconsistent data regarding the prevalence of these anomalies in the general population with a wide range of 0.3% up to 2% [1, 4]. Most reported cases in the literature described a unilateral ectopic ovary diagnosed via imaging or at the time of surgery, while bilateral undescended ovaries represented the minority of patients with one study reporting an incidence of 23% [1].

This unique entity is more commonly seen in conjunction with Müllerian anomalies. One study reported Müllerian anomalies in 73% of patients with ovarian maldescent [1]. Allen et al., 2011 [2], compared the incidence of ovarian maldescent in patients with or without Müllerian anomalies using magnetic resonance imaging (MRI) [2]. Undescended ovaries and fallopian tubes occurred more commonly in association with Müllerian anomalies. Ovarian maldescent was found in 17% and 3% of women with and without Müllerian anomalies respectively [2]. The Müllerian anomalies included hypoplasia, unicornuate, bicornuate, didelphys, and septate uterus [2]. The highest incidence of ovarian maldescent has been reported to occur in patients with unicornuate uterus (up to 42% in cases), followed by Müllerian agenesis (up to 20% of cases) [19].

Dietrich et al., 2007 [1], in a review article of 26 patients with maldescent ovaries, found that 19 patients had Müllerian anomalies, and 12 of those had unicornuate uterus (63.2%) [1]. In patients with unicornuate uterus, the undescended ovary and fallopian tube occurred on the contralateral side. The higher incidence of ovarian maldescent in patients with unicornuate uterus, bicornuate uterus, uterus didelphys, and Müllerian agenesis can be explained on the basis that all such anomalies occur during Müllerian duct migration and uterine body fusion [2]. Such processes may overlap with ovarian descent which is governed by the gubernaculums. The genesis of this association has been presumed to be secondary to the close interrelation of the gubernaculum and the Müllerian ducts; however, these mechanisms are not fully understood [2]. However, ovarian maldescent is not common in patients with anomalies that happen as a result of lack of regression of the septum as governed by apoptosis, such as the case with septate uterus [22]. The latter has nothing to do with ovarian migration [23]. Renal anomalies were associated in up to 23% of patients with undescended ovaries [1]. The most commonly reported anomaly was ipsilateral renal agenesis and less frequently encountered: malposition, malrotation, or kidney duplication [2]. Renal anomalies were found in 23%–24.6% patients with Müllerian anomalies and 36% in patients with both Müllerian anomalies and ovarian maldescent [1, 2].

Current evidence is lacking regarding the connection between undescended ovaries to more subtle Müllerian anomalies, like septate uterus, or other common gynecological pathologies, such as ovarian torsion, polycystic ovaries, premature ovarian failure, or endometriosis. However, an association between obstructive Müllerian anomalies, especially imperforate hymen and obstructed hemivagina and ipsilateral renal anomaly (OHVIRA) and endometriosis has been described in the literature (**Figure 23.4**) [24–26]. In addition, some investigators reported higher incidence of endometriosis and nonobstructive Müllerian anomalies such as unicornuate uterus and uterus didelphys [27]. Furthermore, a limited number of publications reported higher incidence of endometriosis in patients with uterine septum [27–29]. Therefore, it may be a sound idea to rule out endometriosis in patients with maldescent ovaries and Müllerian anomalies, especially if such patients present with abdominal or pelvic pain. The authors of this chapter observed mild endometriosis in three out of five patients with confirmed bilateral maldescent ovaries and Müllerian anomalies utilizing diagnostic laparoscopy and hysteroscopy (**Figure 23.5A,B**; unpublished data). The Müllerian anomalies encountered in these five patients were: Müllerian agenesis (**Figure 23.6**), complete uterine septum, incomplete uterine septum, significant arcuate uterine anomaly, and variant of T-shaped uterus with arcuate uterine anomaly.

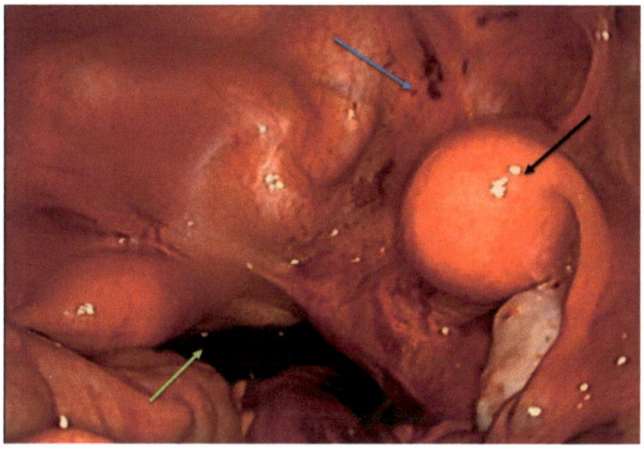

FIGURE 23.4 Laparoscopy of a patient with OHVIRA, illustrating a uterus didelphys with a distended right uterine horn (black arrow) as a result of hematometra secondary to right hemivagina; there is evidence of endometriosis (blue arrow) and slight hematoperitoneum (green arrow).

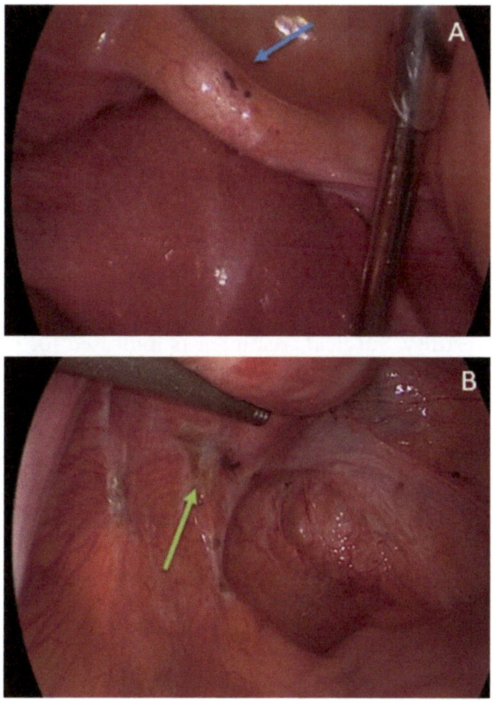


FIGURE 23.5 (A) Minimal endometriosis on the bladder (blue arrow); (B) minimal endometriosis in the Pouch of Douglas (green arrow) in a patient with bilateral maldescent ovaries.

## Clinical presentation

Diagnosis of undescended ovaries can present as a clinical challenge. Several case studies and case series have reported this pathology as a complex condition with a broad spectrum of clinical presentation varying from asymptomatic to complicated abdominal pain [1]. Incidental finding of undescended ovaries was discovered in most cases by imaging or surgery during infertility workup. Some case reports indicate that abdominal pain can be the presenting feature as a result of ovarian cyst formation with inherent complications such as rupture, hemorrhage, or even tumor formation [5, 17, 30, 31]. Common physiologic conditions

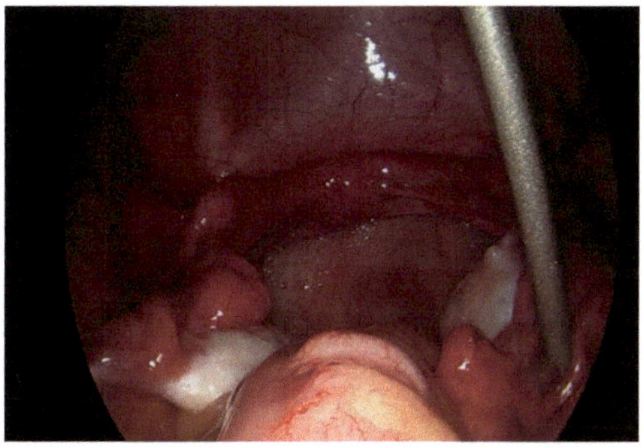

FIGURE 23.6 Subtle bilateral maldescent of the ovaries, more pronounced on the left side, in a patient with Müllerian agenesis.

such as ovulation and also common ovarian pathologies including but not limited to: hemorrhagic corpus luteum, ovarian torsion, or ruptured ovarian cyst can have an unusual presentation of abdominal pain above the true pelvis [12, 32]. This confers a challenge for the clinician at the time of presentation resulting in an extensive evaluation due to a wide differential diagnosis and the possibility of mimicking other abdominal conditions. In the literature, ectopic ovaries have been the cause of suspected gastroenteritis, appendicitis, pancreatitis, cholelithiasis and cholecystitis, nephrolithiasis and pyelonephritis, and inflammatory bowel disease or abdominal tumors [1, 17]. Clinical suspicion could be triggered in a patient who presents with unique features, including: abdominal pain above the true pelvis corresponding with menstrual cycle, history of infertility, history of uterine or other Müllerian anomalies, and renal anomalies.

Maldescent right ovary should always be considered in the differential diagnosis of appendicular mucocel [17, 31]. In addition, patients with maldescent ovaries may present with symptoms of associated renal anomalies. Furthermore, in some patients the presenting feature was that of ectopic pregnancy occurring in an associated undescended noncommunicating fallopian tube after transperitoneal migration of sperm [33].

Maldescent ovary should also be considered in the differential diagnosis of retroperitoneal tumor such as mucinous cyst adenomyoma and intestinal mesenchymoma [9, 34]. Trinidad et al. 2004 [11] suggested that ectopic ovary may be at increased risk of forming tumors, similar to cryptorchidism in males [11]. Trinidad et al., 2004 [11], pointed out to the fact that there was about 12 reported cases of primary retroperitoneal cystadenomas, all in women [11, 34]. These investigators suggested that some of these tumors may have occurred in undiagnosed ectopic ovaries, whether supernumerary or maldescent [11].

In view of findings, higher incidence of maldescent ovaries in patients with Müllerian anomalies compared to those with normal uterine anatomy, a high index of suspicion should be exercised to determine the presence of maldescent ovaries in patients with Müllerian anomalies, especially unicornuate uterus. This should always be borne in mind by gynecologists, despite the rare occurrence of maldescent ovaries. As mentioned above, the authors of this chapter diagnosed five patients with maldescent ovaries and Müllerian anomalies (unpublished data). Three of these patients presented with primary infertility and two of them were found to have stage 1 endometriosis. One of these patients presented with primary amenorrhea secondary to Müllerian agenesis (**Figure 23.6**). The remaining patient presented with severe dysmenorrhea and stage 1 endometriosis (**Figure 23.5A,B**). The authors of this chapter suggest that endometriosis should be ruled out in patients with maldescent ovaries and Müllerian anomalies especially, if such patients present with abdominal or pelvic pain.

## Investigation

The diagnosis of maldescent ovaries can be initially suspected with imaging studies such as hysterosalpingogram, ultrasonography, CT scan, or MRI [1]. A diagnosis of such pathology can be suspected on histosalpingogram (HSG) that demonstrates fallopian tubes to be elongated and pulled upwards with distal ends above the pelvic brim (**Figure 23.7A,B**) [35–37]. Maldescent ovaries may also be suspected when there is difficulty locating one or both ovaries during transvaginal 2D ultrasonography (TV 2D US) [35]. In such situation, the differential diagnosis should include absent ovary (congenital or after surgical removal), pelvic adhesions pulling the ovaries away from its anatomical location, obesity, and bowel disease or conditions that make it difficult to visualize the ovaries [38]. If MRI is performed for other indications like fibroid mapping or suspected Müllerian anomalies, the presence of ovaries above the pelvic brim would suggest maldescent ovaries [2, 13, 37]. MRI may also be considered when both TV 2D US and transabdominal 2D ultrasound (TA 2D US) failed to visualize the ovaries [13]. Ombelet et al., 2003 [13], described the value of MRI after clomiphene citrate ovarian stimulation for the diagnosis of undescended ovaries [13]. The authors pointed out that the multi-follicular growth in the ectopic ovary greatly enhanced MRI diagnosis [13]. It is now well established that MRI is the best noninvasive tool for the diagnosis of maldescent ovaries. In addition, MRI is the best radiologic test for the diagnosis of associated renal and uterine anomalies. Furthermore, it can diagnose extra-peritoneal maldescent ovaries which cannot be detected on laparoscopy.

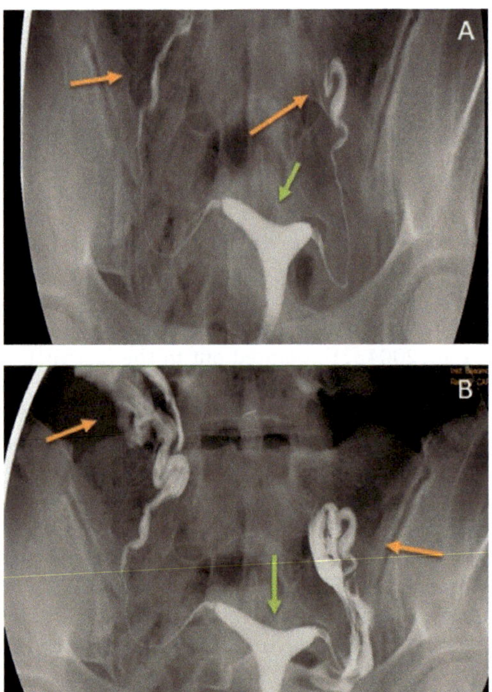


**FIGURE 23.7** (A) HSG showing both fallopian tubes to be pulled upwards toward the pelvic brim (orange arrows); (B) HSG of bilateral localization of the radio opaque material around the tubes (orange arrows). (A) and (B) also illustrate slight fundal depression (green arrows) with differential diagnosis of subtle arcuate versus subtle bicornuate uterus.

Direct visualization during laparoscopy confirms the diagnosis with the findings of ovaries outside their normal location in the ovarian fossa, such as above the pelvic brim.

In a few reports, CT scan was used to evaluate patients presenting with abdominal pain when appendicitis was suspected. In these patients, appendiceal mucocele was suspected [17, 31]. The correct diagnosis of maldescent ovary was made at a time of diagnostic laparoscopy [17, 31].

Dietrich et al., 2007 [1], in a review article of 26 patients with maldescent ovaries showed the diagnosis was made by laparotomy in two patients, by laparoscopy in seven patients, by laparoscopy and other diagnostic modality such as hysteroscopy, HSG, ultrasonography, CT scan, and MRI in six patients, by MRI in six patients, and by a combination of MRI and HSG in one patient [1]. In four patients, in the latter review, the modality by which the diagnosis was made was unknown [1].

## Management

Conservative management is usually adopted in asymptomatic patients with maldescent ovaries. There is no need for surgical removal of a normally appearing undescended ovary. It is important to explain to the patient and her family the benign nature of this rare condition. It is equally important to reassure the patient regarding her reproductive potential, albeit the possible need for assisted methods of conception if the need arise. However, if the patient presents with pain, continuous treatment with oral contraceptives may be indicated, especially in the presence of recurrent ovarian cysts or associated endometriosis. Conservative treatment of associated endometriosis at time of laparoscopy should be attempted in patients with maldescent ovaries and pain and/or infertility. Surgical treatment is indicated for correction of associated uterine septum or significant arcuate anomaly in patients presenting with infertility or recurrent pregnancy loss. In addition, surgical treatment is indicated in the presence of ectopic pregnancy occurring in an associated undescended non-communicating fallopian tube after transperitoneal migration of sperm [33]. Ireo et al., 2018 [30], reported a patient with maldescent ovary with recurrent acute abdomen as a result of recurrent ovarian cyst. The authors performed salpingo oophorectomy of the maldescent ovary and tube with satisfactory outcome [30].

## Implications in infertility

The limited data in the literature indicate that there is no clear association between ovarian maldescent and infertility [4, 13, 37]. Some literature suggest that the majority of cases diagnosed of ovarian maldescent are found during infertility work up, with the remaining of the cases being diagnosed as incidental findings during childhood or adulthood [1]. Current evidence does not show a clear relationship between ovarian maldescent and increased risk of malignant disease. Due to the presence of normal ovarian tissue on an ectopic site, it is not recommended to perform an oophorectomy after diagnosis unless there is a clear suspicion for malignancy [1].

The direct association of the ectopic ovary per se in fecundity and fertility is still unknown [17]. Nevertheless, it is crucial to acknowledge that all the pathologies associated with the undescended ovary can collide and aggregate affecting various phases of the evaluation and treatment of the infertile patient. For instance, a higher prevalence of pregnancy wastage is commonly encountered due to the sole presence of Müllerian anomalies [13, 36].

One of the real challenges that these patients might encounter during evaluation and treatment is visualization of the ovaries on TV 2D US. In such patients, evaluation of ovarian reserve by antral follicle count (AFC) may be very difficult on TV 2D US. In addition, monitoring of follicle growth with TDV 2D US during natural cycle, or during ovulation induction with clomiphene citrate, or aromataze inhibitor such as Letrazole and gonadotropins may prove difficult. In such situations, TA 2D US may be helpful in visualizing the ovaries. However, in such cases, a distended large bowel may interfere with the view.

Similarly, if a patient's fertility treatment encompasses oocyte retrieval, which is usually done under TA 2D US guidance, careful planning for a safe alternative access should be taken into consideration. Ultrasonographic guided percutaneous transabdominal puncture for oocyte retrieval TA 2D US may be performed by an experienced reproductive endocrinologist [39, 40]. In addition, transabdominal transvesical oocyte retrieval can be planned [41]. Alternatively, the original old method of oocyte retrieval under laparoscopic guidance can also be performed, albeit it requires general anesthesia with its inherent risk. It is worth of note that many in vitro fertilization (IVF) centers do not have the facility to perform a laparoscopy [35]. Ectopic ovaries can lie on or near great vessels such as external iliac vessels, viscera, and others. Therefore, in theory, there is a risk of injury to important structures. If an attempt at TV 2D US guided oocyte retrieval is made in the presence of poorly visualized ovaries, there is a real risk of injury to the internal iliac or external iliac vessels. Despite such potential risks, Garg et al., 2016 [37] were able to perform TV 2D US guided oocyte retrieval in a patient with maldescent ovaries without complications, albeit difficulty in reaching the ovaries through this route with the use of transabdominal pressure [37]. Such maneuver is utilized frequently by reproductive surgeons during TV 2D US guided oocyte retrieval when there is difficulty visualizing the ovaries for a variety of reasons, such as obesity or high position of the ovary secondary to pelvic adhesions.

## Conclusion

It is likely that the ectopic ovary is an underreported and/or underdiagnosed pathology. An incidental and isolated finding of abnormally located ovaries should prompt the healthcare provider to educate patients on the possibility and consequences on overall health and fertility. Increased awareness of providers about the possibility of maldescent ovaries in patients presenting with infertility or abdominal pain, especially in the presence of Müllerian anomalies, or renal anomalies, or both, is important for early detection and proper counseling of the patient and her family on this rare entity. MRI, perhaps after ovarian stimulation with clomiphene citrate, is the best noninvasive tool for the diagnosis of maldescent ovaries. Conservative management is the treatment of choice in the majority of cases.

## References


1. Dietrich JE, Hertweck PS, Bond S. Undescended ovaries: a clinical review. *J Pediatr Adol Gynec.* 2007;20(2): 57–60.
2. Allen JW, Cardall S, Kittijarukhajorn M, Siegel CL. Incidence of ovarian maldescent in women with müllerian duct anomalies: evaluation by MRI. *AJR Am J Roentgenol.* 2012;198(4):W381–W385.
3. Baskin LS and Cunha G. Embryology of the genitourinary tract. In: Wein A, Kavoussi L, Partin A, Peters C (eds). *Campbell-Walsh Urology,* 11th edition, 2015. 122 Embryology of the Genitourinary Tract, 282, volume 4, section A 20, 305–340.e4.
4. Verkauf BS and Bernhisel MA. Ovarian maldescent. *Fertil Steril.* 1996;65(1):189–192.
5. Edwards R, McCagg J, Chirico P, Yoost J. The management of an ectopic ovary in an adolescent patient with gastroschisis. *J Pediatr Adol Gynecol.* 2018;31(5):540–542.
6. Castro AA, Morandini F, Calixto CP, Barros WH, Nakatani ET, Castro AA. Ectopic ovary with torsion: uncommon diagnosis made by ultrasound. *Radiol Bras.* 20017;50(1):60–61.
7. Yao L, Mou Y, Wang HX. Sonographic diagnosis of an ovary-containing inguinal hernia with the formation of a corpus luteum in an adult female. *Ultrasound Obstet Gynecol.* Letter to the Editor 2009;34(3):359–360.
8. Laing FC, Townsend BA, Rodriguez JR. Ovary-containing hernia in a premature infant: sonographic diagnosis. *J Ultrasound Med.* 2007;26(7):985–7. https://doi.org/10.7863/jum.2007.26.7.985
9. Pan J, Wang S, Wang H, Fan Z. A rare ectopic ovary mimicking colon sigmoideum mesenchymoma presenting as an intestinal mesenchyoma. *Front Oncol.* 2019;9:580.
10. Lachman MF and Berman MM. The ectopic ovary: A case report and review of the literature. *Arch Pathol Lab Med.* 1991; 115:233–235
11. Trinidad C, Tardáguila F, Fernández GC, Martínez C, Chávarri E, Rivas I. Ovarian maldescent. *Eur Radiol.* 2004;14(5):805–808.
12. Kives SL, Perlman S, Bond S. Ruptured hemorrhagic cyst in an undescended ovary. *J Pediatr Surg.* 2004; 39(11):e4–e6.
13. Ombelet W, Verswijel G, deJonge E. Ectopic ovary and unicornuate uterus. *N Engl J Med.* 2003;348(7):667–668.
14. Nichols DH, Postoloff AV. Congenital ectopic ovary. *Am J Obstet Gynecol* 1951;62:195.
15. McCullough JB, Evans AT, Holley MP. Supernumerary or ectopic ovary: a case report. *Histopathology.* 1992;21(6):582.
16. Rock JA, Parmley T, Murphey AA, et al. Malposition of the ovary associated with uterine anomalies. *Fertil Steril.* 1986;45(4):56.
17. Sinonquel P, Bontinck J, Stevens M. Undescended ovary and fallopian tube presenting as appendiceal mucocele. *Facts Views Vis Obgyn.* 2018;10(1):47–50.
18. Schoenwolf GC, Bleyl SB, Brauer PR, et al. Development of the urogenital system. *Larsens's Human Embryology,* 4th ed, Churchill Livingstone Elsevier, Philadelphia, 2009.
19. Parmley T. The embryology of the female genital tract. In: Verkauf BS. (ed). *Congenital malformations of the female tract and their treatment Norwalk* (CT): Appleton and Lang, 1993.
20. Acién P, del Campo FS, Mayol MJ, Acién M. The female gubernaculum: role in the embryology and development of the genital tract and in the possible genesis of malformations. *Eur J Obstet Gyn R B.* 2011;159(2):426–432.
21. Berek JS, Novak E (eds). In: *Berek and Novak's Gynecology.* Philadelphia: Wolters Kluwer, 2015. Chapter 5. Internet resource.
22. Chan Y, Jayaprakasan K, Zamora J, Thornton JG, Raine-Fenning N, Coomarasamy A. The prevalence of congenital uterine anomalies in unselected and high-risk populations: a systematic review. Hum Reprod Update 2011;17(6):761–771.
23. Lee DM, Osathanondh R, Yep J. Localization of Bcl-2 in the human fetal Müllerian tract. Fertil Steril. 1998;70:135–140.
24. Olive DL, Henderson DY. Endometriosis and Müllerian anomalies. *Obstet Gynecol.* 1987;69:412–415.
25. Sanfilippo JS, Wakim NG, Schikler KN, Yussman MA. Endometriosis in association with uterine anomaly. *Am J Obstet Gynecol.* 1986;154:39–43.
26. Cramer DW, Missmer SA. The epidemiology of endometriosis. *Ann NY Acad Sci.* 2002;955(1):11–22.
27. Nawroth F, Rahimi G, Nawroth C, Foth D, Ludwig M, Schmidt T. Is there an association between septate uterus and endometriosis? *Hum Reprod.* 2006;21(2):542–544.
28. Abuzeid M, Sakhel K, Khedr M, Schwark S, Salem H, Ashraf M. The association between endometriosis and uterine septum. *Hum Reprod.* 2004;supplement:P-610.
29. LaMonica R, Pinto J, Luciano D, Lyapis A, Luciano A. Incidence of septate uterus in reproductive-aged women with and without endometriosis. *J Minim Invasive Gynecol.* 2016;23(4):610–613.